Handbook of Parkinson's Disease

NEUROLOGICAL DISEASE AND THERAPY

Advisory Board

Handbook of Parkinson's Disease

Third Edition

edited by

Rajesh Pahwa
University of Kansas Medical Center
Kansas City, Kansas, U.S.A.

Kelly E. Lyons
University of Kansas Medical Center
Kansas City, Kansas, U.S.A.

William C. Koller
Mount Sinai School of Medicine
New York, New York, U.S.A.

MARCEL DEKKER, INC.   NEW YORK · BASEL

The previous edition was *Handbook of Parkinson's Disease: Second Edition, Revised and Expanded* (William C. Koller, ed.), 1992.

Library of Congress Cataloging-in-Publication Data
A catalog record for this book is available from the Library of Congress.

ISBN: 0-8247-4242-7

This book is printed on acid-free paper.

Headquarters
Marcel Dekker, Inc.
270 Madison Avenue, New York, NY 10016, U.S.A.
tel: 212-696-9000; fax: 212-685-4540

Distribution and Customer Service
Marcel Dekker, Inc.
Cimarron Road, Monticello, New York 12701, U.S.A.
tel: 800-228-1160; fax: 845-796-1772

Eastern Hemisphere Distribution
Marcel Dekker AG
Hutgasse 4, Postfach 812, CH-4001 Basel, Switzerland
tel: 41-61-260-6300; fax: 41-61-260-6333

World Wide Web
http://www.dekker.com

The publisher offers discounts on this book when ordered in bulk quantities. For more information, write to Special Sales/Professional Marketing at the headquarters address above.

We would like to thank our parents, Vidya and Badrinath Pahwa and Thomas and Elaine Lyons, for their many years of continued encouragement, understanding and support throughout our careers.

Foreword

Parkinson's disease is a common neurological condition that is becoming more common as the population ages. It is a chronic condition and can be a source of significant disability. Fortunately, for many decades there has been some understanding of the pathophysiology of Parkinson's disease, and useful therapies have been available. Better therapies and definitive curative therapies, however, are yet to come. For these reasons, Parkinson's disease has been the focus of considerable research effort, and we have seen a virtual explosion of progress in recent years.

The identification of genetic disorders that lead to Parkinson's disease has triggered the rush to research into molecular biology and cell biology of the basal ganglia and neurodegeneration. Imaging has led to greater insights about brain organization and neurotransmitter function. Physiological investigations have told us more about the genesis of the motor disorder of bradykinesia. New emphasis has been placed on the nonmotor aspects of parkinsonian symptomatology, which will help lead to a better quality of life for patients. All this new information has opened the door to new possibilities and to the development of new therapeutics.

However, the new therapies that have appeared in the last decade make the management of the patient with Parkinson's disease more complex, sophisticated, and difficult for the clinician. Which of the various alternatives is best for the individual patient at hand? How should therapy be initiated? Is there anything that will help prevent progression of the disorder as well as ameliorate symptoms? What should be done with agonists, with COMT inhibitors? How should complications, such as dyskinesias, be managed? How should cognitive dysfunction or depression be managed? What is the role of the different surgical options? When should they be employed and which one is best for the individual patient?

To help basic scientists and clinicians to keep up to date, information must be current, authoritative, and cohesively presented. To this end, the third edition of the *Handbook of Parkinson's Disease* is a welcome addition to the literature. It deals with all the aspects of understanding and managing this multifaceted disorder, and should be read from cover to cover and consulted for specific problems. The book will serve as an ideal reference for those working with Parkinson's disease.

Mark Hallett
Chief, Human Motor Control Section
Medical Neurology Branch
National Institute of Neurological Disorders and Stroke
National Institutes of Health
Bethesda, Maryland

Preface

Parkinson's disease is a progressive neurodegenerative condition with often devastating symptoms. In recent years, our knowledge of the disease has increased tremendously. We have achieved a greater understanding of its neurochemistry, neurophysiology, and neuropathology. Genes have been identified that are involved in the pathogenesis of some forms of familial autosomal dominant and autosomal recessive Parkinson's disease. Advancements in neuropsychological and neuroimaging techniques have led to improvements in diagnostic accuracy. Therapeutics have come a long way, too. New medications have been approved, new compounds and therapeutic approaches are under investigation, and we have a better understanding of the use of surgical procedures in Parkinson's disease, particularly deep brain stimulation. In spite of these advances, there continue to be many complications associated with the long-term management of both motor and nonmotor symptoms of the disease and treatment remains a challenge.

We present in this edition of the *Handbook of Parkinson's Disease* the most up-to-date information on the scientific and therapeutic aspects of the disease. The third edition offers a more integrated approach to managing parkinsonian symptoms. There is comprehensive coverage of the latest pharmacological and surgical therapeutics as well as the newest technologies in diagnostic imaging. It is our hope that this volume, in the tradition of the first two editions, will serve as a reference source for physicians, researchers, and other healthcare professionals seeking answers to the many questions related to the understanding and treatment of Parkinson's disease.

We thank each of the authors for their time and commitment in preparing state-of-the-art reviews of the most pertinent aspects of Parkinson's disease. We would also like to thank Jinnie Kim, Ann Pulido, and the other Marcel Dekker, Inc., staff who assisted in the preparation of this book.

Rajesh Pahwa
Kelly E. Lyons
William C. Koller

Contributors

Joseph S. Chung, M.D Division of Movement Disorders, University of Southern California–Keck School of Medicine, Los Angeles, California, U.S.A.

Richard B. Dewey, Jr., M.D. Clinical Center for Movement Disorders, University of Texas Southwestern Medical School, Dallas, Texas, U.S.A.

Dennis W. Dickson, M.D. Department of Pathology, Mayo Clinic, Jacksonville, Florida, U.S.A.

Elmyra V. Encarnacion, M.D. Experimental Therapeutics Branch, Parkinson's Disease and Movement Disorders Center, Neurology Department, University of South Florida and Tampa General Healthcare, Tampa, Florida, U.S.A.

Stewart A. Factor, D.O. Parkinson's Disease and Movement Disorders Center, Albany Medical Center, Albany, New York, U.S.A.

Matthew Farrer, Ph.D. Department of Neuroscience, Mayo Clinic, Jacksonville, Florida, U.S.A. and Mayo Medical School, Rochester, Minnesota, U.S.A.

Christopher G. Goetz, M.D. Department of Neurological Sciences, Rush University, Chicago, Illinois, U.S.A.

Jay M. Gorell, M.D. Department of Neurology, Henry Ford Health Sciences Center, Henry Ford Health System and NIEHS Center for Molecular Toxicology with Human Applications, Wayne State University, Detroit, Michigan, U.S.A.

Ruth Hagestuen, R.N., M.A. The National Parkinson Foundation, Miami, Florida, U.S.A.

Robert A. Hauser, M.D. Division of Movement Disorders, Departments of Neurology, Pharmacology and Experimental Pharmacology, University of South Florida and Tampa General Healthcare, Tampa Florida, U.S.A.

Michael W. Jakowec, Ph.D. Department of Neurology and Department of Cell and Neurobiology, University of Southern California–Keck School of Medicine, Los Angeles, California, U.S.A.

Joseph Jankovic, M.D. Department of Neurology, Baylor College of Medicine, Houston, Texas, U.S.A.

Danna Jennings, M.D Department of Neurology, The Institute for Neurodegenerative Disorders, New Haven, Connecticut, U.S.A.

Marjorie L. Johnson, M.A./C.C.C.-S.L.P. Struthers Parkinson's Center, Minneapolis, Minnesota, U.S.A.

Jorge L. Juncos, M.D. Department of Neurology and Wesley Woods Geriatric Center, Emory University School of Medicine, Atlanta, Georgia, U.S.A.

Anthony E. Lang, M.D., F.R.P.C. Division of Neurology, Department of Medicine, The Toronto Western Hospital, University of Toronto, Toronto, Ontario, Canada

Mark F. Lew, M.D. Department of Neurology, Univesity of Southern California–Keck School of Medicine, Los Angeles, California, U.S.A.

Kelly E. Lyons, Ph.D. Department of Neurology, University of Kansas Medical Center, Kansas City, Kansas, U.S.A.

Kenneth Marek, M.D. Department of Neurology, The Institute for Neurodegenerative Disorders, New Haven, Connecticut, U.S.A.

Deborah C. Mash, Ph.D. Department of Neurology and Molecular and Cellular Pharmacology, University of Miami School of Medicine, Miami, Florida, U.S.A.

Erwin B. Montgomery, Jr., M.D. American Parkinson Disease Association Advanced Center for Research, Departments of Neurology and Neuroscience, Cleveland Clinic Foundation, Cleveland, Ohio, U.S.A.

William Ondo, M.D. Department of Neurology, Baylor College of Medicine, Houston, Texas, U.S.A.

Rajesh Pahwa, M.D. Department of Neurology, University of Kansas Medical Center, Kansas City, Kansas, U.S.A.

Giselle M. Petzinger, M.D. Department of Neurology, University of Southern California–Keck School of Medicine, Los Angeles, California, U.S.A.

Ronald F. Pfeiffer, M.D. Department of Neurology, University of Tennessee Health Science Center, Memphis, Tennessee, U.S.A.

Alex Rajput, M.D. Department of Neurology, University of Saskatchewan, Saskatoon, Saskatchewan, Canada

Ali H. Rajput, M.B.B.S. Department of Neurology, University of Saskatchewan, Saskatoon, Saskatchewan, Canada

Michele Rajput, Ph.D. University of Saskatchewan, Saskatoon, Saskatchewan, Canada

Jayaraman Rao, M.D. Louisiana State University Health Sciences Center, New Orleans, Louisiana, U.S.A.

Benjamin A. Rybicki, Ph.D. Biostatistics and Research Epidemiology, Henry Ford Health Sciences Center, Henry Ford Health System, Detroit, Michigan, U.S.A.

Michael Samuel, B.M.B.Ch., M.R.C.P., M.D. Division of Neurology, Department of Medicine, The Toronto Western Hospital, University of Toronto, Toronto, Ontario, Canada.

Anthony J. Santiago, M.D. Parkinson's Disease and Movement Disorders Center, Albany Medical Center, Albany, New York, U.S.A.

John Seibyl, M.D. Department of Neurology, The Institute for Neurodegenerative Disorders, New Haven, Connecticut, U.S.A.

Kapil D. Sethi, M.D., F.R.C.P. Medical College of Georgia, Augusta, Georgia, U.S.A.

Mark A. Stacy, M.D. Muhammad Ali Parkinson Research Center, Barrow Neurological Institute, Phoenix, Arizona, U.S.A.

Alexander I. Tröster, Ph.D. Departments of Psychiatry and Behavioral Sciences and of Neurological Surgery, University of Washington School of Medicine, Seattle, Washington, U.S.A.

Daryl Victor, M.D. Division of Movement Disorders, Department of Neurology, Columbia University, New York, New York, U.S.A.

Cheryl Waters, M.D., F.R.C.P.(C) Division of Movement Disorders, Department of Neurology, Columbia University, New York, New York, U.S.A.

Ray L. Watts, M.D. Department of Neurology and Wesley Woods Geriatric Center, Emory University School of Medicine, Atlanta, Georgia, U.S.A.

Rosemary L. Wichmann, P.T. Struthers Parkinson's Center, Minneapolis, Minnesota, U.S.A.

Steven Paul Woods, Psy.D. Department of Psychiatry and Behavioral Sciences, University of Washington School of Medicine, Seattle, Washington, U.S.A.

Zbigniew K. Wszolek, M.D. Department of Neurology, Mayo Clinic, Jacksonville, Florida, U.S.A. and Mayo Medical School, Rochester, Minnesota, U.S.A.

Allan D. Wu, M.D. Department of Neurology, Univesity of Southern California–Keck School of Medicine, Los Angeles, California, U.S.A.

Contents

PATHOLOGY AND NEUROCHEMISTRY

ETIOLOGY

MEDICATIONS

SURGICAL THERAPY

OTHER FORMS OF TREATMENT

Handbook of
Parkinson's
Disease

1

Early Iconography of Parkinson's Disease

Christopher G. Goetz
Rush University, Chicago, Illinois, U.S.A.

Parkinson's disease was first described in a medical context in 1817 by James Parkinson, a general practitioner in London. Numerous essays have been written about Parkinson himself and the early history of Parkinson's disease (*Paralysis agitans*), or the shaking palsy. Rather than repeat or resynthesize such prior studies, this introductory chapter focuses on a number of historical visual documents with descriptive legends. Some of these are available in prior publications, but the entire collection has not been presented before. As a group, they present materials from the nineteenth century and will serve as a base on which the subsequent chapters that cover the progress of the twentieth and budding twenty-first centuries are built.

HISTORICAL AND LITERARY PRECEDENTS

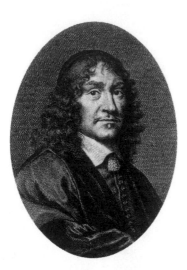

FIGURE 1   **Franciscus de le Böe (1614–1672).** Also known as Sylvius de le Böe and Franciscus Sylvius, this early physician was Professor of Leiden and a celebrated anatomist. In his medical writings he also described tremors, and he may be among the very earliest writers on involuntary movement disorders (1).

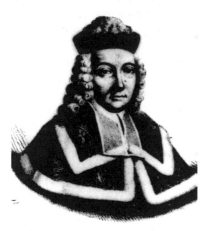

FIGURE 2   **François Boissier de Sauvages de la Croix (1706–1767).** Sauvages was cited by Parkinson himself and described patients with "running disturbances of the limbs," *scelotyrbe festinans*. Such subjects had difficulty walking, moving with short and hasty steps. He considered the problem to be due to diminished flexibility of muscle fibers, possibly his manner of describing rigidity (1,2).

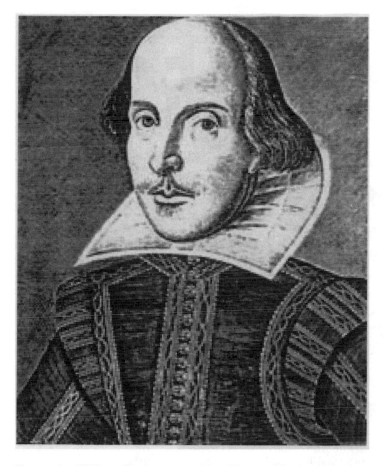

FIGURE 3 **William Shakespeare**. A brilliant medical observer as well as writer, Shakespeare described many neurological conditions, including epilepsy, somnambulism, and dementia. In *Henry VI*, first produced in 1590, the character Dick notices that Say is trembling: "Why dost thou quiver, man," he asks, and Say responds, "The palsy and not fear provokes me" (1). Jean-Martin Charcot frequently cited Shakespeare in his medical lectures and classroom presentations and disputed the concept that tremor was a natural accompaniment of normal aging. He rejected "senile tremor" as a separate nosographic entity. After reviewing his data from the Salpêtrière service where 2000 elderly inpatients lived, he turned to Shakespeare's renditions of elderly figures (3,4): "Do not commit the error that many others do and misrepresent tremor as a natural accompaniment of old age. Remember that our venerated Dean, Dr. Chevreul, today 102 years old, has no tremor whatsoever. And you must remember in his marvelous descriptions of old age (*Henry IV* and *As You Like It*), the master observer, Shakespeare, never speaks of tremor."

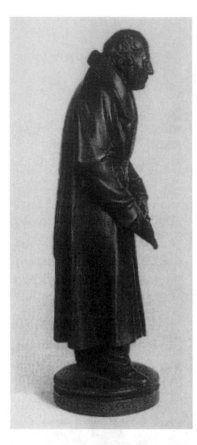

FIGURE 4 Wilhelm von Humboldt (1767–1835). A celebrated academic reformer and writer, von Humboldt, lived in the era of Parkinson and described his own neurological condition in a series of letters, analyzed by Horowski (5). The statue by Friedrich Drake shown in the figure captures the hunched, flexed posture of Parkinson's disease, but von Humboldt's own words capture the tremor and bradykinesia of the disease (6):

> Trembling of the hands ... occurs only when both or one of them is inactive; at this very moment, for example, only the left one is trembling but not the right one that I am using to write. ... If I am using my hands this strange clumsiness starts which is hard to describe. It is obviously weakness as I am unable to carry heavy objects as I did earlier on, but it appears with tasks that do not need strength but consist of quite fine movements, and especially with these. In addition to writing, I can mention rapid opening of books, dividing of fine pages, unbuttoning and buttoning up of clothes. All of these as well as writing proceed with intolerable slowness and clumsiness.

JAMES PARKINSON

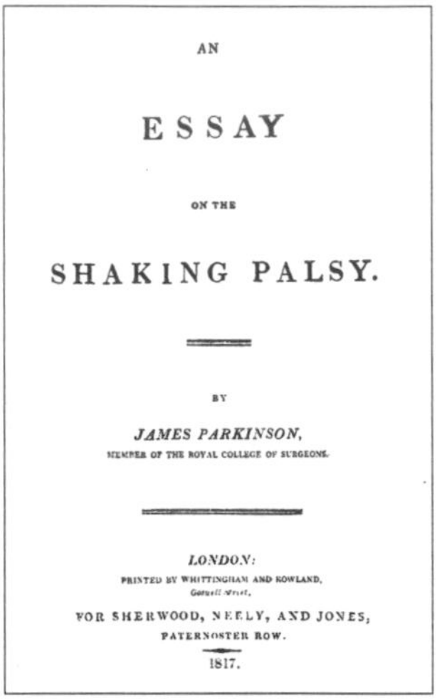

AN

ESSAY

ON THE

SHAKING PALSY.

BY

JAMES PARKINSON,
MEMBER OF THE ROYAL COLLEGE OF SURGEONS.

LONDON:
PRINTED BY WHITTINGHAM AND ROWLAND,
Goswell Street,

FOR SHERWOOD, NEELY, AND JONES,
PATERNOSTER ROW.

1817.

FIGURE 5   Front piece of James Parkinson's *An Essay on the Shaking Palsy*
(from Ref. 7). This short monograph is extremely difficult to find in its original 1817
version, but it has been reproduced many times. In the essay, Parkinson describes
a small series of subjects with a distinctive constellation of features. Although he
had the opportunity to examine a few of the subjects, some of his reflections were
based solely on observation.

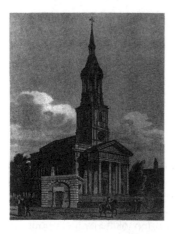

FIGURE 6   St. Leonard's Church (from Ref. 8). The Shoreditch parish church
was closely associated with James Parkinson's life, and he was baptized, married,
and buried there.

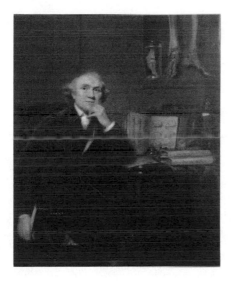

FIGURE 7   (Top) **John Hunter**, painted by J. Reynolds (from Ref. 9). Hunter was admired by Parkinson, who transcribed the surgeon's lectures in his 1833 publication called *Hunterian Reminiscences* (Bottom). In these lectures, Hunter offered observations on tremor. The last sentence of Parkinson's *Essay* reads (7): "... but how few can estimate the benefits bestowed on mankind by the labours of Morgagni, Hunter or Baillie." Currler has posited that Parkinson's own interest in tremor was first developed under the direct influence of Hunter (11).

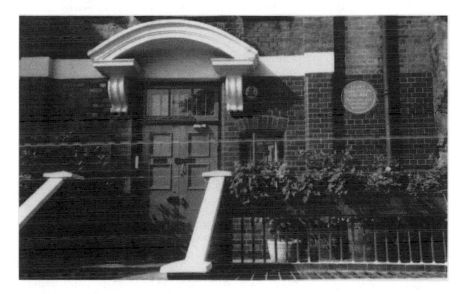

FIGURE 8   James Parkinson's home (from Ref. 12). No. 1 Hoxton Square, London, formerly Shoreditch, today carries a plaque honoring the birthplace of Parkinson.

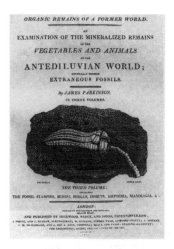

FIGURE 9   James Parkinson as paleontologist (from Ref. 13). An avid geologist and paleontologist, Parkinson published numerous works on fossils, rocks, and minerals. He was an honorary member of the Wernerian Society of Natural History of Edinburgh and the Imperial Society of Naturalists of Moscow.

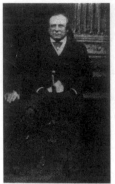

JAMES PARKINSON

FIGURE 10   Counterfeit portrait of James Parkinson (from Ref. 14). To date, no portrait is known to exist of James Parkinson. The photograph of a dentist by the same name was erroneously published and widely circulated in 1938 as part of a *Medical Classics* edition of Parkinson's *Essay*. Because Parkinson died prior to the first daguerreotypes, if a portrait is found, it will be a line drawing, painting, or print. A written description does, however, exist. The paleontologist Mantell wrote (8): "Mr. Parkinson was rather below middle stature, with an energetic intellect, and pleasing expression of countenance and of mild and courteous manners; readily imparting information, either on his favourite science or on professional subjects."

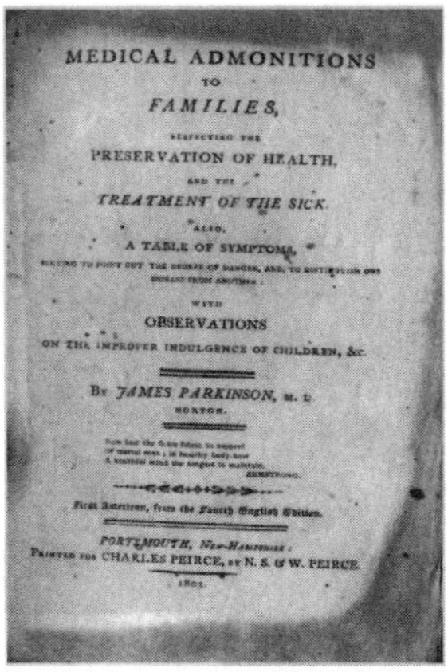

MEDICAL ADMONITIONS
TO
FAMILIES,

PRESERVATION OF HEALTH,

TREATMENT OF THE SICK.

A TABLE OF SYMPTOMS,

OBSERVATIONS

By *JAMES PARKINSON,* M. D.

PORTSMOUTH, New-Hampshire;
PRINTED FOR CHARLES PEIRCE, BY N. S. & W. PEIRCE.

FIGURE 11   One of Parkinson's medical pamphlets (From Ref. 12). An avid writer, Parkinson compiled many books and brochures that were widely circulated on basic hygiene and health. His *Medical Admonitions to Families* and *The Villager's Friend and Physician* were among the most successful, although he also wrote a children's book on safety entitled *Dangerous Sports*, in which he traced the mishaps of a careless child and the lessons he learns through injury (12).

JEAN-MARTIN CHARCOT AND THE SALPÊTRIÈRE SCHOOL

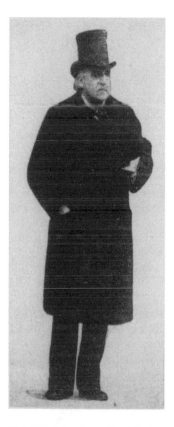

FIGURE 12   **Jean-Martin Charcot**. Working in Paris in the second half of the nineteenth century, Jean-Martin Charcot knew of Parkinson's description and studied the disorder in the large Salpêtrière hospital that housed elderly and destitute women. He identified the cardinal features of Parkinson's disease and specifically separated bradykinesia from rigidity (4,15):

> Long before rigidity actually develops, patients have significant difficulty performing ordinary activities: this problem relates to another cause. In some of the various patients I showed you, you can easily recognize how difficult it is for them to do things even though rigidity or tremor is not the limiting features. Instead, even a cursory exam demonstrates that their problem relates more to slowness in execution of movement rather than to real weakness. In spite of tremor, a patient is still able to do most things, but he performs them with remarkable slowness. Between the thought and the action there is a considerable time lapse. One would think neural activity can only be affected after remarkable effort.

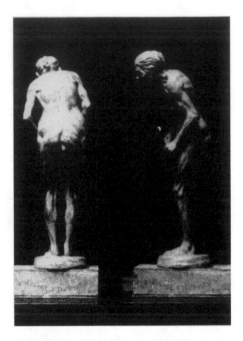

FIGURE 13 **Statue of a parkinsonian woman by Paul Richer** (From Ref. 13). Richer worked with Charcot, and as an artist and sculptor produced several works that depicted the habitus, joint deformities, and postural abnormalities of patients with Parkinson's disease.

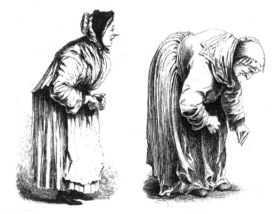

FIGURE 14 **Evolution of parkinsonian disability** (from Ref. 14). The figures drawn by Charcot's student, Paul Richer, capture the deforming posture and progression of untreated Parkinson's disease over a decade.

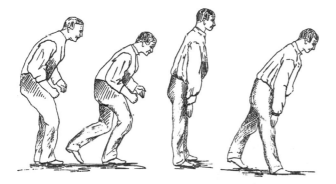

FIGURE 15 **Parkinson's disease and its variants**. Charcot's teaching method involved side-by-side comparisons of patients with various neurological disorders. In one of his presentations on Parkinson's disease, he showed two subjects, one with the typical or archetypal form of the disorder with hunched posture and flexion and another case with atypical parkinsonism, showing an extended posture. The latter habitus is more characteristic of the entity progressive supranuclear palsy, although this disorder was not specifically recognized or labeled by Charcot outside of the term "parkinsonism without tremor" (4).

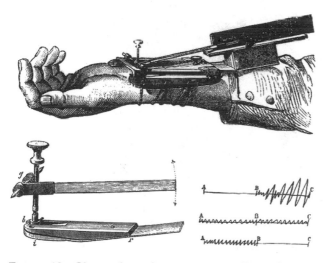

FIGURE 16 **Charcot's early tremor recordings**. Charcot adapted the sphygmograph, an instrument originally used for recording arterial pulsation, to record tremors and movements of the wrist. His resultant tremor recordings (lower right), conducted at rest (A–B) and during activity (B–C), differentiated multiple sclerosis (top recording) from the pure rest tremor (lower recording) or mixed tremor (middle recording) of Parkinson's disease. (From Ref. 18.)

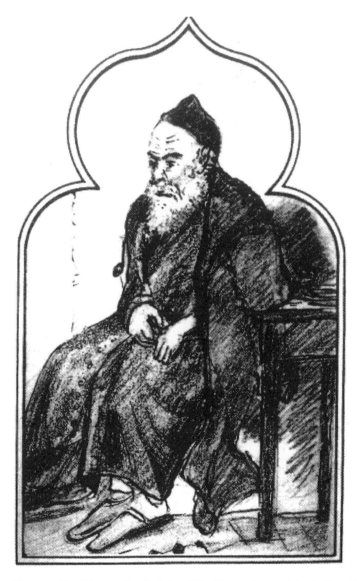

FIGURE 17   Charcot's sketch of Parkinsonian subject. Pencil sketch of a man with Parkinson's disease drawn by Jean-Martin Charcot during a trip to Morocco in 1889 (from Ref. 19). Referring to the highly stereotyped clinical presentation of Parkinson's disease patients, Charcot told his students (3,4): "I have seen such patients everywhere, in Rome, Amsterdam, Spain, always the same picture. They can be identified from afar. You do not need a medical history." Charcot's medical drawings form a large collection, which is housed at the Bibliothèque Charcot at the Hôpital de la Salpêtrière, Paris.

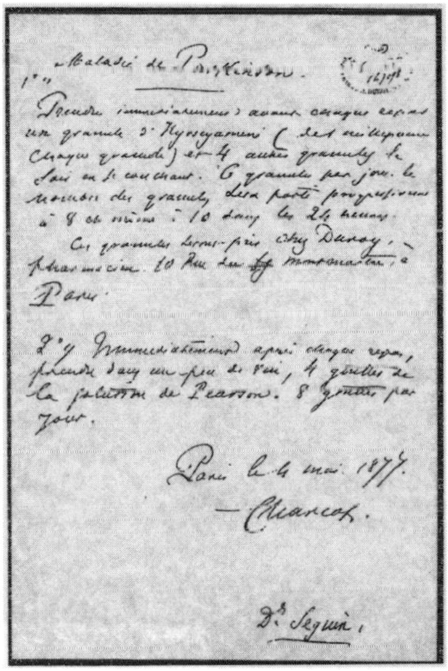

FIGURE 18 **Treatment of Parkinson's disease**. Prescription dated 1877. (From Ref. 20.) In treating Parkinson's disease, Charcot used belladonna alkaloids (agents with potent anticholinergic properties) as well as rye-based products that had ergot activity, a feature of some currently available dopamine agonists (20). Charcot's advice was empiric and preceded the recognition of the well-known dopaminergic/cholinergic balance that is implicit to normal striatal neurochemical activity.

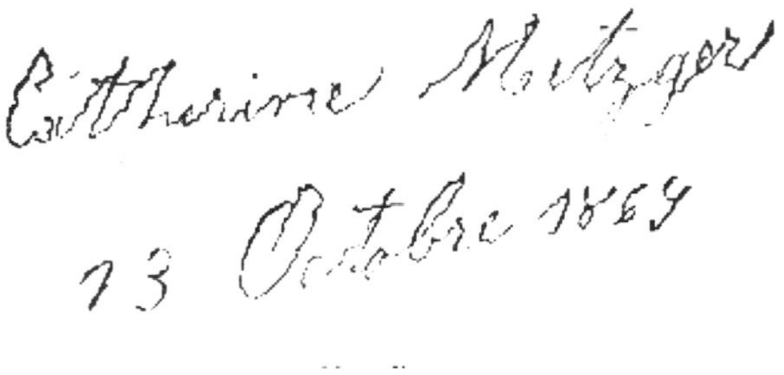

FIGURE 19 **Micrographia and tremorous handwriting** (from Ref. 15). Charcot recognized that one characteristic feature of Parkinson's disease was the handwriting impairment that included tremorous and tiny script. Charcot collected handwriting samples in his patient charts and used them as part of his diagnositic criteria, thereby separating the large and sloppy script of patients with action tremor from the micrographia of Parkinson's disease.

OTHER NINETEENTH-CENTURY CONTRIBUTIONS

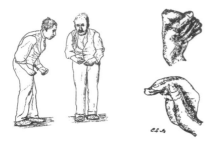

FIGURE 20   William Gower's work. William Gower's *A Manual of Diseases of the Nervous System* shows sketches of patients with Parkinson's disease (left) and diagrams of joint deformities (right) (from Ref. 21). More known for written descriptions than visual images, William Gowers offered one of the most memorable similes regarding parkinsonian tremor: *"the movement of the fingers at the metacarpal-phalangeal joints is similar to that by which Orientals beat their small drums."* His historic textbook, *A Manual of Diseases of the Nervous System*, included sketches of patients with Parkinson's disease as well as diagrams of the characteristic joint deformities.

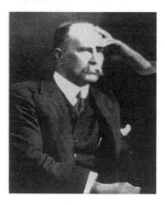

FIGURE 21   William Osler. Osler published his celebrated *Principles and Practice of Medicine* in 1892, one year before Charcot's death. As an internist always resistant to the concept of medical specialization, Osler was influential in propogating information to generalists on many neurological conditions, including Parkinson's disease. Osler was less forthcoming than Charcot in appreciating the distinction between bradykinesia and weakness, and he sided with Parkinson in maintaining that mental function was unaltered. Osler was particularly interested in pathological studies and alluded to the concept of Parkinson's disease as a state of accelerated aging (22).

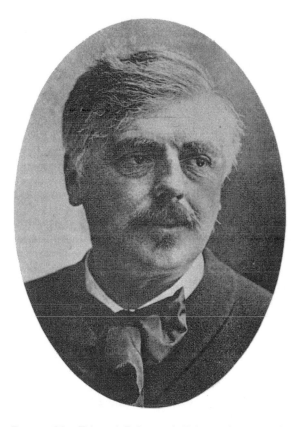

FIGURE 22 **Eduard Brissaud**. Brissaud was a close associate of Charcot and contributed several important clinical observations on Parkinson's disease in the late nineteenth century. Most importantly, however, he brought neuropathological attention to the substantia nigra as the potential cite of disease origin. In discussing a case of a tuberculoma that destroyed the substantia nigra and in association with contralateral hemiparkinsonism, he considered the currently vague knowledge of the nucleus and its putative involvement in volitional and reflex motor control. Extending his thoughts, he hypothesized that "a lesion of the *locus niger* could reasonably be the anatomic basis of Parkinson's disease" (23).

REFERENCES

1. Finger S. Origins of Neuroscience. New York: Oxford University Press, 1994.
2. Sauvages de la Croix FB. Nosologia methodica. Amstelodami: Sumptibus Fratrum de Tournes, 1763.
3. Charcot J-M. Leçons du Mardi: Policlinique: 1887–1888. Paris: Bureaux du Progrès Médical, 1888.

4. Goetz CG. Charcot, the Clinician: The Tuesday Lessons. New York: Raven Press, 1987.
5. Horowski R, Horowski L, Vogel S, Poewe W, Kielhorn F-W. An essay on Wilhelm von Humboldt and the shaking palsy. Neurology 1995; 45:565–568.
6. Leitzmann A. Briefe von Wilhelm von Humboldt an eine Freundin. Leipzig: Inselverlag, 1909.
7. Parkinson J. Essay on the Shaking Palsy. London: Whittingham and Rowland for Sherwood, Neeley and Jones, 1817.
8. Morris AD, Rose FC. James Parkinson: His Life and Times. Boston: Birkhauser, 1989.
9. Allen E, Turk JL, Murley R. The Case Books of John Hunter FRS. London: Royal Society of Medicine, 1993.
10. Parkinson J. Hunterian Reminiscences. London: Sherwood, Gilbert and Piper, 1833.
11. Currier RD. Did John Hunter give James Parkinson an idea? Arch Neurol 1996; 53:377–378.
12. Robert D. Currier Parkinson Archives legged to Christopher G. Goetz.
13. Parkinson J. Organic Remains of a Former World (three volumes). London: Whittingham and Rowland for Sherwood, Neeley and Jones, 1804–1811.
14. Kelly EC. Annotated reprinting: essay on the shaking palsy by James Parkinson. Medical Classics 1938; 2:957–998.
15. Charcot J-M. De la paralysie agitante (leçon 5). Oeuvres Complètes 1:161–188, Paris, Bureaux du Progrès Médical, 1869. In English: On paralysis agitans (Lecture 5). Lectures on the Diseases of the Nervous System, 105–107, translated by G. Sigurson. Philadelphia: HC Lea and Company, 1879.
16. Historical art and document collection, Christopher G. Goetz.
17. Goetz CG, Bonduelle M, Gelfand T. Charcot: Constructing Neurology. New York: Oxford University Press, 1995.
18. Charcot J-M. Tremblements et mouvements choreiforms (leçon 15). Oeuvres Complètes 9:215–228, Paris, Bureaux du Progrès Médical, 1888. In English: Choreiform movements and tremblings. Clinical Lectures on Diseases of the Nervous System, 208–221, translated by E.F. Hurd. Detroit: GS Davis, 1888.
19. Meige H. Charcot Artiste. Nouvelle Iconographie de la Salpêtrière 1898; 11:489–516.
20. Philadelphia College of Physicians, Original manuscript and document collection.
21. Gowers WR. A Manual of Diseases of the Nervous System. London: Churchill, 1886–1888.
22. Osler W. The Principles and Practice of Medicine. New York: Appleton and Company, 1892.
23. Brissaud E. Nature et pathogénie de la maladie de Parkinson (leçon 23, 488–501). Leçons sur les Maladies Nerveuses: la Salpêtrière, 1893–1894. Paris: Masson, 1895.

2

Epidemiology of Parkinsonism

**Ali H. Rajput, Alex Rajput, and
Michele Rajput**
University of Saskatchewan, Saskatoon,
Saskatchewan, Canada

Epidemiology is the study of large numbers of individuals to ascertain incidence, life expectancy, prevalence, time trends, preceding and associated illnesses, and other factors in a disease. Contrasted to laboratory studies in which the experimental conditions can be controlled, epidemiology examines natural events that may have been influenced by health care, economic, and social factors. Epidemiology is broadly divided into four categories—descriptive, analytic, clinical, and experimental—although there is considerable overlap (1).

Descriptive epidemiology deals with incidence, age and sex distribution, life expectancy, and prevalence rates. Analytic epidemiology is aimed at identifying factors that are positively or negatively associated with the illness and hence may be causally linked. Because the events that significantly influence the epidemiology of a disease cannot be controlled, it is important that any bias that may confound the observations be identified and avoided or adjusted for. Clinical epidemiology includes studies that require repeated clinical assessments and/or pathological studies to determine disease profile. Hypotheses generated by descriptive and analytic epidemiology may be tested with these studies. Experimental epidemiology deals with planned large studies designed to determine the impact of intervention on the disease outcome (2,3).

No two epidemiological studies are identical. For many reasons, the methods utilized at one location or at one time may not be possible at another. Also, populations vary by time and place. Epidemiological studies are labor intensive. Patience and thoughtful planning are essential for proper studies, as is teamwork where clinicians work together with those who collect, enter, analyze, and interpret the data. Biostaticians are vital members of the team and should be involved early in the planning of a study. Team members should collectively consider the study design.

Parkinson syndrome (PS) is a clinical diagnosis, and different diagnostic criteria have been used in different studies, therefore, strict comparison of the literature is very difficult (4). A bias may be introduced at any stage—during data collection, analysis, or interpretations. In most studies, the familial PS cases are identified by direct or indirect history; this introduces a significant source of bias. One concordance study of Parkinson's disease (PD) probands and the family members who had a movement disorder revealed that 74% of the secondary cases had PD while the remaining had a different disorder (5). In one family that had several autopsy-verified PD cases, family members were confident that a certain deceased sibling also had PD. He had died in an accident and an autopsy showed no PD pathology(5). Some PS cases may be misclassified as being "old" (5). Thus, it is essential that suspected cases be examined by a neurologist to verify the diagnosis.

It is not uncommon that seemingly similar epidemiological studies arrive at different conclusions. Any study may have only a certain portion that is scientifically valid. Epidemiological reports should be easily comprehensible to an average physician. The best guide is one's own judgment. All analytic epidemiological observations where a certain factor/ event is associated with PS or PD should not be interpreted as indication of a cause for the disease. The cause and effect always coexist, but definite causal linkage requires a considerably higher level of evidence than a mere association.

INCLUSION CRITERIA FOR PARKINSON EPIDEMIOLOGY

The two major considerations for inclusion in PS epidemiology are:

1. Does this individual have PS, normal aging, or another disorder?
2. Does this person have idiopathic PD (6,7) or another variant of PS?

Aging and Parkinsonism

Primitive reflexes that are common in PD are also seen in normal elderly (8–10). Slowed motor functions characteristic of PD are part of normal aging as well (11,12). Paratonia (gegenhalten) in the elderly who cannot hear properly or are unable to follow instructions due to cognitive impairment may be mistaken as parkinsonian rigidity (8,13,14). Arthritis is common in the elderly, and pain during passive movement at the arthritic joint leads to involuntary resistance resembling rigidity. Flexed posture and impaired postural reflexes, the other major features of PS, are also seen in the normal elderly (10,13,15,16). In general, the age-related abnormalities are symmetrical, while PS is often asymmetrical. Rest tremor, a common early feature of PS (17), is not part of normal aging (18) and hence is the single most reliable feature of this disorder.

The most common tremor disorder that is mistaken as PD is essential tremor (ET) (19). Typically, ET is present on positioning a limb against gravity and during activity. ET is usually restricted to the upper limbs and/or head. By contrast, resting tremor is characteristic of PS/PD and may involve the upper and lower limbs. Evolution of ET with time is well known (20). Nearly one third of these patients develop rest tremor during late stages of the disease (19,20) and, therefore, may be mistaken as PS.

For epidemiological surveys, the diagnostic criteria should be simple, consistent through the study interval, and easy to apply. After careful consideration of different diagnostic criteria utilized in epidemiological studies, de Rijk et al. (4) concluded that the most suitable is the presence of two of the three cardinal signs—bradykinesia, rigidity, and tremor. In individuals with preexisting ET, the additional diagnosis of PS should be made only when all three signs are present (19).

Parkinson Variants

The second major consideration is to classify PS cases into different variants. Most neurologists use the term PD for Lewy body disease (6,7). Distinction between different PS variants is difficult, especially during the early stages of the disease. Even in a clinical setting where patients are repeatedly evaluated by experts, accurate clinical diagnosis may not be possible because the telltale features that distinguish other variants from PD may evolve much later or never (7,21,22). Diagnostic criteria applied retrospectively to autopsied cases (23,24) are not practical in epidemiological studies, which are as a rule based on clinical assessment. Classification into possible, probable, and definite PD (25) has limited value in epidemiological studies, which are primarily aimed at measuring the magnitude of the disorder in the population. Some drug-induced PS patients have underlying idiopathic PD (26), and response to levodopa (LD), though valuable, does not always distinguish between different Parkinson syndromes (27). In one study, when the initial clinical diagnosis of PD was made, only 65% of those cases had PD at autopsy (7).

PD is the most common PS variant in clinical (28,29) and pathological series (17). All variants of PS produce significant functional handicap and may improve on the same drugs. Classification into different PS variants is valuable, but it should be recognized that such an exercise would only provide approximate estimates. Autopsy studies to confirm the diagnosis are not possible in epidemiological surveys. Therefore, for descriptive epidemiological studies, all PS variants should be considered. Further classification may then be made based on the best clinical evidence.

DESCRIPTIVE EPIDEMIOLOGY

Incidence of Parkinsonism

Incidence is defined as the number of new cases per year and is usually described per 10^5 population. Incidence can be determined for various categories including gender and age. Incidence studies are difficult because all of the new-onset patients who need to be included may not be recognized until sometime later. In addition, the number of new cases in a community may vary from one year to the next. Consequently, incidence studies require a long period of observation in the same community.

The reported incidence rates of PS vary widely. The lowest incidence in Western countries is reported from Sardinia at $4.9/10^5$ (30). The latest crude annual incidence in Finland is $17.2/10^5$ (31). Based on six general practices in the Netherlands (32), annual incidence was $12/10^5$ for women and $11/10^5$ for men.

In the Western countries, the most reliable incidence studies are from Rochester, Minnesota. Health care in Olmstead County, including Rochester, is provided mainly by the Mayo Clinic–affiliated staff, and the medical records have been carefully compiled since the 1930s. The record linkage system (33) allows the tracking of all Olmstead County residents evaluated at the Mayo Clinic and affiliated hospitals, community physician offices, a community hospital, chronic care institutions, and veteran's hospitals where these patients may be seen. In most PS cases, the diagnosis is confirmed by a qualified neurologist affiliated with the Mayo Clinic (29). Four different incidence reports based on the Rochester, Minnesota, population have been published (28,29,34,35). Drug-induced parkinsonism (DIP) was not known until the early 1960s (36). For the purpose of

TABLE 1   PS-PEP and Other Variants (Excluding Drug-Induced Cases) Diagnosed in Rochester, Minnesota, 1935–1990

	1945–1954 (34)	1935–1966 (35)	1967–1979 (28)	1976–1990 (29)
PEP%	10.7%	6.6%	0	0
All other variants (combined)	89.3%	93.4%	100%	100%
PD (without arteriosclerosis)	60.7%	62.7%	85.5%	>99%
Incidence of PS cases (excluding DIP)	$20.5/10^5$	$18.5/10^5$	$18.2/10^5$	$20.5/10^5$

PEP = postencephalitic parkinsonism;   DIP = drug-induced parkinsonism;   PS = Parkinson syndrome;   PD = Parkinson's disease.

comparison, we excluded DIP from each study. Table 1 shows a summary of incidence rates reported in those studies. There was no significant change in incidence over 55 years. The latest study (29) revealed a PS incidence of 25.6 per 10^5. The PS incidence was $0.8/10^5$ in those 0–29 years of age, $25.6/10^5$ in those 50–59 years, and was more than 11 times higher ($304.8/10^5$) in the 80- to 99-year age group (29). There has been no significant change in age-specific incidence rates during the 55-year interval of these studies (37). However, there is a trend to higher incidence between age 70 and 90 in the most recent study, which is attributed to neuroleptic usage (37). The slightly higher overall incidence of PS in the latest report (29) likely reflects longer life expectancy in the general population, more frequent use of neuroleptics, and improved diagnosis among the demented (29).

An Italian study of persons 65–84 years of age noted an annual incidence of $529.5/10^5$ for PS and $326/10^5$ for PD (38). Some studies have reported a decline in PD incidence after age 79. A northern Manhattan study (39) indicates that the incidence rates of PD consistently increase through age 85. Baldereschi et al. (38) found a continued increase in incidence after age 75, and no decline was noted up to 100 years of age in another study (37). Pathological studies show a progressive increase in the rate of incidental Lewy body (LB) inclusions with advancing age (40,41). These cases are regarded as having preclinical PD. The decline of PS and PD in the very old that has been observed in some studies is attributed to difficulty in ascertaining cases in the presence of comorbid disorders (29). Thus, age remains the single most important risk factor for PS.

Lifetime Risk of Parkinsonism

The current lifetime risk of PS from birth is estimated at 4.4% for men and 3.7% for women (42). Lifetime risk for men 60 years of age is estimated at

4.6% and for women 3.7% (42). This report (42) proposes that at any age, future risk of PD can be calculated (42). The risk of PS in the elderly in an Italian longitudinal study (38) was even higher than that reported from Rochester (42), and men had a higher risk than women (38). Thus far, the highest incidence and risk of PS in the elderly are reported from Italy (38).

Parkinson Variants in the General Population

As noted above, this classification in epidemiological surveys can only be approximate as the final diagnosis may not be possible until after autopsy (7). PS classification has been evolving with time even within the same community (28,29,34,35). Following the first description in 1817 by James Parkinson (43) and the discovery of substantia nigra neuronal loss and LB inclusions, parkinsonism was regarded as a single clinicopathological entity. That concept changed in the 1920s and 1930s. After von Economo encephalitis, an estimated 60% of the victims developed PS, which was classified as postencephalitic parkinsonism (PEP) (44,45). At one time, these patients constituted a large proportion of the PS cases in the general population. No new PEP cases have been reported since the mid-1950s (Table 1). Arteriosclerosis was once reported as a common cause of PS (34,35), but that is a very rare diagnosis now (28,29). This apparent reduction in arteriosclerosis as a cause of PS is due to increased diagnostic accuracy of PS, rather than a dramatic decline in arteriosclerosis in the general population.

Neuroleptic-induced parkinsonism (DIP) was first recognized in the late 1950s and is now a common PS variant (28,29,38) accounting for between 7% (28) and 20% of all PS cases (29). DIP is now the second most common PS variant and is more common in women than men (29).

Large clinicopathological studies of Shy-Drager syndrome (SDS) (46), striatonigral degeneration (SND) (47), and progressive supranuclear palsy (PSP) (48) were first reported in the 1960s, though clinical description of PSP was documented in the nineteenth century (49). Olivopontocerebellar atrophy (OPCA), which often includes some features of PS, has been known since 1900. The current classification includes SND, SDS, and OPCA under the common heading of multiple system atrophy (MSA). Prominent dysautonomia in SDS and akinetic rigid PS features in SND were not fully recognized until 1960 and 1964, respectively, and in all likelihood such cases prior to that were classified as PEP or atypical parkinsonism because they occurred at a relatively young age and had widespread nervous system involvement. In spite of the improved understanding of these uncommon PS variants, the diagnosis is not always possible clinically (7,21,22,50). Autopsy series may be biased because the families of those suffering from the unusual

PS variants may have heightened interest in finding out the nature of the disease and, therefore, be more likely to consent to an autopsy. The true frequency of these variants in the general population is, therefore, not possible to determine. In one epidemiological study, 2.5% of all PS patients were classified as MSA and 4.3% as PSP (29). A previous study from the same community reported PSP diagnosis in 1.4% and MSA diagnosis in 2.1% of PS cases (28). Thus, MSA and PSP each represent less than 5% of the contemporary PS cases in North America.

The most common PS variant in epidemiological studies (28,38,51) is idiopathic PD (6). The proportion of those with PD, however, varies widely in different studies—e.g., 42% (29), 62% (38), and 85% (28). Preponderance of PD is also noted in autopsy studies of unselected PS cases (27,52,53). Dementia with Lewy bodies (DLB) is now a well-recognized entity (54), and extrapyramidal features may also be seen in Alzheimer's disease (AD) (55). One recent PS study (29) noted that 14% of all PS cases had dementia manifesting within one year of PS onset and classified these as "Parkinsonism in dementia." Most of these cases likely had DLB (55). The clinical and pathological classification of PS variants continues to evolve, but the most common variant is still PD (6,7).

Life Expectancy in Parkinsonism

All the PS variants limit mobility. Increased tendency to falls and dysphagia predispose these patients to life-threatening complications (56,57). Life expectancy prior to the widespread use of LD was significantly reduced. In one hospital-based PS series during the 1950s and 1960s, the mean survival after onset was 10.8 years (58). A large proportion of these patients had PEP. The PEP cases had longer survival than other PD cases (58,59). When the PEP cases were excluded, the mean survival in the remaining cases was 9.42 years (58). That study is frequently cited as the yardstick for the pre-LD era life expectancy. Mean survival in the contemporary PS cases cannot be compared with that study. There have been significant social and health care advances leading to longer life in the general population. One would expect that PS patients would share these survival gains. Comparison for PS patients' survival should be made matching for year of birth, gender, and region/country.

Kurtzke et al. (60) noted that patients in the 1980s were, on average, 5 years older at death than those who died in the 1970s, implying that life expectancy since the widespread use of LD has increased by 5 years. Several other studies have also reported longer life expectancy (61,62,63,64), though it remains reduced compared to the general population (64). Some observers, however, remain unconvinced (65,66). At the other extreme are studies that suggest that current PS cases survive longer than the general population (67,68). It is difficult to reconcile that individuals suffering from a progressively disabling disorder would live longer than the matched general population. The most common error in the better-than-expected survival studies is measuring survival from the date of onset assigned several years retrospectively. During that period, the general population would have suffered some death. That gives the PS group an artificial advantage, since they survived at least to diagnosis (67). When we assessed our patients using the date of onset, the PS patients survived longer than the general population (64). The other reason for this error is inclusion of only LD-treated cases (68). For any number of reasons, some patients may not be treated with LD and those destined for longer survival may be treated with LD, which introduces a significant bias. Longer survival has been noted by others if only the LD-treated cases were considered (28). Restricting a study to only clinically diagnosed PD and excluding other variants introduces another source of bias, as the inaccuracy of clinical diagnosis is well known (7,21).

A blinded study withholding modern drugs from one group of matched patients is not possible. In a clinic-based study of 934 PS cases seen between 1968 and 1990 (64,69), survival measured from the date of first assessment was significantly reduced ($p < 0.0001$) in PS (64,69). This study (64,69) also considered the impact of widespread and easy access to LD (regardless of cost) on the survival. The survival remained shorter ($p = 0.029$) than expected for the general population (Fig. 1). Prior to January 1, 1974, LD was available almost exclusively to patients seen at the Movement Disorder Clinic Saskatoon (MDCS). When survival in patients assessed before this date was compared to the expected survival, reduction was even more pronounced ($p < 0.0001$). (Fig. 2) Taken together, these indicate that widespread use of LD has improved survival in PS (64,69). There was no difference in the use of other drugs, which may explain the survival differences (64,69). The survival is negatively impacted in patients with dementia (61,69,70) and in those with a PS diagnosis other than PD. The most favorable prognosis was in the patients diagnosed as PD who had no dementia at initial assessment (64,69).

The timing of treatment with LD indicates that survival benefit is achieved only when patients are treated prior to the loss of postural reflexes (58,64,71). Similar observations of longer survival in patients with early LD treatment have been reported by others (62).

When Figs 1 and 2 are considered together, it is evident that the survival gap between current PS cases and the general population has narrowed ($p = 0.029$ vs. $p < 0.0001$). This gain in life expectancy is attributable exclusively to the better symptomatic control on LD, which

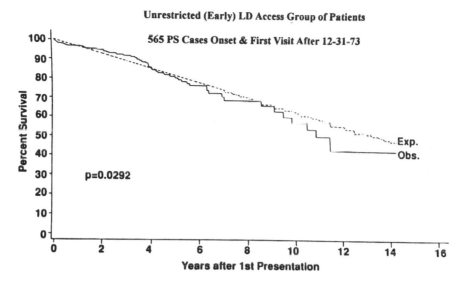

FIGURE 1 Comparison of survival in parkinsonian patients with unrestricted levodopa availability (Obs.) to a sex- and year of birth-matched regional population (Exp.).

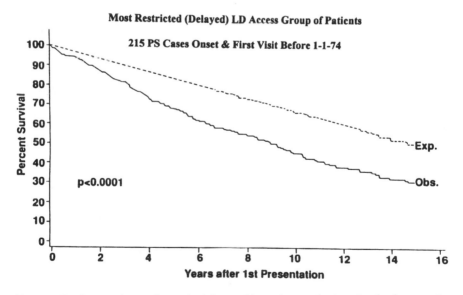

FIGURE 2 Comparison of survival in parkinsonian patients who had severely restricted access to levodopa (Obs.) to a sex- and year of birth-matched regional population (Exp.).

prevents disability and life-threatening complications (56,57). We estimate that an average patient with PD onset at age 62 now lives for approximately 20 years. The survival is shorter in other degenerative diseases associated with PS (17,22). Average survival from onset of PSP is approximately 9 years (72), although rare cases may live for 24 years after onset (22).

Prevalence of Parkinsonism

The prevalence rate is defined as the number of PS patients in the population at a given time and is usually described as cases per 10^5. The term point prevalence implies prevalence rate on a particular date. The two main factors that determine the prevalence rate are the incidence of new cases and the life expectancy. Those issues have been discussed above. If the number of new cases emerged at a constant rate but the life expectancy increased, the prevalence rate would rise.

Several different methods have been used to determine PS prevalence rate. These include review of all the health records in a given community, consumption of antiparkinson drugs (73,74), direct survey of population, and indirect measurement by multiplying incidence rate with mean survival. Although labor intensive, the most reliable method is the door-to-door survey of a community population. The usual procedure involves two steps, an initial survey questionnaire followed by a neurological examination of those whose response is suggestive of PS (75–79). In spite of the considerable efforts, 6–18% of the eligible population cannot be assessed (77,78). The distinction of PS from normal age-related changes and from other systemic and neurological diseases are important considerations for inclusion/ exclusion in such surveys. Door-to-door surveys show that between 35% (78) and 42% (75) of the PS cases identified during the survey were not previously diagnosed. These cases would have been missed in a record review. An undiagnosed PS case would not be receiving antiparkinson drugs, hence the studies based on drug consumption would significantly underestimate the prevalence rate.

Some prevalence studies include only clinically diagnosed PD (31), while others include all PS variants (78). While some studies include all residents of a community and adjust for the age distribution of the population, known as age-adjusted prevalence rate, others restrict the surveys to only persons above a certain age (e.g., 40 years) (75) and describe a crude rate.

In the Caucasian population, the crude prevalence ratios vary from 84/ 10^5 to 775/10^5 population (80,81). The prevalence rates based on door-to-door surveys are $57/10^5$ in China (79), $371.5/10^5$ in Sicily (78), and $775/10^5$ in Australia (83). In a Parsi community from Bombay, India, the prevalence rate was $328/10^5$ (76). In a U.S. community-based study of Copiah County residents, which included only persons over the age of 40 years, the prevalence rate was $347/10^5$ (75). A Dutch study in the early 1990s found a prevalence rate of 1.4% in those aged 55–64 years and 4.3% in an 85- to 95-year age group (82).

In a representative sample of community residents 65 years and older from Canada (83), the prevalence rate was 3% ($3000/10^5$), while in institutionalized persons (84) the rate was 9% ($9000/10^5$). Somewhat comparable figures were reported from Australia (81). They included only PD cases in persons 55 years and older. The prevalence rate of PD was $3600/10^5$ in the community and $4900/10^5$ in the institutionalized persons (81). They estimated that the crude prevalence rate of PD in the entire community was $775/10^5$.

Bennett et al. (10) performed a random sample survey in Boston area residents $\geqslant 65$ years (10) for PS signs. They classified PS as having two of four signs: tremor, bradykinesia, rigidity, and gait abnormality. The prevalence of PS in this study was 14.9% ($14,900/10^5$) in age 65–74 years, 29.5% ($29,500/10^5$) in 75–84 years, and 52.4% ($52,400/10^5$) in those $\geqslant 85$ years (10). This observation represents the highest reported prevalence. It is not clear in this report (10) how many patients were evaluated by a neurologist, and the study has been criticized (29). The age-adjusted (31) 1991 Finnish population PD prevalence rate was $139/10^5$. In a European collaborative study (85) restricted to 65 years and older, the PD overall rate was $1800/10^5$, and in the 85- to 89-year age group, it was $2600/10^5$.

Prevalence rate can also be estimated by multiplying the incidence rate and the mean survival. Most researchers regard Rochester, Minnesota, incidence rates as representative for North America. The latest annual incidence of PS in Rochester is $25.6/10^5$. The survival in PS has increased substantially during the last 3 decades. A conservative estimate of mean survival in contemporary PS is 15 years, though an average PD case would survive longer. Thus, the minimum prevalence rate in the North American general population is estimated at $384/10^5$.

The literature indicates that (1) the age-specific incidence (in Rochester) was unchanged between 1935 and 1990 (37); (2) there is an increase in PS in persons 70–99 years, primarily due to increase in DIP (37); (3) there is large pool of at-risk population, as the general population is living longer; (4) there has been a substantial increase in life expectancy in PS on the current treatment (64,69,86), and (5) the lifetime risk of parkinsonism, which in the 1950s was estimated at 2.4% (34), is now estimated at 3.7% in women and 4.4% in men (42).

Gender and Parkinsonism

A higher incidence of PS in men has been reported in several studies (29,31,38,39,42,87,88), though some reviews conclude that this difference may be artifactual (80). The available evidence indicates that men have a slightly higher risk of parkinsonism than women, with the exception of DIP (29).

Several studies have reported no difference between males and females while other studies have reported a higher prevalence in women (78,89). More recent studies have noted higher incidence and prevalence rates in the males than in females (29,38,76,90,91). The cumulative evidence so far favors a slight male preponderance of PS and PD.

Race, Ethnicity, Skin Color, and Risk of Parkinsonism

Parkinsonism has been reported in all races. Several studies have suggested that those with darker skin have a reduced risk of PD compared to lighter complected individuals (30,92,93,94). However, these differences were attributed to the source of the study—U.S. private hospitals—which at that time African Americans had limited access to (95,96). Studies that included communities with a mixed population did not observe any racial differences (39,75). The risk of parkinsonism is best measured by incidence rates and not by prevalence rates, which are affected by survival rates. In a mixed community, Mayeux et al. (39) observed that the incidence was highest in African American males, but there was higher mortality in this group. There is no evidence that darker skinned persons have a larger number of substantia nigra pigmented neurons or that the vulnerability of these neurons differs in different races. In one dopa-responsive dystonia autopsied case, we discovered markedly hypopigmented substantia nigra, but her skin color and tendency to tan were similar to her other siblings (97). Thus, skin color by itself is not related to the risk of PS or PD.

Geography and Parkinsonism

In most countries, geography and ethnicity are intertwined. In relatively newly settled countries (e.g., the United States and Canada), all racial and ethnic groups live in the same geographic location, which permits better assessment of the role of geographic background in parkinsonism.

The Parkinson-dementia-ALS complex of Guam is unique (98). There are no other large geographic clusters of well-documented PS or PD. The lowest reported prevalence rate is $57/10^5$ population in China (79), followed by $65.6/10^5$ in Sardinia (30), $67/10^5$ in Nigeria (77), $80.6/10^5$ in Japan (99); the highest reported rate is from Australia (81) at $775/10^5$. African

Americans and Caucasians living in the same U.S. communities have similar incidence (39) and prevalence rates (75). The prevalence rate in U.S. African Americans was five times higher than in Nigerians, who presumably share a common genetic background. (77). This difference remained significant when the life expectancy in the general population in the two countries was taken into account (77). It is of note that the same investigator conducted those two studies (75,77) using the same methodology.

Geographic differences among different western Canadian provinces have been reported (100), and a north-south gradient in the United States has been suggested in one study (101) but not confirmed by others (102). Difference in incidence of PS based on the population density in Saskatchewan revealed that those born and raised in smaller communities (population $\leqslant 200$) had an increased risk of parkinsonism (103,104). This study included only those cases that had onset before age 40 years (103). Several other North American and European reports noted a higher risk of PD with rural residence during early age (105–109), but others failed to substantiate this finding (110,111). One Canadian study noted no increase in the risk of PD in those who had previously lived in rural areas or had worked on a farm (112).

In summary, there are geographic differences for the risk of PD, but the risk is not linked to racial or ethnic background. It is attributable to shared geography, which points to a shared environmental exposure.

ANALYTIC AND EXPERIMENTAL EPIDEMIOLOGY OF PD

Epidemiological studies for the causes of PD are difficult to pursue. PD is a clinical diagnosis, and therefore there is significant misclassification bias (5). In addition, reporting of exposure history can be subject to recall bias. A genetic basis for PD has been identified in only a small proportion of cases (see Chapter 14).

Premorbid/Comorbid Disorders and Lifestyle

Clues to PS etiology maybe found in premorbid and comorbid disorders. Several studies have reported that a history of psychoneurosis and psychosomatic illness is more common in PS cases than in matched controls (113,114). A distinctive PD personality—introspective, frugal, stoic, well organized, and adverse to risk—has been suggested (115,116). The significance of these findings is unknown. It may indicate a common pathophysiology or that the individuals with these premorbid disorders have an increased risk of PS.

Lifestyle and Parkinsonism

Several lifestyle issues, including smoking, consumption of coffee, alcohol, and different diets, have been studied (41,117–121) in an effort to determine their relationship to PD. Smoking has been the focus of many studies. Some reports indicate that smoking has a protective effect against PD (117,118,122–130), while others found no relationship (113,119,120,131). Current smoking and past smoking were noted to have a protective effect in some studies (125,127), and only the male smokers had reduced risk in another study (132). No difference in PD risk related to smoking was observed by others (120,131). The cumulative tobacco exposure is reported to reduce PD risk by some (125,129), but no dose effect was found by others (113,119,120,131,133). One recent report of monozygotic PD twins noted that the twins without PD had smoked more ($p = 0.077$) than the co-twins with PD (129).

Lewy body inclusions and marked substantia nigra pigmented neuron loss is the hallmark of PD (6,40,134), and presence of LB observed incidentally at autopsy has been regarded as an indication of preclinical PD (40,134). In one autopsy series of 220 brains, incidental LB inclusions had no relation to ever smoking or current smoking (41), nor was there any association between presence of LB and the pack-years of smoking (41). The risk of LB inclusion correlated with the age of the patient (41). If smoking was protective against PD, one would expect that smokers would have a lower frequency of incidental LB. Smoking benefit to PD risk would also be evident in age of onset and rate of progression. Smokers, in fact, have a younger (113,133) onset age, and the progression is not influenced by continued smoking (119).

In summary, the literature on smoking and risk of PD remains controversial. In spite of several epidemiological studies suggesting a protective effect, as noted above, several critical pieces of evidence do not support this hypothesis. The reported negative association notwithstanding, it is likely that smoking is a marker of the underlying personality trait (119,120).

Studies of the association between PD and the consumption of alcohol have also produced controversial results (120). Lower frequency of PD has been reported in coffee drinkers (117,120). A recent report on diet in twins, on the other hand, indicates that chocolate consumption increases the risk of PD (135). In Western cultures where coffee and alcohol use is common, the incidence of PD is higher than in cultures that do not utilize these substances (77,79). The evidence for coffee, alcohol, or other foods having a protective effect on PD remains weak.

Comorbid Psychiatric Disorders

Depression

Prior to the onset of motor symptoms, depression is more common in PD than in the matched control subjects (114,136–141). Between 30 and 90% of PD patients (142) have been reported to have depression. Depression is frequently unrecognized by patients and caregivers. The available evidence indicates that depression in PD has an endogenous basis in addition to being in reaction to the severity of physical disability (143–146).

Dementia and Parkinsonism

The reported frequency of dementia in PS ranges from 2% (147) to 81% (148), although most were minimally affected in this study. Some cognitive impairment has been reported even in mild early parkinsonian patients (149,150) and is more likely in depressed patients (146). The reported frequency of dementia varies depending on the patient population and the intensity of the search. (151). Several other studies have reported that approximately one third of PS patients at any given time have dementia (147,152–154). Late age of PD onset is associated with increased dementia risk. Dementia was more common in those with onset after age 60 years than the earlier onset (25% vs. 2%) in one study (147) and in those with onset after age 70 years compared to the younger individuals in another study (155).

Dementia evolves at a higher rate in PD than in the matched population. In one case-control study, dementia evolved 3.8 times more often in the patients than in the controls at 5 years (113). In a community-based study, nondemented PD patients (156) were compared with the age-, sex-, and educational level–matched general population. At the end of 4.2 years, the dementia was 5.9 times more common in PD than in the controls (156). One study concluded that by age 85 years, 65% of the surviving cohort had dementia (155). Diagnosis of dementia is associated with significantly reduced survival (60,64,70,157–162).

Other Comorbid Disorders

Literature has produced contradictory evidence on the risk of cancer in PS (58,113,163). Based on available evidence, it is concluded that risk of cancer in PD is not different from the general population. The reported risk of stroke varies considerably. At one time, cerebral ischemia was regarded as a common cause of PD (34,35). Pathological studies indicate that stroke is an extremely rare cause of PS (17). Two recent studies concluded that stroke is less common in parkinsonian patients than in the general population (164,165). One study (165) speculated that dopamine deficiency has a protective effect against ischemic brain damage.

Essential Tremor and Parkinsonism

Several studies found an increased risk of PS in ET patients (166–168), while others could not substantiate this finding (169–172). One reason for the differences is the different patterns of referrals—the most complicated cases attend highly specialized centers. The pathological findings in PD and ET are remarkably different (6,173). In our clinic-based, autopsy-verified ET cases, nearly one third of patients had resting tremor as a natural evolution of the ET (19,20). Of the 21 ET cases, 6 (29%) had clinical evidence of parkinsonism—resting tremor, bradykinesia, and rigidity (19). Only one of those 6 cases had LB pathology. Two had PSP, 2 had DIP, and one had basal ganglia ischemic lesion (20). If the risk of PD were significantly higher in ET patients, we would have expected to see more cases with PD pathology. It is concluded that the risk of PD in ET is not different from that in the general population.

REFERENCES

1. AH Rajput, S Birdi. Epidemiology of Parkinson's disease. Parkinsonism Relat Disord 1997; 3(4):175–186.
2. Parkinson Study Group. DATATOP: a multicenter controlled clinical trial in early Parkinson's disease. Arch Neurol 1989; 46:1052–1060.
3. Parkinson Study Group. Effect of deprenyl on the progression of disability in early Parkinson's disease. N Engl J Med 1989; 821:1364–1371.
4. MC de Rijk, WA Rocca, DW Anderson, MO Melcon, MMB Breteler, DM Maraganore. A population perspective on diagnostic criteria for Parkinson's disease. Neurology 1997; 48:1277–1281.
5. AH Rajput, ME Fenton, D George, A Rajput, W Wilson, L McCulloch. Concordance of common movement disorders among familial cases. Mov Disord 1997; 12(5):747–751.
6. R Duvoisin, LI Golbe. Toward a definition of Parkinson's disease. Neurology 1989; 39:746
7. AH Rajput, B Rozdilsky, AH Rajput. Accuracy of clinical diagnosis in Parkinsonism—a prospective study. Can J Neurol Sci 1991; 18:275–278.
8. LR Jenkyn, AG Reeves, T Warren, RK Whiting, RJ Clayton, WW Moore, A Rizzo, IM Tuzun, JC Bonnet, BW Culpepper. Neurological signs in senescence. Arch Neurol 1985; 42:1154–1157.
9. WC Koller, S Glatt, RS Wilson, JH Fox. Primitive reflexes and cognitive function in the elderly. Ann Neurol 1982; 12:302–304.
10. DA Bennett, LA Beckett, AM Murray, KM Shannon, CG Goetz, DM Pilgrim, DA Evans. Prevalence of parkinsonian signs and associated mortality in a community population of older people. N Engl J Med 1996; 334:71–76.
11. DA Drachman, RR Long, JM Swearer. Neurological evaluation of the elderly patient. In: ML Albert, JE Knoefel, eds. Clinical Neurology of Aging. 2 ed. New York: Oxford University Press, 1994:159–180.

12. G Duncan, JA Wilson. Normal elderly have some signs of PS. Lancet 1989; 1392–1392.
13. AH Rajput. Parkinsonism, aging and gait apraxia. In: MB Stern, WC Koller, eds. Parkinsonian Syndromes. New York: Marcel Dekker, Inc., 1993:511–532.
14. HL Klawans. Abnormal movements in the elderly. Sandorama 1981; 15–18.
15. WJ Weiner, LM Nora, RH Glantz. Elderly inpatients: postural reflex impairment. Neurology 1984; 34:945–947.
16. ME Tinetti, M Speechley, SF Ginter. Risk factors for falls among elderly persons living in the community. N Engl J Med 1988; 319:1701–1707.
17. AH Rajput, R Pahwa, P Pahwa, A Rajput. Prognostic significance of the onset mode in parkinsonism. Neurology 1993; 43:829–830.
18. AH Rajput. Clinical features of tremor in extrapyramidal syndromes. In: LJ Findley, WC Koller, eds. Handbook of Tremor Disorders. New York: Marcel Dekker, Inc., 1994:275–291.
19. AH Rajput, B Rozdilsky, L Ang, A Rajput. Significance of parkinsonian manifestations in essential tremor. Can J Neurol Sci 1993; 20:114–117.
20. A Rajput, C Robinson, AH Rajput. Longitudinal study of essential tremor: 21 autopsy cases. Neurology 2002; 58 (suppl 3):A253–A254.
21. AJ Hughes, SE Daniel, L Kilford, AJ Lees. Accuracy of clinical diagnosis of idiopathic Parkinson's disease: a clinico-pathological study of 100 cases. J Neurol Neurosurg Psychiatry 1992; 55:181–184.
22. S Birdi, AH Rajput, M Fenton, IR Donat, B Rozdilsky, C Robinson, R Macaulay, D George. Progressive supranuclear palsy diagnosis and confounding features—report of 16 autopsied cases. Mov Disord 2001;(in press).
23. AJ Hughes, Y Ben-Shlomo, SE Daniel, AJ Lees. What features improve the accuracy of clinical diagnosis in Parkinson's disease: A clinicopathologic study. Neurology 1992; 42:1142–1146.
24. AJ Hughes, SE Daniel, AJ Lees. Improved accuracy of clinical diagnosis of Lewy body Parkinson's disease. Neurology 2001; 57:1497–1499.
25. DJ Gelb, E Oliver, S Gilman. Diagnostic criteria for Parkinson's disease. Arch Neurol 1999; 56:33–39.
26. AH Rajput, B Rozdilsky, O Hornykiewicz, K Shannak, T Lee, P Seeman. Reversible drug-induced parkinsonism. Clinicopathologic study of two cases. Arch Neurol 1982; 39:644–646.
27. AH Rajput, B Rozdilsky, A Rajput, L Ang. Levodopa efficacy and pathological basis of Parkinson syndrome. Clin Neuropharmacol 1990; 13(6):553–558.
28. AH Rajput, KP Offord, CM Beard, LT Kurland. Epidemiology of parkinsonism: incidence, classification, and mortality. Ann Neurol 1984; 16:278–282.
29. JH Bower, DM Maraganore, SK McDonnell, WA Rocca. Incidence and distribution of parkinsonism in Olmsted County, Minnesota, 1976–1990. Neurology 1999; 52:1214–1220.
30. G Rosati, E Graniere, L Pinna, P De Bastiani, A Pirisi, MC Devoto. The risk of Parkinson's disease in Mediterranean people. Neurology 1980; 32:250–255.

31. AM Kuopio, J Marttila, H Helenius, UK Rinne. Changing epidemiology of Parkinson's disease in southwestern Finland. Neurology 1999; 52:302–308.
32. A Hofman, HJA Collette, AIM Bartelds. Incidence and risk factors of Parkinson's disease in The Netherlands. Neuroepidemiology 1989; 8:296–299.
33. LT Kurland, CA Molgaard. The Patient Record in Epidemiology. Sci Am 1981; 245(4):54–63.
34. LT Kurland. Epidemiology: incidence, geographic distribution and genetic considerations. In: WS Fields, ed. Pathogenesis and Treatment of Parkinsonism. Springfield, IL: Charles C Thomas, 1958:5–43.
35. FT Nobrega, E Glattre, LT Kurland, H Okazaki. Comments on the epidemiology of parkinsonism including prevalence and incidence statistics for Rochester, Minnesota, 1935–1966. In: A Barbeau, JR Brunette, eds. Progress in Neurogenetics. Amsterdam: Excerpta Medica, 1967:474–485.
36. FJ Ayd. A survey of drug-induced extrapyramidal reaction. JAMA 1961; 175:1054–1060.
37. WA Rocca, JH Bower, SK McDonnell, BJ Peterson, DM Maraganore. Time trends in the incidence of parkinsonism in Olmsted County, Minnesota. Neurology 2001; 57:462–467.
38. M Baldereschi, A De Carlo, WA Rocca, P Vanni, S Maggi, E Perissinotto, F Grigoletto, L. Amaducci, D Inzitari, ILSA Working Group. Parkinson's disease and parkinsonism in a longitudinal study. Two-fold higher incidence in men. Neurology 2000; 55:1358–1363.
39. R Mayeux, K Marder, LJ Cote, N Hemenegildo, H Mejia, MX Tang, R Lantigua, D Wilder, B Gurland, A Hauser. The frequency of idiopathic Parkinson's disease by age, ethnic group, and sex in northern Manhattan, 1988–1993. Am J Epidemiol 1995; 142:820–827.
40. WRG Gibb, AJ Lees. The relevance of the Lewy body to the pathogenesis of idiopathic Parkinson's disease. J Neurol Neurosurg Psychiatry 1988; 51:745–752.
41. GW Ross, LR White, H Petrovitch, DG Davis, J Hardman, J Nelson, W Markesbery, DM Morens, A Grandinetti. Lack of association of midlife smoking or coffee consumption with presence of Lewy bodies in the locus ceruleus or substantia nigra at autopsy. Neurology 1999; 52(suppl 2):A539–A540.
42. A Elbaz, JH Bower, DM Maraganore, SK McDonnell, BJ Peterson, JE Ahlskog, DJ Schaid, WA Rocca. Risk tables for parkinsonism and Parkinson's disease. J Clin Epidemiol 2002; 55:25–31.
43. J Parkinson. In: A Bicentenary Volume of Papers Dealing with Parkinson's Disease. M Critchley, WH McMenemey, FMR Walshe, JG Greenfield, eds. London: MacMillan, 1955.
44. RC Duvoisin, MD Yahr. Encephalitis and parkinsonism. Arch Neurol 1965; 12:227–239.
45. JC Krusz, WC Koller, DK Ziegler. Historical review: abnormal movements associated with epidemic encephalitis lethargica. Mov Disord 1987; 3(3):137–141.

46. GM Shy, GA Drager. A neurological syndrome associated with orthostatic hypotension. Arch Neurol 1960; 2:511–527.
47. RD Adams, L van Bogaert, H Van der Eecken. Striato-nigral degeneration. J Neuropathol Exp Neurol 1964; 23:584–608.
48. JC Steele, JC Richardson, J Olszewski. Progressive supranuclear palsy: a heterogeneous degeneration involving the brain stem, ganglia and cerebellum with vertical gaze and pseudobulbar palsy, nuchal dystonia and dementia. Arch Neurol 1964; 10:333–359.
49. CG Goetz. An early photographic case of probable supranuclear palsy. Mov Disord 1996; 11(6):617–618.
50. I Litvan. The clinical and pathologic hallmarks of progressive supranuclear palsy. Curr Opin Neurol 1997; 10:346–350.
51. NI Bohnen, RL Albin, KA Frey, JK Fink. (+)−α−[^{11}C]Dihydrotetrabenzaine PET imaging in familial paroxysmal dystonic choreoathetosis. Neurology 1999; 52:1067–1069.
52. K Jellinger. The pathology of parkinsonism. In: CD Marsden, S Fahn, eds. Movement Disorders 2. London: Butterworths and Co., 1987:124–165.
53. K Jellinger. Pathology of parkinsonism. In: S Fahn, CD Marsden, D Calne, M Goldstein, eds. Recent Developments in Parkinson's Disease. New York: Raven Press, 1986:32–66.
54. IG McKeith, EK Perry, RH Perry, for the Consortium on Dementia with Lewy Bodies. Report of the second dementia with Lewy body international workshop. Neurology 1999; 53:902–905.
55. AR Merdes, LA Hansen, G Ho, D Galasko, CR Hofstetter, LJ Thal, J Corey-Bloom. Diagnostic accuracy for dementia with Lewy bodies. Proceeding of 126th Annual Meeting of the American Neurological Association 2001; 30(abstr).
56. RK Mosewich, AH Rajput, A Shuaib, B Rozdilsky, L Ang. Pulmonary embolism: an under-recognized yet frequent cause of death in parkinsonism. Mov Disord 1994; 9(3):350–352.
57. MK Beyer, K Herlofson, D Arsland, JP Larsen. Causes of death in a community-based study of Parkinson's disease. Acta Neurol Scand 2001; 103(1):7–11.
58. MM Hoehn, MD Yahr. Parkinsonism: onset, progression, and mortality. Neurology 1967; 17:427–442.
59. DD Webster Critical analysis of disability in Parkinson's disease. Mod Treat 1968; 5(2):257–282.
60. JF Kurtzke, TP Flaten, FM Murphy. Death rates from Parkinson's disease in Norway reflect increased survival. Neurology 1991; 41:1665–1667.
61. RJ Uitti, JE Ahlskog, DM Maraganore, MD Muenter, EJ Atkinson, RH Cha, PC O'Brien. Levodopa therapy and survival in idiopathic Parkinson's disease: Olmsted County project. Neurology 1993; 43:1918–1926.
62. CH Markham, SG Diamond. Long-term follow-up of early dopa treatment in Parkinson's disease. Ann Neurol 1986; 19:365–372.

63. SG Diamond, CH Markham. Mortality of Parkinson patients treated with Sinemet. In: LJ Pooirier, TL Sourkes, PJ Bedard, eds. Advances in Neurology, Vol. 24. New York: Raven Press, 1979:489–497.
64. AH Rajput. Levodopa prolongs life expectancy and is non-toxic to substantia nigra. Parkinsonism Relat Disord 2001; 8:95–100.
65. J Jankovic. Levodopa strengths and weaknesses. Neurology 2002; 58(suppl 1):S19–S32.
66. CE Clarke. Does levodopa therapy delay death in Parkinson's disease? A review of the evidence. Mov Disord 1995; 10(3):250–256.
67. RAC Roos, JCF Jongen, EA Van der Velde. Clinical course of patients with idiopathic Parkinson's disease. Mov Disord 1996; 11(3):236–242.
68. SG Diamond, CH Markham. Present mortality in Parkinson's disease: the ratio of expected to observed deaths with a method to calculate expected deaths. J Neural Transm 1976; 88:259–269.
69. AH Rajput, RJ Uitti, A Rajput, KP Offord. Timely levodopa (LD) administration prolongs survival in Parkinson's disease. Parkinsonism Relat Disord 1997; 8(3):159–165.
70. RJ Uitti, AH Rajput, JE Ahlskog, KP Offord, DR Schroeder, MM Ho, M Prasad, A Rajput, P Basran. Amantadine treatment is an independent predictor of improved survival in Parkinson's disease. Neurology 1996; 46:1551–1556.
71. S Fahn, RL Elton, UPDRS Development Committee. Unified Parkinson's disease rating scale. In: S Fahn, CD Marsden, D Calne, M Goldstein, eds. Recent Developments in Parkinson's disease. 2 ed. Florham Park, NJ: Macmillan Healthcare Information, 1987:153–305.
72. A Rajput, AH Rajput. Progressive supranuclear palsy. Clinical features, pathophysiology and management. Drugs Aging 2002; 18(12):913–925.
73. F Menniti-Ippolito, S Spila-Alegiani, N Vanacore, V Bonifati, G. Diana, G Meco, R Raschetti. Estimate of parkinsonism prevalence through drug prescription histories in the Province of Rome, Italy. Acta Neurol Scand 1995; 92(1):49–54.
74. D Strickland, JM Bertoni, RF Pfeiffer. Descriptive epidemiology of Parkinson's disease through proxy measures. Can J Neurol Sci 1996; 23:279–284.
75. BS Schoenberg, DW Anderson, AF Haerer. Prevalence of Parkinson's disease in the biracial population of Copiah County, Mississippi. Neurology 1985; 35(6):841–845.
76. NE Bharucha, EP Bharucha, AE Bharucha, AV Bhise, BS Schoenberg. Prevalence of Parkinson's disease in the Parsi Community of Bombay, India. Arch Neurol 1988; 45:1321–1323.
77. BS Schoenberg, BO Osuntokun, AOG Adejua, O Bademosi, V Nottidge, DW Anderson, AF Haerer. Comparison of the prevalence of Parkinson's disease in black populations in the rural United States and in rural Nigeria: door-to-door community studies. Neurology 1988; 38:645–646.

78. L Morgante, WA Rocca, AE Di Rosa, P De Domenico, F. Grigoletto, F Meneghini, A Reggio, G Savettieri, MG Castiglione, F Patti, R DiPerri. Prevalence of Parkinson's disease and other types of parkinsonism: a door-to-door survey in three Sicilian municipalities. Neurology 1992; 42:1901–1907.

79. SC Li, BS Schoenberg, CC Wang, XM Cheng, DY Rui, CL Bolis, DG Schoenberg. A prevalence survey of Parkinson's disease and other movement disorders in the People's Republic of China. Arch Neurol 1985; 42:655–657.

80. RJ Marttila. Epidemiology. In: WC Koller, ed. Handbook of Parkinson's Disease Second Edition—Revised and Expanded. New York: Marcel Dekker, Inc., 1992:35–57.

81. DKY Chan, M Dunne, A Wong, E Hu, WT Hung, RG Beran. Pilot study of prevalence of Parkinson's disease in Australia. Neuroepidemiology 2001; 20:112–117.

82. MC de Rijk, MMB Breteler, GA Graveland, A Ott, DE Grobbee, FGA Van der Meche, A Hofman. Prevalence of Parkinson's disease in the elderly: The Rotterdam study. Neurology 1995; 45:2143–2146.

83. S Moghal, AH Rajput, C D'Arcy, R Rajput. Prevalence of movement disorders in elderly community residents. Neuroepidemiology 1994; 13:175–178.

84. S Moghal, AH Rajput, R Meleth, C D'Arcy, R Rajput. Prevalence of movement disorders in institutionalized elderly. Neuroepidemiology 1995; 14:297–300.

85. MC de Rijk, LJ Launer, K Berger, MMB Breteler, JF Dartigues, M Baldereschi, L Fratiglioni, A Lobo, J Martinez-Lage, C Trenkwalder, A Hofman, Neurologic Dis Elderly Res Grp. Prevalence of Parkinson's disease in Europe: a collaborative study of population-based cohorts. Neurology 2000; 54:S21–S23.

86. C Joseph, JB Chassan, ML Koch. Levodopa in Parkinson's disease: a long-term appraisal of mortality. Ann Neurol 1978; 3:116–118.

87. JH Bower, DM Maraganore, SK McDonnell, WA Rocca. Influence of strict, intermediate, and broad diagnostic criteria on the age- and sex-specific incidence of Parkinson's disease. Mov Disord 2000; 15:819–825.

88. LM Nelson, SK Van Den Eeden, CM Tanner, RD Fross, AL Bernstein, LA Paroubeck, ME Sorel, MK Miller. Incidence of Idiopathic Parkinson's disease (PD) in a health maintenance organization (HMO): variations by age gender and race/ethnicity. Neurology 1997; 48(suppl 2):A334.

89. AH Rajput, W Stern, A Christ. Early Onset Parkinsonism, unpublished, 1983.

90. N Vanacore, V Bonifati, A Bellatreccia, F Edito, G Meco. Mortality Rates for Parkinson's disease and Parkinsonism in Italy (1969–1987). Neuroepidemiology 1992; 11:65–73.

91. SG Diamond, CH Markham, MM Hoehn, FH McDowell, MD Muenter. An examination of male-female differences in progression and mortality of Parkinson's disease. Neurology 1990; 40:763–766.

92. II Kessler. Epidemiology study of Parkinson's disease. Am J Epidemiol 1972; 96:242–254.

93. MR Lerner, RS Goldman. Skin colour, MPTP, and Parkinson's disease. Lancet 1987; 212.

94. II Kessler. Epidemiologic studies of Parkinson's disease, II. A hospital based survey. Am J Epidemiol 1972; 95(4):308–318.

95. LT Kurland, PH Darrell, RW Darrell. Epidemiologic and genetic characteristics of parkinsonism: a review. Int J Neurol 1961; 2(1)11–24.

96. DE Lilienfeld. An epidemiological overview of amyotrophic lateral sclerosis, Parkinson's disease, and dementia of the Alzheimer type. In: DB Calne, ed. Neurodegenerative Diseases. Philadelphia: W.B. Saunders Co., 1993:399–425.

97. AH Rajput, WRG Gibb, XH Zhong, KS Shannak, S Kish, LG Chang, O Hornykiewicz. Dopa-responsive dystonia: pathological and biochemical observations in a case. Ann Neurol 1994; 35:396–402.

98. A Hirano, N Malamud, LT Kurland. Parkinsonism-dementia complex, an endemic disease on the island of Guam. Brain 1961; 84:662–679.

99. H Harada, S Nishikawa, K Takahashi. Epidemiology of Parkinson's disease in a Japanese city. Arch Neurol 1983; 40:151–154.

100. LW Svenson. Regional disparities in the annual prevalence rates of Parkinson's disease in Canada. Neuroepidemiology 1991; 10:205–210.

101. WE Lux, JF Kurtzke. Is Parkinson's disease acquired? Evidence from a geographic comparison with multiple sclerosis. Neurology 1987; 87:467–471.

102. DE Lilienfeld, D Sekkor, S Simpson, D Perl, J Ehland, G. Marsh, E Chan, J Godbold, P Landrigan. Parkinsonism death rates by race, sex and geography: a 1980's update. Neuroepidemiology 1990; 9:243–247.

103. AH Rajput, RJ Uitti, W Stern, W Laverty. Early onset Parkinson's disease in Saskatchewan. Can J Neurol Sci 1986; 13:312–316.

104. AH Rajput, RJ Uitti, W Stern, W Laverty, K O'Donnell, D O'Donnell, WK Yuen, A Dua. Geography, drinking water chemistry, pesticides and herbicides and the etiology of Parkinson's disease. Can J Neurol Sci 1987; 14:414–418.

105. C Hertzman, M Wiens, D Bowering, B Snow, D Calne. Parkinson's disease: a case-control study of occupational and environmental risk factors. Am J Indust Med 1990; 17:349–355.

106. W Koller, B Vetere-Overfield, C Gray, C Alexander, T Chin, J Dolezal, R Hassanein, C Tanner. Environmental risk factors in Parkinson's disease. Neurology 1990; 40:1218–1221.

107. CM Tanner, B Chen, W Wang, M Peng, Z Liu, X Liang, L Kao, DW Gilley, BS Schoenberg. Environmental factors in the etiology of Parkinson's disease. Can J Neurol Sci 1987; 14:419–423.

108. JP Hubble, T Cao, RES Hassanein, JS Neuberger, WC Koller. Risk factors for Parkinson's disease. Neurology 1993; 43:1693–1697.

109. SM Ludin, HP Ludin. Is Parkinson's disease of early onset a separate disease entity? J Neurol 1989; 236:203–207.

110. A Seidler, W Hellenbrand, B-P Robra, P Vieregge. Possible environmental, occupational, and other etiologic factors for Parkinson's disease: a case-control study in Germany. Neurology 1996; 46:1275–1284.

111. CM Tanner, B Chen, W Wang, M Peng. Environmental factors and Parkinson's disease: a case-control study in China. Neurology 1989; 39(5):660–664.
112. KM Semchuk, EJ Love, RG Lee. Parkinson's disease and exposure to agricultural work and pesticide chemicals. Neurology 1992; 42:1328–1335.
113. AH Rajput, KP Offord, CM Beard, LT Kurland. A case control study of smoking habits, dementia and other illnesses in idiopathic Parkinson's disease. Neurology 1987; 87:226–232.
114. M Shiba, JH Bower, DM Maraganore, SK McDonnell, BJ Peterson, JE Ahlskog, DJ Schaid, WA Rocca. Anxiety disorders and depressive disorders preceding Parkinson's disease: a case-control study. Mov Disord 2000; 15:669–677.
115. CJ Todes, AJ Lees. The premorbid personality of patients with Parkinson's disease. J Neurol Neurosurg Psychiatry 1985; 48:97–100.
116. MA Menza, LI Golbe, RA Cody, NE Forman. Dopamine-related personality traits in Parkinson's disease. Neurology 1993; 43:505–508.
117. A Paganini-Hill. Risk factors for Parkinson's disease: the Leisure World Cohort Study. Neuroepidemiology 2001; 20:118–124.
118. DM Morens, A Grandinetti, D Reed, LR White, GW Ross. Cigarette smoking and protection from Parkinson's disease: False association or etiologic clue. Neurology 1995; 45:1041–1051.
119. LI Golbe, RA Cody, RC Duvoisin. Smoking and Parkinson's disease. Search for a dose-response relationship. Arch Neurol 1986; 43:774–778.
120. MD Benedetti, JH Bower, DM Maraganore, SK McDonnell, BJ Peterson, JE Ahlskog, DJ Schaid, WA Rocca. Smoking, alcohol, and coffee consumption preceding Parkinson's disease—a case-control study. Neurology 2000; 55:1350–1358.
121. JM Gorrell, CC Johnson, BA Rybicki. Parkinson's disease and its comorbid disorders: an analysis of Michigan mortality date, 1970 to 1990. Neurology 1994; 44:1865–1868.
122. EC Hammond. Smoking in relation to the death of one million men and women. In: Epidemiologic Approaches to the Study of Cancer and Other Chronic Diseases. National Cancer Institute Monography No. 19. Washington, DC: U.S. Government Printing Office, 1966:127–204.
123. HA Kahn. The Dorn Study of Smoking and Mortality Among U.S. Veterans: Report on eight and one-half years of observation. In: Epidemiologic Approaches to the Study of Cancer and Other Chronic Diseases. National Cancer Institute Monograph No. 19. Washington, DC: U.S. Government Printing Office, 1966:1–125.
124. MD Nefzinger, FA Quadfasel, VC Karl. A retrospective study of smoking and Parkinson's disease. Am J Epidemiol 1968; 88:149–158.
125. A Grandinetti, DM Morens, D Reed, D MacEachern. Prospective study of cigarette smoking and the risk of developing idiopathic Parkinson's disease. Am J Epidemiol 1994; 139:1129–1138.

126. DM Morens, A Grandinetti, D Reed, LR White. Smoking-associated protection from Alzheimer's and Parkinson's disease. Lancet 1994; 343:356–357.

127. RJ Baumann, HD Jameson, HE McKean, DG Haack, LM Weisberg. Cigarette smoking and Parkinson's disease. A comparison of cases with matched neighbors. Neurology 1980; 80:839–843.

128. RB Godwin-Austen, PN Lee, MG Marmot, GM Stern. Smoking and Parkinson's disease. J Neurol Neurosurg Psychiatry 1982; 85:577–581.

129. CM Tanner, SM Goldman, DA Aston, R Ottman, J Ellenberg, R Mayeux, JW Langston. Smoking and Parkinson's disease in twins. Neurology 2002; 58:581–588.

130. MA Hernan, SM Zhang, AM Rueda-deCastro, GA Colditz, FE Speizer, A Ascherio. Cigarette smoking and the incidence of Parkinson's disease in two prospective studies. Ann Neurol 2001; 50(6):780–786.

131. R Mayeux, MX Tang, K Marder, LJ Cote, Y Stern. Smoking and Parkinson's disease. Mov Disord 1994; 9(2):207–212.

132. PA Wolf, RG Feldman, M Saint-Hilaire, M Kelly-Hayes, FJ Tores, P Mosbach, CS Kase, RB D'Agostino. Precursors and natural history of Parkinson's disease: The Framingham Study. Neurology 1991; 41(1):371.

133. DG Haack, RJ Baumann, HE McKean, HD Jameson, JA Turbeck. Nicotine exposure and Parkinson's disease. Am J Epidemiol 1981; 114:191–200.

134. WR Gibb. Idiopathic Parkinson's disease and the Lewy body disorders. Neuropathol Appl Neurobiol 1986; 12:223–234.

135. SM Goldman, M Kusumi, D Aston, JW Langston, CM Tanner. Dietary intake of isoquinoline derivatives (IQs) and PD: a study in twins (abstr). Neurology 2002; 58(suppl 3):A409.

136. SE Starkstein, TJ Preziosi, ML Berthier, PL Bolduc, HS Mayberg, RG Robinson. Depression and cognitive impairment in Parkinson's disease. Brain 1989; 112:1141–1153.

137. SE Starkstein, ML Berthier, PL Bolduc, TJ Preziosi, RG Robinson. Depression in patients with early versus late onset of Parkinson's disease. Neurology 1989; 39:1441–1445.

138. G Dooneief, E Mirabello, K Bell, K Marder, Y Stern, R Mayeux. An estimate of the incidence of depression in idiopathic Parkinson's disease. Arch Neurol 1992; 49:305–307.

139. SE Starkstein, G Petracca, E Chemerinski, M Merello. Prevalence and correlates of parkinsonism in patients with primary depression. Neurology 2001; 57:553–555.

140. BE Levin, MM Llabre, WJ Weiner. Parkinson's disease and depression: psychometric properties of the Beck Depression Inventory. J Neurol Neurosurg Psychiatry 1988; 51:1401–1404.

141. The Global Parkinson's Disease Survey (GPDS) Steering Committee. Factors impacting on quality of life in Parkinson's disease: results from an international survey. Mov Disord 2002; 17(1):60–67.

142. SJ Huber, DL Freidenberg, GW Paulson, EC Shuttleworth, JA Christy. The pattern of depressive symptoms varies with progression of Parkinson's disease. J Neurol Neurosurg Psychiatry 1990; 53:275–278.

143. AE Taylor, JA Saint-Cyr, AE Lang, FT Kenny. Parkinson's disease and depression. A critical re-evaluation. Brain 1986; 109:279–292.

144. AE Taylor, JA Saint-Cyr, AE Lang. Idiopathic Parkinson's disease: revised concepts of cognitive and affective status. Can J Neurol Sci 1988; 15:106–113.

145. A-M Gotham, RG Brown, CD Marsden. Depression in Parkinson's disease: a quantitative and qualitative analysis. J Neurol Neurosurg Psychiatry 1986; 49:381–389.

146. SE Starkstein, PL Bolduc, HS Mayberg, TJ Preziosi, RG Robinson. Cognitive impairments and depression in Parkinson's disease: a follow up study. J Neurol Neurosurg Psychiatry 1990; 53:597–602.

147. M Hietanen, H Teravainen. The effect of age of disease onset on neuropsychological performance in Parkinson's disease. J Neurol Neurosurg Psychiatry 1988; 51:244–249.

148. WE Martin, RB Loewenson, JA Raesch, AB Baker. Parkinson's disease: clinical analysis of 100 patients. Neurology 1973; 23:783–790.

149. BE Levin, MM Llabre, WJ Weiner. Cognitive impairments associated with early Parkinson's disease. Neurology 1989; 39:557–561.

150. WP Goldman, JD Baty, VD Buckles, S Sahrmann, JC Morris. Cognitive and motor functioning in Parkinson disease—subjects with and without questionable dementia. Arch Neurol 1998; 55:674–680.

151. RJ Marttila, UK Rinne. Dementia in Parkinson disease. Acta Neurol Scand 1976; 54:431–441.

152. AH Rajput, B Rozdilsky. Parkinsonism and dementia: effects of L-dopa. Lancet 1975; 1:108.

153. SJ Huber, EC Shuttleworth, JA Christy, DW Chakeres, A Curtin, GW Paulson. Magnetic resonance imaging in dementia of Parkinson's disease. J Neurol Neurosurg Psychiatry 1989; 52:1221–1227.

154. RG Brown, CD Marsden. How common is dementia in Parkinson's disease? Lancet 1984; 2:1262–1265.

155. R Mayeux, Y Stern, R Rosenstein, K Marder, A Hauser, L Cote, S Fahn. An estimate of the prevalence of dementia in idiopathic Parkinson's disease. Arch Neurol 1988; 45:260–262.

156. D Aarsland, K Andersen, JP Larsen, A Lolk, H Nielsen, P Kragh-Sorensen. Risk of dementia in Parkinson's disease. A community-based, prospective study. Neurology 2001; 56:730–736.

157. IG McKeith, D Galasko, K Kosaka, EK Perry, DW Dickson, LA Hansen, DP Salmon, J Lowe, SS Mirra, EJ Byrne, G Lennox, NP Quinn, JA Edwardson. Consensus guidelines for the clinical and pathologic diagnosis of dementia with Lewy body(DLB): report of the consortium on DLB international workshop. Neurology 1996; 47:1113–1124.

158. OL Lopez, SR Wisnieski, JT Becker, F Boller, ST DeKosky. Extrapyramidal signs in patients with probable Alzheimer disease. Arch Neurol 1997; 54(8):969–975.

159. HI Hurtig, JQ Trojanowski, J Galvin, D Ewbank, ML Schmidt, VMY Lee, CM Clark, G Glosser, MB Stern, SM Gollomp, SE Arnold. Alpha-synuclein cortical Lewy bodies correlate with dementia in Parkinson's disease. Neurology 2000; 54:1916–1921.

160. JR Gulcher, P Jónsson, A Kong, K Kristjánsson, ML Frigge, A Kárason, IE Einarsdóttir, H Stefánsson, AS Einarsdóttir, S Sigurdardóttir, S Baldursson, S Björnsdóttir, SM Hrafnkelsdóttir, F Jakobsson, J Benedickz, K Stefánsson. Mapping of a familial essential tremor gene, FET1, to chromosome 3q13. Nature Genet 1997; 17:84–87.

161. G Levy, M-X Tang, ED Louis, LJ Cote, B Alfaro, H Mejia, Y Stern, K Marder. The contribution of incident dementia to mortality in PD (abstr). Neurology 2002; 58 (suppl 3):A408.

162. AH Rajput, W Stern, WH Laverty. Chronic low dose therapy in Parkinson's disease: an argument for delaying levodopa therapy. Neurology 1984; 34(8):991–996.

163. B Jansson, J Jankovic. Low cancer rates among patients with Parkinson's disease. Ann Neurol 1995; 17:505–509.

164. LK Struck, RL Rodnitzky, JK Dobson. Stroke and its modification in Parkinson's disease. Stroke 1990; 21:1395–1399.

165. A Korten, J Lodder, F Vreeling, A Boreas, L Van Raak, F Kessels. Stroke and idiopathic Parkinson's disease: Does a shortage of dopamine offer protection against stroke? Mov Disord 2001; 16:119–123.

166. JJ Geraghty, J Jankovic, WJ Zetusky. Association between essential tremor and Parkinson's disease. Ann Neurol 1985; 17:329–333.

167. A Barbeau, M Roy. Familial subsets in idiopathic Parkinson's disease. Can J Neurol Sci 1984; 11:144–150.

168. RW Hornabrook, JT Nagurney. Essential tremor in Papua, New Guinea. Brain 1976; 99:659–672.

169. AH Rajput, KP Offord, CM Beard, LT Kurland. Essential tremor in Rochester, Minnesota: a 45-year study. J Neurol Neurosurg Psychiatry 1984; 47:466–470.

170. AF Haerer, DW Anderson, BS Schoenberg. Prevalence of essential tremor: results from the Copiah County study. Arch Neurol 1982; 89:750–751.

171. L Cleeves, LJ Findley, W Koller. Lack of association between essential tremor and Parkinson's disease. Ann Neurol 1988; 24:23–26.

172. RJ Marttila, I Rautakorpi, UK Rinne. The relation of essential tremor to Parkinson's disease. J Neurol Neurosurg Psychiatry 1984; 47:734–735.

173. AH Rajput. Pathological and neurochemical basis of essential tremor. In: WC Koller, LJ Findley, eds. Handbook of Tremor Disorders. New York: Marcel Dekker, Inc., 1994:233–244.

3

Differential Diagnosis of Parkinsonism

Kapil D. Sethi
Medical College of Georgia, Augusta,
Georgia, U.S.A.

Parkinsonism refers to a clinical syndrome characterized by a variable combination of tremor, bradykinesia or akinesia, rigidity, and postural instability. In general, two of these four features must be present to make a diagnosis of parkinsonism. However, the situation is complicated by rare cases of pure akinesia in the absence of tremor and rigidity that have the classic pathology of Parkinson's disease (PD) (1). Within the rubric of parkinsonism there are a myriad of disorders, some yet unclassified (Table 1).

The most common cause of parkinsonism is PD. Pathologically, PD is characterized by nigral cell loss and Lewy bodies in the remaining neurons, and the term "Lewy body parkinsonism" is sometimes used synonymously with PD. Some researchers consider it most appropriate to refer to even the pure clinical picture of PD as "Parkinson's syndrome" on the premise that PD may not be one disease. Whereas the purists demand the presence of Lewy bodies at autopsy to diagnose PD, these inclusions may not be present in some inherited forms of otherwise classical PD. Currently, one such condition, the "parkin parkinsonism" has been mapped to chromosome 6 (2). This autosomal recessive parkinsonism of juvenile onset differs pathologically from sporadic disease in that no Lewy bodies are found in

TABLE 1   Classification of Parkinsonism

Primary Parkinson's disease
  Sporadic
  Familial
Secondary Parkinsonism
  Drug-induced parkinsonism (DIP)
  Toxin-induced parkinsonism
  Infectious
    Creutzfeld-Jakob disease (CJD)
  Metabolic
  Structural
    Tumor
    Subdural hematoma
  Vascular
Other Degenerative Disorders
  Progressive supranuclear palsy (Steele-Richardson-Olzewaski syndrome) (PSP)
  Multiple-system atrophy (MSA)
    Shy-Drager syndrome (SDS)
    Olivopontocerebellar atrophy (OPCA)
    Striatonigral disease (SND)
  Cortical basal ganglionic degeneration (CBGD)
  Dementia with Lewy bodies (DLB)
  Hereditary degenerative diseases
  Spinocerebellar ataxias (SCA)
  Hallervorden-Spatz disease
  Huntington's disease
  Neuroacanthocytosis
  Wilson's disease
  X-linked dystonia-parkinsonism (Lubag)

the substantia nigra at autopsy. The clinical picture can be similar to idiopathic PD, including the presence of tremor (3). Two other forms of inherited parkinsonism, one with the locus on the long arm of chromosome 4 and the other with the locus on chromosome 2p13, have been described where typical Lewy body pathology is found (4,5).

In the absence of a known biological marker, the challenge facing the clinician is to make an accurate diagnosis of PD and differentiate it from other similar conditions. This review will give a practical approach to the differential diagnosis of parkinsonism and examine the diagnostic accuracy of PD. Because PD is the most common cause of parkinsonism, it is useful to review the typical clinical picture of PD.

THE TYPICAL CLINICAL PICTURE OF PD

The onset of PD is gradual and the course slowly progressive, albeit at different rates in different individuals. In most series, 65–70% of the patients present with an asymmetrical tremor, especially of the upper extremity (6). After a variable delay, the disorder progresses to the other side with bilateral bradykinesia and gait difficulty that takes the form of festination and, in advanced cases, freezing. Postural instability and falls tend to be a late feature. Eye movements may show saccadic pursuit, and the upgaze may be limited, especially in the elderly. Downgaze is normal. Autonomic disturbances are common but in early disease are not severe. Depression may occur early in the disease, but dementia as a presenting manifestation is not a feature of PD. Several signs should ring alarm bells when considering a diagnosis of PD. These include early severe dementia, early severe autonomic dysfunction, gaze difficulty (especially looking down), upper motor neuron or cerebellar signs, stepwise deterioration, and apraxia (Table 2).

CONDITIONS MIMICKING PARKINSONISM

The first step is to differentiate other conditions that may be confused with parkinsonism. Essential tremor (ET) is more common than PD and results in tremor that affects the head and neck and the upper extremities (7). The tremor is absent at rest except in most severe cases and is increased by maintained posture and voluntary movement. Mild cogwheeling may be present, but bradykinesia is not a feature (Table 3). The confusion occurs when a patient with a long history of ET begins to develop signs of bradykinesia or a rest tremor. Patients with PD may have a prominent action tremor adding to the diagnostic uncertainty. In addition there are elderly patients with ET who exhibit mild bradykinesia (8). Whether patients with ET are at an increased risk to develop PD is debatable (9). Psychomotor slowing in a severely depressed individual may resemble PD, but there is no tremor and patients improve with antidepressant therapy. Frequently depression and PD coexist.

Drug-Induced Parkinsonism

Drug-induced parkinsonism (DIP) is a common complication of antipsychotic drug use, with a reported prevalence of 15–60% (10). In one study,

TABLE 2 Features Indicating an Alternate Diagnosis to Parkinson's Disease

Early or predominant feature	Disease
Young onset	Drug- or toxin-induced parkinsonism, Wilson's disease, Hallervorden-Spatz disease
Minimal or absent tremor	PSP, vascular parkinsonism
Atypical tremor	CBGD, MSA
Postural instability	PSP, MSA
Ataxia	MSA
Pyramidal signs	MSA, vascular parkinsonism
Amyotrophy	MSA, parkinsonism dementia of Guam
Symmetric onset	PSP, MSA
Myoclonus	CBGD, CJD, MSA
Dementia	DLB
Apraxia, cortical sensory loss	CBGD
Alien limb sign	CBGD
Gaze palsies	PSP, OPCA, CBGD, DLB, PSG
Dysautonomia	MSA
Hallucinations (non–drug related)	DLB
Acute onset	Vascular parkinsonism, toxin-induced, psychogenic
Stepwise deterioration	Vascular parkinsonism

PSP = progressive supranuclear palsy; CBGD = cortiobasal ganglionic degeneration; MSA = multiple system atrophy; CJD = Creutzfeld-Jakob disease; DLB = dementia with Lewy bodies; OPCA = olivopontocerebellar atrophy; PSG = progressive subcortical gliosis.

TABLE 3 Differentiating Essential Tremor from Parkinson's Disease

	Essential tremor	Parkinson's disease
Body parts affected	Arms > Head > Voice > Legs	Arms > Jaw > Legs
Rest tremor	−	+++
Postural tremor	+++	+
Kinetic tremor	+++	±
Tremor frequency	7–12 Hz	4–6 Hz
Bradykinesia	−	++
Cogwheel rigidity	±	++
Family history	++	±
Response to beta blockers	+	−
Response to levodopa	−	++
Postural instability	−	+

51% of 95 patients referred for evaluation to a geriatric medicine service had parkinsonism associated with prescribed drugs (11). Frequently these patients are misdiagnosed as PD and treated with dopaminergic drugs without any benefit. In a community study, 18% of all cases initially thought to be PD were subsequently diagnosed as DIP (12).

The symptoms of DIP may be indistinguishable from PD. DIP is often described as symmetrical, whereas PD is often asymmetrical. However, one series found asymmetry of signs and symptoms in DIP in 30% of patients (13). Patients with DIP are as varied in their clinical manifestations as patients with PD. Some patients have predominant bradykinesia, while in others tremor is dominant. Postural reflexes may be impaired. Festination is uncommon and freezing is rare (13,14).

When the patient is on a dopamine blocking agent (DBA), it is difficult to distinguish underlying PD from DIP. If possible, the typical DBAs should be stopped or substituted with atypical antipsychotics and the symptoms and signs of DIP should resolve within a few weeks to a few months. In fact, it could take up to 6 months or more for signs and symptoms to resolve completely (15). If there is urgency in making the diagnosis, cerebrospinal fluid dopamine metabolites may be studied. These are low in untreated PD but are relatively normal or increased in DIP. However, this test may not always be helpful clinically (16). One study utilizing 6-fluorodopa positron emission tomography (PET) scanning showed that a normal PET scan predicted good recovery from DIP upon cessation of DBA and an abnormal PET scan was associated with persistence of signs in some but not all patients (17). DIP should be considered, and inquiry should be made about intake of antipsychotic drugs and other DBAs like metoclopramide (Table 4).

Progressive Supranuclear Palsy

Progressive supranuclear palsy (PSP), also known as Steele-Richardson-Olszewski syndrome, is easy to diagnose in advanced stages (18,19). However, diagnostic confusion may occur early in the disease and in cases that have atypical features. Typically, the disorder presents with a gait disturbance with resultant falls in over half the cases (20). Measurable bradykinesia in the upper extremities may not be present initially. The clinical features of PSP consist of supranuclear gaze palsy, especially involving the downgaze, with nuchal extension and predominant truncal extensor rigidity. Varying degrees of bradykinesia, dysphagia, personality changes, and other behavioral disturbances coexist. Patients often exhibit a motor recklessness and get up abruptly out of a chair (Rocket sign), even if this results in a fall.

TABLE 4 Drugs Known to Cause Parkinsonism

Generic name	Trademark
Chlorpromazine	Thorazine
Thiordazine	Mellaril
Mesoridazine	Serentil
Chlorprothixine	Taractan
Triflupromazine hydrochloride	Vesprin
Carphenazine maleate	Proketazine
Acetophenazine maleate	Tindal
Prochlorperazine	Compazine
Piperacetazine	Quide
Butaperazine maleate	Repoise maleate
Perphenazine	Tilafon
Molindone hydrochloride	Moban
Thiothixene	Navane
Trifluoperazine hydrochloride	Stelazine
Haloperidol	Haldol
Fluphenazine hydrochloride	Prolixin
Amoxapine	Asendin
Loxapine	Loxitane, Daxolin
Metoclopramide	Reglan
Promazine	Sparine
Promethazine	Phenergan
Thiethylperazine	Torecan
Trimeprazine	Temaril
Combination drugs	Etrafon, Triavil

Extraocular movement (EOM) abnormalities are very characteristic but may not be present at the onset of the illness or for several years. Rarely a patient with PSP may die without developing EOM abnormalities (21). EOM abnormalities consist of square wave jerks, instability of fixation, slow or hypometric saccades, and predominantly a downgaze supranuclear palsy (22,23). Generation of a saccade in the direction opposite to a stimulus (antisaccade test) is frequently abnormal in PSP (23). The oculocephalic responses are present in early disease but may be lost with advancing disease, suggesting a nuclear element to the gaze palsy. Bell's phenomenon may be lost in advanced cases. Some patients with PSP have a limb dystonia that can be asymmetrical (24). This can cause confusion with corticobasal ganglionic degeneration (CBGD), which will be discussed subsequently. Rest tremor is rare but has been reported in pathologically confirmed PSP (25).

PSP differs from PD radiologically in that in advanced cases there is atrophy of the mid-brain tectum and tegmentum with resultant diminution of the anteroposterior (AP) diameter of the midbrain (26,27). There may be dilatation of the posterior third ventricle and sometimes a signal alteration may be seen in the tegmentum of the midbrain (28). PET scanning utilizing 6-fluorodopa may distinguish PSP from PD in that the uptake diminished equally in both the caudate and putamen, whereas in PD the abnormalities are largely confined to the putamen (29). PET scan using raclopride binding shows that the D2 receptor sites are diminished in PSP, whereas in PD these are normal (30).

Clinically CBGD, dementia with Lewy bodies (DLB), progressive subcortical gliosis (PSG), multiple system atrophy (MSA), and even prion diseases have been misdiagnosed as PSP because of the presence of supranuclear gaze palsies (31–34). PSP also needs to be distinguished from other causes of supranuclear gaze palsy including cerebral Whipple's disease, adult-onset Niemann-Pick type C, and multiple cerebral infarcts (35–37). The presence of prominent early cerebellar symptoms or early, unexplained dysautonomia would favor MSA over PSP (38), and the presence of alien limb syndrome, cortical sensory deficits, focal cortical atrophy on MRI would favor CBGD (39). The clinical diagnostic criteria proposed by Litvan et al. may be helpful (40,41).

Multiple System Atrophy

This term, originally coined by Graham and Oppenheimer (42), refers to a variable combination of parkinsonism, autonomic, pyramidal, or cerebellar symptoms and signs. MSA can be subdivided into three types: striatonigral degeneration (SND), olivopontocerebellar atrophy (OPCA), and Shy-Drager syndrome (SDS) (43). All subtypes of MSA may have parkinsonian features. It is especially difficult to differentiate PD from SND. SND was originally described by Van Eecken et al. (44). The parkinsonian features of MSA consist of progressive bradykinesia, rigidity, and postural instability (43). In a clinicopathological report, one of four patients had a rest tremor characteristic of PD (45). Although symptoms are usually bilateral, unilateral presentations have been described (46). Useful clinical clues for the diagnosis of MSA include disproportionate anterocollis and the presence of cold blue hands. The autonomic failure is more severe than that seen in idiopathic PD and occurs early in MSA.

The response to levodopa is usually not as dramatic or sustained in MSA as in PD (47). However, it must be noted that several patients with MSA may initially respond to levodopa, but the benefit usually declines within one or 2 years of treatment (48). Levodopa-induced dyskinesias may occur in MSA. These dyskinesias typically involve the face and neck but may involve the extremities as well (49,50). It is clear, therefore, that the presence of levodopa dyskinesias cannot be used to make a definite diagnosis of PD. The situation is further complicated by the fact that patients with PD may develop autonomic dysfunction including postural hypotension, urinary problems, constipation, impotence, and sweating disturbances. This autonomic dysfunction in PD may be worsened by dopaminergic therapy. Autonomic dysfunction tends to be severe in MSA and occurs early (51). Stridor can occur early in MSA but not in PD (52). Urinary symptoms are very common in MSA. On urodynamic testing, there is a combination of detrusor hyperreflexia and urethral sphincter weakness (53). In addition, neurogenic anal and urethral sphincter abnormalities are very common in MSA (54). However, this finding is not diagnostic and may occur in other conditions like PSP (55). Neuroimaging may show nonspecific abnormalities like diffuse hypointensity involving the putamen, but more specific findings include a strip of lateral putaminal hyperintensity or pontine atrophy with an abnormal cross sign in the pons. (56).

Dementia with Lewy Bodies

In this disorder, Lewy bodies are found in widespread areas of the neocortex as well as the brain stem and diencephalic neurons (57). Some of these patients may have associated neurofibrillary tangles consistent with coincidental Alzheimer's disease. The parkinsonian syndrome of DLB may be indistinguishable from PD. However, these patients have early-onset dementia and may have hallucinations, delusions, and even psychosis in the absence of dopaminergic therapy (58,59). Another characteristic feature is wide fluctuations in cognitive status. Rarely, the patients with DLB may develop supranuclear gaze palsy, resulting in confusion with PSP (31,32). Some patients respond partially and temporarily to dopaminergic therapy. Occasionally the response to levodopa is robust. The electroencephalographic (EEG) recording in DLB may be abnormal with background posterior slowing and frontally dominant burst activity that is not a feature of PD.

Corticobasal Ganglionic Degeneration

Rebeiz et al. initially described this disorder as corticodentatonigral degeneration with neuronal achromasia (60). CBGD typically presents in the 6th or 7th decade with slowly progressive unilateral, tremulous, apraxic, and rigid upper limb (61). The disorder tends to be gradually progressive with progressive gait disturbances, cortical sensory loss, and stimulus sensitive myoclonus resulting in a "jerky useless hand" (62–64). Jerky useless lower extremity is uncommon but may occur. Rarely these patients may develop Babinski signs and supranuclear gaze palsy.

When typical, the clinical picture is distinct and easily recognizable. However, atypical cases may be confused with PSP, and the myoclonic jerking may be confused with the rest tremor of PD. The gait disturbance typically consists of slightly wide based apraxic gait rather than the typical festinating gait of PD. Fixed limb dystonia may be prominent and strongly suggests CBGD, but some patients with PSP may also have asymmetrical limb dystonia (24). Patients with CBGD do not benefit from levodopa, and the course is relentlessly progressive.

Rare cases of the parietal form of Pick's disease may be confused with CBGD (65). The clinical spectrum of CBGD has recently been expanded to include early-onset dementia and aphasia (66), but in general these patients have a conspicuous absence of cognitive deficits. The magnetic resonance image (MRI) in CBGD shows focal atrophy especially in the parietal areas (67), and the PET scan shows asymmetrical decrease of regional cerebral metabolic rates for glucose utilization (68).

Frontotemporal Dementia with Parkinsonism

Frontotemporal dementia (FTD) is characterized by profound behavioral changes and an alteration in personality and social conduct with relative preservation of memory (69,70). Extrapyramidal symptoms are common, and parkinsonism occurs in 40% of patients (71). Akinesia, rigidity, and a shuffling gait are the most common signs with typical tremor being rare (72). PET scan reveals an equal decrease in fluorodopa uptake in the caudate and the putamen as opposed to PD, where putamen is preferentially involved. (72). This disorder should be easy to distinguish from PD but may be confused with DLB and other disorders causing dementia and parkinsonism. Tables 5 and 6 summarize some of the differential diagnostic features.

Toxin-Induced Parkinsonism

In general, these disorders are uncommon and may pose less of a differential diagnostic problem. 1-Methyl-4-phenyl-1,2,3,6-tetrahydopyridine (MPTP)-induced parkinsonism is distinct from DIP in that it is irreversible and is due to the destruction of the substantia nigra neurons (73). The clinical features have some similarities to PD, except that the onset is abrupt and the affected individuals are younger than typical PD (74,75). These patients respond to levodopa with early levodopa-induced fluctuations (76). The patients may worsen gradually even in the absence of continued exposure to the toxin

TABLE 5   Differential Diagnosis of Parkinson's Disease

	PD	PSP	MSA	CBGD	DLB
Symmetry of deficit	+	+++	+++	−	+
Axial rigidity	+	+++	++	+	+
Limb dystonia	+	+	+	++	+
Postural instability	++	+++	++	+	++
Vertical gaze palsy	+	+++	+	++	+
Dysautonomia	+	−	++	−	+
Levodopa response	+++	−	+	−	++
Asymmetrical cortical atrophy	−	−	−	++	−
Hallucinations (nondrug)	−	−	−	−	+

PD = Parkinson's disease; PSP = progressive supranuclear palsy; MSA = multiple system atrophy; CBGD = corticobasal ganglionic degeneration; DLB = dementia with Lewy bodies.

TABLE 6   MRI Features of Some Cases of Parkinsonism

	PD	PSP	MSA (OPCA)	MSA (SND)	CBGD
Cortical atrophy	+	+	±	+	++
Putaminal atrophy	−	−	−	++	−
Pontine atrophy	−	+	+++	−	−
Midbrain atrophy	−	++	+	−	−
Cerebellar atrophy	−	−	++	−	−
High putaminal iron	−	−	+	+	−

PD = Parkinson's disease; PSP = progressive supranuclear palsy; MSA = multiple system atrophy; OPCA = olivopontocerebellar atrophy; SND = striatonigral degeneration; CBGD = corticobasal ganglionic degeneration.

(77). In manganese poisoning, the patients may have symptoms very similar to PD, including soft speech, clumsiness, and impaired dexterity; however, the patients have a peculiar cock-walk gait in which they swagger on their toes (78,79). They may also have limb and truncal dystonia that is very unusual in untreated PD. Dementia and cerebellar dysfunction may occur, and these patients do not respond well to dopaminergic drugs. Patients with manganese exposure who develop otherwise typical PD had an earlier age of onset as compared to controls (80).

Parkinsonism as a result of carbon monoxide intoxication has been well described (81,82). The parkinsonism may be delayed after the acute episode. These patients often show a slow shuffling gait, loss of arm swing, retropulsion, bradykinesia, rigidity, and, occasionally, a rest tremor. The pull test tends to be markedly abnormal. The computerized tomography (CT) scan or MRI scan may show necrotic lesions of the globus pallidus (83,84). There may also be associated white matter lesions that may progress without further exposure to carbon monoxide (85). Other toxins that have been reported to cause parkinsonism include carbon disulfide (86), cyanide (87,88), and methanol (89,90). These patients often have an acute onset and in some cases show basal ganglia lesions on neuroimaging. Posthypoxic parkinsonism has an acute evolution following a bout of severe prolonged hypoxia. A variable degree of intellectual deterioration often accompanies posthypoxic parkinsonism, and the patients usually do not have rest tremor.

Posttraumatic Parkinsonism

Isolated head trauma is rarely a cause of parkinsonism (91). Parkinsonism may be seen in the setting of diffuse severe cerebral damage after brain injury (92). However, repeated minor trauma to the head, as in boxers (dementia pugilistica), may be complicated by the late onset of dementia, parkinsonism, and other clinical features (93,94). Obviously, the boxers are not immune to developing PD as they get older. However, the onset of parkinsonism and dementia in a professional boxer would be very suggestive of dementia pugulistica. The imaging studies may show a cavum septum pellucidum and cerebral atrophy. A PET study using 6-fluorodopa showed damage to both the caudate and the putamen in posttraumatic parkinsonism, whereas in PD the putamen is more severely involved.

Multi-Infarct Parkinsonism

Arteriosclerotic or multi-infarct parkinsonism is a debatable entity (95). Patients typically have predominant gait disturbance with slightly wide-based gait with some features of gait apraxia and frequent freezing (96).

These patients have lower-body parkinsonism, and they usually lack the typical rest tremor or signs in the upper extremity (97). The gait disorder may not be distinct from senile gait, and a similar gait disorder may also be seen in patients with Binswanger's disease (98,99). Levodopa responsiveness is uncommon but has been demonstrated occasionally in patients with pathologically confirmed multi-infarct parkinsonism.

The proposed criteria for the diagnosis of vascular parkinsonism include acute or subacute onset with a stepwise evolution of akinesia and rigidity along with vascular risk factors (100). This should be supplemented by at least two or more infarcts in the basal ganglia on neuroimaging. In some cases there may be more widespread MRI white matter abnormalities. Spontaneous improvement in symptoms and signs without dopaminergic therapy is suggestive of vascular parkinsonism.

Some patients with multiple cerebral infarction have a clinical picture characterized by gaze palsies, akinesia, and balance difficulties consistent with PSP. In fact, one study found that 19 out of 58 patients with a clinical diagnosis of PSP had radiographic evidence of multiple small infarcts in the deep white matter and the brainstem (35).

Parkinsonism with Hydrocephalus

Patients with hydrocephalus have varying degrees of hypomimia, bradykinesia, and rigidity in the absence of tremor. This may occur in high-pressure as well as in normal-pressure hydrocephalus (NPH) (101). High-pressure hydrocephalus rarely poses any diagnostic difficulties because of the relatively acute onset in the presence of signs of raised intracranial pressure. However, NPH may be more difficult to distinguish from PD in some cases. The classic triad of NPH includes a subacute onset of dementia, gait difficulty, and urinary incontinence (102). The gait is slightly wide based with features of gait apraxia or slight ataxia. Rarely, levodopa responsiveness has been demonstrated (103). In some patients the gait might improve over the next few hours to days by the removal of cerebral spinal fluid (104).

Parkinsonism Due to Structural Lesions of the Brain

Blocq and Merinesco were the first to report a clinicopathological correlation of midbrain tuberculoma involving the substantia nigra and contralateral parkinsonism (105,106). In most cases the responsible lesions have been tumors, chiefly gliomas and meningiomas. Interestingly, these are uncommon in the striatum and have usually involved the frontal or parietal lobes. Subdural hematoma may present with subacute onset of parkinsonism, with some pyramidal signs at times (107). Other rare causes of parkinsonism and structural lesions have included striatal abscesses (108) and vascular malformations. However, the structural lesions are easily confirmed by neuroimaging. Occasionally parkinsonism has been reported in patients with basal ganglia calcifications that usually occur in primary hypoparathyroidism. The calcification should be obvious on neuroimaging (109).

Infectious and Postinfectious Causes of Parkinsonism

The classic postencephalitic parkinsonism is now exceedingly uncommon. It was characterized by a combination of parkinsonism and other movement disorders. Particularly characteristic were "oculogyric crises," which resulted in forceful and painful ocular deviation lasting minutes to hours. Other causes of oculogyric crises are Tourette's syndrome, neuroleptic induced acute dystonia, paroxysmal attacks in multiple sclerosis, and possibly conversion reaction. The parkinsonism may improve with levodopa, but response deteriorates quickly. Parkinsonism rarely occurs as a sequelae of other sporadic encephalitides. Human immunodeficiency virus (HIV) dementia has also been reported with parkinsonian features. Other infectious causes include striatal abscesses and neurosyphilis.

Psychogenic Parkinsonism

Compared to other psychogenic movement disorders like tremor, psychogenic parkinsonism is uncommon (110). A tremor of varying rates with marked distractibility along with inconsistent slowness and the presence of feigned weakness and numbness might lead to the correct diagnosis.

PARKINSONISM IN YOUNG ADULTS

The onset of parkinsonism under the age of 40 is usually called young-onset parkinsonism. When symptoms begin under the age of 20, the term "juvenile parkinsonism" is sometimes used (111). Under the age of 20, parkinsonism typically occurs as a component of a more widespread degenerative disorder. However, Parkin parkinsonism may present with dystonia and parkinsonism in patients under the age of 20.

Dopa-Responsive Dystonia

There is a significant overlap in young patients with dystonia and parkinsonism. Patients with young-onset parkinsonism manifest dystonia that may be responsive to dopamingeric drugs (112). However, the response may deteriorate upon long-term follow-up. Patients with hereditary dopa-responsive dystonia have an excellent and sustained response to low doses of levodopa (113). In addition, PET scan shows markedly reduced 6-fluorodopa uptake in patients with young-onset PD, whereas the fluorodopa uptake is normal in patients with dopa-responsive dystonia (114). Patients with dopa-responsive dystonia have a guanosine triphosphate (GTP)–cyclohydrolase deficiency that is not a feature of PD in young adults.

Wilson's Disease

Wilson's disease may present primarily with a neuropsychiatric impairment. It should be considered in every case of young-onset parkinsonism because it is eminently treatable and the consequences of nonrecognition can be grievous. Most common neurological manifestations are tremor, dystonia, rigidity, dysarthria, drooling, and ataxia. A combination of parkinsonism and ataxia is particularly indicative of neurological Wilson's disease (115). Parkinsonism is the most prevalent motor dysfunction, whereas about 25% of the patients present with disabling cerebellar ataxia, tremor, or dysarthria (116). Typically, the tremor involves the upper limbs and the head and rarely the lower limbs. It can be present at rest, with postural maintenance, and may persist with voluntary movements. The classic tremor is coarse and irregular and present during action. Holding the arms forward and flexed horizontally can emphasize that the proximal muscles are active (wing-beating tremor). Less commonly, tremor may affect just the tongue and the orofacial area (117). Dystonia is also quite common. The characteristic feature is an empty smile due to facial dystonia. Dysarthria is very common and may take the form of a dystonic or a scanning dysarthria. Approximately 30% of the patients present with behavioral and mental status changes (118). The psychiatric disorder may take the form of paranoid symptoms sometimes accompanied by delusional thinking and hallucinations. Early presentation may be a decline in memory and school performance. Patients may develop anxiety, moodiness, disinhibited behavior, and loss of insight. A characteristic feature is inappropriate laughter. Although eye movements are typically normal, some cases of Wilson's disease may show a saccadic pursuit, gaze distractibility, or difficulty in fixation (119). Macrosaccadic oscillations have been personally observed in a patient with Wilson's disease, and the abnormal eye movements disappeared after successful therapy. Kayser-Fleischer (KF) rings due to copper deposition in the cornea may be easy to recognize in patients with a light-colored iris, but in patients with brown irides these rings may be very difficult to see. Usually the ring is golden-brown in color and involves the whole circumference of the cornea. However, in the early stages the ring may be more apparent in the upper than the lower pole. Rarely these rings can be unilateral. KF rings are best appreciated by a careful slit-lamp examination done by a competent neur-ophthalmologist. Typically the absence of KF rings on the slit-lamp examination rules out neurological Wilson's disease. However, there are reports of patients with typical Wilson's disease without any KF rings (120,121).

Radiologically, advanced cases of Wilson's disease may have cavitation of the putamen (122). However, putaminal lesions are not specific for Wilson's disease. Other causes of putaminal cavitation or lesions include hypoxic ischemic damage, methanol poisoning, mitochondrial encephalomyopathy, and wasp sting encephalopathy. Nearly half the patients with neurological Wilson's disease have hypodensities of the putamina on CT scans in contrast to patients with hepatic disease, who frequently have normal CT scans (123). MRI is more sensitive, and almost all patients with neurological features have some disturbance on T_2-weighted images in the basal ganglia with a pattern of symmetrical, bilateral, concentric-laminar T_2 hyperintensity, and the involvement of the pars compacta of the substantia nigra, periaqueductal gray matter, the pontine tegmentum, and the thalamus (124). The hepatic component of Wilson's disease may cause increased T_1 signal intensity in the globus pallidus (125). In the adult age group, the basal ganglia lesions may be different from those in the pediatric group; the putaminal lesions may not be present; the globus pallidus and substantia nigra may show increased hypointensity on T_2-weighted images. Cortical and subcortical lesions may also be present with a predilection to the frontal lobe. However, rare cases of neurological Wilson's disease may have normal MRI (126). PET scanning may show a reduction of 6-fluroudopa uptake (127).

The most useful diagnostic test is serum ceruloplasmin and a 24-hour urinary copper excretion supplemented by a slit-lamp examination for KF rings. Unfortunately, not all patients with Wilson's disease have a low ceruloplasmin level (128). Measurement of liver copper concentration makes a definitive diagnosis. Normally, it is between 50–100 µg/g of tissue, and in patients with Wilson's disease it may be over 200 µg/g (129).

Hallervorden-Spatz Disease

Hallervorden-Spatz disease (HSD) is usually a disease of children, but young adults may be affected. Typically, the disease occurs before the age of 20. Facial dystonia tends to be prominent, coupled with gait difficulty and postural instability. Patients may have night blindness progressing to visual loss secondary to retinitis pigmentosa. Other extrapyramidal signs include choreoathetosis and a tremor that has been poorly characterized. Cognitive problems include impairment of frontal tasks and memory disturbances. Psychiatric manifestations have been reported in HSD. CT scans in HSD are often normal, but low-density lesions have been described in the globus pallidus. MRI, especially using a high field strength magnet, shows decreased signal intensity in the globus pallidus with a central hyperintensity. We have termed it the "eye of the tiger sign" (130).

Juvenile Huntington's Disease

This autosomal dominant neurodegenerative disorder typically presents with chorea, difficulty with gait, and cognitive problems. However, the "Westphal variant" of the disease affecting the young may manifest bradykinesia, tremulousness, myoclonic jerks, and occasionally seizures and cognitive disturbances (131). Eye movement abnormalities including apraxia of eye movements can be remarkable in this setting. When coupled with a lack of family history, these young patients may be confused with young-onset PD, but neuroimaging and gene testing should easily distinguish the two.

Hemiparkinsonism Hemiatrophy Syndrome

These patients have a longstanding hemiatrophy of the body and develop a progressive bradykinesia and dystonic movements around the age of 40 (132,133). Ipsilateral corticospinal tract signs may be found, which are not a feature of PD. Neuroimaging reveals brain asymmetry with atrophy of the contralateral hemisphere with compensatory ventricular dilatation. Regional cerebral metabolic rates are diminished in the hemisphere contralateral to the clinical hemiatrophy in the putamen and the medial frontal cortex, whereas in idiopathic PD the regional cerebral metabolic rates are normal or increased contralateral to the clinically affected side (134).

X-Linked Dystonia Parkinsonism (Lubag)

This inherited disorder usually occurs in the Philippines. However, rare cases are seen in other parts of the world (135). Typical age of presentation is around the age of 30–40 years. Focal dystonia or tremor is the initial finding followed by other parkinsonian features. Rarely parkinsonian features may precede dystonia. Clinically this disorder is differentiated from idiopathic PD by the presence of marked dystonia and the pattern of inheritance.

Neuroacanthocytosis

This is a rare cause of parkinsonism and typically presents with a hyperkinetic movement disorder including chorea, tic-like features, and polyneuropathy. MRI shows a characteristic atrophy of the caudate and a hyperintensity in the putamen on T_2-weighted images, and acanthocytes are revealed on a fresh blood smear (136).

DIAGNOSTIC CRITERIA FOR PARKINSON'S DISEASE

From the preceding discussion it is obvious that there are a large number of disorders that can be confused with PD. In an effort to improve diagnostic accuracy, several sets of clinical diagnostic criteria for PD have been proposed (137–140). Table 7 lists the UK Parkinson's Disease Society Brain Bank clinical diagnostic criteria (UKPDBBCDC).

The first clinicopathological study found that only 69–75% of the patients with the autopsy-confirmed diagnosis of PD had at least two of the three cardinal manifestations of PD: tremor, rigidity, and bradykinesia (140). Furthermore, 20–25% of patients who showed two of these cardinal features had a pathological diagnosis other than PD. Even more concerning, 13–19% of patients who demonstrated all three cardinal features typically associated with a clinical diagnosis of PD had another pathological diagnosis.

Rajput et al. reported autopsy results in 59 patients with parkinsonian syndromes (141). After a long-term follow-up period, the clinical diagnosis of PD was retained in 41 of 59 patients. However, only 31 of 41 (75%) patients with clinically determined PD showed histopathological signs of PD at autopsy examination.

A third series was comprised of 100 patients with a clinical diagnosis of PD, who had been examined during their life by different neurologists using poorly defined diagnostic criteria. When autopsies were performed (mean interval between symptom onset and autopsy = 11.9 years), PD was found in 76 patients. The authors reviewed the charts of these patients and then applied the accepted UKPDBBCDS clinical criteria for PD requiring bradykinesia and at least one other feature, including rigidity, resting tremor, or postural instability, and focusing on clinical progression, asymmetry of onset, and levodopa response. Sixteen additional exclusion criteria were also applied (Table 7). With the application of these diagnostic criteria, 89 of the original 100 patients were considered to have PD, but, again, only 73 (82%) were confirmed to have PD at autopsy. When the authors reexamined the patients with all three cardinal features (excluding the postural instability), only 65% of patients with an autopsy diagnosis of PD fit this clinical category.

The authors have reexamined the issue. They studied another 100 patients with a clinical diagnosis of PD that came to neuropathological examination. Ninety fulfilled pathological criteria for PD. Ten were

TABLE 7   United Kingdom Parkinson's Disease Society Brain Bank Clinical
Diagnostic Criteria

Inclusion criteria	Exclusion criteria	Supportive criteria
Bradykinesia (slowness of initiation of voluntary movement with progressive reduction in speed and amplitude of repetitive actions) Plus at least one of the following • Muscular rigidity: • 4–6 Hz rest tremor • Postural instability not caused by primary visual, vestibular, cerebellar, or proprioceptive dysfunction	• History of repeated strokes with stepwise progression of parkinsonian features • History of repeated head injury • History of definite encephalitis • Oculogyric crises • Neuroleptic treatment at onset of symptoms • More than one affected relative • Sustained remission • Strictly unilateral features after 3 years • Supranuclear gaze palsy • Cerebellar signs • Early severe autonomic involvement • Early severe dementia with disturbances of memory, language, and praxis • Babinski sign • Presence of cerebral tumour or communicating hydrocephalus on CT scan • Negative response to large doses of levodopa (if malabsorption excluded) • MPTP exposure	(Three or more required for diagnosis of definite PD.) • Unilateral onset • Rest tremor present • Progressive disorder • Persistent asymmetry affecting side of onset most • Excellent response (70–100%) to levodopa • Severe levodopa-induced chorea • Levodopa response for 5 years or more • Clinical course of 10 years or more

misdiagnosed: MSA (six), PSP (two), postencephalitic parkinsonism (one), and vascular parkinsonism (one). They next examined the accuracy of diagnosis of parkinsonian disorders in a specialist movement disorders service (144). They reviewed the clinical and pathological features of 143 cases of parkinsonism, likely including many of the patients previously reported (143). They found a surprisingly high positive predictive value (98.6%) of clinical diagnosis of PD among the specialists. In fact, only 1 of 73 patients diagnosed with PD during life was found to have an alternate diagnosis. This study demonstrated that the clinical diagnostic accuracy of PD may be improved by utilizing stringent criteria and a prolonged follow up

REFERENCES

1. Quinn NP, Luthert P. Hanover M, Marsden CD. Pure akinesia due to Lewy body. Parkinson's disease: a case with pathology. Move Disord 1989; 4:885–892.
2. Rajput AH. Pathologic and biochemical studies of juvenile parkinsonism linked to chromosome 6q. Neurology 1999; 53(6):1375.
3. Klein C, Pramstaller PP, Kis B, Page CC, Kann M, Leung J, Woodward H, Castellan CC, Scherer M, Vieregge P, Breakefield XO, Kramer PL, Ozelius LJ. Parkin deletions in a family with adult-onset, tremor-dominant parkinsonism: expanding the phenotype. Ann Neurol 2000; 48(1):65–71.
4. Polymeropoulos MH. Autosomal dominant Parkinson's disease and alpha-synuclein. Ann Neurol 1998; 44(3 suppl 1):S63–64.
5. Gasser T. Genetics of Parkinson's disease. Ann Neurol 1998; 4(3 suppl 1):S53–71.
6. Paulson HL, Stern MB. Clinical manifestations of Parkinson's disease. In: Watts RL, Koller WC, eds. Movement Disorders: Neurological Principles and Practice. New York: McGraw-Hill, 1997:183–199.
7. Findley LJ, Koller WC. Essential tremor. Clin Neuropharm 1989; 12:453–482.
8. Montgomery EB, Baker KB, Koller WC, Lyons K. Motor initiation and execution in essential tremor and Parkinson's disease. Mov Disord 2000; 3:511–515.
9. Pahwa R, Koller WC. Is there a relationship between Parkinson's disease and essential tremor? Clin Neuropharm 1993; 16:30–35.
10. Hardie RJ, Lees AJ. Neuroleptic induced Parkinson's syndrome. Clinical features and results of treatment with levodopa. Neurology 1987; 37:850–854.
11. Stephen PJ, Williams J. Drug-induced parkinsonism in the elderly. Lancet 1987; 2:1082.
12. Mutch WJ, Dingwall-Fordyce I, Downie AW, et al. Parkinson's disease in a Scottish city. Br Med J 1986; 292:534–536.
13. Sethi KD, Zamrini EY. Asymmetry in clinical features of drug-induced parkinsonism. J Neuropsych Clin Neurosci 1990; 2:64–66.

14. Giladi N, Kao R, Fahn S. Freezing phenomenon in patients with parkinsonian syndromes. Mov Disord 1997; 12(3):302–305.
15. Klawans HL, Bergan D, Bruyn GW. Prolonged drug induced parkinsonism. Confin Neurol 1973; 35:368–377.
16. LeWitt PA, Galloway MP, Matson W, Milbury P, McDermott M, Srivatsva DK, Oakes D. Markers of dopamine metabolism in Parkinson's disease. Neurology 1992; 42:2111–2117.
17. Burn DJ, Brooks DJ. Nigral dysfunction in drug-induced parkinsonism: an [18]flurodopa PET study. Neurology 1993; 43:552–556.
18. Steele JC, Richardson JC, Olszewski J. Progressive supranuclear palsy. Arch Neurol 1964; 10:333–359.
19. Steele JC. Progressive supranuclear palsy. Brain 1972; 95:693–704.
20. Golbe LI, Davis PH, Schoenberg BS, Duvoisin RC. Prevalence and natural history of progressive supranuclear palsy. Neurology 1988; 38:1031–1034.
21. Nuwer MR. Progressive supranuclear palsy despite normal eye movements. Arch Neurol 1981; 38:784.
22. Troost B, Daroff R. The ocular motor defects in progressive supranuclear palsy. Ann Neurol 1977; 2:397–403.
23. Vidailhet M, Rivaud S, Gouider-Khouja N, et al. Eye movements in parkinsonian syndromes. Ann Neurol 1994; 35:420–426.
24. Barclay CL, Lang AE. Dystonia in progressive supranuclear palsy. J Neurol Neurosurg Psychiatry 1997; 62(4):352–356.
25. Masucci EF, Kurtzke JF. Tremor in progressive supranuclear palsy. Acta Neurol Scand 1989; 80:296–300.
26. Schonfeld SM, Golbe LI, Sage JI, Safer JN, Duvoisin RC. Computed tomographic findings in progressive supranuclear palsy: correlation with clinical grade. Mov Disord 1987; 2:263–278.
27. Savoiardo M, Girotti F, Strada L, Cieri E. Magnetic resonance imaging in progressive supranuclear palsy and other parkinsonian disorders. J Neural Transm Suppl 1994; 42:93–110.
28. Yagishita A, Oda M. Progressive supranuclear palsy: MRI and pathological findings. Neuroradiology 1996; 38(suppl 1):S60–66.
29. Brooks DJ, Ibanez V, Sawle GV, et al. Differing patterns of striatal F-dopa uptake in Parkinson's disease, multiple system atrophy, and progressive supranuclear palsy. Ann Neurol 1990; 28:547–555.
30. Brooks DJ, Ibanez V, Sawle GV, et al. Striatal D2 receptor status in patients with Parkinson's disease, striatonigral degeneration, and progressive supranuclear palsy, measures with C-raclopride and positron emission tomography. Ann Neurol 1992; 31:184–192.
31. Fearnley JM, Revesz T, Brooks DJ, Frackowiak RS, Lees AJ. Diffuse Lewy body disease presenting with a supranuclear gaze palsy. J Neurol Neurosurg Psychiatry 1991; 54:159–161.
32. De Bruin VM, Lees AJ, Daniel SE. Diffuse Lewy body disease presenting with supranuclear gaze palsy, parkinsonism, and dementia: a case report. Mov Disord 1992; 7:355–358.

33. Foster NL, Gilman S, Berent S, et al. Progressive subcortical gliosis and progressive supranuclear palsy can have similiar clinical and PET abnormalities. J Neurol Neurosurg Psychiatry 1992; 55:707–713.

34. Lees AJ, Gibb W, Barnard RO. A case of progressive subcortical gliosis presenting clinically as Steele-Richardson Olszewski syndrome. J Neurol Neurosurg Psychiatry 1988; 51:1224–1227.

35. Dubinsky RM, Jankovic J. Progressive supranuclear palsy and a multi-infarct state. Neurology 1987; 37:570–576.

36. Winikates J, Jankovic J. Vascular progressive supranuclear palsy. J Neural Transm Suppl 1994, 42.189–201.

37. Fink JK, Filling- Katz MR, Sokol J et al. Clinical spectrum of Niemann-Pick disease type C Neurology 1989; 39:1040–1049.

38. Quinn N. Multiple system atrophy. In: Marsden C, Fahn S, eds. Movement Disorders. Newton, MA: Butterworth-Heinemann, 1994:262–281.

39. Gibb WR, Luthert PJ, Marsden CD. Corticobasal degeneration. Brain 1989; 112:1171–1192.

40. Litvan I, Agid Y, Jankovic J, et al. Accuracy of clinical criteria for the diagnosis of progressive supranuclear palsy (Steele-Richardson-Olszcwski syndrome). Neurology 1996; 46:922–930.

41. Litvan I, Agid Y, Calne D, Campbell G et al. Clinical research criteria for the diagnosis of progressive supranuclear palsy (Steele-Richardson-Olszewski syndrome) report of the NINDS-SPSP international workshop. Neurology 1996; 47:1–9.

42. Graham JG, Oppenheimer DR. Orthostatic hypotension and nicotine sensitivity in a case of multiple system atrophy. J Neurol Neurosurg Psych 1969; 32:28–34.

43. Wenning GK, Ben Shlomo Y, Magalhaes M, Daniel SE, Quinn NP. Clinical features and natural history of multiple system atrophy; an analysis of 100 cases. Brain 1994; 117:835–845.

44. Van Eecken H, Adams RD, and Van Bogaert, L. Striopallidal-nigral degeneration. J Neuropathol Exp Neurol 1960; 19:159–166.

45. Adams RA, Van Bogaert L, Van der Eecken H. Striato-nigral degeneration. J Neuropathol Exp Neurol 1964; 23:584–608.

46. Wenning GK, Tison F, Ben-Shlomo Y, Daniel SE, Quinn NP. Multiple system atrophy: a review of 203 pathologically proven cases. Mov Disord 1997; 12:133–147.

47. Rajput AH, Kazi KH, Rozdilsky B. Striatonigral degeneration, response to levodopa therapy. J Neurol Sci 1972; 16:331–341.

48. Hughes AJ, Colosimo C, Kleedorfer B, Daniel SE, Lees AJ. The dopaminergic response in multiple system atrophy. J Neurol Neurosurg Psych 1992; 55:1009–1013.

49. Lang AE, Birnbaum A, Blair RDG, Kierans C. Levodopa related response fluctuations in presumed olivopontocerebellar atrophy. Mov Disord 1986; 1:93–102.

50. Quinn NP. Unilateral facial dystonia in multiple system atrophy. Mov Disord 1992; 7(suppl):79.
51. Shy GM, Drager GA. A neurologic syndrome associated with orthostatic hypotension. Arch Neurol 1960; 2:511–527.
52. Wu YR, Chen CM, Ro LS, Chen ST, Tang LM. Vocal cord paralysis as an initial sign of multiple system atrophy in the central nervous system. J Formosan Med Assoc 1996; 95(10):804–806.
53. Bonnet AM, Pichon J, Vidailhet M, Gouider-Khouja N, Robain G, Perrigot M, Agid Y. Urinary disturbances in striatonigral degeneration and Parkinson's disease: clinical and urodynamic aspects. Mov Disord 1997; 12(4):509–513.
54. Kirby R, Fowler C, Gosling J, Bannister R. Urethro-vesical dysfunction in progressive autonomic failure with multiple system atrophy. J Neurol Neurosurg Psychiatry 1986; 49:554–562.
55. Valldeoriola F, Valls-Sole E, Tolosa S, Marti MJ. Striated anal sphincter denervation in patients with progressive supranuclear palsy. Mov Disord 1995; 10(5):550–555.
56. Schrag A, Good CD, Miszkiel K, et al. Differentiation of atypical parkinsonian syndromes with routine MRI. Neurology 2000; 54:697–702.
57. McKeith IG, Galasko D, Kosaka K, et al. Consensus guidelines for the clinical and pathological diagnosis of dementia with Lewy bodies (DLB): report of the Consortium on DLB International Workshop. Neurology 1996; 47:1113–1124.
58. Mega MS, Masterman DL, Benson DF, Vinters HV, Tomiyasu U, Craig AH, Foti DJ, Kaufer D, Scharre DW, Fairbanks L, Cummings JL. Dementia with Lewy bodies: reliability and validity of clinical and pathologic criteria. Neurology 1996; 47(6):1403–1409.
59. Ala TA, Yang KH, Sung JH, Frey WH. Hallucinations and signs of Parkinsonism help distinguish patients with dementia and cortical Lewy bodies from patients with Alzheimer's disease at presentation: a clinicopathological study. J Neurol Neurosurg Psychiatry 1997; 62(1):16–21.
60. Rebeiz JJ, Kolodny EH, Richardson EP. Corticodentatonigral degeneration with neuronal achromasia. Arch Neurol 1968; 18:220–223.
61. Riley De, Lang AE, Lewis A, et al. Cortical-basal ganglionic degeneration. Neurology 1990; 40:1203–1212.
62. Rinne Jo, Lee MS, Thompson PD, Marsden CD. Corticobasal degeneration: a clinical study of 36 cases. Brain 1994; 117:1183–1196.
63. Chen R, Ashby P, Lang AE. Stimulus-sensitive myoclonus in akinetic-rigid syndromes. Brain 1992; 115:1875–1888.
64. Litvan I, Agid Y, Gostz C, et al. Accuracy of the clinical diagnosis of corticobasal degeneration: a clinicopathological study. Neurology 1997; 48:119–125.
65. Lang AE, Bergeron C, Pollanen MS, Ashby P. Parietal Pick's disease mimicking cortical-basal ganglionic degeneration. Neurology 1994; 44:1436–1440.

66. Katai S, Maruyama T, Nakamura A, Tokuda T, Shindo M, Yanagisawa N. A case of corticobasal degeneration presenting with primary progressive aphasia. Rinsho Shinkeigaku Clin Neurol 1997; 37(3):249 252.

67. Grisoli M, Fetoni V, Savoiardo M, Girotti F, Bruzzone MG. MRI in corticobasal degeneration. Eur J Neurol 1995; 2:547–552.

68. Nagasawa H, Tanji H, Nomura H, Saito H, Itoyama Y, Kimura I, Tuji S, Fujiwara T, Iwata R, Itoh M, Ido T. PET study of cerebral glucose metabolism and fluorodopa uptake in patients with corticobasal degeneration. J Neurol Sci 1996; 139(2):210–217.

69. Neary D, Snowden J, Gustafsson L, et al. Frontotemporal lobar degeneration: a consensus on clinical diagnostic criteria. Neurology 1998; 51:1546–1554.

70. Gustaffson L. The clinical picture of frontal lobe degeneration of non-Alzheimer type. Dementia 1993; 4:143–148.

71. Pasqueir F, Lebert F, Lavenu I, Guillaume B. The clinical picture of frontotemporal dementia: diagnosis and follow-up. Geriatr Cogn Disord 1999; 109(suppl 1):10–14.

72. Rinne JO, Laine M, Kaasinen V, et al. Striatal dopamine transporter and extrapyramidal symptoms in frontotemporal dementia. Neurology 2002; 58:1489–1493.

73. Davis GC, Williams AC, Markey SP, et al. Chronic parkinsonism secondary intravenous injection of meperidine analogues. Psychiatry Res 1979; 1:249–254.

74. Langston JW, Ballard P, Tetrud J, Irwin I. Chronic Parkinsonism in humans due to a product of meperidine-analog synthesis. Science 1983; 219:979–980.

75. Tetrud JW, Langston JW, Garbe PL, Ruttenber JA. Early parkinsonism in persons exposed to 1-methyl-4-phenyl-1,2,3,6-tetrahydropyridine (MPTP). Neurology 1989; 39:1482–1487.

76. Langston JW, Ballard PA. Parkinsonism induced by 1-methyl-4-phenyl-1,2,3,6-tetrahydropyridine (MPTP): implications for treatment and the pathogenesis of Parkinson's disease. Can J Neurol Sci 1984; 11:160–165.

77. Langston JW. MPTP-induced parkinsonism: How good a model is it? In: Fahn S, Marsden CD, Teychenne P, Jenner P, eds. Recent advances in Parkinson's disease. New York: Raven Press, 1986:119–126.

78. Huang CC, Chu NS, Song C, Wang JD. Chronic manganese intoxication. Arch Neurol 1989; 46:1104–1112.

79. Barbeau A. Manganese and extrapyramidal disorders. Neurotoxicology 1984; 5:113–136.

80. Racette BA, McGee- Minnich L, Moerlein SM, Mink JW, Videen TO, Perlmutter JS. Welding-related parkinsonism: clinical features, treatment, and pathophysiology. Neurology 2001; 56(1):8–13.

81. Min SK. A brain syndrome associated with delayed neuro-psychiatric sequelae following acute carbon monoxide intoxication. Acta Psychiatr Scand 1986; 73:80–86.

82. Lee MS, Marsden CD. Neurological sequelae following carbon monoxide poisoning: Clinical course and outcome according to the clinical types and brain computed tomography scan findings. Mov Disord 1994; 9:550–558.

83. Miura T, Mitomo M, Kawai R, Harada. CT of the brain in acute carbon monoxide intoxication. Characteristic features and prognosis. AJNR 1985; 6:739–742.

84. Kobayashi K, Isaki K, Fukutani Y, et al. CT findings of the interval form of carbon monoxide poisoning compared with neuropathological findings. Eur Neurol 1984; 23:34–43.

85. Vieregge P, Klostermann W, Blumm RG, Borgis KJ. Carbon monoxide poisoning: clinical, neurophysiological and brain imaging observations in acute phase and follow up. J Neurol 1989; 239:478–481.

86. Peters HA, Levine RL, Matthews CG, Chapman LJ. Extrapyramidal and other neurological manifestations associated with carbon disulfide fumigant exposure. Arch Neurol 1988; 45:537–540.

87. Uitti RJ, Rajput AH, Aashenhurst EM, Rozkilsky B. Cyanide-induced parkinsonism: a clinicalopathologic report. Neurology 1985; 35:921–925.

88. Rosenberg NL, Myers JA, Wayne WR. Cyanide-induced parkinsonism: clinical, MRI, and 6-fluorodopa PET studies. Neurology 1989; 39:142–144.

89. Guggenheim MA, Couch JR, Weinberg W. Motor dysfunction as a permanent complication of methanol ingestion. Arch Neurol 1971; 24:550–554.

90. Mclean DR, Jacobs H, Mielki BW. Methanol poisoning a clinical and pathological study. Ann Neurol 1980; 8:161–167.

91. Factor SA, Sanchez-Ramos J, Weiner WJ. Trauma as an etiology of parkinsonism: a historical review of the concept. Mov Disord 1988; 3:30–36.

92. Factor SA. Posttraumatic parkinsonism. In: Stern MB, Koller WC, eds. Parkinsonian Syndromes. New York: Marcel Dekker, 1993:95–110.

93. Critchley M. Medical aspects of boxing, particularly from a neurological standpoint. Br Med J 1957; 1:357–362.

94. Martland HS. Punch drink. J Am Med Assoc 1928; 91:1103–1107.

95. Critchley M. Arteriosclerotic parkinsonism. Brain 1929; 52:23–83.

96. Fitzgerald PM, Jankoic J. Lower body parkinsonism: evidence for a vascular etiology. Mov Disord 1989; 4:249–260.

97. Parkes JD, Marsden CD, Rees JE, et al. Parkinson's disease: Cerebral arteriosclerosis and senile dementia. Q J Med 1974; 43:49–61.

98. Thompson PD, Marsden CD. Gait disorder of subcortical arteriosclerotic encephalopathy: Binswanger's disease. Mov Disord 1987; 2:1–8.

99. Mark MH, Sage JI, Walters AS, et al. Binswanger's disease presenting as L-dopa-responsive parkinsonism: clinicopathologic study of three cases. Mov Disord 1995; 10:450–454.

100. Hurtig HI. Vascular parkinsonism. In: Stern MB, Koller WC, eds. Parkinsonian Syndromes. New York: Marcel Dekker, 1993:81–93.

101. Krauss JK, Regel JP, Droste DW, Orszag M, Boremanns JJ, Vach W. Movement disorders in adult hydrocephalus. Mov Disord 1997; 12:53–60.

102. Hakim S, Adams RD. The special clinical problem of symptomatic hydrocephalus with normal cerebrospinal fluid hydrodynamics. J Neurol Sci 1965; 2:307–327.

103. Jacobs L, Conti D, Kinkel WR, Manning EEG. A Normal pressure hydrocephalus: relationship of clinical and radiographic findings to improvement following shunt surgery. JAMA 1976; 235(5):510–512.

104. Ahlberg J, Norlen L, Blomstrand C, Wikkelso C. Outcome of shunt operation on urinary incontinence in normal pressure hydrocephalus predicted by lumbar puncture. J Neurol Neurosurg Psychiatry 1988; 51:105–108.

105. Waters CH. Structural lesions and parkinsonism. In: Stern MB, Koller WC, eds. Parkinsonian syndromes. New York: Marcel Dekker, 1993:137–144.

106. Blocq, Marinesco G. Sur un cas tremblement parkinsonien hemiplegique symptomatique dune tumeur de pedoncule cerebral. Cr Soc Biol 1893; 45:105–111.

107. Samiy E. Chronic subdural hematoma presenting a parkinsonian syndrome. J Neurosurg 1963; 20:903.

108. Adler CH, Stern MB, Brooks ML. Parkinsonism secondary to bilateral striatal fungal abscesses. Mov Disord 1989; 4:333–337.

109. Murphy MJ. Clinical correlations of CT scan-detected calcification of the basal ganglia. Ann Neurol 1979; 6:507–511.

110. Lang AE, Koller WC, Fahn S. Psychogenic parkinsonism. Arch Neurol 1995; 52:802–810.

111. Quinn N, Critchley P, Marsden CD. Young onset Parkinson's disease. Mov Disord 1987; 2:73–91.

112. Gershanik OS. Early-onset parkinsonism. In: Jankovic J, Tolosa E, eds. Parkinson's Disease and Movement Disorders. Baltimore: Williams & Wilkins, 1993:235–252.

113. Nygaard TG, Marsden CD, Fahn S. Dopa-responsive dystonia: long-term treatment response and prognosis. Neurology 1991; 41:174–181.

114. Snow BJ, Nygaard TG, Takahashi H, Calne DB. Positron emission tomographic studies of dopa-responsive dystonia and early-onset idiopathic parkinsonism. Ann Neurol 1993; 34:733–738.

115. Dobyns WB, Goldstein NNP, Gordon H. Clinical spectrum of Wilson's disease (hepatolenticular degeneration). Mayo Clin Proc 1979; 54:35–42.

116. Walshe JM, Yealland M. Wilson's disease: the problem of delayed diagnosis. J Neurol Neurosurg Psychiatry 1992; 55:692–696.

117. Topaloglu H, Gucuyener K, Orkun C, Renda Y. Tremor of tongue and dysarthria as the sole manifestation of Wilson's disease. Clin Neurol Neurosurg 1990; 92:295–296.

118. Cheinberg IH, Sternlieb I, Richman J. Psychiatric manifestations of Wilson's disease. Birth defects. Orig Art Ser 1968; 4:85–86.

119. Wilson SAK. Progressive lenticular degeneration: a familial nervous disease associated with cirrhosis of the liver. Brain 1912; 34:295–509.

120. Weilleit J, Kiechl SG. Wilson's disease with neurological impairment but no Kayser-Fleischer rings. Lancet 1991; 337:1426.

121. Demirkiran M, Jankovic J, Lewis RA, Cox DW. Neurologic presentation of Wilson disease without Kayser-Fleischer rings. Neurology 1996; 46(4):1040–1043.
122. Nelson RF, Guzman DA, Grahovaac Z, Howse DCN. Computerized tomography in Wilson's disease. Neurology 1979; 29:866–868.
123. Dettori P, Rochelle MB, Demalia L, et al. Computerized cranial tomography in presymptomatic and hepatic form of Wilson's disease. Eur Neurol 1984; 23:56–63.
124. King AD, Walshe JM, Kendall BE, Chinn RJ, Paley MN, Wilkinson ID, Halligan S, Hall-Craggs MA. Cranial MR imaging in Wilson's disease. Am J Roentgenol 1996; 167(6):1579–1584.
125. Steindl P, Ferenci P, Dienes HP, Grimm G, Pabinger I, Madl C, Maier-Dobersberger T, Herneth A, Dragosics B, Meryn S, Knoflach P, Granditsch G, Gangl A. Wilson's disease in patients presenting with liver disease: a diagnostic challenge. Gastroenterology 1997; 113(1):212–218.
126. Saatci I, Topcu M, Baltaoglu FF, Kose G, Yalaz K, Renda Y, Besim A. Cranial MR findings in Wilson's disease. Acta Radiol 1997; 38(2):250–258.
127. Snow BJ, Bhatt M, Martin WR, et al. The nigrostriatal dopaminergic pathway in Wilson's disease studied with positron emission tomography. J Neurol Neurosurg Psychiatry 1991; 54:12–17.
128. Scheinberg IH, Sternlieb I. Wilson's disease: Major Problems in Internal Medicine. Vol. 23. Philadelphia: W. B. Saunders, 1984.
129. Brewer GJ, Yuzbasiyan-Gurkan V. Wilson's disease. Medicine 1992; 71:139–164.
130. Sethi KD, Adams RJ, Loring DW, EL Gammal T. Hallervorden-Spatz syndrome: clinical and magnetic resonance imaging correlations. Ann Neurol 1988; 24:692–694.
131. Adams P, Falek A, Arnold J. Huntington's disease in Georgia: age at onset. Am J Hum Genet 1988; 43:695–704.
132. Klawans HL. Hemiparkinsonism as a late complication of hemiatrophy: a new syndrome. Neurology 1981; 31:625–628.
133. Buchman AS, Christopher GG, Goetz MD, Klawans HI. Hemiparkinsonism with hemiatrophy. Neurology 1988; 38:527–530.
134. Przedborski S, Giladi N, Takikawa S, et al. Metabolic topography of the hemiparkinsonism-hemiatrophy syndrome. Neurology 1994; 44:1622–1628.
135. Waters CH, Faust PL, Powers J, et al. Neuropathology of lubag (X-linked dystonia-parkinsonism). Mov Disord 1993; 8:387–390.
136. Spitz MC, Jankovic J, Killian JM. Familial tic disorder, parkinsonism, motor neuron disease and acanthocytosis: a new syndrome. Neurology 1985; 35:366–370.
137. Hughes AJ, Ben-Shlomo Y, Daniel SE, Lees AJ. What features improve the accuracy of clinical diagnosis in Parkinson's disease: a clinicopathologic study. Neurology 1992; 42:1142–1146.
138. Gelb DJ, Oliver E, Gilman S. Diagnostic criteria for Parkinson disease. Arch Neurol 1999; 56:33–39.

139. Gibb WR, Lees AJ. The relevance of the Lewy body to the pathogenesis of idiopathic Parkinson's disease. J Neurol Neurosurg Psychiatry 1988; 51:745–752.

140. Ward C, Gibb W. Research diagnostic criteria for Parkinson's disease. In: Streifler M, Korczyn A, Melamed E, Youdim M, eds. Advances in Neurology: Parkinson's Disease: Anatomy, Pathology, and Therapy. New York: Raven Press, 1990.

141. Rajput AH, Rozdilsky B, Rajput A. Accuracy of clinical diagnosis in parkinsonism prospective study. Can J Neurol Sci 1991; 18:275–278.

142. Hughes AJ, Daniel SE, Kilford L, Lees AJ. Accuracy of clinical diagnosis of idiopathic Parkinson's disease: a clinico-pathological study of 100 cases. J Neurol Neurosurg Psychiatry 1992; 55:181–184.

143. Hughes AJ, Daniel SE, Lees AJ. Improved accuracy of clinical diagnosis of Lewy body Parkinson's disease. Neurology 2001; 57:1497–1499.

144. Hughes AJ, Daniel SE, Ben-Shlomo Y, Lees AJ. The accuracy of diagnosis of parkinsonian syndromes in a specialist movement disorder service. Brain 2002; 125:861–870.

4

Pathophysiology and Clinical Assessment of Parkinsonian Symptoms and Signs

Joseph Jankovic
Baylor College of Medicine, Houston,
Texas, U.S.A.

In his 1817 "An Essay on the Shaking Palsy," James Parkinson recorded many features of the condition that now bears his name (1). Parkinson emphasized the tremor at rest, flexed posture, festinating gait (Fig. 1), dysarthria, dysphagia, and constipation. Charcot and others later pointed out that the term paralysis agitans used by Parkinson was inappropriate, because in Parkinson's disease (PD) the strength was usually well preserved and many patients with Parkinson's disease did not shake.

Although traditionally regarded as a motor system disorder, PD is now considered to be a much more complex syndrome involving the motor as well as the nonmotor systems. For example, oily skin, seborrhea, pedal edema, fatigability, and weight loss are recognized as nonspecific but nevertheless typical parkinsonian features. The autonomic involvement is responsible for orthostatic hypotension, paroxysmal flushing, diaphoresis, problems with thermal regulation, constipation, and bladder, sphincter, and sexual disturbances. The involvement of the thalamus and the spinal

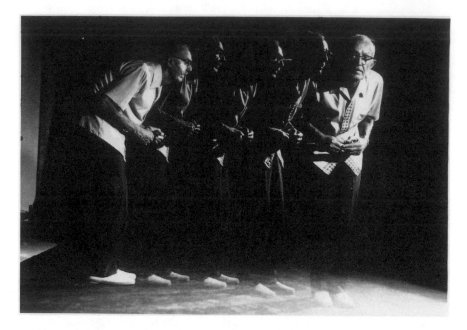

FIGURE 1   A 74-year-old man with 9 years of bilateral parkinsonism demonstrated by hypomimia, hand tremor and posturing, stooped posture, and a shuffling gait.

dopaminergic pathway may explain some of the sensory complaints, such as pains, aches, and burning-tingling paresthesias (2). The special sensory organs may also be involved in PD and cause visual, olfactory, and vestibular dysfunction (3).

A large number of studies have drawn attention to the protean neurobehavioral abnormalities in PD, such as apathy, fearfulness, anxiety, emotional lability, social withdrawal, increasing dependency, depression, dementia, bradyphrenia, a type of anomia termed the "tip-of-the-tongue phenomenon," visual-spatial impairment, sleep disturbance, psychosis, and other psychiatric problems (4,5).

The rich and variable expression of PD often causes diagnostic confusion and a delay in treatment. In the early stages, parkinsonian symptoms are often mistaken for simple arthritis or bursitis, depression, normal aging, Alzheimer's disease, or stroke (Fig. 2). PD often begins on one side of the body, but usually becomes bilateral within a few months or years. However, parkinsonism may remain unilateral, particularly when it is a late sequela of posttraumatic hemiatrophy or when it is due to a structural lesion in the basal ganglia (6). In a survey of 181 treated PD patients, Bulpitt

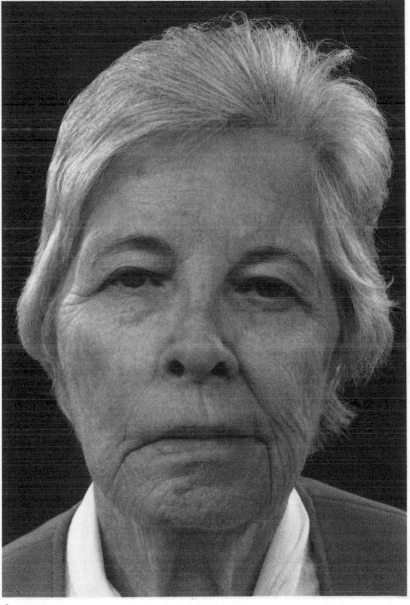

A

FIGURE 2 (A) 74-year-old woman with facial asymmetry and right hemiatrophy for 5 years associated with right hemiparkinsonism. (B) Voluntary facial contraction reveals no evidence of right facial weakness.

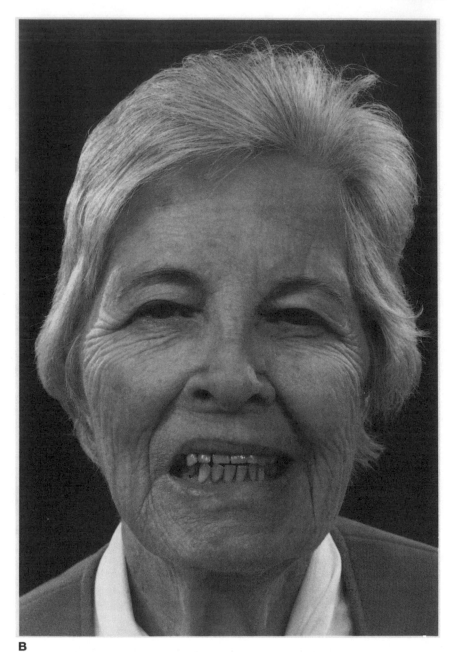

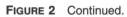

FIGURE 2 Continued.

et al. (7) found at least 45 different symptoms attributable to PD. However, only 9 of these symptoms were reported by the patients, with more than fivefold excess compared with those of a control population of patients randomly selected from a general practice. These common symptoms included being frozen or rooted to a spot, grimacing, jerking of the arms and legs, shaking hands, clumsy hands, salivation, poor concentration, severe apprehension, and hallucinations. However, even these frequent symptoms are relatively nonspecific and do not clearly differentiate PD patients from diseased controls. In many cases, a follow up for several years is needed before the diagnosis becomes apparent. Gonera et al. (8) found that 4–6 years prior to the onset of classic PD symptoms patients experience a prodromal phase characterized by more frequent visits to general practitioners and specialists as compared to normal controls. During this period PD patients, compared to normal controls, had a higher frequency of mood disorder, "fibromyalgia," and shoulder pain.

Different diagnostic criteria for PD, based on clinical and pathological findings, have been proposed, but their reliability has not been vigorously tested. In one study of 800 patients diagnosed clinically as PD and prospectively followed by trained parkinsonologists from early, untreated stages, the final diagnosis after a mean of 7.6 years of follow-up was considered to be other than PD in 8.1% of cases (9). In a study of 143 cases of parkinsonism who came to autopsy and had a clinical diagnosis made by neurologists, the positive predictive value of the clinical diagnosis of PD was 98.6%, and for the other parkinsonian syndromes it was 71.4% (10).

While systemic, mental, sensory, and other nonmotor symptoms of PD are often quite disabling, PD patients are usually most concerned about the symptoms that relate to their disturbance of movement (11). Several studies have demonstrated that patients who predominantly manifest "axial" symptoms, such as dysarthria, dysphagia, loss of equilibrium, and freezing, are particularly disabled by their disease as compared to those who have predominantly limb manifestations (12). The poor prognosis of patients in whom these symptoms predominate is partly due to a lack of response of these symptoms to dopaminergic drugs.

The specific mechanisms underlying the various PD symptoms are poorly understood. An accurate assessment of the disorder's motor signs should help to differentiate them from the motor changes associated with normal aging. Normal elderly subjects may have a mild extrapyramidal impairment, including slow movement and a shuffling gait. Other signs often attributed to PD also have been described with increased frequency among normal elderly subjects. These include disinhibition of the nuchocephalic reflex, glabellar blink reflex, snout reflex, head-retraction reflex, and the presence of paratonia, impaired vertical glaze, and cogwheel visual pursuit (13). Although these signs occur more frequently in parkinsonian patients than other aged individuals, they are not specific for PD. However, they may indicate an age-dependent loss of striatal dopamine and dopamine receptors (14). The receptor loss may explain why these age-related motor signs do not improve with levodopa treatment (15).

This chapter will focus on these motor manifestations. The emphasis will be on the pathophysiology and clinical assessment of the cardinal signs of PD: bradykinesia, tremor, rigidity, and postural instability (Table 1).

TABLE 1   Motor Features of Parkinsonism

Tremor at rest[a]
Rigidity[a]
Bradykinesia[a]
Loss of postural reflexes[a]
Hypomimia (masked facies)
Speech disturbance (hypokinetic dysarthria)
Hypophonia
Dysphagia
Sialorrhea
Respiratory difficulties
Loss of associated movements
Shuffling, short-step gait
Festination
Freezing
Micrographia
Difficulty turning in bed
Slowness in activities of daily living
Stooped posture, kyphosis, and scoliosis,
Dystonia, myoclonus, orofacial dyskinesia
Neuro-ophthalmological findings
Impaired visual contrast sensitivity
Visuospatial impairment
Impaired upward gaze, convergence, and smooth pursuit
Impaired vestibuloocular reflex
Hypometric saccades
Decreased blink rate
Spontaneous and reflex blepharospasm (glabellar or Myerson's sign)
Lid apraxia (opening or closure)
Motor findings related to dopaminergic therapy
Levodopa-induced dyskinesias (chorea, dystonia, myoclonus, tic)

[a]Cardinal signs.

BRADYKINESIA

Bradykinesia, or slowness of movement, if often used interchangeably with hypokinesia (poverty of movement) and akinesia (absence of movement). Bradykinesia is the most characteristic symptom of basal ganglia dysfunction in PD (16,17). It may be manifested by a delay in the initiation, and by slowness of execution, of a movement. Other aspects of bradykinesia include a delay in arresting movement, decrementing amplitude and speed of repetitive movement, and an inability to execute simultaneous or sequential actions. In addition to whole body slowness and impairment of fine motor movement, other manifestations of bradykinesia include drooling due to impaired swallowing of saliva (18), monotonous (hypokinetic) dysarthria, loss of facial expression (hypomimia), and reduced arm swing when walking (loss of automatic movement). Micrographia has been postulated to result from an abnormal response due to reduced motor output or weakness of agonist force coupled with distortions in visual feedback (19). The term bradyphrenia refers to slowness of thought, but bradyphrenia does not always correlate with bradykinesia, and therefore different biochemical mechanisms probably underlie these two parkinsonian disturbances (20).

After recording electromyographic (EMG) patterns in the antagonistic muscles of parkinsonian patients during a brief ballistic elbow flexion, Hallett and Khoshbin (21) concluded that the most characteristic feature of bradykinesia was the inability to "energize" the appropriate muscles to provide a sufficient rate of force required for the initiation and the maintenance of a large, fast (ballistic) movement. Therefore, PD patients need a series of multiple agonist bursts to accomplish a larger movement. Micrographia, a typical PD symptom, is an example of a muscle-energizing defect (21). The impaired generation and velocity of ballistic movement can be ameliorated with levodopa (22,23).

Bradykinesia, more than any other cardinal sign of PD, correlates well with striatal dopamine deficiency. Measuring brain dopamine metabolism of rats running on straight and circular treadmills, Freed and Yamamoto (24) found that dopamine metabolism in the caudate nucleus was more affected by posture and direction of movement. Dopamine metabolism in the nucleus accumbens was more linked to the speed and direction of the antagonists, appears to be normal in PD, and is probably more under cerebellar than basal ganglia control (21,25). In other words, in PD the simple motor program to execute a fast ballistic movement is intact, but it fails because the initial agonist burst is insufficient. The degree of bradykinesia correlates well with a reduction in the striatal fluorodopa uptake measured by positron emission tomography (PET) scans and in turn with nigral damage (26). Studies performed initially in monkeys made parkinsonian with the toxin 1-methyl-4-phenyl-1,2,3,6-tetrahydropyridine (MPTP) (27) and later in patients with PD provide evidence that bradykinesia results from excessive activity in the subthalamic nucleus (STN) and the internal segment of globus pallidus (GPi) (28). Thus, there is both functional and biochemical evidence of increased activity in the outflow nuclei, particularly STN and GPi, in patients with PD. As a result of the abnormal neuronal activity at the level of the GPi, the muscle discharge in patients with PD changes from the normal high (40 Hz) to pulsatile (10 Hz) contractions. These muscle discharges can be auscultated with a stethoscope (29). More recent studies suggest that the observed 15–30 Hz oscillations of the STN may reflect synchronization with cortical beta oscillation via the cortico-subthalamic pathway and may relate to mechanisms of bradykinesia since stimulation at the 15 Hz rate worsens bradykinesia and dopaminergic drugs promote faster oscillations (about 70 Hz) and improve bradykinesia, similar to the high-frequency stimulation associated with deep brain stimulation (DBS) (30,31).

Bradykinesia, like other parkinsonian symptoms, is dependent on the emotional state of the patient. With a sudden surge of emotional energy, the immobile patient may catch a ball or make other fast movements. This curious phenomenon, called "kinesia paradoxica," demonstrates that the motor programs are intact in PD, but that patients have difficulty utilizing or accessing the programs without the help of an external trigger (32). Therefore, parkinsonian patients are able to make use of prior information to perform an automatic or a preprogrammed movement, but they cannot use this information to initiate or select a movement. Another fundamental defect in PD is the inability to execute learned sequential motor plans automatically (33). This impairment of normal sequencing of motor programs probably results from a disconnection between the basal ganglia and the supplementary motor cortex, an area that subserves planning function for movement. The supplementary motor cortex receives projections from the motor basal ganglia (via the globus pallidus and ventrolateral thalamus) and, in turn, projects to the motor cortex. In PD, the early component of the premovement potential (Bereitschaftpotential) is reduced, probably reflecting inadequate basal ganglia activation of the supplementary motor area (34,35). Recording from the motor cortex of MPTP monkeys, Tatton et al. (36) showed markedly increased gain of the long-latency (M2) segments of the mechanoreceptor-evoked responses. This and other findings indicate that PD patients have an abnormal processing of sensory input necessary for the generation and execution of movement.

Most of the neurophysiological and neurobehavioral studies in PD have concluded that the basal ganglia (and possibly the supplementary motor cortex) play a critical role in planning and in sequencing voluntary movements (37). For example, when a patient arises from a chair, he or she may "forget" any one of the sequential steps involved in such a seemingly simple task: to flex forward, place hands on the arm rests, place feet under the chair, and then push out of the chair into an erect posture. Similar difficulties may be encountered when sitting down, squatting, kneeling, turning in bed, and walking. Lakke (32) suggests that since the patient can readily perform these activities under certain circumstances, such as when emotionally stressed ("kinesia paradoxica"), the intrinsic program is not disturbed, and therefore these axial motor abnormalities are a result of apraxia. Thus, the PD patient has an ability to "call up" the axial motor program on command.

The inability to combine motor programs into complex sequences seems to be a fundamental motor deficit in PD. The study of reaction time (RT) and velocity of movement provide some insight into the mechanisms of the motor deficits at an elementary level. Evarts et al. (38) showed that both RT and movement times (MT) are independently impaired in PD. In patients with asymmetrical findings, the RT is slower on the more affected side (39). The RT is influenced not only by the degree of motor impairment, but also by the interaction between the cognitive processing and the motor response. This is particularly evident when choice RT is used and compared to simple RT (20). Bradykinetic patients with PD have more specific impairment in choice RT, which involves a stimulus categorization and a response selection, and reflects disturbance at more complex levels of cognitive processing (40). Bereitschaftspotential, a premovement potential, has been found to be abnormal in PD patients and to normalize with levodopa (41). The MT, particularly when measured for proximal muscles, is less variable than the RT and more consistent with the clinical assessment of bradykinesia. Both MT and RT are better indicators of bradykinesia than the speed of rapid alternating movements. Ward et al. (42) attempted to correlate the median MT and RT with tremor, rigidity, or manual dexterity in 10 patients rated on a 0–4 modified Columbia scale. The only positive correlations were found between MT and rigidity and between RT and manual dexterity. Of the various objective assessments of bradykinesia, the MT correlates best with the total clinical score, but it is not as sensitive an indicator of the overall motor deficit as is the clinical rating. Ward et al. (42) concluded that although MT was a useful measurement, it alone did not justify the use of elaborate and expensive technology. The clinical rating scale probably more accurately reflects the patient's disability because it includes more relevant observations.

TREMOR

Tremor, while less specific than bradykinesia, is one of the most recognizable symptoms of PD. However, only half of all patients present with tremor as the initial manifestation of PD, and 15% never have tremor during the course of the illness (43). Although tremor at rest (4–6 Hz) is the typical parkinsonian tremor, most patients also have tremor during activity, and this postural tremor (5–8 Hz) may be more disabling than the resting tremor. Postural tremor without parkinsonian features and without any other known etiology is often diagnosed as essential tremor (Table 2). Isolated postural tremor clinically identical to essential tremor, however, may be the initial presentation of PD, and it may be found with higher-than-

TABLE 2   Differential Diagnosis of Parkinson and Essential Tremor

	Essential tremor	Parkinsonian tremor
Age at onset (years)	10–80	55–75
Sex	M ≤ F	M ≥ F
Family history	+++	+
Site of involvement	Hands, head, voice	Hands, legs, jaw, chin, tongue
Characteristics	Flexion-extension	Supination-pronation
Influencing factors		
Rest	↓	↑
Action	↑	↓
Mental concentration walking	↓	↑
Frequency (Hz)	8–12	4–7
Electromyography contractions	Simultaneous	Alternating
Associated features		
Cogwheel rigidity	± (cogwheel without rigidity)	+
Dystonia	+	++
Hereditary neuropathy	+	0
Neuropathology	No discernible pathology	Nigrostriatal degeneration, Lewy bodies
Treatment	Alcohol, beta-blockers, primidone, botulinum toxin	Anticholinergics amantadine dopaminergic drugs surgery

expected frequency in relatives of patients with PD (44). The two forms of postural tremor can be differentiated by a delay in the onset of tremor when arms assume an outstretched position. While most patients with Parkinson's tremor have a latency of a few seconds (up to a minute) before the tremor reemerges during postural holding, hence "reemergent tremor," postural tremor of ET usually appears immediately after arms assume a horizontal posture (45). Since the reemergent tremor has similar frequency to that of rest tremor and both tremors generally respond to dopaminergic drugs, we postulate that the reemergent tremor represents a variant of the more typical rest tremor. It has been postulated that the typical tremor at rest results from nigrostriatal degeneration and consequent disinhibition of the pacemaker cells in the thalamus (46). These thalamic neurons discharge rhythmically at 5–6 Hz, a frequency similar to the typical parkinsonian tremor at rest (47,48). Some support for the thalamic pacemaker theory of PD tremor also comes from the studies of Lee and Stein (49), which show that the resting 5 Hz tremor is remarkably constant and relatively resistant to resetting by mechanical perturbations. Furthermore, during stereotactic thalamotomy, 5 Hz discharges are usually recorded in the nucleus ventralis intermedius of the thalamus in parkinsonian as well as in normal subjects, even in the absence of visible tremor (50). This rhythmic bursting is not abolished by deafferentation or paralysis (16). Because the frequency (6 Hz) of the postural (action) tremor is the same as the frequency of the cogwheel phenomenon elicited during passive movement, some authors have suggested that the postural tremor and cogwheel phenomenon have similar pathophysiologies (51) (Fig. 3).

The biochemical defect underlying either resting or postural parkinsonian tremor is unknown. Bernheimer and colleagues (52) showed that the severity of tremor paralleled the degree of homovanillic acid (HVA) reduction in the pallidum. In contrast, bradykinesia correlated with dopamine depletion in the caudate nucleus. In an experimental monkey model of parkinsonian tremor, a pure lesion in the ascending dopaminergic nigrostriatal pathway is not sufficient to produce the alternating rest tremor (53). Experimental parkinsonian tremor requires nigrostriatal disconnection combined with a lesion involving the rubrotegmentospinal and the dentatorubrothalamic pathways. A typical PD tremor is observed in humans and in experimental animals exposed to MPTP, a neurotoxin that presumably affects, rather selectively, the nigrostriatal dopaminergic system (54,55). However, the cerebellorubrothalamic system has not been examined in detail in this MPTP model. Furthermore, in MPTP subjects, a prominent action tremor was more typically seen than a tremor at rest.

In the early studies, mechanical and optic devices were used to record tremor (56). Electromyography (EMG) recordings and accelerometers,

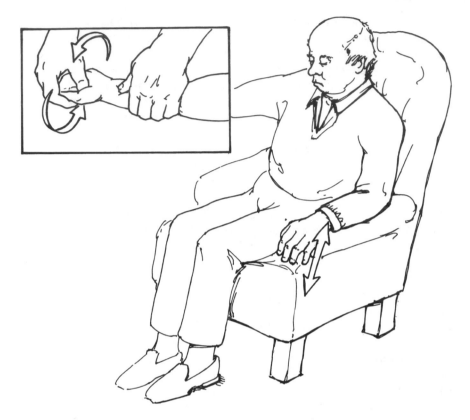

FIGURE 3 Parkinsonian cogwheel rigidity elicited by passive rotation of the wrist is enhanced by voluntary repetitive movement of the contralateral hand.

assisted by computer analysis, have been utilized to measure the characteristics of tremor. However, most accelerometers record tremor in a single plane. By using computed triaxial accelerometry, we recorded the distortion of the normal motion characteristics in patients with PD and ET during voluntary arm abduction-adduction movement (22). There was a good correlation between the reduction in the distortion and the clinical improvement in response to medications. However, the quantitative recordings of tremor, although accurate, are time consuming, costly, and influenced by the emotional state of the patient. Moreover, it is questionable whether such recordings provide a reliable index of a meaningful therapeutic response.

RIGIDITY AND POSTURAL ABNORMALITIES

Rigidity is less variable than tremor, and it probably better reflects the patient's functional disability. Rigidity may contribute to subjective stiffness and tightness, a common complaint in patients with PD. However, there is relatively poor correlation between the sensory complaints experienced by most patients and the degree of rigidity (57,58). In mild cases, cogwheel rigidity can be brought out by a passive rotation of the wrist or flexion-extension of the forearm while the patient performs a repetitive voluntary movement in the contralateral arm (59) (Fig. 3). Rigidity may occur proximally (e.g., neck, shoulders, and hips) and distally (e.g., wrists and ankles). At times it can cause discomfort and actual pain. Painful shoulder, probably due to rigidity but frequently misdiagnosed as arthritis, bursitis, or rotator cuff, is one of the most frequent initial manifestations of PD (60). Rigidity is often associated with postural deformity resulting in flexed neck and trunk posture and flexed elbows and knees. Some patients develop ulnar deviation of hands ("striatal hand"), which can be confused with arthritis (61). Other skeletal abnormalities include neck flexion ("dropped head" or "bent spine") (62) and trunkal flexion ("camptocormia") (63,64) (Figs. 4, 5). Duvoisin and Marsden (65) studied 20 PD patients with scoliosis and found that 16 of the patients tilted away from the side with predominant parkinsonian symptoms. However, subsequent studies could not confirm this observation (66).

The neurophysiological mechanisms of rigidity are still poorly understood. Spinal monosynaptic reflexes are usually normal in PD. Recordings from muscle spindle afferents revealed an activity in rigid parkinsonian patients not seen in normal controls. This suggested an increased fusimotor drive due to hyperactivity of both alpha and gamma motor neurons. However, this fusimotor overactivity probably is an epiphenomenon, reflecting the inability of PD patients to relax fully. Passive shortening of a rigid muscle, due to PD or seen in tense subjects, produces an involuntary contraction called the Westphal phenomenon. While the mechanism of this sign is unknown, it probably is the result of excessive supraspinal drive on normal spinal mechanism. This shortening reaction may be abolished by procaine infiltration of the muscle. Thus, there is no convincing evidence of a primary defect of fusimotor function in parkinsonian rigidity (67).

The measurement of torque or of resistance during passive flexion-extension movement has been used most extensively as an index of rigidity. Utilizing these techniques, it has been demonstrated that rigidity correlated with increased amplitude of the long-latency (transcerebral) responses to sudden stretch. These long-latency stretch reflexes represent a positive

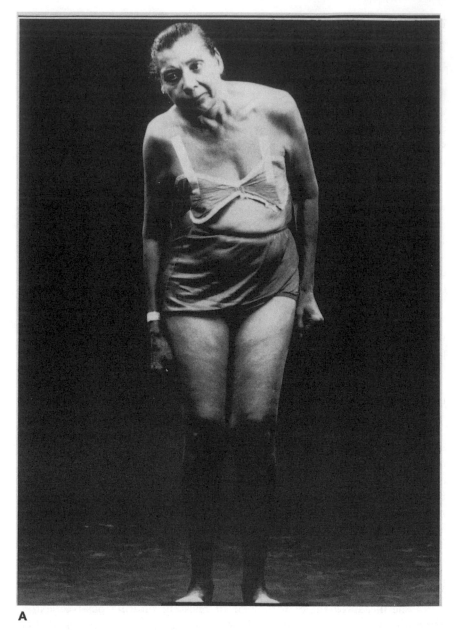

A

FIGURE 4   A 63-year-old woman with progressive scoliosis to the right side for 20 years and left hemiparkinsonism manifested by hand and leg tremor, rigidity, and bradykinesia: (A) front view; (B) back view.

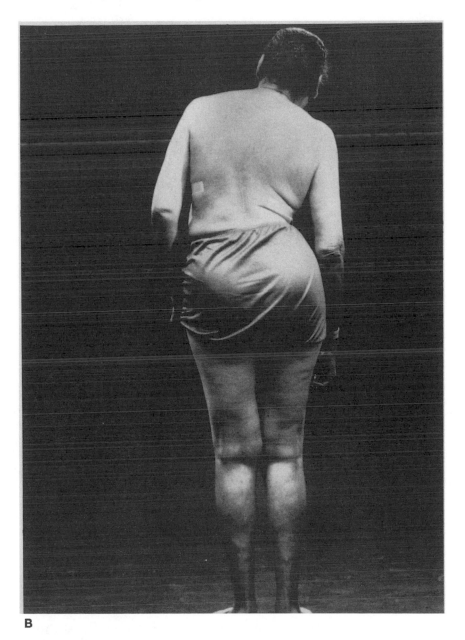

B

FIGURE 4 Continued.

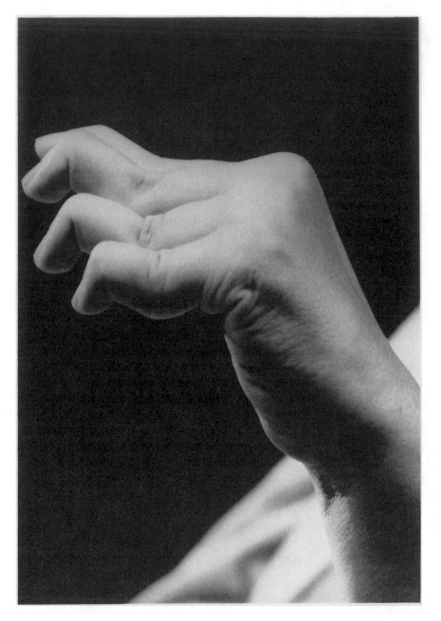

FIGURE 5   A 44-year-old woman with PD showing typical dystonic ("striatal") hand with flexion at the metacarpophalangeal joints, extension at the proximal interphalangeal joints, and flexion of the distal interphalangeal joints. The dystonia completely resolved with levodopa (61).

(release) phenomenon, mediated by motor pathways that do not traverse the basal ganglia. The earlier techniques of passively flexing and extending the limbs were later refined by Mortimer and Webster (68), who designed a servocontrolled electronic device to move the limb at a constant angular velocity. They and others (69–71) demonstrated a close relationship between the enhanced long-latency stretch reflexes and the degree of activated rigidity. The opposite is true in Huntington's disease, in which these long-latency stretch reflexes are diminished or absent. Using measurements of the tonic stretch reflex as an index of rigidity, Meyer and Adorjani (72) found an inverse correlation between the "dynamic sensitivity" (ratio between the increase in reflex EMG at a high versus low angular velocity) and the severity of parkinsonian rigidity. On the other hand, the "static" component of the tonic stretch reflex (the maximum reflex activity at greatest stretch or at sustained stretch) positively correlated with the severity of rigidity. Both the dynamic and the static components of the tonic stretch reflex may be reduced by antiparkinson drugs (72). Although Lee and Tatton (70) showed diminution of the amplitude of the reflex after treatment, correlating it with improvement in rigidity, the measurement of long-latency responses is quite cumbersome, time consuming, and possibly unreliable (73). Moreover, a marked overlap in the long-latency response between PD and normal subjects has been noted (74).

POSTURAL INSTABILITY

The loss of balance associated with propulsion and retropulsion is probably the least specific, but most disabling, of all parkinsonian symptoms. Purdon-Martin (75), after studying nine brains of patients with postencephalitic parkinsonism, concluded that the globus pallidum degeneration was most responsible for the loss of righting reflexes and of postural instability in parkinsonian patients. Reichert et al. (3) correlated postural instability in PD patients with reduced or absent vestibular responses. Traub et al. (76) studied postural reflexes in 29 PD patients by recording anticipatory postural responses in the legs (triceps surae) in response to perturbations of one of the arms. In normal subjects, a burst of activity can be recorded from the calf muscles at a latency of 80 msec after the perturbation. This postural adjustment occurs even before any movement can be recorded in the legs (latency, 150 msec). Therefore, this reflex adjustment is anticipatory and centrally generated. In PD, the anticipatory postural reflexes are absent or markedly diminished. Such abnormalities were present in 10 of the 18 patients with moderately severe PD and in 2 of 11 Parkinson's disease patients without obvious postural instability. Since some patients with normal anticipatory reflexes can still fall, it is likely that other mechanisms contribute to the falls of parkinsonian patients (77,78). Furthermore, patients with progressive supranuclear palsy, who are much more prone to falling than PD patients, have normal anticipatory postural responses (76). Weiner et al. (79) found moderate or severe loss of balance in response to a standing postural perturbation in 68% of 34 patients in a geriatric care facility. They suggested that a postural reflex dysfunction was largely responsible for the unexplained falls in the elderly.

Loss of postural reflexes usually occurs in more advanced stages of the disease and, along with freezing (see below), is the most common cause of falls, often resulting in hip fractures. The loss of protective reactions further contributes to fall-related injuries. Many patients with postural instability, particularly when associated with flexed trunkal posture, have festination, manifested by faster and faster walking as if chasing its center of gravity in order to prevent falling. When combined with axial rigidity and bradykinesia, loss of postural reflexes causes the patient to collapse into the chair when attempting to sit down. The "pull test" (pulling the patient by the shoulders) is commonly used to determine the degree of a patient's retropulsion or propulsion.

FREEZING AND OTHER GAIT ABNORMALITIES

The slow, shuffling, narrow-based gait is one of the most characteristic features of PD (80). The parkinsonian gait reveals certain features that overlap with the gait disturbance associated with normal pressure hydrocephalus (81,82). In a study of 50 subjects older than 70 years, Sudarsky and Ronthal (83) established a principal cause of the gait disorder in all but seven subjects ("essential gait disorder"). They, but not others (84), suggested that this senile gait is related to normal pressure hydrocephalus. The gait and postural problems associated with PD probably result from a combination of bradykinesia, rigidity, loss of anticipatory proprioceptive reflexes, loss of protective reaction to a fall, gait and axial apraxia, ataxia, vestibular dysfunction, and orthostatic hypotension. When gait disorder, with or without freezing and postural instability, is the dominant motor dysfunction, than "lower body" parkinsonism should be considered in the differential diagnosis (85). This syndrome is thought to represent a form of "vascular" parkinsonism associated with a multi-infarct state. Furthermore, gait disorder and postural instability are typically associated with progressive supranuclear palsy (86,87).

One of the most disabling symptoms of PD "freezing," also referred to as "motor blocks", is a form of akinesia (loss of movement) (88,89). The observation that some patients even with severe bradykinesia have no freezing and other patients have a great deal of freezing but minimal or no bradykinesia suggests that the two signs have different pathophysiologies. Furthermore, that bradykinesia usually responds well to levodopa whereas freezing does not indicate that freezing may be a manifestation of a nondopaminergic disturbance. Freezing consists of a sudden, transient (a few seconds) inability to move. It typically causes "start hesitation" when initiating walking, as well as a sudden inability to move the feet (as if "glued to the ground") when turning or walking through narrow passages (such as the door or the elevator), crossing streets with heavy traffic, or approaching a destination (target hesitation). Patients often learn a variety of tricks to overcome the freezing attacks, including marching to command ("left, right, left, right"), visual cues such as stepping over objects (end of a walking stick, pavement stone, cracks in the floor, etc.), walking to music or a metronome, shifting body weight, and rocking movements (85,90,91). When freezing occurs early in the course of the disease or is the predominant symptom, a diagnosis other than PD should be considered. Disorders associated with prominent freezing include progressive supranuclear palsy, multiple system atrophy, and vascular ("lower body") parkinsonism (85,92).

OTHER MOTOR MANIFESTATIONS

There are many other motor findings in PD (Table 1), most of which are directly related to one of the cardinal signs. For example, the loss of facial expression (hypomimia, masked facies) and the bulbar symptoms (dysarthria, hypophonia, dysphagia, and sialorrhea) result from orofacial-laryngeal bradykinesia and rigidity (93,94). Respiratory difficulties result from a variety of mechanisms, including a restrictive component due to rigid respiratory muscles and levodopa-induced respiratory dyskinesias (95,96).

Of the various oculomotor problems characteristically seen in PD, the following are most common: impaired saccadic and smooth pursuit, limitation of upward gaze and convergence, oculogyric crises, spontaneous and reflex blepharospasm, apraxia of lid opening (involuntary levator inhibition), and apraxia of eyelid closure (97,98). Although supranuclear ophthalmoplegia is often used to differentiate progressive supranuclear palsy from Parkinson's disease, this oculomotor abnormality has also been described in otherwise typical parkinsonism (99).

ASSESSMENT OF DISABILITY

The assessment of PD is difficult because the movement disorder is expressed variably in an individual patient (intrapatient variability) at different times, and it is influenced by emotional state, response to medication, and other variables. Moreover, there is a marked interpatient variability of symptoms and signs. To study this heterogeneity and to determine possible patterns of clinical associations, we analyzed the clinical findings in 334 patients with idiopathic PD. We identified at least two distinct clinical populations of parkinsonian patients (100). One subtype was characterized by a prominent tremor, an early age at onset, and a greater familiar tendency. Another subtype was dominated by postural instability and gait difficulty (PIGD) and was associated with greater degree of dementia, bradykinesia, functional disability, and a less favorable long-term prognosis.

These findings are supported by the results of an analysis of 800 patients with untreated PD included in the multicenter trial of Deprenyl and Tocopherol Antioxidative Therapy of Parkinson's Disease (DATA-TOP). The PIGD group had greater occupational disability and more intellectual impairment, depression, lack of motivation, and impairment in activities of daily living than a corresponding group of patients with tremor-dominant PD (12). Based on the analysis of clinical correlates in this cohort of patients, the investigators concluded that patients with older age of onset and a presentation with PIGD and with bradykinesia are more likely to have a more aggressive course than those whose symptoms being early and are dominated by tremor (101). In order to determine the overall rate of functional decline and to assess the progression of different signs of PD, we prospectively followed 297 patients (181 males) with clinically diagnosed PD for at least 3 years (101). Data from 1731 visits over an average period of 6.36 years (range: 3–17) were analyzed. The annual rate of decline in the total Unified Parkinson's Disease Rating Scale (UPDRS) scores was 1.34 units (when assessed during "on") and 1.58 (when assessed during "off"). Patients with older age at onset had a more rapid progression of disease than those with younger age at onset. Furthermore, the older onset group had significantly more progression in mentation, freezing, and parts I and II UPDRS subscores. Handwriting was the only component of the UPDRS that did not significantly deteriorate during the observation period. Regression analysis of 108 patients, whose symptoms were rated during their "off" state, showed faster rate of cognitive decline as age at onset increased. The slopes of progression in UPDRS scores, when adjusted for age at initial visit, were steeper for the PIGD group of patients as compared to the tremor-dominant group. These findings, based on longitudinal follow-up data, provide evidence for a variable course of progression of the different PD symptoms, thus implying different biochemical or degenerative mechanisms for the various clinical features associated with PD.

Thus, PD should not be considered a unitary disorder, but a syndrome with characteristic patterns of symptoms, course, response to therapy, and different etiologics. The different subsets of PD may have different pathogenesis and even different genetic predisposition. Tremor-dominant PD may be related to an autosomal dominant essential tremor (44).

The accurate and reliable evaluation of motor dysfunction is essential for an objective assessment of the efficacy of potentially useful drugs. Various mechanical, electrophysiological, and clinical methods have been utilized to measure the motor findings in PD objectively. Some of the techniques are designed to measure the frequency, amplitude, force, velocity, acceleration of contraction, and other quantitative parameters of the abnormal movement. However, such measurements may have little relevance to the actual functional disability of the patient.

In assessing the motor symptoms and signs of PD, two approaches have been used, both of which strive to quantitate the motor findings (73). One method utilizes neurological history and an examination with subjective rating of symptoms, signs and functional disability, and the other method utilizes timing of specific tasks or neurophysiological tests of particular motor disturbances. While the latter method is considered to be more "objective" and "scientific," it is not necessarily more accurate, reliable, or relevant than the clinical rating. However, both approaches have certain advantages and disadvantages, and, when combined, they may provide a useful method of assessing the severity of the disability and the response to therapy.

Most of the subjective methods of assessment of parkinsonian disability utilize rating scales of various symptoms and disabilities. Probably the most widely used method of staging PD is the Hoehn-Yahr scale (102). While this staging scale is useful in comparing populations of PD patients, it is relatively insensitive to changes in a patient's clinical state. Therefore, the Hoehn-Yahr scale is not useful in monitoring the response of individual patients to therapy.

Thus, it is important that the severity of the disease is objectively assessed in the context of the individual's goals and needs. Although a variety of neurophysiological and computer-based methods have been proposed to quantitate the severity of the various parkinsonian symptoms and signs, most studies rely on clinical rating scales, particularly the UPDRS (103–107) (see Appendix). In some studies the UPDRS is supplemented by more objective timed tests, such as the Purdue Pegboard test and movement and reaction times (17). There are also many scales, such as the Parkinson's Disease Questionnaire-39 (PDQ-39) and the Parkinson's Disease Quality of Life Questionnaire (PDQL), that attempt to assess the overall health related quality of life (108).

REFERENCES

1. Parkinson J. An Essay on the Shaking Palsy. London: Sherwood, Neely, and Jones, 1817.
2. Ford B, Louis ED, Greene P, Fahn S. Oral and genital pain syndromes in Parkinson's disease. Mov Disord 1996; 11:421–426.
3. Reichert WH, Doolittle J, McDowell FM. Vestibular dysfunction in Parkinson's disease. Neurology 1982; 32:1 133–1138.
4. Aarsland D, Andersen K, Larsen JP, et al. Risk of dementia in Parkinson's disease. A community-based, prospective study. Neurology 2001; 56:730–736.
5. Dubois B, Pillon B. Cognitive and behavioral aspects of basal ganglia disorders. In: Jankovic J, Tolosa E, eds. Parkinson's Disease and Movement Disorders. 4th ed. Philadelphia: Lippincott Williams and Wilkins, 2002.
6. Giladi N, Burke RE, Kostic V, et al. Hemiparkinsonism-hetniatrophy syndrome: clinical and neuroradiologic features. Neurology 1990; 40: 1731–1734.
7. Bulpitt CJ, Shaw K, Clifton P, Stenn G, Davies JB, Reid IL. The symptoms of patients treated for Parkinson's disease. Clin Neuropharmacol 1985; 8:175–183.
8. Gonera EG, van't Hof M, Berger HJC, et al. Symptoms and duration of the prodromal phase in Parkinson's disease. Mov Disord 1997; 12:871–876.
9. Jankovic J, Rajput AH, McDermott MP, Perl DP. The evolution of diagnosis in early Parkinson disease. Arch Neurol 2000; 57:369–372.
10. Hughes AJ, Daniel SE, Ben-Shlomo Y, Lees AJ. The accuracy of diagnosis of parkinsonian syndromes in a specialist movement disorder service. Brain 2002; 125:861–870.
11. Jankovic J. Clinical aspects of Parkinson's disease. In: Marsden CD, Fahn, S, eds. New Trends in the Treatment of Parkinson's Disease. Carnforth, England: Parthenon Publishing, 1991:53–76.
12. Jankovic J, McDermott M, Carter J, et al. Variable expression of Parkinson's disease: a base-line analysis of the DATATOP cohort. Neurology 1990; 40:1529–1534.
13. Jenkyn LR, Reeves AG, Warren T, et al. Neurologic signs in senescence. Arch Neurol 1984; 42:1154–1157.
14. Wagner HN. Probing the chemistry of the mind. N Engl J Med 1985; 312:44–46.
15. Newman RP, LeWitt PA, Jaffe M, Calne DB, Larsen TA. Motor function in the normal aging population: treatment with levodopa. Neurology 1985; 35:571–573.
16. Marsden CD. The pathophysiology of movement disorders. Neurol Clin North Am 1984; 2:435–459.
17. Jankovic J, Ben-Arie L, Schwartz K, Chen K, Kahn K, Lai EC, Krauss JK, Grossman R. Movement and reaction times and fine coordination tasks following pallidotomy. Mov Disord 1999; 14:57–62.

18. Bagheri H, Damase-Michel C, Lapeyre-Mestre M, et al. A study of salivary secretion in Parkinson's disease. Clin Neuropharm 1999; 22213–22215.

19. Teulings H-L, Contreras-Vidal JL, Stelmach GE, Adler CH. Adaptation of handwriting size under distorted visual feedback in patients with Parkinson's disease and elderly and young controls. J Neurol Neurosurg Psychiatry 2002; 72:315–324.

20. Rafal RD, Posner MI, Walker JA, Friedrich FJ. Cognition and the basal ganglia: separating mental and motor components of performance in Parkinson's disease. Brain 1984; 107:1083–1094.

21. Hallett M, Khoshbin S. A physiological mechanism of bradykinesia. Brain 1980; 103:301–314.

22. Jankovic J, Frost JD. Quantitative assessment of parkinsonian and essential tremor: clinical application of triaxial accelerometry. Neurolory 1981; 31:1235–1240.

23. Baroni A, Benvenuti F, Fantini L, Pantaleo T, Urbani F. Human ballistic arm abduction movements: effects of L-dopa treatment in Parkinson's disease. Neurology 1984; 34:868–876.

24. Freed CR, Yamamoto BK. Regional brain dopamine metabolism: a marker for the speed, direction, and posture of moving animals. Science 1985; 229:62–65.

25. Ito M. The Cerebellum and Neural Control. New York: Raven Press, 1984.

26. Vingerhoets FJG, Schulzer M, Calne DB, et al. Which clinical sign of Parkinson's disease best reflects the nigrostriatal lesion? Ann Neurol 1997; 41:58–64.

27. Bergman H, Wichmann T, DeLong MR. Reversal of experimental parkinsonism by lesions of the subthalamic nucleus. Science 1990; 249:1436–1438.

28. Dostrovsky JO, Hutchinson WD, Lozano AM. The globus pallidus, deep brain stimulation and Parkinson's disease. Neuroscientist 2002; 8:284–290.

29. Brown P. Muscle sounds in Parkinson's disease. Lancet 1997; 349:533–535.

30. Farmer S. Neural rhythms in Parkinson's disease. Brain 2002; 125:1175–1176.

31. Levy R, Ashby P, Hutchison WD, Lang AE, Lozano AM, Dostrovsky JO. Dependence of subthalamic nucleus oscillations on movement and dopamine in Parkinson's disease. Brain 2002; 125:1196–1209.

32. Lakke JPWF. Axial apraxia in parkinson's disease. J Neurol Sci 1985; 69:37–46.

33. Marsden CD. The mysterious motor function of the basal ganglia. Neurology 1982; 32:514–539.

34. Schultz W. Recent physiological and pathophysiological aspects of parkinsonian movement disorders. Life Sci 1984; 34:2213–2223.

35. Dick JPR, Rothwell JC, Day BL, et al. The Bereitschaftpotential is abnormal in Parkinson's disease. Brain 1989; 112:233–244.

36. Tatton WG, Eastovan MJ, Bedingham W, Verrier MC, Bruce IC. Defective utilization of sensory input as the basis for bradykinesia, rigidity and

decreased movement repertoire in parkinson's disease: a hypothesis. Can J
Neurol Sci 1984; 11:136–147.

37. Stern Y, Mayeux R, Rosen J, Illson J. Perceptual motor dysfunction in
Parkinson's disease: a deficit in sequential and predictive voluntary movement.
J Neurol Neurosurg Psychiatry 1983; 46:145–151.

38. Evarts EV, Teravainen M, Calne DB. Reaction time in Parkinson's disease.
Brain 1981; 104:167–1861.

39. Yokochi F, Nakamura R, Narabayashi H. Reaction time of patients with
Parkinson's disease with reference to asymmetry of neurological signs.
J Neurol Neurosurg Psychiatry 1985; 48:702–705.

40. Pirozzolo FJ, Jankovic J, Mahurin RK. Differentiation of choice reaction
time performance in Parkinson's disease on the basis of motor symptoms.
Neurology 1985; 35(suppl 1):222.

41. Dick PJR, Cantello R, Buruma O, et al. The Bereitschaftspotential, L-dopa
and Parkinson's disease. Electroencephalogr Clin Neurophysiol 1987; 66:263–
274.

42. Ward CD, Sanes JN, Dambrosia JM, Calne DB. Methods for evaluating
treatment in Parkinson's disease. In: Fahn S, CaIne DB, Shoulson I, eds.
Experimental Therapeutics of Movement Disorders. New York: Raven Press,
1983:1–7.

43. Martin WE, Loewenson RB, Resch JA, Baker AB. Parkinson's disease.
Clinical analysis of 100 patients. Neurology 1983; 23:783–790.

44. Jankovic J. Essential tremor: a heterogeneous disorder. Mov Disord 2002 (in
press).

45. Jankovic J, Schwartz, KS, Ondo W. Re-emergent tremor of Parkinson's
disease. J Neurol Neurosurg Psychiatry 1999; 67:646–650.

46. Findley LJ, Gresty MA. Tremor and rhythmical involuntary movements in
Parkinson's disease. In: Findley LJ, Capildeo R, eds. Movement Disorders:
Tremors. New York: Oxford University Press, 1984:295–304.

47. Llinas R, Jahnsen H. Electrophysiology of mammalian thalamic neurons in
vitro. Nature 1982; 297:406–408.

48. Lamarre Y. Animal models of physiological, essential and parkinsonian-like
tremors. In: Findley LJ, Capildeo R, eds. Movement Disorders: Tremor. New
York: Oxford University Press, 1984:183–194.

49. Lee RG, Stein RB. Resetting of tremor by mechanical perturbations: a
comparison of essential tremor and parkinsonian tremor. Ann Neurol 1981;
10:523–531.

50. Kelly PJ, Ahlskog JE, Goerss SJ, et al. Computer-assisted stereotactic
ventralis lateralis thalamatomy with microelectrode recording control in
patients with Parkinson's disease. Mayo Clin Proc 1987; 62:655–664.

51. Findley LJ, Gresty MA, Halmagyi GM. Tremor, the cogwheel phenomenon
and clonus in Parkinson's disease. J Neurol Neurosurg Psychiatry 1981;
44:534–546.

52. Bernheimer H, Birkmayer W, Horrnykiewicz O, Jellinger K, Seitelberger F.
Brain dopamine and the syndromes of Parkinson and Huntington: clinical

morphological and neurochemical correlations. J Neurol Sci 1973; 20:415–455.
53. Pechadre JC, Larochelle I, Poirier LJ. Parkinsonian akinesia, rigidity and tremor in the monkey. Histopathological and neuropharmacological study. J Neurol Sci 1976; 28:147–157.
54. Ballard PA, Tetrud JW, Laneston JW. Permanent human parkinsonism due to 1-methyl-4-phenyl-1,2,3,6-tetrahydropyridine (MPTP): seven cases. Neurology 1985; 35:949–956.
55. Snyder SH, D'Amato RI. MPT: A neurotoxin relevant to the pathophysiology of Parkinson's disease. Neurology 1986; 36:250–258.
56. Holmes G. Clinical symptoms of cerebellar disease and their interpretation. Lancet 1922; 1:1231–1237.
57. Snider SR, Fahn S, Isgreen WP, et al. Primary sensory symptoms in parkinsonism. Neurology 1979; 26:423–429.
58. Koller WC. Sensory symptoms in Parkinson's disease. Neurology 1984; 34:957–959.
59. Matsumoto K, Rossomann F, Lin TH, Cooper IS. Studies on induced exacerbation of parkinsonian rigidity. The effect of contralateral voluntary activity. J Neurol Neurosurg Psychiatry 1963; 26:27–32.
60. Riley D, Lang AE, Blair RDG, et al. Frozen shoulder and other disturbances in Parkinson's disease. J Neurol Neurosurg Psychiatry 1989; 52:63–66.
61. Jankovic J, Tintner R. Dystonia and parkinsonism. Parkinson's Dis Relat Disord 2001; 8:109–121.
62. Askmark H, Edebol Eeg-Olofsson K, Johnsson A, et al. Parkinsonism and neck extensor myopathy. A new syndrome or coincidental findings? Arch Neurol 2001; 58:232–237.
63. Djaldetti R, Mosberg-Galili R, Sroka H, et al. Camptocormia (bent spine) in patients with Parkinson's disease—characterization and possible pathogenesis of an unusual phenomenon. Mov Disord 1999; 14:443–447.
64. Jankovic J, Fahn S. Dystonic disorders. In: Jankovic J, Tolosa E, eds. Parkinson's Disease and Movement Disorders. 4th ed. Philadelphia: Lippincott Williams and Wilkins, 2002.
65. Duvoisin RC, Marsden CD. Note on the scoliosis of parkinsonism. J Neurol Neurosurg Psychiatry 1975; 38:787–793.
66. Grimes JD, Hassan MN, Trent G, Halle D, Armstrong GW. Clinical and radiographic features of scoliosis in Parkinson's disease. Adv Neurol 1987; 45:353–355.
67. Burke D. Pathophysiologic aspects of rigidity and dystonia. In: Benecke R, Conrad B, Marsden CD, eds. Motor Disturbances I. London: Academic Press, 1987:87–100.
68. Mortimer JA, Webster D. Evidence for a quantitative association between EMG stretch responses and parkinsonian rigidity. Brain Res 1979; 162:169–173.
69. Berardelli A, Sabra AF, Hallett M. Physiologic mechanisms of rigidity in Parkinson's disease. J Neurol Neurosurg Psychiatry 1983; 46:45–53.

70. Lee RG, Tatton WG. Motor responses to sudden limb displacements in primates with specific CNS lesions and in human patients with motor system disorders. Can J Neurol Sci 1975; 2:285–293.

71. Rothwell JL, Obeso JA, Traub MM, et al. The behavior of the long-latency stretch reflex n patients with Parkinson's disease. J Neurol Neurosurg Psychiatry 1983; 76:35–44.

72. Meyer M, Adorjani C. Quantification of the effects of muscle relaxant drugs in man by tonic stretch reflex. In: Desmedt JE, ed. Motor Control Mechanisms in Health and Disease. New York: Raven Press, 1983:997–1012.

73. Marsden CD, Schachter M. Assessment of extrapyramidal disorders. Br J Clin Pharmacol 1981; 11:129–151.

74. Teräväinen H, CaIne DB. Quantitative assessment of parkinsonian deficits. In: Rinne UK, Klingler M. Stamm G, eds. Parkinson's Disease. Current Progress, Problems and Management. Amsterdam: Elsevier/North-Holland, 1980:145–164.

75. Purdon-Martin J. The Basal Ganglia and Posture. Philadelphia: JB Lippincott, 1967.

76. Traub MM, Rothwell JC, Marsden CD. Anticipatory postural reflexes in Parkinson's disease and other akinetic-rigid syndromes and in cellular ataxia. Brain 1980; 103:393–412.

77. Aita JF. Why patients with Parkinson's disease fall. JAMA 1982; 247:515–516.

78. Koller WC, Glatt S, Vetere-Overfield B, Hassanein R. Falls in Parkinson's disease. Clin Neuropharmacol 1989; 12:98–105.

79. Weiner WJ, Nora LM, Glantz RH. Elderly inpatients: postural reflex impairment. Neurology 1984; 34:945–947.

80. Jankovic J, Nutt JG, Sudarsky L. Classification, diagnosis and etiology of gait disorders. In: Ruzicka E, Hallett M, Jankovic J, eds. Gait Disorders. Philadelphia: Lippincott Williams & Wilkins, 2001:119–134.

81. Fisher CM. Hydrocephalus as a cause of disturbance of gait in the elderly. Neurology 1982; 32:1358–1363.

82. Knutsson E, Lying-Tunell M. Gait apraxia in manual-pressure hydrocephalus: problems of movement and muscle activation. Neurology 1985; 35:155–160.

83. Sudarsky L, Ronthal M. Gait disorders among elderly patients. A survey study of 50 patients. Arch Neurol 1983; 40:740–743.

84. Koller WC, Wilson RS, Glatt SL, Huckman MS, Fox JR. Senile gait: correlation with computed tomographic scans. Ann Neurol 1983; 13:343–344.

85. FitzGerald PM, Jankovic J. Lower body parkinsonism: evidence for vascular etiology. Mov Disord 1989; 4(3):249–260.

86. Jankovic J, Friedman D, Pirozzolo FJ, McCrary JA. Progressive supranuclear palsy: clinical, neurobehavioral, and neuro-ophthalmic findings. Adv Neurol 1990; 53:293–304.

87. Winikates J, Jankovic J. Clinical correlates of vascular parkinsonism. Arch Neurol 1999; 56:98–102.

88. Giladi N, Kao R, Fahn S. Freezing phenomenon in patients with parkinsonian syndromes. Mov Disord 1997; 12:302–305.
89. Giladi N, McDermott MP, Fahn S, et al. Freezing of gait in PD. Prospective assessment of the DATATOP cohort. Neurology 2001; 56:1712–1721.
90. Dietz MA, Goetz CG, Stebbins GT. Evaluation of a modified inverted walking stick as a treatment for parkinsonian freezing episodes. Mov Dis 1990; 5:243–247.
91. Marchese R, Diverio M, Zucchi F, et al. The role of sensory cues in the rehabilitation of parkinsonian patients: A comparison of two physical therapy protocols. Mov Disord 2001; 15:879–883.
92. Elble RJ, Cousins R, Leffler K, Hughes L. Gait initiation by patients with lower-half parkinsonism. Brain 1996; 119:1705–1716.
93. Critchley M. Speech disorders of parkinsonism: a review. J Neurol Neurosurg Psychiatry 1981; 44:757–758.
94. Hunker CJ, Abbs JH, Barlow SM. The relationship between parkinsonian rigidity and hypokinesia in the orofacial system: a quantitative analysis. Neurology 1982; 32:749–755.
95. Jankovic J. Respiratory dyskinesia in Parkinson's disease. Neurology 1986; 36:303–304.
96. Rice JE, Antic R, Thompson PD. Disordered respiration as a levodopa-induced dyskinesia in Parkinson's disease. Mov Disord 2002; 17:524–527.
97. Jankovic J. Clinical features, differential diagnosis and pathogenesis of blepharospasm and cranial-cervical dystonia. In: Bosniak SL, ed. Blepharospasm. New York: Pergamon Press, 1985:67–82.
98. Leport FE, Duvoisin RC. Apraxia of eyelid opening: an involuntary levator inhibition. Neurology 1985; 35:423–427.
99. Guiloff RJ, George RJ, Marsden CD. Reversible supranuclear ophthalmoplegia associated with parkinsonism. J Neurol Neurosurg Psychiatry 1980; 43:552–554.
100. Zetusky WJ, Jankovic I, Pirozzolo FJ. The heterogeneity of Parkinson's disease: clinical and prognostic implications. Neurology 1985; 35:522–526.
101. Jankovic J, Kapadia AS. Functional decline in Parkinson's disease. Arch Neurol 2001; 58:1611–1615.
102. Hoehn MM, Yahr MD. Parkinsonism: onset, progression and mortality. Neurology 1967; 17:427–442.
103. Fahn S, Elton RL. Members of the UPDRS Development Committee: Unified Parkinson's Disease Rating Scale. In: Fahn S, Marsden CD, Calne DB, Lieberman A, eds. Recent Developments in Parkinson's Disease. Vol. II. Florham Park, NJ: Macmillan Health Care Information, 1987:153–163.
104. Goetz CG, Stebbins GT, Shale HM, et al. Utility of an objective dyskinesia rating scale for Parkinson's disease: inter- and intrarater reliability assessment. Mov Disord 1994; 9:390–394.
105. Goetz CG, Stebbins GT, Chmura TA, et al. Teaching tape for the motor section of the Unified Parkinson's Disease Rating Scale. Mov Disord 1995; 10:263–266.

106. Bennett DA, Shannon KM, Beckett LA, et al. Metric properties of nurses' ratings of parkinsonian signs with a modified Unified Parkinson's Disease Rating Scale. Neurology 1997; 49:1580–1587.
107. Stebbins GT, Goetz CG, Lang AE, Cubo E. Factor analysis of the motor section of the Unified Parkinson's Disease Rating Scale during the off-state. Mov Disord 1999; 14:585–589.
108. Marinus J, Ramaker C, Van Hilten JJ, Stiggelbout AM. Health related quality of life in Parkinson's disease: a systematic review of disease specific instruments. J Neurol Neurosurg Psychiatry 2002; 72:241–248.

APPENDIX: UNITED RATING SCALE FOR PARKINSONISM (103), DEFINITIONS OF 0–4 SCALE

Mentation, Behavior, and Mood

1. Mentation

   0 = None.

   1 = Mild. Consistent forgetfulness with partial recollection of events and no other difficulties.

   2 = Moderate memory loss, with disorientation and moderate difficulty handling complex problems. Mild but definite impairment of function at home with need of occasional prompting.

   3 = Severe memory loss with disorientation as to time and often place. Severe impairment in handling problems.

   4 = Severe memory loss with orientation preserved to person only. Unable to make judgments or solve problems. Requires much help with personal care. Cannot be left alone at all.

2. Thought Disorder (due to dementia or drug intoxication)

   0 = None.

   1 = Vivid dreaming.

   2 = "Benign" hallucinations with insight retained.

   3 = Occasional to frequent hallucinations or delusions, without insight, could interfere with daily activities.

   4 = Persistent hallucinations, delusions, or florid psychosis. Not able to care for self.

3. Depression

   0 = Not present.

   1 = Periods of sadness or guilt greater than normal, never sustained for days or weeks.

2 = Sustained depression (one week or more).

3 = Sustained depression with vegetative symptoms (insomnia, anorexia, weight loss, loss of interest).

4 = Sustained depression with vegetative symptoms and suicidal thoughts or intent.

4. Motivation/Initiative

0 = Normal.

1 = Less assertive than usual; more passive.

2 = Loss of initiative or disinterest in elective (nonroutine) activities.

3 = Loss of initiative or disinterest in day-to-day (routine) activities.

4 = Withdrawn, complete loss of motivation.

Activities of Daily Living

5. Speech

0 = Normal.

1 = Mildly affected. No difficulty being understood.

2 = Moderately affected. Sometimes asked to repeat statements.

3 = Severely affected. Frequently asked to repeat statements.

4 = Unintelligible most of the time.

6. Salivation

0 = Normal.

1 = Slight but definite excess of saliva in mouth; may have nighttime drooling.

2 = Moderately excessive saliva with some drooling.

3 = Marked excess of saliva with some drooling.

4 = Marked drooling, requires constant tissue or handkerchief.

7. Swallowing

0 = Normal.

1 = Rare choking.

2 = Occasional choking.

3 = Requires soft food.

4 = Requires NG tube or gastrotomy feeding.

8. Handwriting

0 = Normal.

1 = Slightly slow or small.

2 = Moderately slow or small; all words are legible.

3 = Severely affected; not all words are legible.

4 = The majority of words are not legible.

9. Cutting Food

0 = Normal.

1 = Somewhat slow and clumsy, but no help needed.

2 = Can cut most food, although clumsy and slow, some help needed.

3 = Food must be cut by someone, but can still feed slowly.

4 = Needs to be fed.

10. Dressing

0 = Normal.

1 = Somewhat slow, but no help needed.

2 = Occasional assistance with buttoning, getting arms in sleeves.

3 = Considerable help required but can do some things alone.

4 = Helpless.

11. Hygiene

0 = Normal.

1 = Somewhat slow, but no help needed.

2 = Needs help to shower or bathe; or very slow in hygienic care.

3 = Requires assistance for washing, brushing teeth, combing hair, going to bathroom.

4 = Foley catheter or other mechanical aids.

12. Turning in Bed

0 = Normal.

1 = Somewhat slow and clumsy, but no help needed.

2 = Can turn alone or adjust sheets, but with great difficulty.

3 = Can initiate, but not turn or adjust sheets alone.

4 = Helpless.

13. Falling

0 = Normal.

1 = Rare falling.

2 = Occasionally falls, less than once per day.

3 = Falls an average of once daily.

4 = Falls more than once daily.

14. Freezing

   0 = None.
   1 = Rare freezing when walking, may have start-hesitation.
   2 = Occasional freezing when walking.
   3 = Frequent freezing. Occasionally falls from freezing.
   4 = Frequent falls from freezing.

15. Walking

   0 = Normal.
   1 = Mild difficulty. May not swing arms or may tend to drag leg.
   2 = Moderate difficulty, but requires little or no assistance.
   3 = Severe disturbance of walking, requiring assistance.
   4 = Cannot walk at all, even with assistance.

16. Tremor

   0 = Absent.
   1 = Slight and infrequently present.
   2 = Moderate; bothersome to patient.
   3 = Severe; interferes with many activities.
   4 = Marked, interferes with most activities.

17. Sensory Symptoms

   0 = None.
   1 = Occasionally has numbness, tingling, or mild aching.
   2 = Frequently, has numbness, tingling or aching, not distressing.
   3 = Frequent painful sensations.
   4 = Excruciating pain.

Motor Examination (single point in time)

18. Speech

   0 = Normal.
   1 = Slight loss of expression, diction, and/or volume.
   2 = Monotone, slurred but understandable; moderately impaired.
   3 = Marked impairment, difficult to understand.
   4 = Unintelligible.

19. Facial Expression

   0 = Normal.
   1 = Minimal hypomimia, could be normal "poker face."

2 = Slight but definitely abnormal diminution of facial expression.

3 = Moderate hypomimia, lips parted some of the time.

4 = Masked or fixed facies with severe or complete loss of facial expression, lips parted 1/4 inch or more.

20. Tremor at Rest

0 = Absent.

1 = Slight and infrequently present.

2 = Mild in amplitude and persistent. Or moderate in amplitude, but only intermittently present.

3 = Moderate in amplitude and present most of the time.

4 = Marked in amplitude and present most of the time.

21. Action Tremor

0 = Absent.

1 = Slight; present with action.

2 = Moderate in amplitude; present with action.

3 = Moderate in amplitude, with posture holdings as well as action.

4 = Marked in amplitude, interferes with feeding.

22. Rigidity (judged on passive movement of major points with patient relaxed in sitting position; cogwheeling to be ignored)

0 = Absent.

1 = Slight or detectable only when activated by mirror or other movements.

2 = Mild to moderate.

3 = Marked, but full range of motion easily achieved.

4 = Severe, range of motion achieved with difficulty.

23. Finger Taps (patient taps thumb with index finger in rapid succession with widest amplitude possible, each hand separately)

0 = Normal.

1 = Mild slowing and/or reduction in amplitude.

2 = Moderately impaired. Definite and early fatiguing. May have occasional arrests in movement.

3 = Severely impaired. Frequent hesitation in initiating movements or arrests in ongoing movement.

4 = Can barely perform the task.

24. Hand Movements (patient opens and closes hands in rapid succession with widest amplitude possible, each hand separately)

   0 = Normal.
   1 = Mild slowing and/or reduction in amplitude.
   2 = Moderately impaired. Definite and early fatiguing. May have occasional arrests in movement.
   3 = Severely impaired. Frequent hesitation in initiating movements or arrests in ongoing movement.
   4 = Can barely perform the task.

25. Hand Pronation-Supination (pronation-supination movements of hands, vertically or horizontally, with as large as amplitude as possible, both hands simultaneously)

   0 = Normal.
   1 = Mild slowing and/or reduction in amplitude.
   2 = Moderately impaired. Definite and early fatiguing. May have occasional arrests in movement.
   3 = Severely impaired. Frequent hesitation in initiating movements or arrests in ongoing movement.
   4 − Can barely perform the task.

26. Leg Agility (patient taps heel on ground in rapid succession, picking up entire leg. Amplitude should be about three inches)

   0 = Normal.
   1 = Mild slowing and/or reduction in amplitude.
   2 = Moderately impaired. Definite and early fatiguing. May have occasional arrests in movement.
   3 = Severely impaired. Frequent hesitation in initiating movements or arrests in ongoing movement.
   4 = Can barely perform the task.

27. Arising from Chair (patient attempts to arise from a straight-back wood or metal chair with arms folded across chest)

   0 = Normal.
   1 = Slow, or may need more than one attempt.
   2 = Pushes self up from arms of seat.
   3 = Tends to fall back and may have to try more than one time, but can get up without help.
   4 = Unable to arise without help.

28. Posture

0 = Normal.
1 = Not quite erect, slightly stooped posture; could be normal for older person.
2 = Moderately stooped posture, definitely abnormal; can be slightly leaning to one side.
3 = Severely stooped posture with kyphosis; can be moderately leaning to one side.
4 = Marked flexion with extreme abnormality of posture.

29. Gait

0 = Normal.
1 = Walks slowly, may shuffle with short steps, but no festination or propulsion.
2 = Walks with difficulty, but requires little or no assistance; may have some festination, short steps, or propulsion.
3 = Severe disturbance of gait, requiring assistance.
4 = Cannot walk at all, even with assistance.

30. Postural Stability (response to sudden posterior displacement produced by pull on shoulders while patient erect with eyes open and feet slightly apart. Patient is prepared)

0 = Normal.
1 = Retropulsion, but recovers unaided.
2 = Absence of postural response, would fall if not caught by examiner.
3 = Very unstable, tends to lose balance spontaneously.
4 = Unable to stand without assistance.

31. Body Bradykinesia (combining slowness, hesitancy, decreased armswing, small amplitude, and poverty of movement in general)

0 = None.
1 = Minimal slowness, giving movement a deliberate character; could be normal for some persons. Possibly reduced amplitude.
2 = Mild degree of slowness, giving and poverty of movement which is definitely abnormal. Alternatively, some reduced amplitude.
3 = Moderate slowness, poverty or small amplitude of movement.
4 = Marked slowness, poverty or small amplitude movement.

Complications of Therapy

Score these items to represent the status of the patient in the week prior to the examination.

Dyskinesias

32. Duration: What proportion of the walking day are dyskinesias present? (Historical information)

    0 = None
    1 = 1–25% of day
    2 = 26–50% of day
    3 = 51–75% of day
    4 = 76–100% of day

33. Disability: How disabling are the dyskinesias? (historical information; may be modified by office examination)

    0 = Not disabling
    1 = Mildly disabling
    2 = Moderately disabling
    3 = Severely disabling
    4 = Completely disabling

34. Pain: How painful are the dyskinesias?

    0 = No painful dyskinesia
    1 = Slight
    2 = Moderate
    3 = Severe
    4 = Marked

35. Presence of Early Morning Dystonia (historical Information)

    0 = No
    1 = Yes

Clinical Fluctuations

36. "Off" Duration: What proportion of the waking day is the patient "off" on average?

    0 = None
    1 = 1–25% of day
    2 = 26–50% of day
    3 = 51–75% of day
    4 = 76–100% of day

37. "Off" Predictable: Are any "off" periods predictable as to timing after a dose of medication?

    0 = No
    1 = Yes

38. "Off" Unpredictable: Are any "off" periods unpredictable as to timing after a dose of medication?

    0 = No
    1 = Yes

39. "Off" Sudden: Do any of the "off" periods come on suddenly, e.g., over a few seconds?

    0 = No
    1 = Yes

Other Complications

40. Anorexia, Nausea, Vomiting: Does the patient have anorexia, nausea, or vomiting?

    0 = No
    1 = Yes

41. Sleep Disturbances: Does the patient have any sleep disturbances, e.g., insomnia or hypersomnolence?

    0 = No
    1 = Yes

42. Symptomatic Orthostasis: Does the patient have symptomatic orthostasis?

    0 = No
    1 = Yes

Modified Hoehn and Yahr Staging

Stage 0 = No signs of disease
Stage I = Unilateral disease
Stage I.5 = Unilateral disease plus axial involvement
Stage II = Bilateral disease, without impairment of balance
Stage II.5 = Mild bilateral disease, with recovery on pull test
Stage III = Mild to moderate bilateral disease; some postural instability; physically independent

Stage IV = Severe disability; still able to walk or stand unassisted
Stage V = Wheel chair bound or bedridden unless aided

Modified Schwab and England Activities of Daily Living Scales

100%—Completely independent. Able to do all chores without slowness, difficulty or impairment. Essentially normal. Unaware of any difficulty.

90%—Completely independent. Able to do all chores with some degree of slowness, difficulty and impairment. Might take twice as long. Beginning to be aware of difficulty.

80%—Completely independent in most chores. Takes twice as long. Conscious of difficulty and slowness.

70%—Not Completely independent. More difficulty some chores. Three to four times as long in some. Must spend a large part of the day with chores.

60%—Some dependency. Can do most chores, but exceeding slowly and with much effort. Errors; some impossible.

50%—More dependent. Help with half, slower, etc. Difficulty with everything.

40%—Very dependent. Can assist with all chores, but few alone.

30%—With effort, now and then does a few chores alone or begins alone. Much help needed.

20%—Nothing alone. Can be a slight help with some chores. Severe invalid.

10%—Totally dependent, helpless. Complete invalid.

0%—Vegetative functions such as swallowing, bladder and bowel functions are not

5

Nonmotor Symptoms of Parkinson's Disease

Richard B. Dewey, Jr.
University of Texas Southwestern Medical School,
Dallas, Texas, U.S.A.

INTRODUCTION

Parkinson's disease is generally thought of first and foremost as a disorder of motor control. The cardinal signs of PD are all motor defects, which generally respond favorably to dopaminergic stimulation. While the most obvious pathological change in PD is degeneration of pigmented neurons in the substantia nigra, many other neuronal pathways not involved in motor function (such as the noradrenergic locus ceruleus, the serotonergic raphe nuclei, and the cholinergic nucleus basalis of Meynert) also degenerate in this disease (1). It is not surprising, therefore, that nonmotor symptoms abound in this patient population (Table 1). In this chapter we will consider the most common and important nonmotor symptoms seen in PD and, where possible, discuss therapeutic options for these problems.

TABLE 1   Nonmotor Symptoms of Parkinson's Disease

Dementia
Depression
Anxiety
Psychosis (medication-induced)
Olfactory dysfunction
Pain and sensory disturbances
Autonomic dysfunction
Seborrhea
Sleep disorders

DEMENTIA

Incidence and Prevalence

Estimates of the incidence and prevalence of dementia in PD vary widely due in part to differing operational definitions of dementia and to varying study designs. Cross-sectional studies of clinic or hospital cohorts (2–4) have generally produced lower estimates (around 15–20%) due possibly to a referral bias in which demented patients are seen less frequently in PD follow-up clinics and instead are either institutionalized, lost to follow-up, or treated in Alzheimer's disease clinics. Community-based prevalence studies (5–7) reveal that the proportion of PD patients with dementia ranges from 30 to 40%. The incidence of dementia in a community-based cohort of PD patients was found to be 95.3 per 1000 person-years, which amounted to a sixfold greater risk of dementia in PD versus normal controls (8). Most studies have shown that older age at onset of PD, longer duration of PD, and greater severity of motor symptoms are positive predictors of the development of dementia.

Pathology

The pathological findings in demented PD patients have been quite varied and inconsistent. This variability is due in part to selection bias (clinically unusual cases are more likely to come to autopsy) and in part to varying histopathological techniques used to study these brains. A consistent feature of the older pathological studies of PD dementia is a significant loss of neurons in the nucleus basalis of Meynert associated with extensive reductions of choline acetyltransferase in cortical regions (9,10). These findings suggest that the dementia of PD is in part related to the same cholinergic defect that is seen in Alzheimer's disease. Further supporting a relationship between the dementia of PD and Alzheimer's pathology are studies showing extensive cortical plaques and tangles in these patients (11,12). However, the plaque and tangle counts did not correlate precisely with the presence or absence of dementia or with the degree of depopulation of the nucleus basalis.

More recent pathological studies have focused on the association of cortical Lewy bodies with dementia in PD. The advent of ubiquitin immunohistochemistry led to the recognition that the number of cortical Lewy bodies correlated positively with the degree of cognitive impairment (13). The discovery of the alpha-synuclein gene mutation in an Italian PD kindred (14) led rapidly to the development of alpha-synuclein immunohistochemistry, which even more reliably identifies both cortical and brainstem Lewy bodies. Recent studies have now shown that cortical Lewy bodies positive for alpha-synuclein are the most sensitive and specific markers for dementia in PD, with amyloid plaques and neurofibrillary tangles being present only inconsistently (15,16). One group has calculated that cortical Lewy bodies (as identified with alpha-synuclein immunostaining) are 91% sensitive and 90% specific for dementia in PD (15).

Apaydin et al. have recently attempted to better characterize the syndrome of PD dementia by reviewing brain autopsy specimens and the clinical histories of patients with PD who later developed dementia (17). They used the Mayo Health Sciences Research Database to identify all patients seen between 1976 and 1997 who had definite PD (defined as two of three cardinal features and a levodopa response) and who later (after at least 4 years from onset of PD) developed dementia. Thirteen such patients had brain autopsy material available; one patient was found to have progressive supranuclear palsy, and the other 12 had findings consistent with diffuse or transitional Lewy body disease. Of great importance, the histories of these patients revealed that while most had a favorable response to levodopa early in the clinical course, the benefit from this drug was later lost as the dementia became severe later in life. The authors have demonstrated that for the most common scenario of PD dementia in which dementia develops late in the clinical course and is associated with a relative diminution of the levodopa response, the pathological substrate is widespread cortical Lewy bodies.

Clinical Presentation

In light of the presence of both Lewy body and Alzheimer pathology in the brains of demented PD patients, some authors have suggested that PD and AD are not really different diseases but merely extremes of a spectrum of neurodegeneration (18). They raised the intriguing possibility that those patients who are classified as having AD with "extrapyramidal signs" may differ from those diagnosed as PD with dementia only in that the former are followed in AD clinics and the latter in PD clinics. Regardless of whether this view is correct, it is clear that the timing of symptom onset and severity of dementia and parkinsonism factor heavily into the clinical diagnosis assigned during life. At the risk of oversimplifying the situation, patients presenting early with dementia who later develop mild to moderate parkinsonism are usually diagnosed with AD (after other identifiable causes of senile dementia are excluded) while the converse presentation (early prominent levodopa-responsive parkinsonism with later onset of dementia) fits with a clinical diagnosis of Parkinson's disease. Diffuse Lewy body disease (DLB) is diagnosed when dementia and parkinsonism develop together with fluctuating cognitive status and formed visual hallucinations (19).

Classically, the dementia of PD has been described as a "subcortical" dementia in which psychomotor retardation, memory abnormalities, cognitive impairment, and mood disturbances are considered cardinal features (20). A number of studies comparing patients with PD dementia to those with AD matched for dementia severity have suggested important differences in the clinical features of the dementia in these two conditions. Litvan et al. found that semantic and episodic memory were impaired in both groups of patients but that these defects were more severe in AD patients (21). They also reported that demented PD patients were more impaired on executive tasks than AD patients. Cummings et al. compared 16 patients with PD dementia to 10 with AD and found that the AD group had much greater language dysfunction (anomia, decreased speech content), whereas the PD-dementia group had more prominent motor speech abnormalities (22). Others have been less impressed with these differences and have suggested that the dementia of PD has substantial "cortical" features in common with AD (23).

A major problem with such comparative studies is the inherent difficulty in matching the groups for dementia severity. If scores on neuropsychometric testing are used to match the groups, then obviously no differences in the test results will be found. Similarly, it is difficult to match the groups on disability because the motor defects seen in PD patients contribute to disability, making it difficult to tease out the contribution of the dementia per se to the overall disability of the patient. In light of the considerable clinical and pathological overlap between PD dementia and AD with extrapyramidal features, the temporal profile of development of dementia with respect to the onset and severity of parkinsonism remains the most useful clinical criterion for distinguishing between these conditions.

Treatment

While there are no published studies evaluating the effects of cholinesterase inhibitors on the dementia of PD, several recent reports have looked at this class of drugs in patients with diffuse Lewy body disease. Since recent pathological studies now suggest that the dementia in PD is due mainly to diffuse cortical Lewy bodies, these studies might be relevant to the treatment of PD dementia.

Samuel et al. looked at 16 patients prospectively identified as having AD ($n = 12$) or DLB ($n = 4$); both groups were given donepezil 5 mg daily and assessed at 6 months with the mini-mental state examination (MMSE) (24). They found that scores on the MMSE improved to a significantly greater degree in the 4 patients with DLB compared to those with typical AD. They also observed among all study patients that those with "extrapyramidal features" experienced improvement in the MMSE compared to those without signs of parkinsonism, in whom the score declined.

McKeith et al. reported the results of a double-blind, placebo-controlled study of 120 patients with DLB treated with rivastigmine up to 12 mg daily or placebo for 20 weeks (25). They found that the percentage of patients with a 30% or greater improvement in the NPI-4 (a subscale of the neuropsychiatric inventory evaluating delusions, hallucinations, apathy, and depression) was 47.5% in the rivastigmine group and 27.9% in the placebo group in the intent-to-treat population, a difference that reached statistical significance at the $p = 0.03$ level. Of even greater interest was the observation that UPDRS motor scores did not change in either group whether randomized to placebo or rivastigmine. These data argue against the conventional wisdom that cholinergic agents might worsen the motor function of PD patients and suggest that this class of drugs should be considered as a therapeutic option for PD dementia. Clear recommendations for such therapy, however, will require prospective, randomized controlled trials in this patient population.

DEPRESSION

Prevalence

As is the case with dementia, prevalence estimates of depression in PD vary considerably. Slaughter et al. performed a review of the literature and determined an overall prevalence of depression (gleaned from analyzing 45 earlier studies) of 31% (26). In those studies in which DSM-III or DSM-III-R criteria for depression were strictly followed, the prevalence was higher at 42.4%. Dysthymic disorder is even more common, prompting some to suggest that this might be an intrinsic property of PD itself (27).

Pathophysiology

The depression of PD is said to occur in a bimodal distribution, with most depressed patients having either early or advanced disease (28). Those with moderate symptoms of PD have less depression. This observation fits the notion that depression in PD is a reactive depression, which develops when patients find out that they have a degenerative brain disease at the time of diagnosis and again late in the course when disease symptoms are worse. A study comparing the frequency of depression in PD and arthritis showed no difference, which also supports this reactive depression model (29). However, other studies have shown a higher incidence of depression compared to other chronic disabling diseases, calling the reactive depression hypothesis into question (30).

The alternative view is that the neurodegenerative process in PD is the proximate cause of depression through depletion of brain monoamines. Support for this view is found in studies showing that depression is more common among those PD patients with a significant decline in cognitive function in a 12-month period (31) and those studies demonstrating loss of dopaminergic neurons in the ventral tegmental area in patients with parkinsonism, dementia, and depression (32). Maricle et al. showed in a double-blind, placebo-controlled study that intravenous infusions of levodopa resulted in improvement in mood and anxiety in fluctuating PD patients, which supports the concept that endogenous dopamine depletion in PD leads to depressed mood (33). Mayeux et al. reported that the major metabolite of serotonin, 5-hydroxyindoleacetic acid (5HIAA), is reduced in the cerebrospinal fluid (CSF) of PD patients with both major depression and dysthymic disorder, which suggests that the serotonin hypothesis of depression might also be relevant to PD depression (34). However, reduced CSF 5HIAA was also seen in some PD patients without depression, indicating that this biochemical change is not sufficient to cause depression but might create a susceptibility to depressive illness.

Clinical Features

Recognizing the clinical features of depression in PD patients is a challenge, mainly because several key features of depression, such as loss of appetite, concentration difficulties, sleep disturbances, and slowness of movement, are features of PD itself (35). A recent study showed that during the course of routine follow-up visits for PD, neurologists with special expertise in movement disorders correctly made the diagnosis of depression in only 35% of patients who were known to have depressed mood, as shown by a Beck Depression Inventory score (BDI) greater than 10 (36). The routine use of validated screening instruments for depression in this population may therefore be indicated to improve diagnosis.

PD related depression presents with dysphoria characterized by the presence of hopelessness, pessimism, and decreased motivation. Negative features such as guilt and feelings of worthlessness are not often seen (29). Several studies have shown that dysphoria increases in association with parkinsonian off states (37,38) and that mood and anxiety improve following dopaminergic stimulation (33,37). In spite of the high prevalence of depression in PD, for unclear reasons suicide is no more common in PD patients than in the general population (39).

Treatment

In light of the high prevalence of depression in PD, it is surprising that few well-designed studies of drug therapy for PD depression have been reported. Klaassen et al. published a meta-analysis of therapy trials for depression in PD in 1995, and they concluded that while several small trials of tricyclic antidepressants were positive, methodological limitations of these studies were such that clear recommendations for treatment could not be made (40). In a small study of bupropion in PD, the drug was found to result in a 30% improvement in parkinsonism, while only 5 of 12 depressed PD patients experienced improvement in mood (41).

There have been no properly controlled studies on the selective serotonin reuptake inhibitors (SSRIs) in the depression of PD. One study of 14 nondepressed PD patients treated with 20 mg daily of fluoxetine showed that scores on the Montgomery-Asburg Depression Rating Scale fell significantly after one month of treatment (42). Sertraline was evaluated in an open-label study of 15 depressed PD patients at a dose of 50 mg per day and was found to produce a significant improvement in the BDI without affecting motor scores (43). While several case reports have suggested a potential for SSRI antidepressants to worsen parkinsonism (44,45), these events are considered to be quite uncommon (46).

When data from controlled clinical trials are lacking, expert opinion may be of some use. Richard and Kurlan surveyed 71 members of the Parkinson Study Group (who together followed over 23,000 patients with PD) regarding antidepressant use in depressed PD patients (47). The results were that SSRIs were selected as first-line agents most frequently, with tricyclics being less popular choices. Those who favored initiation with SSRIs considered these drugs more effective and less likely to produce side effects compared to tricyclic antidepressants.

In cases where depression does not remit following appropriate drug trials, electroconvulsive therapy (ECT) should be considered. ECT has long been considered to be effective in drug-refractory cases of depression, and several reports have found an antidepressant effect in depressed PD patients. Douyon et al. showed benefits for mood after ECT in all 7 patients studied, and in those for whom pre- and post-Hamilton Depression Scale scores were available ($n = 4$), a mean improvement of 50% was seen on this measure (48). Additionally, significant improvement in parkinsonian motor function was seen in 5 of 7 patients after only two treatments. Other reports have appeared confirming this finding but have emphasized a particular sensitivity of these patients to ECT-induced delirium (49,50). Most authors noted that this delirium resolves within 2–3 weeks, though they offered varying explanations for this phenomenon ranging from structural changes in the caudate nucleus (49) to dopaminergic psychosis owing to increased permeability of the blood-brain barrier resulting from ECT (51,52). Those advocating the latter hypothesis reported that post-ECT delirium was largely prevented by reducing the dose of dopaminergic drugs by one third to one half of the typical dosage before starting ECT. In light of the powerful antidepressant effects of ECT together with the beneficial effect on parkinsonian motor function, clinicians should consider this treatment modality if several drug trials for depression prove ineffective or poorly tolerated.

ANXIETY

Prevalence

Anxiety is common in PD, occurring about as frequently as depression. Stein et al. found that 9 of 24 patients (38%) with PD suffered from a significant anxiety disorder and that anxiety did not correlate with the severity of parkinsonism or with antiparkinsonian drug exposure (53). Vazquez et al. observed panic attacks in 30 of 131 (23%) PD patients treated with levodopa and stated that 90% of the time, these attacks occurred in the off phase and were relieved by administration of levodopa (54). A comparison of the frequency of anxiety in PD with that seen in other disabling medical conditions showed that anxiety occurred in 29% of PD patients and in only 5% of disabled osteoarthritis patient controls (55). This finding was interpreted as indicating that the anxiety seen in PD is not merely a reaction to the disability inherent in this condition but is more likely related to the underlying neuropathology of the disease.

Pathophysiology

The causes of the various anxiety disorders associated with PD are unknown. While dopaminergic drug therapy could potentially cause anxiety, the observations that anxiety occurs most commonly in the off state (54) and is reversible following a dose of levodopa (37) argue for the opposite conclusion that the dopaminergic deficiency state of PD is in part responsible for anxiety.

Several lines of research support the view that the intrinsic dopaminergic deficiency in PD may be causally related to anxiety. Cash et al. found that in the brains of nondemented PD patients norepinephrine content in the locus ceruleus (LC) was normal while dopamine levels in this region were reduced by 42% (56). Since it is known that dopaminergic projections inhibit the firing of noradrenergic neurons of the LC, and since excess noradrenergic tone correlates with anxiety, Iruela et al. have postulated that the link between anxiety and PD can be at least partially explained by a mechanism in which degeneration of dopaminergic projections to the LC results in disinhibition of LC neurons, which in turn causes anxiety by excess production of norepinephrine (57). Richard et al. showed in a small pilot study that yohimbine (which activates noradrenergic neurons by blockade of the alpha$_2$-adrenergic autoreceptor) triggered panic attacks in three of five PD patients with a history of anxiety, a frequency similar to that seen in psychiatric patients with panic disorder (58). This observation supports the notion that PD is associated with a state of increased noradrenergic sensitivity that could be related to anxiety.

Another possible contributing cause to anxiety seen in PD is autonomic dysfunction. Berrios et al. compared 32 randomly selected PD patients with 32 age-matched healthy controls and found that the PD group had significantly less beat-to-beat variation in heart rate with respiration, a lower Valsalva ratio, and a larger postural drop in blood pressure than the control group, suggesting the presence of autonomic dysfunction in the PD group (59). They also noted a significant correlation between autonomic complaints and anxiety within the PD group. They concluded that anxiety and depression in some PD patients may represent a "behavioral phenocopy" caused by autonomic failure.

Clinical Features

In their review of anxiety in PD, Richard et al. point out that many different anxiety disorders have been reported in this patient population including generalized anxiety disorder, panic disorder, simple phobia, social phobia, agoraphobia, obsessive-compulsive disorder, and anxiety disorder not otherwise specified (60). No adequate studies exist of sufficiently large populations to establish the relative frequencies of the various anxiety disorders in PD.

Treatment

There have been no randomized controlled clinical trials of pharmacotherapy for the anxiety of PD. Thus, treatment recommendations are based on anecdotal reports and expert opinion. When panic attacks occur coincident with off states, the most rational treatment approach is to modify dopaminergic drugs to reduce the number and duration of off states. This can be accomplished by shortening the interdose interval of levodopa, adding a dopamine agonist, initiating therapy with a COMT inhibitor, or utilizing subcutaneous injections of apomorphine (61).

In those patients with generalized anxiety disorder or panic attacks unrelated to motor fluctuations, benzodiazepines such as alprazolam, lorazepam, or clonazepam are recommended (62). Others have been careful to point out that elderly patients are particularly sensitive to benzodiazepines with regard to sedation and risk of falls and that therefore these agents should be used for short periods only (63). Buspirone at doses of 5–20 mg per day can also be useful (62), but high-dose therapy (100 mg/day) is not recommended due to a worsening of the motor features of PD (64). Patients who do not respond to benzodiazepines may benefit from low-dose tricyclic antidepressant therapy with agents such as nortriptyline, desipramine, and imipramine (62).

Psychological therapies using strategies including cognitive therapy, behavioral training, and relaxation techniques are recommended to help patients cope with stressful elements of the disease (63). One study showed that scores on the Beck Anxiety Inventory diminished significantly following surgery for PD (pallidotomy, thalamotomy, and pallidal deep brain stimulation), indicating that those patients who are candidates for brain surgery on the basis of their motor dysfunction might experience amelioration of their anxiety disorder postoperatively as well (65).

AUTONOMIC DYSFUNCTION

Prevalence

Determining the prevalence of autonomic dysfunction in idiopathic PD is difficult because early in the clinical course, PD can be easily mistaken for multiple systems atrophy (MSA, Shy-Drager syndrome) in which autonomic failure is universal. Generally, as the diseases progress, MSA patients become less and less responsive to levodopa and their autonomic failure becomes increasingly severe. By contrast, PD patients continue to respond favorably to levodopa throughout their lifetime and autonomic failure is relatively less severe when compared to MSA. Magalhaes et al. retrospectively reviewed clinical records for autonomic symptoms of 33 patients with autopsy-proven MSA for comparison with 135 patients with pathologically proven PD (66). They found that clinically significant orthostatic hypotension was present in 30% of patients with PD and 88% of those with MSA. Other autonomic problems were also less common in PD than in MSA, respectively: bladder dysfunction 32% vs. 82%, constipation 36% vs. 57%, stridor or apnea 2% vs. 42%, and dysphagia 7% vs. 30%. From these data, one can observe that clinically important autonomic failure occurs in about a third of patients with PD.

Clinical Features and Pathology

The autonomic problems seen in PD patients cover the entire spectrum of autonomic dysfunction and include orthostatism, constipation, dysphagia, drooling, excessive sweating, heat intolerance, urinary disturbances, and male sexual dysfunction (67). While levodopa is known to produce an acute hypotensive response, autonomic testing performed before and after clinically effective doses of levodopa in patients chronically taking this drug did not reveal differences in orthostatic, Valsalva's, or cold pressor responses (68), which suggests that the underlying neuropathology of PD, not drug treatment, is the major cause of these problems. Wakabayashi and Takahashi in their review of the neuropathology of autonomic dysfunction in PD point out that Lewy bodies and cell loss are seen in the hypothalamus, intermediolateral nucleus of the spinal cord (sympathetic preganglionic neurons), sympathetic ganglia, dorsal motor nucleus of the vagus (parasympathetic preganglionic neurons), and the myenteric and submucosal plexuses of the gastrointestinal tract from the upper esophagus to the rectum (69).

The major clinical challenge is differentiating between PD with autonomic failure and MSA, which is important for counseling the patient regarding prognosis. Generally, late onset of autonomic signs and mild severity favors a diagnosis of PD over MSA. However, in a large clinicopathological study of autonomic failure in parkinsonism, one third of pathologically confirmed cases of MSA were misdiagnosed as having PD during life (66). In this group of MSA patients, the age at onset of the disease was later and autonomic signs were absent at presentation, features that typically favor a diagnosis of PD rather than MSA. Importantly, however, at the time of death the severity of autonomic failure in this group of MSA patients was the same as that in the larger group of MSA patients who were correctly diagnosed during life. This suggests that very severe autonomic failure, even late in the clinical course of parkinsonism, should raise clinical suspicion of MSA.

Treatment

Of the various autonomic features seen in PD, orthostatic hypotension is one of the most disabling. Nevertheless, this problem is frequently treatable. Most authorities recommend physical measures first, such as sleeping with the head of the bed elevated 30 degrees, liberalization of dietary salt, and the use of support hose. In patients with mild symptoms of orthostatism these measures may suffice. For more severe cases, fludrocortisone 0.1 mg daily should be added while monitoring potassium levels and supplementing with potassium when needed. Doses greater than 0.3 mg/day do not offer any additional benefit. When these measures fail, therapy with pressors is indicated. Jankovic et al. found that midodrine (2.5–10 mg) produced a 10 mm or greater increase in standing systolic blood pressure one hour after dosing in 11 of 16 (69%) patients (70). The usual recommended dose of midodrine is 10 mg three times daily. Similar beneficial effects on standing blood pressure have been seen with ergotamine/caffeine in a retrospective study of autonomic failure in parkinsonian patients (71). In that study, this agent resulted in long-term improvement in both standing blood pressure and symptoms of orthostatism in four of eight patients.

Other autonomic problems can be treated as well. One study found that the excessive sweating seen in the face and neck of some PD patients could be corrected by dosing with levodopa (68). Constipation can usually be managed by liberalizing fluid intake and adding fiber to the diet. Nocturia and urinary incontinence often respond to agents such as oxybutynin and tolterodine. Excessive salivation, which is due to swallowing dysfunction, not oversecretion of saliva, may respond to administration of glycopyrrolate.

PAIN

Pain is a common problem in PD, affecting as many as 46% of patients, and can be either primary or secondary to motor dysfunction (72). Severe rigidity or off-period dystonia are common causes of secondary pain, which can often be addressed by optimization of dopaminergic medication. Primary pain is poorly understood but is most commonly seen in the off state. Limb burning sensations, lancinating facial pain, abdominal pain, and generalized pain have all been described (73,74). Primary pain syndromes associated with Parkinson's disease respond poorly to analgesic medications and are best addressed by modifying antiparkinsonian drugs in an effort to reduce or eliminate off time (75). In one case, subcutaneous apomorphine injections were found to be dramatically effective when other dopaminergic agents and a myriad of analgesic drugs failed (73).

OLFACTORY DYSFUNCTION

It has long been recognized that most patients with PD have a diminished sense of smell and that this may be present in very early or undiagnosed patients (76,77). Berendse et al. studied olfactory function in relatives of PD patients and then compared SPECT using a dopamine transporter ligand on 25 hyposmic relatives of PD patients with 23 normosmic relatives used as controls (78). They found a reduction in dopamine transporter binding in 4 of the 25 hyposmic relatives (2 of whom later developed clinical parkinsonism) and in none of the normosmic controls. This study indicated that impaired olfaction can precede the onset of motor symptoms and could conceivably be used to screen patients for presymptomatic PD. The pathological substrate for PD-related anosmia appears to be neuronal loss with Lewy body formation in the anterior olfactory nucleus (79).

REFERENCES

1. Jellinger KA. Pathology of Parkinson's disease. Changes other than the nigrostriatal pathway. Mol Chem Neuropathol 14:153–197, 1991.
2. Friedman A, Barcikowska M. Dementia in Parkinson's disease. Dementia 5:12–16, 1994.
3. Girotti F, Soliveri P, Carella F, Piccolo I, Caffarra P, Musicco M, Caraceni T. Dementia and cognitive impairment in Parkinson's disease. J Neurol Neurosurg Psychiatry 51:1498–1502, 1988.
4. Mayeux R, Stern Y, Rosenstein R, Marder K, Hauser A, Cote L, Fahn S. An estimate of the prevalence of dementia in idiopathic Parkinson's disease. Arch Neurol 45:260–262, 1988.
5. Mayeux R, Denaro J, Hemenegildo N, Marder K, Tang MX, Cote LJ, Stern Y. A population-based investigation of Parkinson's disease with and without dementia. Relationship to age and gender. Arch Neurol 49:492–497, 1992.
6. Marder K, Tang MX, Cote L, Stern Y, Mayeux R. The frequency and associated risk factors for dementia in patients with Parkinson's disease. Arch Neurol 52:695–701, 1995.
7. Aarsland D, Tandberg E, Larsen JP, Cummings JL. Frequency of dementia in Parkinson disease. Arch Neurol 53:538–542, 1996.

8. Aarsland D, Andersen K, Larsen JP, Lolk A, Nielsen H, Kragh-Sorensen P. Risk of dementia in Parkinson's disease: a community-based, prospective study. Neurology 56:730–736, 2001.

9. Perry EK, Curtis M, Dick DJ, Candy JM, Atack JR, Bloxham CA, Blessed G, Fairbairn A, Tomlinson BE, Perry RH. Cholinergic correlates of cognitive impairment in Parkinson's disease: comparisons with Alzheimer's disease. J Neurol Neurosurg Psychiatry 48:413–421, 1985.

10. Whitehouse PJ, Hedreen JC, White CL, 3rd, Price DL. Basal forebrain neurons in the dementia of Parkinson disease. Ann Neurol 13:243–248, 1983.

11. Gaspar P, Gray F. Dementia in idiopathic Parkinson's disease. A neuropathological study of 32 cases. Acta Neuropathol 64:43–52, 1984.

12. Boller F, Mizutani T, Roessmann U, Gambetti P. Parkinson disease, dementia, and Alzheimer disease: clinicopathological correlations. Ann Neurol 7:329–335, 1980.

13. Mattila PM, Roytta M, Torikka H, Dickson DW, Rinne JO. Cortical Lewy bodies and Alzheimer-type changes in patients with Parkinson's disease. Acta Neuropathol (Berl) 95:576–582, 1998.

14. Polymeropoulos MH, Lavedan C, Leroy E, Ide SE, Dehejia A, Dutra A, Pike B, Root H, Rubenstein J, Boyer R, Stenroos ES, Chandrasekharappa S, Athanassiadou A, Papapetropoulos T, Johnson WG, Lazzarini AM, Duvoisin RC, Di Iorio G, Golbe LI, Nussbaum RL. Mutation in the alpha-synuclein gene identified in families with Parkinson's disease. Science 276:2045–2047, 1997.

15. Hurtig HI, Trojanowski JQ, Galvin J, Ewbank D, Schmidt ML, Lee VM, Clark CM, Glosser G, Stern MB, Gollomp SM, Arnold SE. Alpha-synuclein cortical Lewy bodies correlate with dementia in Parkinson's disease. Neurology 54:1916–1921, 2000.

16. Mattila PM, Rinne JO, Helenius H, Dickson DW, Roytta M. Alpha-synuclein-immunoreactive cortical Lewy bodies are associated with cognitive impairment in Parkinson's disease. Acta Neuropathol (Berl) 100:285–290, 2000.

17. Apaydin H, Ahlskog JE, Parisi JE, Boeve BF, Dickson DW. Parkinson disease neuropathology: later-developing dementia and loss of the levodopa response. Arch Neurol 59:102–112, 2002.

18. Perl DP, Olanow CW, Calne D. Alzheimer's disease and Parkinson's disease: distinct entities or extremes of a spectrum of neurodegeneration? Ann Neurol 44 (suppl 1):S19–31, 1998.

19. McKeith IG, Galasko D, Kosaka K, Perry EK, Dickson DW, Hansen LA, Salmon DP, Lowe J, Mirra SS, Byrne EJ, Lennox G, Quinn NP, Edwardson JA, Ince PG, Bergeron C, Burns A, Miller BL, Lovestone S, Collerton D, Jansen EN, Ballard C, de Vos RA, Wilcock GK, Jellinger KA, Perry RH. Consensus guidelines for the clinical and pathologic diagnosis of dementia with Lewy bodies (DLB): report of the consortium on DLB international workshop. Neurology 47:1113–1124, 1996.

20. Cummings JL. The dementias of Parkinson's disease: prevalence, characteristics, neurobiology, and comparison with dementia of the Alzheimer type. Eur Neurol 28 (suppl 1):15–23, 1988.

21. Litvan I, Mohr E, Williams J, Gomez C, Chase TN. Differential memory and executive functions in demented patients with Parkinson's and Alzheimer's disease. J Neurol Neurosurg Psychiatry 54:25–29, 1991.

22. Cummings JL, Darkins A, Mendez M, Hill MA, Benson DF. Alzheimer's disease and Parkinson's disease: comparison of speech and language alterations. Neurology 38.680–684, 1988.

23. Ross HF, Hughes TA, Boyd JL, Biggins CA, Madeley P, Mindham RH, Spokes EG. The evolution and profile of dementia in Parkinson's disease. Adv Neurol 69:343–347, 1996.

24. Samuel W, Caligiuri M, Galasko D, Lacro J, Marini M, McClure FS, Warren K, Jeste DV. Better cognitive and psychopathologic response to donepezil in patients prospectively diagnosed as dementia with Lewy bodies: a preliminary study. Int J Geriatr Psychiatry 15:794–802, 2000.

25. McKeith I, Del Ser T, Spano P, Emre M, Wesnes K, Anand R, Cicin-Sain A, Ferrara R, Spiegel R. Efficacy of rivastigmine in dementia with Lewy bodies: a randomised, double-blind, placebo-controlled international study. Lancet 356:2031–2036, 2000.

26. Slaughter JR, Slaughter KA, Nichols D, Holmes SE, Martens MP. Prevalence, clinical manifestations, etiology, and treatment of depression in Parkinson's disease. J Neuropsychiatry Clin Neurosci 13:187–196, 2001.

27. Yamamoto M. Depression in Parkinson's disease: its prevalence, diagnosis, and neurochemical background. J Neurol 248 (suppl 3):5–11, 2001.

28. Starkstein SE, Preziosi TJ, Bolduc PL, Robinson RG. Depression in Parkinson's disease. J Nerv Ment Dis 178:27–31, 1990.

29. Gotham AM, Brown RG, Marsden CD. Depression in Parkinson's disease: a quantitative and qualitative analysis. J Neurol Neurosurg Psychiatry 49:381–389, 1986.

30. Robins AH. Depression in patients with Parkinsonism. Br J Psychiatry 128:141–145, 1976.

31. Starkstein SE, Mayberg HS, Leiguarda R, Preziosi TJ, Robinson RG. A prospective longitudinal study of depression, cognitive decline, and physical impairments in patients with Parkinson's disease. J Neurol Neurosurg Psychiatry 55:377–382, 1992.

32. Torack RM, Morris JC. The association of ventral tegmental area histopathology with adult dementia. Arch Neurol 45:497–501, 1988.

33. Maricle RA, Nutt JG, Valentine RJ, Carter JH. Dose-response relationship of levodopa with mood and anxiety in fluctuating Parkinson's disease: a double-blind, placebo-controlled study. Neurology 45:1757–1760, 1995.

34. Mayeux R, Stern Y, Cote L, Williams JB. Altered serotonin metabolism in depressed patients with parkinson's disease. Neurology 34:642–646, 1984.

35. Tandberg E, Larsen JP, Aarsland D, Cummings JL. The occurrence of depression in Parkinson's disease. A community-based study. Arch Neurol 53:175–179, 1996.
36. Shulman LM, Taback RL, Rabinstein AA, Weiner WJ. Non-recognition of depression and other non-motor symptoms in Parkinson's disease. Parkinsonism Relat Disord 8:193–197, 2002.
37. Maricle RA, Nutt JG, Carter JH. Mood and anxiety fluctuations in Parkinson's disease associated with levodopa infusion: preliminary findings. Mov Disord 10:329–332, 1995.
38. Brown RG, Marsden CD, Quinn N, Wyke MA. Alterations in cognitive performance and affect-arousal state during fluctuations in motor function in Parkinson's disease. J Neurol Neurosurg Psychiatry 47:454–465, 1984.
39. Stenager EN, Wermuth L, Stenager E, Boldsen J. Suicide in patients with Parkinson's disease. An epidemiological study. Acta Psychiatr Scand 90:70–72, 1994.
40. Klaassen T, Verhey FR, Sneijders GH, Rozendaal N, de Vet HC, van Praag HM. Treatment of depression in Parkinson's disease: a meta-analysis. J Neuropsychiatry Clin Neurosci 7:281–286, 1995.
41. Goetz CG, Tanner CM, Klawans HL. Bupropion in Parkinson's disease. Neurology 34:1092–1094, 1984.
42. Montastruc JL, Fabre N, Blin O, Senard JM, Rascol O, Rascol A. Does fluoxetine aggravate Parkinson's disease? A pilot prospective study. Mov Disord 10:355–357, 1995.
43. Hauser RA, Zesiewicz TA. Sertraline for the treatment of depression in Parkinson's disease. Mov Disord 12:756–759, 1997.
44. Steur EN. Increase of Parkinson disability after fluoxetine medication. Neurology 43:211–213, 1993.
45. Jimenez-Jimenez FJ, Tejeiro J, Martinez-Junquera G, Cabrera-Valdivia F, Alarcon J, Garcia-Albea E. Parkinsonism exacerbated by paroxetine. Neurology 44:2406, 1994.
46. Caley CF, Friedman JH. Does fluoxetine exacerbate Parkinson's disease? J Clin Psychiatry 53:278–282, 1992.
47. Richard IH, Kurlan R. A survey of antidepressant drug use in Parkinson's disease. Parkinson Study Group. Neurology 49:1168–1170, 1997.
48. Douyon R, Serby M, Klutchko B, Rotrosen J. ECT and Parkinson's disease revisited: a "naturalistic" study. Am J Psychiatry 146:1451–1455, 1989.
49. Figiel GS, Hassen MA, Zorumski C, Krishnan KR, Doraiswamy PM, Jarvis MR, Smith DS. ECT-induced delirium in depressed patients with Parkinson's disease. J Neuropsychiatry Clin Neurosci 3:405–411, 1991.
50. Oh JJ, Rummans TA, O'Connor MK, Ahlskog JE. Cognitive impairment after ECT in patients with Parkinson's disease and psychiatric illness. Am J Psychiatry 149:271, 1992.
51. Fink M, Zervas IM. ECT and delirium in Parkinson's disease. J Neuropsychiatry Clin Neurosci 4:231–232, 1992.

52. Faber R. More on ECT and delirium in Parkinson's disease. J Neuropsychiatry Clin Neurosci 4:232, 1992.

53. Stein MB, Heuser IJ, Juncos JL, Uhde TW. Anxiety disorders in patients with Parkinson's disease. Am J Psychiatry 147:217–220, 1990.

54. Vazquez A, Jimenez-Jimenez FJ, Garcia-Ruiz P, Garcia-Urra D. "Panic attacks" in Parkinson's disease. A long-term complication of levodopa therapy. Acta Neurol Scand 87:14–18, 1993.

55. Menza MA, Robertson-Hoffman DE, Bonapace AS. Parkinson's disease and anxiety: comorbidity with depression. Biol Psychiatry 34:465–470, 1993.

56. Cash R, Dennis T, L'Heureux R, Raisman R, Javoy-Agid F, Scatton B. Parkinson's disease and dementia: norepinephrine and dopamine in locus ceruleus. Neurology 37:42–46, 1987.

57. Iruela LM, Ibanez-Rojo V, Palanca I, Caballero L. Anxiety disorders and Parkinson's disease. Am J Psychiatry 149:719–720, 1992.

58. Richard IH, Szegethy E, Lichter D, Schiffer RB, Kurlan R. Parkinson's disease: a preliminary study of yohimbine challenge in patients with anxiety. Clin Neuropharmacol 22:172–175, 1999.

59. Berrios GE, Campbell C, Politynska BE. Autonomic failure, depression and anxiety in Parkinson's disease. Br J Psychiatry 166:789–792, 1995.

60. Richard IH, Schiffer RB, Kurlan R. Anxiety and Parkinson's disease. J Neuropsychiatry Clin Neurosci 8:383–392, 1996.

61. Dewey RB, Jr., Hutton JT, LeWitt PA, Factor SA. A randomized, double-blind, placebo-controlled trial of subcutaneously injected apomorphine for parkinsonian off-state events. Arch Neurol 58:1385–1392, 2001.

62. Lieberman A. Managing the neuropsychiatric symptoms of Parkinson's disease. Neurology 50 (suppl 6):S33–38, 1998.

63. Walsh K, Bennett G. Parkinson's disease and anxiety. Postgrad Med J 77:89–93, 2001.

64. Ludwig CL, Weinberger DR, Bruno G, Gillespie M, Bakker K, LeWitt PA, Chase TN. Buspirone, Parkinson's disease, and the locus ceruleus. Clin Neuropharmacol 9:373–378, 1986.

65. Higginson CI, Fields JA, Troster AI. Which symptoms of anxiety diminish after surgical interventions for Parkinson disease? Neuropsychiatry Neuropsychol Behav Neurol 14:117–121, 2001.

66. Magalhaes M, Wenning GK, Daniel SE, Quinn NP. Autonomic dysfunction in pathologically confirmed multiple system atrophy and idiopathic Parkinson's disease—a retrospective comparison. Acta Neurol Scand 91:98–102, 1995.

67. Appenzeller O, Goss JE. Autonomic deficits in Parkinson's syndrome. Arch Neurol 24:50–57, 1971.

68. Goetz CG, Lutge W, Tanner CM. Autonomic dysfunction in Parkinson's disease. Neurology 36:73–75, 1986.

69. Wakabayashi K, Takahashi H. Neuropathology of autonomic nervous system in Parkinson's disease. Eur Neurol 38 (suppl 2):2–7, 1997.

70. Jankovic J, Gilden JL, Hiner BC, Kaufmann H, Brown DC, Coghlan CH, Rubin M, Fouad-Tarazi FM. Neurogenic orthostatic hypotension: a double-blind, placebo-controlled study with midodrine. Am J Med 95:38–48, 1993.

71. Dewey RB, Jr., Rao SD, Holmburg SL, Victor RG. Ergotamine/caffeine treatment of orthostatic hypotension in parkinsonism with autonomic failure. Eur J Neurol 5:593–599, 1998.

72. Goetz CG, Tanner CM, Levy M, Wilson RS, Garron DC. Pain in Parkinson's disease. Mov Disord 1:45–49, 1986.

73. Factor SA, Brown DL, Molho ES. Subcutaneous apomorphine injections as a treatment for intractable pain in Parkinson's disease. Mov Disord 15:167–169, 2000.

74. Hillen ME, Sage JI. Nonmotor fluctuations in patients with Parkinson's disease. Neurology 47:1180–1183, 1996.

75. Quinn NP, Koller WC, Lang AE, Marsden CD. Painful Parkinson's disease. Lancet 1:1366–1369, 1986.

76. Doty RL, Stern MB, Pfeiffer C, Gollomp SM, Hurtig HI. Bilateral olfactory dysfunction in early stage treated and untreated idiopathic Parkinson's disease. J Neurol Neurosurg Psychiatry 55:138–142, 1992.

77. Hawkes CH, Shephard BC, Daniel SE. Olfactory dysfunction in Parkinson's disease. J Neurol Neurosurg Psychiatry 62:436–446, 1997.

78. Berendse HW, Booij J, Francot CM, Bergmans PL, Hijman R, Stoof JC, Wolters EC. Subclinical dopaminergic dysfunction in asymptomatic Parkinson's disease patients' relatives with a decreased sense of smell. Ann Neurol 50:34–41, 2001.

79. Pearce RK, Hawkes CH, Daniel SE. The anterior olfactory nucleus in Parkinson's disease. Mov Disord 10:283–287, 1995.

6

Neuropsychological Aspects of Parkinson's Disease and Parkinsonian Syndromes

Alexander I. Tröster and Steven Paul Woods
University of Washington School of Medicine, Seattle, Washington, U.S.A.

INTRODUCTION

Consistent with the clinical focus of this volume, this chapter first acquaints the reader with basic distinctions between the clinical "brain-behavior" disciplines, namely neuropsychology, behavioral neurology, and neuropsychiatry. After describing the most common approaches to neuropsychological evaluation and the goals of neuropsychological evaluation in Parkinson's disease (PD), the chapter highlights the cognitive alterations most frequently accompanying PD and those that occur in and differentiate dementias seen in PD from other neurodegenerative conditions. A discussion of the impact of emotional comorbidity on cognition makes clear the importance of treating anxiety, depression, and psychiatric symptoms in optimizing the afflicted person's functioning and quality of life. Both medical and surgical treatments, the latter enjoying a renaissance after a protracted, relative absence from the treatment armamentarium after the introduction of levodopa, have the potential to impact cognition. Only a sparse literature devotes itself to treatment-related neurobehavioral complications and less frequent improvements. The chapter concludes with a brief comparison of the most common cognitive alterations accompanying parkinsonian and related syndromes, such as multiple system atrophy, progressive supranuclear palsy (Steele-Richardson-Olzewski syndrome), and essential tremor. Although the neuropsychological features in parkinsonian syndromes probably lack the specificity and sensitivity to be of differential diagnostic utility, the neurobehavioral differences observed among groups of patients with various disorders can guide diagnostic hypotheses and inform about the plural neurobehavioral roles of the basal ganglia.

Neuropsychology, Behavioral Neurology, and Neuropsychiatry

Sir William Osler first used the term neuropsychology in 1913; however, neuropsychology, at least as a clinical endeavor, did not emerge as a subdiscipline of psychology until the 1940s, largely in response to demands for the assessment and rehabilitation of brain-injured soldiers in World War II (1). Neuropsychology shares with behavioral neurology and neuropsychiatry the goal of relating behavior to underlying brain structure and function, but it differs from its two sister disciplines in several dimensions (2). Neuropsychology's principal clinical method, namely its standardized, quantitative, norm-referenced approach to the evaluation of cognition and behavior, is perhaps the characteristic that most clearly distinguishes it from behavioral neurology and neuropsychiatry.

Common Approaches to Neuropsychological Evaluation

Neuropsychological assessment approaches fall broadly into three categories: (1) the *fixed battery* (or cognitive-metric) approach; (2) the *process* (or hypothesis-testing) approach; and (3) the *flexible battery* approach. These approaches can readily be conceptualized as differing along two dimensions: test selection and administration/interpretation. Test selection may be fixed or flexible; administration and interpretation are characterized, respectively, as standardized and actuarial at one extreme, and as nonstandardized and qualitative at the other extreme. Each approach has strengths and weaknesses (see Table 1).

The *fixed battery* approach falls at the extremes of fixed test selection, standardized administration, and actuarial interpretation. It is best exemplified by the Halstead-Reitan Battery (HRB) (3). The *process*, or hypothesis-testing, approach emphasizes qualitative aspects of neuropsychological functions that are founded in developmental and cognitive psychology. Champions of the process approach, most notably Edith Kaplan, promote "testing the limits" with patients and assessing the component processes of cognition rather than relying exclusively upon

TABLE 1 Advantages and Disadvantages of Three Major Approaches to Neuropsychological Assessment

	Fixed	Flexible	Process
Comprehensiveness	−	+/−	+
Ease of administration	+	−	−
Compatibility with research database	+	−	−
Ease of training technical personnel	+	−	−
Cost	−	+	+/−
Time required	−	+	+/−
Information about cognitive mechanisms underlying impairment	−	+	+
Normative data	+/−	+/−	+/−
Ease of incorporating new technical developments	−	+	+
Information redundancy	+	−	−
Comparability of scores across tests	+/−	+/−	−

+, advantage/strength; −, disadvantage/weakness; +/−, test battery dependent.

summary scores. In other words, the process approach sees as critical "how" a task is solved and how the solution unfolds over time, rather than the achievement score quantifying the quality of the end-product.

Although the fixed battery and process approaches dominated neuropsychology initially, the *flexible battery* has recently emerged as the most commonly used approach to neuropsychological evaluation (4). Flexible batteries benefit from the strengths of the fixed battery and process approaches by striving to quantify the qualitative aspects of cognition and task performance (5). In this way, the flexible battery approach capitalizes on advances in cognitive neuroscience while remaining firmly grounded in psychometric theory. In addition, the flexible battery approach incorporates a standard battery of tests from which the clinician can tailor his or her evaluation to address particular clients needs and explore given domains of function in greater detail as desired. Many clinicians, in the tradition of Benton, will utilize a small fixed battery and then elaborate this battery depending upon the referral question, the patient's ability to cooperate with certain tasks, patient and family concerns, and presenting diagnoses.

The particular components and length of a neuropsychological evaluation will vary across clinical settings, but typically include the following:

- A clinical interview and review of records to ascertain relevant biopsychosocial background information
- Informal observations regarding patient behavior, cognition, and affect
- The administration of psychometric tests to measure intelligence, attention and executive functions, language, learning and memory, visuospatial perception, praxis, motor and sensory-perception, mood state, quality of life, and personality/coping variables (see Table 2 for a sample of tests and the domains of functioning they evaluate)
- An integration of findings and recommendations into oral and/or written feedback that is provided to the patient, family, and healthcare providers

THE ROLE OF NEUROPSYCHOLOGY IN THE MANAGEMENT OF PARKINSON'S DISEASE

Neuropsychology provides an important contribution to the management of patients with PD. A neuropsychological evaluation delineates the nature and extent of cognitive changes, if any, and a profile of relative neuropsychological strengths and weaknesses. Such knowledge is helpful in:

- The determination of the most probable etiology of mild and new-onset cognitive changes
- Development and formulation of strategies or treatments to ameliorate the impact of cognitive deficits on functioning
- Guidance of the patient and family in making and requesting adaptive changes in the patient's home, leisure, and work environments that enhance functioning and minimize handicap
- Decision making about the appropriateness of medical and neurosurgical interventions for a patient;

ASSESSMENT OF COMPETENCE TO CONSENT TO TREATMENT

Financial, Legal, and Placement Planning

Given the noteworthy prevalence of cognitive and behavioral changes in PD, every patient would, in ideal circumstances, receive a baseline evaluation when first diagnosed with PD. Such a baseline neuropsychological evaluation would facilitate the accurate detection and diagnosis of subsequent neurobehavioral changes and permit the evaluation of treatment effects. This, however, occurs rarely and probably reflects cost-effectiveness issues in a managed care environment, and the reluctance of many patients, and some physicians, to contemplate in the early disease stages the threat of

TABLE 2 Commonly Used Neuropsychological Tests by Cognitive Domain Assessed

Cognitive domain	Test
Premorbid Estimates	Barona Demographic Equations; North American Adult Reading Test (NAART); Wechsler Test of Adult Reading (WTAR); Wide Range Achievement Test (WRAT)
Neuropsychological screening	Mattis Dementia Rating Scale (DRS); Repeatable Battery for the Assessment of Neuropsychological Status (RBANS)
Intelligence	Kaufman Brief Intelligence Test (KBIT); Raven's Progressive Matrices; Wechsler Abbreviated Scale of Intelligence (WASI); Wechsler Adult Intelligence Scale (WAIS)
Attention and working memory	Auditory Consonant Trigrams (ACT); Brief Test of Attention (BTA); Continuous Performance Tests (CPT); Digit and Visual Spans; Paced Auditory Serial Addition Test (PASAT); Stroop Test
Executive function	Cognitive Estimation Test (CET); Delis-Kaplan Executive Function Scale (DKEFS); Halstead Category Test; Trailmaking Test (TMT)[a]; Wisconsin Card Sorting Test (WCST)
Memory	Benton Visual Retention Test (BVRT-R); California Verbal Learning Test (CVLT); Rey Auditory Verbal Learning Test (RAVLT); Rey Complex Figure Test (RCFT)[a]; Wechsler Memory Scale (WMS)[a]
Language	Boston Naming Test (BNT); Controlled Oral Word Association Test (COWAT); Sentence Repetition; Token Test; Complex Ideational Material
Visuoperception	Benton Facial Recognition Test; Benton Judgment of Line Orientation (JLO); Hooper Visual Organization Test (VOT)
Motor and sensory perception	Finger Tapping[a]; Grooved Pegboard[a]; Hand Dynamometer[a]; Sensory-Perceptual Examination
Mood state and personality	Beck Anxiety Inventory (BAI); Beck Depression Inventory (BDI); Hamilton Depression Scale (HDS); Minnesota Multiphasic Personality Inventory (MMPI); Profile of Mood States (POMS); State-Trait Anxiety Inventory (STAI)
Quality of life, coping, and stressors	Parkinson's Disease Questionnaire (PDQ); Coping Responses Inventory (CRI); Ways of Coping Questionnaire; Life Stressors and Social Resources Inventory (LISRES)

[a] Test may not be appropriate for patients with marked motor impairment.
Source: Adapted from Ref. 96.

later, possibly significant, cognitive compromise. In the absence of an early baseline evaluation, a neuropsychological evaluation in the context of cognitive morbidity relies on less accurate, probabilistic estimation of premorbid functioning to detect and estimate the extent of impairments.

Accordingly, if a full evaluation is not indicated or cannot be achieved soon after diagnosis, a cognitive screening should be contemplated as an alternative. Such screening can be readily achieved in the neurologist's office using the Mattis Dementia Rating Scale (DRS) (6) or comparable instruments. Likewise, the administration of brief self-report measures of mood state and quality of life [e.g., the Beck Depression (7) and Anxiety Inventories (8) and Parkinson's Disease Questionnaire 8-item short form (9)], are invaluable in screening for mood disturbance and the extent to which treatments impact quality of life. Affective disturbances are crucial to screen for on a regular basis considering the high prevalence of anxiety and depression in patients with PD (10) and the high likelihood of these entities going undiagnosed in routine neurologic practice (11). The optimization of quality of life, from the patient's perspective, facilitates a patient–physician collaboration and treatment adherence.

A more comprehensive neuropsychological evaluation that supplements screening should be strongly considered under the following circumstances:

- If the patient, caregiver, and/or clinician suspect changes in the patient's ability to carry out fundamental and/or instrumental activities of living that are unlikely to be related to motor dysfunction.
- If there is concern regarding a possible evolving dementia related to depression, PD, Alzheimer's disease (AD), or any other medical and/or psychiatric condition.
- If the neurologist suspects that brief cognitive screening tests [e.g., the Mini Mental State Exam (12)] are not sufficiently sensitive to detect possible changes in cognitive functions; indeed, screening measures designed to detect cognitive decline in AD are typically poorly sensitive to mild subcortical dementias as often seen in PD (13).
- If the patient is being considered for surgical treatment of PD. In fact, recently published guidelines emphasize the need for neuropsychological evaluation in this regard (14). Such evaluation facilitates patient selection and provides a baseline against which to evaluate potential post-surgical neurobehavioral changes and their implications.
- If a patient experiences difficulties at work likely unrelated to motor symptoms and signs.

- When issues and questions arise regarding a person's competence to manage financial affairs, prepare an advanced directive or living will, or consent to treatment (15).
- When questions arise about the most appropriate environment for the continued care of the patient.
- When patient and/or family report that the patient experiences emotional changes and/or is withdrawing from social roles, to determine whether this is associated with cognitive changes.
- Once a patient has experienced delirium or hallucinosis, given that such phenomena may be harbingers of dementia (16).

Prior to making a referral for neuropsychological evaluation, it is important to determine whether neuropsychological evaluation is appropriate to address the specific question the clinician or patient might have. Of equal importance is that the referring clinician carefully articulates the referral question, which allows the neuropsychologist to tailor evaluative procedures accordingly, and that the neuropsychologist clearly communicates findings and their possible implications to the referring clinician, patient, and family, while specifically addressing the referral question.

NEUROPSYCHOLOGICAL FINDINGS IN PARKINSON'S DISEASE

James Parkinson (17) contended that patients with shaking palsy did not exhibit significant intellectual changes; however, by the late 1800s, investigators had begun to recognize the presence of cognitive deficits in patients with PD (18). Mild neuropsychological changes are now widely accepted to occur in early PD; such changes are evident in about 20% of persons with PD (19) and most often include deficient information-processing speed, visuospatial abilities, verbal fluency, recall, and frontal/executive functions (20,21). The neuropsychological dysfunction associated with early PD is hypothesized to reflect nigrostriatal dopamine (DA) depletion and the resultant disruption of frontal-subcortical pathways. More pronounced cognitive dysfunction is evident only later in the disease and is probably attributable to neurochemical changes extending beyond the dopaminergic systems (22–24), in addition to structural neuropathology. The dementia (prevalence of about 30%), or perhaps more accurately dementias, observed in PD probably reflect diverse neuropathological entities. At autopsy, dementia in clinically diagnosed PD most often reveals AD or Lewy body dementia (LBD) pathology or some combination of pathologies associated with these two conditions. Consequently, although dementia in PD generally conforms neurobehaviorally to a "subcortical dementia" profile early in its course, the dementia in PD is neuropsychologically heterogeneous across individuals and, almost invariably, later in its course has both cortical and subcortical features. Nonetheless, many cognitive features of early dementia in PD represent an exacerbation of the cognitive changes observable in PD without dementia.

Neuropsychological Dysfunction in Parkinson's Disease Without Dementia

In reviewing the PD literature, Lieberman (25) reported that approximately 19% (range 17–53%) of treated and untreated PD patients without dementia demonstrate cognitive dysfunction. Unfortunately, few of the studies reviewed reported formal criteria for determining what did or did not constitute dementia, thus making it difficult to determine whether patients were in the early stages of dementia. When present in early PD, cognitive dysfunction is typically mild and most commonly involves bradyphrenia (a slowness of thought) and subtle deficits in executive functions, recall, and/or visuoperceptual/spatial functions (26).

Attention and Executive Functions

Attention and executive deficits in PD are most often ascribed to frontal lobe dysfunction secondary to striato-frontal deafferentation and, in particular, pathophysiological alterations in the basal ganglionic-dorsolateral frontal loops (with medial nigral dopamine depletion impacting the caudate and its frontal projections) (27). Performance on simple tasks of attention, for example, forward digit span, is most often preserved in patients with PD (28). On the other hand, deficits on tasks requiring complex attention, planning, reasoning, abstraction, conceptualization, and cognitive flexibility are more readily identified in PD. Deficits are most apparent on tasks that require spontaneous, self-directed information-processing strategy formulation and deployment (29). Executive dysfunction may account for some of the deficits observed on recall, verbal fluency, and visuoperceptual tasks (30), but it is unlikely that executive deficits alone can explain the range of cognitive changes observable in PD (31,32).

Language

Hypophonia and dysarthria sometimes characterize speech in patients with PD. As compared to patients with AD, aphasia and paraphasic errors are rarely observed in PD, though production and comprehension of complex syntax may be reduced on occasion (33–35). Comprehension of written material and writing (limited by motor impairments) are also relatively preserved in PD. More common are deficits on verbal fluency tasks requiring, within time constraints, the oral generation of words belonging to semantic categories or beginning with certain letters of the alphabet (36,37). Verbal fluency decrements are not universally observed in PD but, when present, probably reflect deficient use of word-retrieval strategies such as clustering and/or switching (37), meaning grouping of words by component sound or category, and moving efficiently between sounds and categories.

Learning and Memory

Deficits in memory are not a characteristic of PD. Patients with PD display difficulty retrieving newly learned information from memory stores, as indicated by mild impairments in free recall, but relatively intact recognition and cued recall (38). Patients with PD may also show an increased reliance on serial encoding (recalling words in the order they are presented) and reduced semantic encoding (recalling words according to their semantic category) (39). Although retrieval and semantic encoding deficits are evident in group studies of PD, there is diversity in memory profiles of individual patients with PD (40). Remote memory is generally preserved in early PD (41). Findings regarding performance on measures of nondeclarative memory, which refers to "knowing how" and is a form of remembering that can be expressed only through the performance of task operations, appear to be task-dependent (42). Thus, impairments in the learning of new motor, perceptual, and cognitive skills may or may not be evident (43–46), while priming is typically intact (44,47).

Visuospatial Perception

Visuoperceptual impairments are thought to occur in early PD, even when motoric task demands are minimized (48,49); however, some argue that visuoperceptual impairments are secondary to deficits in set-shifting, spatial memory, bradyphrenia, and dexterity (30,50). Visuospatial impairments do not appear to improve with dopamine replacement and do not reliably vary with motor "on" and "off" periods. Thus, if dopamine impacts visuoperceptual abnormalities in PD, it is probably in conjunction with other neurochemical or pathophysiological processes (51).

Neuropsychological Dysfunction in Parkinson's Disease with Dementia

The annual incidence of clinically diagnosed dementia in PD (PDD) is about 3% for individuals younger than 60 years and 15% or less for those 80 years and older (52,53). Estimates of PDD prevalence vary between 9% and 93%, depending on which diagnostic criteria, ascertainment methods, and sampling methods are implemented (20), but most commonly range from

30 to 50%. Dementia is very rarely present early in the disease course; moreover, dementia that precedes or accompanies the evolution of motor symptoms should raise concern that the dementia might be related to factors other than PD, for example AD, LBD, or depression. Indeed, recent consensus criteria and recommendations (54) propose that the clinical diagnostic term "PD with dementia" be reserved for individuals who have a clinical diagnosis of PD and have had only motor symptoms for at least 12 months (admittedly an arbitrary period) before developing fluctuating cognition and other neuropsychiatric symptoms such as hallucinations. When the neuropsychiatric presentation precedes any extrapyramidal signs, the differential diagnoses include LBD, AD, and vascular dementia. Whether PDD and LBD turn out to be neuropathologically distinct entities remains to be resolved, as does the issue of whether PDD and LBD are neuropsychologically distinct.

Dementia in PD, like other dementias, involves multiple cognitive impairments and a related decline in day-to-day functioning. Cummings's (55) categorization of dementia as "cortical" and "subcortical" on the basis of neurobehavioral features has been criticized on neuroanatomical grounds, but nevertheless remains a useful clinical heuristic. While recent work suggests that the cognitive profile of dementia in PD is likely heterogeneous (perhaps reflecting variability in neuropathological findings) at the group level, the neuropsychological deficits evident in PDD resemble those of the "subcortical" dementias. Perhaps the most striking features of the "subcortical" dementias, including PDD, are bradyphrenia, memory-retrieval deficits, executive dysfunction, diminished spontaneity, and depression. Features of the "cortical" dementias such as AD (e.g., aphasia, agnosia, and apraxia) are typically absent in PDD, often even later in the course of dementia.

Attention and Executive Functions

Performance on more complex attentional tasks—i.e., those that require the self-allocation of attentional resources, divided attention, and selective attention—is impaired in PDD (56,57). As the disease progresses, patients with PDD may show difficulty even on those attentional tasks in which external cues are provided (58).

Executive functions are tied to frontal-striatal-thalamic circuit integrity, especially to the dorsolateral circuit (59). Frontal lobe dysfunction in PDD most likely stems from nigrostriatal dopaminergic deficits (60) resulting in a striato-cortical deafferentation effect, although cholinergic dysfunction secondary to neuronal loss in the septal and basal nuclei likely also plays a role in executive dysfunction (61). Executive deficits are particularly evident on tasks that require patients to develop, deploy, and maintain efficient information-processing strategies. It has been hypothesized that the basal ganglia and frontal-subcortical circuits function as a subcognitive, internal navigational system that limit PDD patients' available options for efficient problem solving (60,62).

Poor performance on tasks that require coordination of complex mental and motor functions (e.g., operation of an automobile) may be conditioned by visuospatial deficits leading to the defective planning and execution of strategies to accomplish a task (e.g., turning a corner while walking or driving) (63).

Language

Verbal fluency findings in PDD are inconsistent. In general, patients with PDD are impaired comparably to patients with AD on lexical and semantic verbal fluency tasks (64), and in some cases verbal fluency deficits may be even more severe in PDD (24). Impairment in visual confrontation naming, most often measured by the Boston Naming Test, is less pronounced in PDD than in AD, if present at all (65).

Memory

Memory deficits are evident in PDD, although the profile of memory impairment in PDD is both qualitatively and quantitatively different than is observed in patients with AD. As in patients with PD, the memory deficit in early PDD is typically characterized by deficits in retrieval, rather than consolidation. That is, patients with early PDD are sufficiently able to retain information over time, but show deficits in retrieving the information from memory in free recall trials, i.e., without the aid of recognition or cueing. As the dementia becomes more severe, patients with PDD display broader memory deficits, including deficient encoding and consolidation that is comparable to patients with AD (16). While remote memory is typically intact early in PDD, deficits in this area become increasingly evident as the dementia progresses (49,66). However, the remote memory impairment is milder in PDD than in AD. Also, in contrast to AD, in which more remote memories are relatively preserved, PDD affects recall of the various decades of a patient's life similarly (67). In contrast to nondemented patients with PD, patients with PDD typically perform poorly on most nondeclarative memory tasks (44).

Visuoperceptual Functions

Impaired visuospatial and visuoconstructive functions have been found consistently in PDD relative to nondemented patients and healthy controls, even when tasks minimize or eliminate motor demands (68–70). Findings from studies comparing the visuoperceptual abilities of PD and AD groups are not conclusive. However, it appears that patients with LBD show more prominent visuoconstructional and visuospatial deficits than do patients with AD (71,72).

Affect and Emotion

In contrast to AD, depression is much more frequent in PDD. In fact, the presence of depression is often considered an important distinguishing feature between subcortical and cortical dementia syndromes.

Depression has been found to exacerbate cognitive dysfunction in PD, an issue discussed in greater detail below. Patients with PDD and LBD, in particular, experience hallucinations more commonly than do patients with AD (73).

Risk Factors for Dementia in Parkinson's Disease

Various demographic and disease variables predict dementia in PD (see Table 3). More recent work suggests that neuropsychological evaluation may also facilitate early identification of PDD. Jacobs et al. (74) and Mahieux et al. (75) noted that poorer performance by patients with PD on verbal fluency, attentional, and visuospatial tasks was associated with subsequent development of dementia. Woods and Tröster (76) found that nondemented PD patients who met criteria for dementia at one-year follow-up evaluation demonstrated poorer baseline performance on measures of word list learning and recognition, complex auditory attention, and executive function relative to PD patients who did not develop a dementia.

IMPACT OF DEPRESSION AND ANXIETY ON COGNITION IN PARKINSON'S DISEASE

Affective disturbances such as anxiety and depression are common in patients with PD. What follows is a review of findings concerning the impact of affective symptoms on neuropsychological functions in PD.

TABLE 3 Risk Factors for Dementia in Parkinson's Disease

Demographic variables	Disease variables	Neurobehavioral variables
Greater age	Later onset	Depression
Lower education	Disease duration	Diminished cognitive test
Lower socioeconomic	Disease severity	performance:
status	Susceptibility to	Executive/attention
Family history of	levodopa-induced	Verbal fluency
Parkinson's dementia	psychosis or confusion	Visuoperceptual
		List learning

Depression

Symptoms of depression are commonly observed in patients with PD. Prevalence rates for depression in PD range from 7 to 90% (although 40% is the most frequently cited estimate). Approximately one half of PD patients become depressed at some point during the disease course (77), with about half of these patients developing minor depression, while the other half develops major depression. Depression is a known risk factor for PD and PD-related dementia (52,78) and has been shown to adversely impact functional ability (79,80) and accelerate the progression of cognitive decline in PD (81,82).

Depression in PD is unique in that, unlike in other neurodegenerative conditions such as AD, it significantly affects cognition (83). Executive functions and memory are foremost among the neuropsychological abilities impaired by depression (84–86). The negative impact of depression on cognition is more readily evident in the latter stages of PD, and depression must be of at least moderate severity before it markedly impacts cognition (87,88).

In light of depression's detrimental effect on cognition, an important clinical question with treatment implications is whether cognitive and/or functional decline in PD is a dementia due to neurodegeneration or due to depression. Little literature addresses the incidence and prevalence of dementia due to depression in PD and whether dementia in patients with comorbid depression improves with treatment and resolution of depressive symptomatology (89). Etiological inferences about an individual PD patient's dementia, when the dementia is accompanied by marked depression, should probably be deferred until such time as the depression has been adequately treated and neuropsychological revaluation has been performed. Recent attention has also been drawn to the need to distinguish depression from apathy in PD (90). Apathy may occur in as many as 45% of patients with PD and, like depression, may be associated with executive deficits (91).

Anxiety

Anxiety disorders are seen in approximately 40% of patients with PD (92). Despite their frequent occurrence and contribution to morbidity and caregiver burden (10), anxiety symptoms in PD have received relatively little attention, perhaps because they overlap with symptoms of depression and medication effects and are thus difficult to measure (93). The relationship between anxiety and cognition in PD has received virtually no attention. Ryder et al. (94) found that self-reported symptoms of anxiety, but not depression, were related to cognitive functioning in a small sample of male patients with PD. Self-reported trait anxiety was negatively related to performance on a neuropsychological screening battery, accounting for approximately 70% of the variance. The authors posit that anxiety may partly explain the association between depression and cognition in PD, although replication of their findings and additional large-scale studies are needed.

EFFECT OF PHARMACOLOGICAL AND SURGICAL TREATMENTS ON COGNITIVE FUNCTIONS IN PARKINSON'S DISEASE

Modern treatment algorithms for patients with PD consist of both pharmacological and surgical intervention strategies (95). Neuropsychological evaluation can facilitate objective measurement of cognitive, neurobehavioral, emotional, and quality-of-life outcomes associated with treatment as well as aid in determinations regarding treatment (96).

Pharmacological Treatments

Anticholinergics and Cholinesterase Inhibitors

Anticholinergic medications used to treat motor symptoms in PD potentially produce adverse effects on memory, executive functions, as well as global cognitive abilities. In placebo-controlled studies, Bedard and colleagues found anticholinergics to induce executive deficits in PD but not in control participants (97,98). Although anticholinergic-induced memory decrements are observable even in patients without preexisting cognitive impairments (99), Saint-Cyr (100) found that confusional states are more likely to be induced by anticholinergics in patients with preexisting cognitive impairment. Thus, anticholinergics should be avoided in elderly patients who are susceptible to developing confusional states (101).

Cholinesterase inhibitors were initially used sparingly and rarely in PDD and LBD. There is increasing recognition that cholinesterase inhibitors such as rivastigmine may improve not only cognition, but also neuropsychiatric symptoms in both conditions, and that these agents are well tolerated by patients with PD (102,103).

Levodopa and Dopamine Agonists

Findings concerning the impact of levodopa on cognitive functions are inconsistent, with studies showing improvement, decrements, and an absence of significant cognitive changes associated with levodopa therapy or its withdrawal (104). Despite these inconsistent findings, evidence is accumulating that levodopa has short-term effects on certain aspects of memory and executive functions, perhaps as mediated by disease stage. For example, Kulisevsky and colleagues (105) reported short-term improvements in learning and memory, visuoperception, and certain executive functions associated with dopamine-replacement therapies but stated that these cognitive improvements were not maintained over time. Relatedly, Owen et al. (106) found that only certain aspects of executive functioning (i.e., planning accuracy) were improved with levodopa therapy early in the disease, whereas other aspects (response latency) remained relatively unaffected. That levodopa affects only certain components of cognitive functions is consistent with the findings of Fournet and colleagues (107), who reported poorer performance only on working memory tasks in patients with PD after withdrawal from levodopa, and of Lange et al. (108), who also found that levodopa withdrawal impacted performance on only a minority of executive function measures. Levodopa's rather selective effects on working memory and certain executive functions may be related to its mediation of dorsolateral frontal cortex blood flow in response to executive task activation (109).

Selegiline

Selegiline, a selective monoamine oxidase-B inhibitor, has been hypothesized to exert a neuroprotective effect in PD by way of reducing physiological stress associated with MAO-B oxidation of dopamine. Along with improvement in motor functions, several small, uncontrolled studies have found selegiline to be associated with improved global cognitive functioning, P300 latencies, and/or memory in patients with PD (110–113). In contrast, selegiline was reported not to significantly impact cognition in a large sample of untreated patients with early PD (114).

Surgical Interventions

Ablative Surgeries

Ablative surgical interventions for treatment of PD involve stereotactic procedures in which lesions are placed in the globus pallidus, thalamus, or subthalamic nucleus to reduce motor symptoms. Cognitive and emotional outcomes after ablative procedures for PD in the 1950s and 1960s are sparsely documented. Wilkinson and Tröster (115) pointed out that outcomes in early and more recent studies are difficult to compare for a variety of reasons. In general, however, modern studies reveal that ablative procedures such as pallidotomy, thalamotomy, and subthalamotomy (especially unilateral) are relatively safe from a cognitive perspective.

With regard to unilateral pallidotomy, declines in verbal fluency performance have been reported in approximately 75% of outcome studies that included a measure of verbal fluency (48,116–118). Postoperative decrements on measures of attention, memory, and executive functions (typically mild and transient) have been reported occasionally, and significant cognitive complications even more rarely (for review, see Refs. 119, 120). Preexisting cognitive impairment, advanced age, and dominant hemisphere surgery have been proposed as increasing the risk for postoperative cognitive decline.

Few formal neuropsychological studies of bilateral pallidotomy have been undertaken, despite the observation that the most frequent adverse events among such patients are declines in speech and cognition (120). Remarkably, despite their small number, these studies yield inconsistent findings. While some suggest that cognitive declines after bilateral pallidotomy may be limited in scope and severity (121,122) or, indeed, that some gains in memory might be observed (123), others report marked morbidity (124,125).

Although early studies examining outcomes after thalamotomy reported decrements in language and memory with regularity (see Ref. 96 for review), modern thalamotomy is associated with minimal risk of cognitive morbidity (126,127). Initial reports of the apparent cognitive safety of subthalamotomy (128,129) remain to be confirmed by larger, controlled studies.

Deep Brain Stimulation

Nonablative surgical procedures for the treatment of PD involve either unilateral or bilateral implantation of high-frequency stimulation electrodes into deep brain nuclei. Studies detailing neuropsychological outcomes after unilateral pallidal (GPi) deep brain stimulation (DBS) have supported the neurobehavioral safety of this technique (see Refs. 96, 130 for reviews), although a few studies have demonstrated minor postoperative declines in verbal fluency (131–133). The majority of studies indicate that even bilateral GPi stimulation is cognitively well tolerated (134–136), although in isolated cases cognitive declines can occur (125,137).

There remain few studies evaluating cognitive outcomes after thalamic DBS, but preliminary findings suggest that this procedure is associated with minimal cognitive morbidity soon after (138,139) and up to one year after surgery (140). Indeed, subtle and limited cognitive improvements might be witnessed after thalamic DBS.

The majority of DBS procedures now target the subthalamic nucleus (STN). Modest decrements in verbal fluency are the most commonly reported adverse cognitive sequelae associated with STN DBS. Findings regarding possible postoperative declines and/or improvements in global cognitive abilities, memory, attention, and executive functions are inconsistent (see Refs. 96, 141 for reviews). When considered in the context of the considerable benefits of surgery on motor functions, mood state, and quality of life (142), the cost of possible minor and/or transient cognitive declines in a minority of well-selected patients seems to be overshadowed by the benefits. Preliminary evidence indicates that elderly patients (>69 years), as well as those patients displaying presurgical cognitive deficits, might be at greater risk for neurobehavioral morbidity after STN DBS.

Transplantation

Fetal mesencephalic tissue transplantation studies have indicated variability in neurocognitive outcomes among individual patients, but given small sample sizes, the source of variability is difficult to identify (see Ref. 96 for review).

NEUROPSYCHOLOGICAL ASPECTS OF PARKINSON-PLUS SYNDROMES AND ESSENTIAL TREMOR

"Parkinson-plus syndromes" traditionally include progressive supranuclear palsy (PSP), multiple system atrophy (MSA), and corticobasal ganglionic degeneration (CBGD). Although sparse, preliminary neuropsychological studies indicate that the cognitive impairment profiles likely differ across the parkinson-plus syndromes (see Ref. 143 for review). A summary of key differences is presented in Table 4.

Progressive Supranuclear Palsy

Prevalence rates of dementia in PSP range between 50 and 80%, although some authors contend that these numbers reflect overdiagnosis due to bradyphrenia, emotional problems, and visual dysfunction that accompany PSP. Cognitive deficits are seen in approximately 50% of patients with PSP (143), with the neuropsychological profile in PSP being typical of diseases with subcortical involvement, including slowed information processing, executive dysfunction, and information-retrieval deficits (144). As compared to patients with PD, cognitive slowing and executive dysfunction in PSP emerge earlier in the disease course, are more severe, and progress more rapidly (145–148), and this differential executive dysfunction may reflect radiographically demonstrated differences in frontal atrophy between the

TABLE 4 Comparison of Neurobehavioral Features of Parkinson's Disease with Dementia (PDD), Lewy Body Dementia (LBD), Corticobasal Ganglionic Degeneration (CBGD), Progressive Supranuclear Palsy (PSP), and Multiple System Atrophy (MSA)

	PDD	LBD	CBGD	PSP	MSA
Attention	-	—	-	-	—
Executive (e.g., problem solving, conceptualization, planning, flexibility)	—	—	-	—	0/-
Language					
Letter fluency	—	—	-	-/—	-
Category Fluency	—	—	-	-	-
Visual confrontation naming	0/-	-/—	0/-	0	0
Memory for new information					
Recall	—	-/—	0/-	0/-	0/-
Recognition	0/-	-	0	0	0
Memory for old information	-	?	?	0	0
Praxis	0/-	0/-	—	0/-	0
Alien-hand sign	0	0	-/—	0	0
Visuoperceptual/ constructional functions	-	—	-	-	-
Depression	—	—	-	0/-	0/-
Apathy	-	-	-	—	—
Fluctuating cognition	0/-	—	0	0	0

0, impairment absent; -, mild to moderate impairment; —, moderate to severe impairment.

two conditions (149). Executive dysfunction in PSP may also differ qualitatively from that in PD (150). Memory and attention are relatively intact in PSP, although retrieval deficits and accelerated rates of forgetting may be present (151,152). The early presence of cognitive impairment distinguishes PSP from MSA (153).

Multiple System Atrophies

The MSA nomenclature includes several different diseases, including olivopontocerebellar atrophy (OPCA), striatonigral degeneration (SND), and Shy-Drager syndrome (SDS). Cognitive deficits are relatively mild in most forms of MSA, and dementia is not a common feature of these conditions (154), except perhaps in OPCA, in which 40–60% of patients may develop dementia, with dementia prevalence greater in familial forms of the disease (155). Mild executive and memory deficits have been reported in MSA (SND and SDS) (156) but are considered to be of similar severity to those observed in nondemented patients with PD (147,157). Patients with MSA may show more pronounced attentional impairments and longer reaction times than patients with PD (157,158).

Corticobasal Ganglionic Degeneration

The prevalence of cognitive impairment and/or dementia in CBGD is not established. Neuropsychological functions appear to be relatively preserved in the early stages of CBGD (at least within an average of 5 years of diagnosis (159), with dementia emerging as a more common feature later in the disease course (160). While the neuropsychological profile of CBGD reveals both cortical and subcortical features (161), it is possible to differentiate CBGD from AD and PSP at the group level (147,162). The neuropsychological profile associated with CBGD is marked by significant executive dysfunction, which is comparable in severity to PSP, but relatively milder than is observed in patients with AD. Also evident in CBGD is asymmetric apraxia (not evident in PSP or AD), alien-hand sign (not reported in PSP or AD), impairment in motor programming and speed (similar to PSP but unlike AD), attentional dysfunction, and deficits in verbal fluency (comparable to AD). Memory impairment in CBGD is characterized by deficient retrieval—a finding comparable to PSP, but qualitatively and quantitatively different from AD, which is more likely to be marked by deficient consolidation and retention of information over time. Recall on remote memory tests is impaired, but unlike in AD, recognition is intact (163).

Essential Tremor

Recent findings raise the possibility that patients with essential tremor (ET) may display deficits in complex attention, verbal fluency, and executive functions, perhaps related to disruption of cerebello-thalamo-cortical circuits (164–167). Although the neuropsychological dysfunctions of ET and PD overlap, those in PD are more widespread.

REFERENCES

1. MD Lezak. Neuropsychological Assessment, 3rd ed. New York: Oxford University Press, 1995.
2. MF Mendez, W VanGorp, JL Cummings. Neuropsychiatry, neuropsychology, and behavioral neurology—a critical comparison. Neuropsychiatry Neuropsychol Behav Neurol 8:297–302, 1995.

3. RM Reitan, D Wolfson. The Halstead-Reitan Neuropsychological Test Battery. Tucson: Neuropsychology Press, 1985.
4. JJ Sweet, PJ Moberg, Y Suchy. Ten-year follow-up survey of clinical neuropsychologists: part I. Practices and beliefs. Clin Neuropsychologist 14:18–37, 2000.
5. AM Poreh. The quantified process approach: an emerging methodology to neuropsychological assessment. Clin Neuropsychologist 14:212–222, 2000.
6. S Mattis. Dementia Rating Scale. Odessa: Psychological Assessment Resources, 1988.
7. AT Beck, RA Steer. Beck Depression Inventory. San Antonio: Psychological Corporation, 1987.
8. AT Beck, RA Steer. Beck Anxiety Inventory. San Antonio: The Psychological Corporation, 1993.
9. C Jenkinson, R Fitzpatrick, V Peto. The Parkinson's Disease Questionnaire: User Manual for the PDQ-39, PDQ-8 and PDQ Summary Index. Oxford: Health Services Research Unit, Department of Public Health, Oxford University, 1998.
10. L Marsh. Anxiety disorders in Parkinson's disease. Int Rev Psychiatry 12:307–318, 2000.
11. LM Shulman, RL Taback, AA Rabinstein, WJ Weiner. Non-recognition of depression and other non-motor symptoms in Parkinson's disease. Park Rel Disord 8:193–197, 2002.
12. MF Folstein, SE Folstein, PR McHugh. "Mini-mental state." A practical method for grading the cognitive state of patients for the clinician. J Psychiatr Res 12:189–198, 1975.
13. IG McKeith, D Burn. Spectrum of Parkinson's disease, Parkinson's dementia, and Lewy body dementia. Neurol Clin 18:865–902, 2000.
14. JM Bronstein, A DeSalles, MR DeLong. Stereotactic pallidotomy in the treatment of Parkinson disease: an expert opinion. Arch Neurol 56:1064–1069, 1999.
15. MP Dymek, P Atchison, L Harrell, DC Marson. Competency to consent to medical treatment in cognitively impaired patients with Parkinson's disease. Neurology 56:17–24, 2001.
16. Y Stern, K Marder, MX Tang, R Mayeux. Antecedent clinical features associated with dementia in Parkinson's disease. Neurology 43:1690–1692, 1993.
17. J Parkinson. An Essay on the Shaking Palsy. London: Sherwood, Neely & Jones, 1817.
18. JM Charcot. Lectures on Diseases of the Nervous System. 1. London: New London Society, 1878.
19. BE Levin, HL Katzen. Early cognitive changes and nondementing behavioral abnormalities in Parkinson's disease. In: WJ Weiner, AE Lang, eds. Advances in Neurology, Vol. 65. Behavioral Neurology of Movement Disorders. New York: Raven Press, 1995, pp 85–95.

20. DM Jacobs, Y Stern, R Mayeux. Dementia in Parkinson's disease, Huntington's disease, and other degenerative conditions. In: MJ Farah, TE Feinberg, eds. Patient-Based Approaches to Cognitive Neuroscience. Cambridge, MA: MIT Press, 2000, pp 375–384.

21. BE Levin, MM Llabre, WJ Weiner. Cognitive impairments associated with early Parkinson's disease. Neurology 39:557–561, 1989.

22. B Dubois, B Pillon. Cognitive and behavioral aspects of movement disorders. In: J Jankovic, E Tolosa, eds. Parkinson's Disease and Movement Disorders, 3rd ed. Baltimore: Williams & Wilkins, 1998, pp 837–858.

23. S McPherson, JL Cummings. Neuropsychological aspects of Parkinson's disease and parkinsonism. In: I Grant, KM Adams, eds. Neuropsychological Assessment of Neuropsychiatric Disorders, 2nd ed. New York: Oxford University Press, 1996, pp 288–311.

24. Y Stern, M Richards, M Sano, R Mayeux. Comparison of cognitive changes in patients with Alzheimer's and Parkinson's disease. Arch Neurol 50:1040–1045, 1993.

25. A Lieberman. Managing the neuropsychiatric symptoms of Parkinson's disease. Neurology 50 (Suppl. 6):533–538, 1998.

26. MW Bondi, AI Tröster. Parkinson's disease: neurobehavioral consequences of basal ganglia dysfunction. In: PD Nussbaum, ed. Handbook of Neuropsychology and Aging. New York: Plenum, 1997, pp 216–245.

27. JL Cummings. Frontal-subcortical circuits and human behavior. Arch Neurol 50:873–880, 1993.

28. AI Tröster, JA Fields, WC Koller. Parkinson's disease and parkinsonism. In: CE Coffey, JL Cummings, eds. Textbook of Geriatric Neuropsychiatry, 2nd ed. Washington, DC: American Psychiatric Press, 2000, pp 559–600.

29. AE Taylor, JA Saint-Cyr. The neuropsychology of Parkinson's disease. Brain Cogn 28:281–296, 1995.

30. MW Bondi, AW Kaszniak, KA Bayles, KT Vance. Contributions of frontal system dysfunction to memory and perceptual abilities in Parkinson's disease. Neuropsychology 7:89–102, 1993.

31. ED Stefanova, VS Kostic, LJ Ziropadja, GG Ocic, M Markovic. Declarative memory in early Parkinson's disease: serial position learning effects. J Clin Exp Neuropsychol 23:581–591, 2001.

32. AI Tröster, JA Fields. Frontal cognitive function and memory in Parkinson's disease: toward a distinction between prospective and declarative memory impairments? Behav Neurol 8:59–74, 1995.

33. M Grossman, S Carvell, MB Stern, S Gollomp, HI Hurtig. Sentence comprehension in Parkinson's disease: the role of attention and memory. Brain Lang 42:347–384, 1992.

34. P Lieberman, J Friedman, LS Feldman. Syntax comprehension deficits in Parkinson's disease. J Nerv Ment Dis 178:360–365, 1990.

35. RL Skeel, B Crosson, SE Nadeau, J Algina, RM Bauer, EB Fennell. Basal ganglia dysfunction, working memory, and sentence comprehension in patients with Parkinson's disease. Neuropsychologia 39:962–971, 2001.

36. FM Lewis, LL Lapointe, BE Murdoch. Language impairment in Parkinson's disease. Aphasiology 12:193–206, 1998.

37. AK Troyer, M Moscovitch, G Winocur, L Leach, M Freedman. Clustering and switching on verbal fluency tests in Alzheimer's and Parkinson's disease. J Int Neuropsychol Soc 4:137–143, 1998.

38. B Pillon, B Deweer, Y Agid, B Dubois. Explicit memory in Alzheimer's, Huntington's, and Parkinson's diseases. Arch Neurol 50:374–379, 1993.

39. EL Buytenhuijs, HJ Berger, KP Van Spaendonck, MW Horstink, GF Borm, AR Cools. Memory and learning strategies in patients with Parkinson's disease. Neuropsychologia 32:335–342, 1994.

40. JV Filoteo, LM Rilling, B Cole, BJ Williams, JD Davis, JW Roberts. Variable memory profiles in Parkinson's disease. J Clin Exp Neuropsychol 19:878–888, 1997.

41. B Leplow, C Dierks, P Herrmann, N Pieper, R Annecke, G Ulm. Remote memory in Parkinson's disease and senile dementia. Neuropsychologia 35:547–557, 1997.

42. M Sarazin, B Deweer, A Merkl, N Von Poser, B Pillon, B Dubois. Procedural learning and striatofrontal dysfunction in Parkinson's disease. Mov Disord 17:265–273, 2002.

43. FR Ferraro, DA Balota, LT Connor. Implicit memory and the formation of new associations in nondemented Parkinson's disease individuals and individuals with senile dementia of the Alzheimer type: a serial reaction time (SRT) investigation. Brain Cogn 21:163–180, 1993.

44. WC Heindel, DP Salmon, CW Shults, PA Walicke, N Butters. Neuropsychological evidence for multiple implicit memory systems: a comparison of Alzheimer's, Huntington's, and Parkinson's disease patients. J Neurosci 9:582–587, 1989.

45. M Huberman, M Moscovitch, M Freedman. Comparison of patients with Alzheimer's and Parkinson's disease on different explicit and implicit tests of memory. Neuropsychiatry Neuropsychol Behav Neurol 7:185–193, 1994.

46. BJ Knowlton, JA Mangels, LR Squire. A neostriatal habit learning system in humans. Science 273:1399–1402, 1996.

47. MW Bondi, AW Kaszniak. Implicit and explicit memory in Alzheimer's disease and Parkinson's disease. J Clin Exp Neuropsychol 13:339–358, 1991.

48. M Alegret, V Pere, C Junqué, F Valldeoriola, E Tolosa. Visuospatial deficits in Parkinson's disease assessed by judgment of line orientation test: error analyses and practice effects. J Clin Exp Neuropsychol 23:592–598, 2001.

49. SJ Huber, EC Shuttleworth, GW Paulson. Dementia in Parkinson's disease. Arch Neurol 43:987–990, 1986.

50. RG Brown, CD Marsden. Visuospatial function in Parkinson's disease. Brain 109:987–1002, 1986.

51. B Pillon, B Dubois, AM Bonnet, M Esteguy, J Guimaraes, JM Vigouret, F Lhermitte, Y Agid. Cognitive slowing in Parkinson's disease fails to respond to levodopa treatment: the 15-objects test. Neurology 39:762–768, 1989.

52. K Marder, MX Tang, L Cote, Y Stern, R Mayeux. The frequency and associated risk factors for dementia in patients with Parkinson's disease. Arch Neurol 52:695–701, 1995.

53. R Mayeux, J Chen, E Mirabello, K Marder, K Bell, G Dooneief, L Cote, Y Stern. An estimate of the incidence of dementia in idiopathic Parkinson's disease. Neurology 40:1513–1517, 1990.

54. IG McKeith, D Galasko, K Kosaka, EK Perry, DW Dickson, LA Hansen, DP Salmon, J Lowe, SS Mirra, FJ Byrne, G Lennox, NP Quinn, JA Edwardson, PG Ince, C Bergeron, A Burns, BL Miller, S Lovestone, D Collerton, EN Jansen, C Ballard, RA de Vos, GK Wilcock, KA Jellinger, RH Perry. Consensus guidelines for the clinical and pathologic diagnosis of dementia with Lewy bodies (DLB): report of the consortium on DLB international workshop. Neurology 47:1113–1124, 1996.

55. JL Cummings. Subcortical dementia. Neuropsychology, neuropsychiatry, and pathophysiology. Br J Psychiatry 149:682–697, 1986.

56. RG Brown, CD Marsden. Internal versus external cues and the control of attention in Parkinson's disease. Brain 111:323–345, 1988.

57. MJ Wright, RJ Burns, GM Geffen, LB Geffen. Covert orientation of visual attention in Parkinson's disease: an impairment in the maintenance of attention. Neuropsychologia 28:151–159, 1990.

58. T Yamada, M Izyuuinn, M Schulzer, K Hirayama. Covert orienting attention in Parkinson's disease. J Neurol Neurosurg Psychiatry 53:593–596, 1990.

59. MS Mega, JL Cummings. Frontal-subcortical circuits and neuropsychiatric disorders. J Neuropsychiatry Clin Neurosci 6:358–370, 1994.

60. AE Taylor, JA Saint-Cyr, AE Lang. Memory and learning in early Parkinson's disease: evidence for a "frontal lobe syndrome." Brain Cogn 13:211–232, 1990.

61. B Dubois, B Pilon, F Lhermitte, Y Agid. Cholinergic deficiency and frontal dysfunction in Parkinson's disease. Ann Neurol 28:117–121, 1990.

62. C Robertson, KA Flowers. Motor set in Parkinson's disease. J Neurol Neurosurg Psychiatry 53:583–592, 1990.

63. CD Marsden. The mysterious motor function of the basal ganglia: the Robert Wartenberg Lecture. Neurology 32:514–539, 1982.

64. AI Tröster, JA Fields, JA Testa, RH Paul, CR Blanco, KA Hames, DP Salmon, WW Beatty. Cortical and subcortical influences on clustering and switching in the performance of verbal fluency tasks. Neuropsychologia 36:295–304, 1998.

65. AI Tröster, JA Fields, AM Paolo, R Pahwa, WC Koller. Visual confrontation naming in Alzheimer's disease and Parkinson's disease with dementia (abstr) Neurology 46 (suppl): A292–293, 1996.

66. M Freedman, P Rivoira, N Butters, DS Sax, RG Feldman. Retrograde amnesia in Parkinson's disease. Can J Neurol Sci 11:297–301, 1984.

67. RH Paul, JR Graber, DC Bowlby, JA Testa, MJ Harnish, WW Beatty. Remote memory in neurodegenerative disease. In: AI Tröster, ed. Memory in

Neurodegenerative Disease: Biological, Cognitive, and Clinical Perspectives. Cambridge: Cambridge University Press, 1998, pp 184–196.

68. M Globus, B Mildworf, E Melamed. Cerebral blood flow and cognitive impairment in Parkinson's disease. Neurology 35:1135–1139, 1985.

69. SJ Huber, DL Freidenberg, EC Shuttleworth, GW Paulson, JA Christy. Neuropsychological impairments associated with severity of Parkinson's disease. J Neuropsychiatry Clin Neurosci 1:154–158, 1989.

70. B Pillon, B Dubois, F Lhermitte, Y Agid. Heterogeneity of cognitive impairment in progressive supranuclear palsy, Parkinson's disease, and Alzheimer's disease. Neurology 36:1179–1185, 1986.

71. KK Gnanalingham, EJ Byrne, A Thornton, MA Sambrook, P Bannister. Motor and cognitive function in Lewy body dementia: comparison with Alzheimer's and Parkinson's diseases. J Neurol Neurosurg Psychiatry 62:243–252, 1997.

72. Z Walker, RL Allen, S Shergill, CL Katona. Neuropsychological performance in Lewy body dementia and Alzheimer's disease. Br J Psychiatry 170:156–158, 1997.

73. LA Klatka, ED Louis, RB Schiffer. Psychiatric features in diffuse Lewy body disease: a clinicopathologic study using Alzheimer's disease and Parkinson's disease comparison groups. Neurology 47:1148–1152, 1996.

74. DM Jacobs, K Marder, LJ Cote, M Sano, Y Stern, R Mayeux. Neuropsychological characteristics of preclinical dementia in Parkinson's disease. Neurology 45:1691–1696, 1995.

75. F Mahieux, G Fenelon, A Flahault, MJ Manifacier, D Michelet, F Boller. Neuropsychological prediction of dementia in Parkinson's disease. J Neurol Neurosurg Psychiatry 64:178–183, 1998.

76. SP Woods, AI Tröster. Prodromal frontal/executive dysfunction predicts incident dementia in Parkinson's disease. J Int Neuropsychol Soc 9:17–24, 2003.

77. G Dooneief, E Mirabello, K Bell, K Marder, Y Stern, R Mayeux. An estimate of the incidence of depression in idiopathic Parkinson's disease. Arch Neurol 49:305–307, 1992.

78. JP Hubble, T Cao, RE Hassanein, JS Neuberger, WC Koller. Risk factors for Parkinson's disease. Neurology 43:1693–1697, 1993.

79. SA Cole, JL Woodard, JL Juncos, JL Kogos, EA Youngstrom, RL Watts. Depression and disability in Parkinson's disease. J Neuropsychiatry Clin Neurosci 8:20–25, 1996.

80. SE Starkstein, HS Mayberg, R Leiguarda, TJ Preziosi, RG Robinson. A prospective longitudinal study of depression, cognitive decline, and physical impairments in patients with Parkinson's disease. J Neurol Neurosurg Psychiatry 55:377–382, 1992.

81. M Sano, Y Stern, J Williams, L Cote, R Rosenstein, R Mayeux. Coexisting dementia and depression in Parkinson's disease. Arch Neurol 46:1284–1286, 1989.

82. SE Starkstein, TJ Preziosi, PL Bolduc, RG Robinson. Depression in Parkinson's disease. J Nerv Ment Dis 178:27–31, 1990.

83. JA Fields, S Norman, KA Straits-Tröster, AI Tröster. The impact of depression on memory in neurodegenerative disease. In: AI Tröster, ed. Memory in Neurodegenerative Disease: Biological, Cognitive, and Clinical Perspectives. New York: Cambridge University Press, 1998, pp 314–337.

84. G Kuzis, L Sabe, C Tiberti, R Leiguarda, SE Starkstein. Cognitive functions in major depression and Parkinson disease. Arch Neurol 54:982–986, 1997.

85. S Norman, AI Tröster, JA Fields, R Brooks. Effects of depression and Parkinson's disease on cognitive functioning. J Neuropsychiatry Clin Neurosci 14:31–36, 2002.

86. AI Tröster, AM Paolo, KE Lyons, SL Glatt, JP Hubble, WC Koller. The influence of depression on cognition in Parkinson's disease: a pattern of impairment distinguishable from Alzheimer's disease. Neurology 45:672–676, 1995.

87. F Boller, P Marcie, S Starkstein, L Traykov. Memory and depression in Parkinson's disease. Eur J Neurol 5:291–295, 1998.

88. SE Starkstein, PV Rabins, ML Berthier, BJ Cohen, MF Folstein, RG Robinson. Dementia of depression among patients with neurological disorders and functional depression. J Neuropsychiatry Clin Neurosci 1:263–268, 1989.

89. T Klaassen, FR Verhey, GH Sneijders, N Rozendaal, HC de Vet, HM van Praag. Treatment of depression in Parkinson's disease: a meta-analysis. J Neuropsychiatry Clin Neurosci 7:281–286, 1995.

90. LM Shulman. Apathy in patients with Parkinson's disease. Int Rev Psychiatry 12:298–306, 2000.

91. V Isella, P Melzi, M Grimaldi, S Iurlaro, R Piolti, C Ferrarese, L Frattola, I Appollonio. Clinical, neuropsychological, and morphometric correlates of apathy in Parkinson's disease. Mov Disord 17:366–371, 2002.

92. IH Richard, RB Schiffer, R Kurlan. Anxiety and Parkinson's disease. J Neuropsychiatry Clin Neurosci 8:383–392, 1996.

93. CI Higginson, JA Fields, WC Koller, AI Tröster. Questionnaire assessment potentially overestimates anxiety in Parkinson's disease. J Clin Psychol Med Set 8:95–99, 2001.

94. KA Ryder, ST Gontkovsky, KL McSwan, JG Scott, KJ Bharucha, WW Beatty. Cognitive function in Parkinson's disease: association with anxiety but not depression. Aging Neuropsychol Cogn 9:77–84, 2002.

95. CW Olanow, RL Watts, WC Koller. An algorithm (decision tree) for the management of Parkinson's disease (2001): treatment guidelines. Neurology 56:S1–S88, 2001.

96. AI Tröster, JA Fields. The role of neuropsychological evaluation in the neurosurgical treatment of movement disorders. In: D Tarsy, JL Vitek, AM Lozano, eds. Surgical Treatment of Parkinson's Disease and Other Movement Disorders. Totowa, NJ: Humana Press, 2003, pp 213–240.

97. MA Bedard, B Pillon, B Dubois, N Duchesne, H Masson, Y Agid. Acute and long-term administration of anticholinergics in Parkinson's disease: specific effects on the subcortico-frontal syndrome. Brain Cogn 40:289–313, 1999.

98. MA Bedard, S Lemay, JF Gagnon, H Masson, F Paquet. Induction of a transient dysexecutive syndrome in Parkinson's disease using a subclinical dose of scopolamine. Behav Neurol 11:187–195, 1998.

99. WC Koller. Disturbance of recent memory function in parkinsonian patients on anticholinergic therapy. Cortex 20:307–311, 1984.

100. JA Saint-Cyr, AE Taylor, AE Lang. Neuropsychological and psychiatric side effects in the treatment of Parkinson's disease. Neurology 43(Suppl. 5):S47–52, 1993.

101. M Pondal, T Del Ser, F Bermejo. Anticholinergic therapy and dementia in patients with Parkinson's disease. J Neurol 243:543–546, 1996.

102. I McKeith, T Del Ser, P Spano, M Emre, K Wesnes, R Anand, A Cicin-Sain, R Ferrara, R Spiegel. Efficacy of rivastigmine in dementia with Lewy bodies: a randomised, double-blind, placebo-controlled international study. Lancet 356:2031–2036, 2000.

103. PJ Reading, AK Luce, IG McKeith. Rivastigmine in the treatment of parkinsonian psychosis and cognitive impairment: preliminary findings from an open trial. Mov Disord 16:1171–1174, 2001.

104. J Kulisevsky. Role of dopamine in learning and memory: implications for the treatment of cognitive dysfunction in patients with Parkinson's disease. Drugs Aging 16:365–379, 2000.

105. J Kulisevsky, C Garcia-Sánchez, ML Berthier, M Barbanoj, B Pascual-Sedano, A Gironell, A Estévez-González. Chronic effects of dopaminergic replacement on cognitive function in Parkinson's disease: a two-year follow-up study of previously untreated patients. Mov Disord 15:613–626, 2000.

106. AM Owen, BJ Sahakian, JR Hodges, BA Summers, CE Polkey, TW Robbins. Dopamine-dependent fronto-striatal planning deficits in early Parkinson's disease. Neuropsychology 9:126–140, 1995.

107. N Fournet, O Moreaud, JL Roulin, B Naegele, J Pellat. Working memory functioning in medicated Parkinson's disease patients and the effect of withdrawal of dopaminergic medication. Neuropsychology 14:247–253, 2000.

108. KW Lange, TW Robbins, CD Marsden, M James, AM Owen, GM Paul. L-Dopa withdrawal in Parkinson's disease selectively impairs cognitive performance in tests sensitive to frontal lobe dysfunction. Psychopharmacology 107:394–404, 1992.

109. R Cools, E Stefanova, RA Barker, TW Robbins, AM Owen. Dopaminergic modulation of high-level cognition in Parkinson's disease: the role of the prefrontal cortex revealed by PET. Brain 125:584–594, 2002.

110. SN Dixit, M Behari, GK Ahuja. Effect of selegiline on cognitive functions in Parkinson's disease. J Assoc Physicians India 47:784–786, 1999.

111. G Finali, M Piccirilli, GL Piccinin. Neuropsychological correlates of L-deprenyl therapy in idiopathic parkinsonism. Prog Neuropsychopharmacol Biol Psychiatry 18:115–128, 1994.

112. MH Hietanen. Selegiline and cognitive function in Parkinson's disease. Acta Neurol Scand 84:407–410, 1991.

113. M Tarczy, I Szirmai. Failure of dopamine metabolism: borderlines of parkinsonism and dementia. Acta Biomed Ateneo Parmense 66:93–97, 1995.

114. K Kieburtz, M McDermott, P Como, J Growdon, J Brady, J Carter, S Huber, B Kanigan, E Landow, A Rudolph. The effect of deprenyl and tocopherol on cognitive performance in early untreated Parkinson's disease. Parkinson Study Group. Neurology 44.1756–1759, 1994.

115. SB Wilkinson, AI Tröster. Surgical interventions in neurodegenerative disease: impact on memory and cognition In: AI Tröster, ed. Memory in Neurodegenerative Disease: Biological, Cognitive, and Clinical Perspectives. Cambridge, UK: Cambridge University Press, 1998, pp 362–376.

116. DA Cahn, EV Sullivan, PK Shear, G Heit, KO Lim, L Marsh, B Lane, P Wasserstein, GD Silverberg. Neuropsychological and motor functioning after unilateral anatomically guided posterior ventral pallidotomy. Preoperative performance and three-month follow-up. Neuropsychiatry Neuropsychol Behav Neurol 11:136–145, 1998.

117. RM de Bie, PR Schuurman, DA Bosch, RJ de Haan, B Schmand, JD Speelman. Outcome of unilateral pallidotomy in advanced Parkinson's disease: cohort study of 32 patients. J Neurol Neurosurg Psychiatry 71:375–382, 2001.

118. J Green, WM McDonald, JL Vitek, M Haber, H Barnhart, RA Bakay, M Evatt, A Freeman, N Wahlay, S Triche, B Sirockman, MR DeLong. Neuropsychological and psychiatric sequelae of pallidotomy for PD: Clinical trial findings. Neurology 58:858–865, 2002.

119. MK York, HS Levin, RG Grossman, WJ Hamilton. Neuropsychological outcome following unilateral pallidotomy. Brain 122:2209–2220, 1999.

120. RM de Bie, RJ de Haan, PR Schuurman, RA Esselink, DA Bosch, JD Speelman. Morbidity and mortality following pallidotomy in Parkinson's disease: a systematic review. Neurology 58:1008–1012, 2002.

121. R Scott, R Gregory, N Hines, C Carroll, N Hyman, V Papanasstasiou, C Leather, J Rowe, P Silbum, T Aziz. Neuropsychological, neurological and functional outcome following pallidotomy for Parkinson's disease. A consecutive series of eight simultaneous bilateral and twelve unilateral procedures. Brain 121:659–675, 1998.

122. RB Scott, J Harrison, C Boulton, J Wilson, R Gregory, S Parkin, PG Bain, C Joint, J Stein, TZ Aziz. Global attentional–executive sequelae following surgical lesions to globus pallidus interna. Brain 125:562–574, 2002.

123. RP Iacono, JD Carlson, S Kuniyoshi, A Mohamed, C Meltzer, S Yamada. Contemporaneous bilateral pallidotomy [electronic manuscript]. Neurosurg Focus 2:Manuscript 5, 1997.

124. J Ghika, F Ghika-Schmid, H Fankhauser, G Assal, F Vingerhoets, A Albanese, J Bogousslavsky, J Favre. Bilateral contemporaneous poster-oventral pallidotomy for the treatment of Parkinson's disease: neuropsycho-

logical and neurological side effects. Report of four cases and review of the literature. J Neurosurg 91:313–321, 1999.

125.   LL Trépanier, R Kumar, AM Lozano, AE Lang, JA Saint-Cyr. Neuropsychological outcome of GPi pallidotomy and GPi or STN deep brain stimulation in Parkinson's disease. Brain Cogn 42:324–347, 2000.

126.   M Fukuda, S Kameyama, M Yoshino, R Tanaka, H Narabayashi. Neuropsychological outcome following pallidotomy and thalamotomy for Parkinson's disease. Stereotact Funct Neurosurg 74:11–20, 2000.

127.   K Hugdahl, K Wester. Neurocognitive correlates of stereotactic thalamotomy and thalamic stimulation in Parkinsonian patients. Brain Cogn 42:231–252, 2000.

128.   L Alvarez, R Macias, J Guridi, G Lopez, E Alvarez, C Maragoto, J Teijeiro, A Torres, N Pavon, MC Rodriguez-Oroz, L Ochoa, H Hetherington, J Juncos, MR DeLong, JA Obeso. Dorsal subthalamotomy for Parkinson's disease. Mov Disord 16:72–78, 2001.

129.   RJ McCarter, NH Walton, AF Rowan, SS Gill, M Palomo. Cognitive functioning after subthalamic nucleotomy for refractory Parkinson's disease. J Neurol Neurosurg Psychiatry 69:60–66, 2000.

130.   JA Fields, AI Tröster. Cognitive outcomes after deep brain stimulation for Parkinson's disease: a review of initial studies and recommendations for future research. Brain Cogn 42:268–293, 2000.

131.   M Merello, MI Nouzeilles, G Kuzis, A Cammarota, L Sabe, O Betti, S Starkstein, R Leiguarda. Unilateral radiofrequency lesion versus electrostimulation of posteroventral pallidum: a prospective randomized comparison. Mov Disord 14:50–56, 1999.

132.   AI Tröster, JA Fields, SB Wilkinson, R Pahwa, E Miyawaki, KE Lyons, WC Koller. Unilateral pallidal stimulation for Parkinson's disease: neurobehavioral functioning before and 3 months after electrode implantation. Neurology 49:1078–1083, 1997.

133.   G Vingerhoets, C van der Linden, E Lannoo, V Vandewalle, J Caemaert, M Wolters, D Van den Abbeele. Cognitive outcome after unilateral pallidal stimulation in Parkinson's disease. J Neurol Neurosurg Psychiatry 66:297–304, 1999.

134.   C Ardouin, B Pillon, E Peiffer, P Bejjani, P Limousin, P Damier, I Arnulf, AL Benabid, Y Agid, P Pollak. Bilateral subthalamic or pallidal stimulation for Parkinson's disease affects neither memory nor executive functions: a consecutive series of 62 patients. Ann Neurol 46:217–223, 1999.

135.   JA Fields, AI Tröster, SB Wilkinson, R Pahwa, WC Koller. Cognitive outcome following staged bilateral pallidal stimulation for the treatment of Parkinson's disease. Clin Neurol Neurosurg 101:182–188, 1999.

136.   B Pillon, C Ardouin, P Damier, P Krack, JL Houeto, H Klinger, AM Bonnet, P Pollak, AL Benabid, Y Agid. Neuropsychological changes between "off" and "on" STN or GPi stimulation in Parkinson's disease. Neurology 55:411–418, 2000.

137. K Dujardin, P Krystkowiak, L Defebvre, S Blond, A Destee. A case of severe dysexecutive syndrome consecutive to chronic bilateral pallidal stimulation. Neuropsychologia 38:1305–1315, 2000.

138. D Caparros-Lefebvre, S Blond, N Pécheux, F Pasquier, H Petit. Evaluation neuropsychologique avant et après stimulation thalamique chez 9 parkinsoniens. Rev Neurol 148:117–122, 1992.

139. AI Tröster, SB Wilkinson, JA Fields, K Miyawaki, WC Koller. Chronic electrical stimulation of the left ventrointermediate (Vim) thalamic nucleus for the treatment of pharmacotherapy-resistant Parkinson's disease: a differential impact on access to semantic and episodic memory? Brain Cogn 38:125–149, 1998.

140. SP Woods, JA Fields, KE Lyons, WC Koller, SB Wilkinson, R Pahwa, AI Tröster. Neuropsychological and quality of life changes following unilateral thalamic deep brain stimulation in Parkinson's disease: a 12-month follow-up. Acta Neurochir 143:1273–1278, 2001.

141. SP Woods, JA Fields, AI Tröster. Neuropsychological sequelae of subthalamic nucleus deep brain stimulation in Parkinson's disease: a critical review. Neuropsychol Rev 12:111–126, 2002.

142. P Martinez-Martin, F Valldeoriola, E Tolosa, M Pilleri, JL Molinuevo, J Rumià, E Ferrer. Bilateral subthalamic nucleus stimulation and quality of life in advanced Parkinson's disease. Mov Disord 17:372–377, 2002.

143. F Stocchi, L Brusa. Cognition and emotion in different stages and subtypes of Parkinson's disease. J Neurol 247(suppl 2):II114–121, 2000.

144. MH Mark. Lumping and splitting the Parkinson plus syndromes: dementia with Lewy bodies, multiple system atrophy, progressive supranuclear palsy, and cortical-basal ganglionic degeneration. Neurol Clin 19:607–627, 2001.

145. B Dubois, B Pillon, F Legault, Y Agid, F Lhermitte. Slowing of cognitive processing in progressive supranuclear palsy. A comparison with Parkinson's disease. Arch Neurol 45:1194–1199, 1988.

146. ER Maher, EM Smith, AJ Lees. Cognitive deficits in the Steele-Richardson-Olszewski syndrome (progressive supranuclear palsy). J Neurol Neurosurg Psychiatry 48:1234–1239, 1985.

147. B Pillon, N Gouider-Khouja, B Deweer, M Vidailhet, C Malapani, B Dubois, Y Agid. Neuropsychological pattern of striatonigral degeneration: comparison with Parkinson's disease and progressive supranuclear palsy. J Neurol Neurosurg Psychiatry 58:174–179, 1995.

148. P Soliveri, D Monza, D Paridi, F Carella, S Genitrini, D Testa, F Girotti. Neuropsychological follow up in patients with Parkinson's disease, striatonigral degeneration-type multisystem atrophy, and progressive supranuclear palsy. J Neurol Neurosurg Psychiatry 69:313–318, 2000.

149. NJ Cordato, C Pantelis, GM Halliday, D Velakoulis, SJ Wood, GW Stuart, J Currie, M Soo, G Olivieri, GA Broe, JG Morris. Frontal atrophy correlates with behavioural changes in progressive supranuclear palsy. Brain 125:789–800, 2002.

150. TW Robbins, M James, AM Owen, KW Lange, AJ Lees, PN Leigh, CD Marsden, NP Quinn, BA Summers. Cognitive deficits in progressive supranuclear palsy, Parkinson's disease, and multiple system atrophy in tests sensitive to frontal lobe dysfunction. J Neurol Neurosurg Psychiatry 57:79–88, 1994.

151. B Dubois, B Deweer, B Pillon. The cognitive syndrome of progressive supranuclear palsy. Adv Neurol 69:399–403, 1996.

152. J Grafman, I Litvan, M Stark. Neuropsychological features of progressive supranuclear palsy. Brain Cogn 28:311–320, 1995.

153. D Testa, D Monza, M Ferrarini, P Soliveri, F Girotti, G Filippini. Comparison of natural histories of progressive supranuclear palsy and multiple system atrophy. Neurol Sci 22:247–251, 2001.

154. N Quinn, G Wenning. Multiple system atrophy. Curr Opin Neurol 8:323–326, 1995.

155. J Berciano. Olivopontocerebellar atrophy. A review of 117 cases. J Neurol Sci 53:253–272, 1982.

156. K Deguchi, H Takeuchi, I Sasaki, M Tsukaguchi, T Touge, M Nishioka. Impaired novelty P3 potentials in multiple system atrophy—correlation with orthostatic hypotension. J Neurol Sci 190:61–67, 2001.

157. G Meco, M Gasparini, F Doricchi. Attentional functions in multiple system atrophy and Parkinson's disease. J Neurol Neurosurg Psychiatry 60:393–398, 1996.

158. Z Pirtosek, M Jahanshahi, G Barrett, AJ Lees. Attention and cognition in bradykinetic-rigid syndromes: an event-related potential study. Ann Neurol 50:567–573, 2001.

159. JO Rinne, MS Lee, PD Thompson, CD Marsden. Corticobasal degeneration. A clinical study of 36 cases. Brain 117:1183–1196, 1994.

160. DA Grimes, AE Lang, CB Bergeron. Dementia as the most common presentation of cortical-basal ganglionic degeneration. Neurology 53:1969–1974, 1999.

161. NP Stover, RL Watts. Corticobasal degeneration. Semin Neurol 21:49–58, 2001.

162. PJ Massman, KT Kreiter, J Jankovic, RS Doody. Neuropsychological functioning in cortical-basal ganglionic degeneration: differentiation from Alzheimer's disease. Neurology 46:720–726, 1996.

163. WW Beatty, JG Scott, DA Wilson, JR Prince, DJ Williamson. Memory deficits in a demented patient with probable corticobasal degeneration. J Geriatr Psychiatry Neurol 8:132–136, 1995.

164. M Gasparini, V Bonifati, E Fabrizio, G Fabbrini, L Brusa, GL Lenzi, G Meco. Frontal lobe dysfunction in essential tremor: a preliminary study. J Neurol 248:399–402, 2001.

165. LH Lacritz, R Dewey, Jr., C Giller, CM Cullum. Cognitive functioning in individuals with "benign" essential tremor. J Int Neuropsychol Soc 8:125–129, 2002.

166. WJ Lombardi, DJ Woolston, JW Roberts, RE Gross. Cognitive deficits in patients with essential tremor. Neurology 57:785–790, 2001.
167. AI Tröster, SP Woods, JA Fields, KE Lyons, R Pahwa, CI Higginson, WC Koller. Neuropsychological deficits in essential tremor: an expression of cerebello-thalamo-cortical pathophysiology? Eur J Neurol 9:143–151, 2002.

7

Management of Neurobehavioral Symptoms in Parkinson's Disease

Jorge L. Juncos and Ray L. Watts
Emory University School of Medicine, Atlanta, Georgia, U.S.A.

INTRODUCTION

Idiopathic Parkinson's disease (PD) is a neurodegenerative disorder that affects over 1 million individuals in the United States and Canada (1). It is considered a movement disorder based on the motor symptoms that herald its onset and dominate its early course. These motor symptoms are typically what bring patients to the doctor and are the target of most modern medical and surgical therapies. According to recent surveys that examined quality of life issues in PD, depression and other psychiatric symptoms have a higher impact on quality of life than the motor symptoms (2,3). Similarly, as the disease advances, it is the psychiatric symptoms, especially drug-induced hallucinations and delusions, that most contribute to the risk of nursing home placement (4).

The symptoms of PD are mediated by the progressive loss of aminergic neurons in the brainstem. These include dopaminergic, serotonergic, and noradrenergic neurons. Parkinsonian motor symptoms are due to the progressive loss of dopaminergic neurons in the substantia nigra that innervate the striatum. Dopamine denervation is by far the most severe, best studied, and most closely associated with the motor symptoms of PD. In contrast, it appears that the less severe serotonergic and noradrenergic denervation may mediate the frequent psychiatric symptoms of PD such as depression and anxiety. Once present, these symptoms may become a source of major disability. Psychotic symptoms may be mediated by the chronic effects of dopaminomimetic therapy superimposed on slowly accumulating cortical Lewy body pathology (5,6).

COGNITIVE IMPAIRMENT

Mild to moderate cognitive dysfunction affects may nondemented patients with PD. Although this dysfunction has been termed bradyphrenia, the cognitive equivalent of bradykinesia, it is now clear that the dysfunction extends beyond a mere slowing of cognition to include aspects of working memory, attention, mental flexibility, visuospatial function, word fluency, and executive functions. The latter include anticipation, planning, initiation, and the monitoring of goal-directed behaviors. The biochemical basis for these deficits is thought to be, at least in part, due to denervation of the dopaminergic and noradrenergic inputs to the frontal lobes. Other factors include basal ganglia dysfunction, which can independently impair selected aspects of attention and mental flexibility.

Iatrogenic factors that can affect cognition in PD include the use of dopaminomimetic therapy to treat motor symptoms. This drug effect is complex and variable, with levodopa being unable to compensate for all the cognitive deficits observed in PD (7). It depends on the duration of illness, the severity of motor signs, the presence of dementia, sleep disturbances, and possibly depression. For instance, in the early stages of PD, levodopa treatment can improve executive functions normally regulated by the prefrontal cortex. However, this improvement is incomplete and task specific. As the disease advances, patients with a stable clinical response to levodopa fail to exhibit a notable improvement in vigilance and executive function, and patients who exhibit motor fluctuations tend to exhibit transient deterioration in these functions (8). Finally, the effect of these drugs in patients with PD and dementia is likely to be more notable and complex.

Other negative iatrogenic influences on cognitive function in PD include the use of drugs like anticholinergics and amantadine, often used to treat tremor and dyskinesias, and psychotropics used to treat sleep disturbances and affective symptoms. These drugs can negatively affect different aspects of memory and attention, particularly in already demented patients. Like these drug effects, many intercurrent medical illnesses and depression can adversely yet reversibly affect cognitive function, thereby making their early recognition and treatment important.

DEMENTIA: THE PD/AD/LBD OVERLAP SYNDROMES

Dementia occurs in approximately 20–30% of PD patients. It represents a major risk factor for the development of many behavioral disturbances, including psychotic symptoms. Dementia appears to be associated with the combined effect of age and the severity of extrapyramidal symptoms (9). Pathologically, up to 40% of autopsy cases with a primary diagnosis of PD have comorbid findings consistent with senile dementia of the Alzheimer's type (SDAT) (10,11). Conversely, up to 30–40% of patients with SDAT have comorbid parkinsonian features and harbor Lewy body pathology that extends beyond the dopamine neurons in the brainstem to involve the frontal cortex, hippocampus, amygdala, and basal forebrain (12). These defects conspire with aminergic deficits to increase disability and the incidence of psychotropic-induced side effects. They also contribute to the progression of parkinsonian motor symptoms by narrowing the therapeutic window of all antiparkinsonian agents.

Lewy body dementia (LBD) is an increasingly recognized syndrome in which dementia is accompanied by spontaneous parkinsonian features, depressive features, and apathy (5,13). Unlike SDAT, this form of dementia exhibits significant fluctuations in arousal ranging from "narcoleptic-like" sleep attacks to delirium in advanced cases. Sleep is often disrupted by sleep fragmentation due to rapid eye movement (REM)–related behavioral disorders. Patients have spontaneous features of PD and are extremely sensitive to drug-induced parkinsonism. Although parkinsonism associated with LBD can be indistinguishable from idiopathic PD, several clinical features tend to help differentiate the two. The course of LBD is more rapid than that of idiopathic PD (5–7 vs. 15–20 years); postural tremor is often more prominent than rest tremor, and the response to levodopa therapy tends to be short-lived. Compared to SDAT patients, LBD patients have spontaneous and drug-induced visual hallucinations early in the course of the illness and frequently exhibit fixed delusions. Although memory is clearly impaired in both conditions, visuospatial and frontal neuropsychological functions are more prominently affected in LBD than in SDAT.

BEHAVIORAL AND PSYCHOLOGICAL SYMPTOMS OF DEMENTIA IN PARKINSONIAN SYNDROMES

Disturbances of behavior, mood, and perception are common in patients with dementia. These so-called behavioral psychological symptoms of dementia (BPSD) are a major source of distress for patients and their caregivers. Clinically they include symptoms prominent in Alzheimer's disease including apathy, depression, delusional jealousy, paranoia, auditory hallucinations, screaming, and agitation (14). Before DSM-IV helped codify these symptoms as a defined clinical entity, they were thought to be secondary to the distress associated with the dementing process (15). The mechanisms mediating this heterogeneous group of symptoms are poorly understood, but in Alzheimer's disease and LBD, they appear to be linked to the accumulating cholinergic pathology (16). Clinical and research assessment methods are now being developed to assess these symptoms (17). The aim is to organize the complex array of symptoms of BPSD into logical and empiric clusters that can help guide research and, ultimately, treatment.

Several such symptom clusters have been identified: apathy, aggression and agitation, depression, psychosis, and possibly dementia-associated delirium. It should be apparent that these symptoms are not limited to demented patients, nor are they necessarily independent of each other. For instance, patients with PD can have drug-induced visual hallucinations without being demented, and patients with depression are often apathetic. BPSD-associated apathy and agitation are discussed in this section. Depression and psychosis are discussed under other psychiatric symptoms below.

It should be noted that most of the information above on BPSD comes from studies of patients with Alzheimer's disease and vascular dementia. Nonetheless, there is ample evidence that these symptoms may be as prominent and disabling in PD with dementia, particularly in LBD (18–20). The major difference between patients with Alzheimer's disease and PD-dementia syndromes is that, in the latter, these symptoms are as likely to be caused by the medications used to treat the motor symptoms as they are by the illness.

Apathy is characterized by lack of interest, diminished motivation, emotional indifference, flat affect, lack of concern, and social inactivity. Apathetic patients exhibit diminished overt behavioral, cognitive, and emotional components of goal-directed behavior, a change not attributable to level of consciousness or acute emotional distress. It is a major source of caregiver distress, as it is perceived as a personality change in the patient resulting in "no longer caring or appreciating the sacrifices being made on his or her behalf." Apathy can be the result of drug therapy (particularly antipsychotics), metabolic illnesses (e.g., hypothyroidism), and environmental factors such as institutionalization. Apathy can be a feature of depression but can be differentiated from it. For instance, most depressed patients exhibit increased emotional distress, whereas the typical apathetic patient exhibits decreased emotional distress and a lack of emotional response to others. Apathy is also a major feature of dementia, particularly in LBD, where it is presumed to be related to the well-established frontal lobe dysfunction. In depressed patients apathy responds to antidepressants, and in demented patients it can respond to acetylcholinesterase inhibitors (21,22).

Agitation and aggression are perhaps the most distressing BPSD symptoms and a critical factor in the decision to institutionalize patients with LBD or PD-SDAT. Clinically the behaviors can take the form of motor restlessness, verbal outbursts, and verbal or physical aggression. These symptoms are often comorbid with psychosis and depression, yet psychosis and depression are surprisingly uncommon predictors of aggressive behaviors (23). Although more prominent in patients with advanced dementia, in patients chronically treated with dopaminomimetic agents, they can appear in the early stages of dementia.

Agitation and aggression require careful interpretation of the semiology and individualized treatment approaches, particularly in patients who can no longer effectively communicate their needs. For instance many patients become agitated because they are in pain that they cannot explain or localize; they may be uncomfortable due to severe constipation or urinary retention, or because they have developed an acute medical illness like a urinary tract infection. Also important are psychosocial factors, which include caregiver exhaustion and stress, or for those in chronic care facilities, possible institutional mistreatment. Management consists of eliminating or treating acute medical conditions and modifying the triggering psychosocial factor whenever possible. Treatment of depression and psychosis as appropriate are also important. These treatments are discussed below.

In patients not responding to these approaches, anticonvulsants are being used with increasing frequency but variable success (24). In a 6-week, placebo-controlled study of divalproex sodium (mean dose 826 ± 126 mg/day titrated over weeks) for agitation in dementia (mostly SDAT), 68% of 56 nursing home patients showed reduced agitation compared to 52% in the placebo group ($p = 0.06$) (25). However, side effects occurred in 68% of the divalproex group compared to 33% of the placebo group. This high rate of side effects is of particular concern given the fact that valproic acid can cause reversible tremor and other parkinsonian features in demented patients without PD (26,27). It remains an open question whether these doses are effective in patients receiving ongoing treatment with dopaminomimetics and how long it can be tolerated. Experience with using alternative anticonvulsants like carbamazepine, lamotrigine, and topiramate in this population is virtually nonexistent.

There is little evidence to support the long-term use of benzodiazepines in the treatment of BPSD-associated agitation. In the acute setting, short-acting benzodiazepines with few active metabolites, like lorazepam, may be helpful in controlling agitated behaviors until more definitive measures can be taken. Because many of the patients with agitation in the setting of PD and LBD are probably already taking an atypical antipsychotic and several antiparkinsonian agents, it is important to anticipate the profound effects on blood pressure and arousal that may result from the combination.

PSYCHIATRIC SYMPTOMS

Depression

Depression affects up to 50% of patients and may be present at any stage of the illness or even precede the onset of motor symptoms (28,29). Although depression correlates poorly with the severity of motor symptoms (30), it is probably the single most important contributor to poor quality of life in PD (2,3). Depression can also have a negative impact on cognition and motor function even in the face of optimally treated motor symptoms (31–34). A common etiology for the subacute (i.e., days to weeks) loss of response to antiparkinsonian drug therapy is the development of depression. Depression in PD may be difficult to recognize because many of its symptoms overlap those of PD. This overlap includes psychomotor retardation, loss of energy, decreased motivation, social withdrawal, poor sleep, and somatic complaints (29). Personality changes in the form of apathy, lack of assertiveness, and indecisiveness are also common, further obscuring the differential. It is important to rule out other medical conditions like hypothyroidism, vitamin deficiencies (e.g., B_{12}), or cerebrovascular disease, which may contribute to negative symptoms and depression. Testosterone deficiency can be associated with otherwise refractory depression, loss of libido, fatigue, and other nonmotor symptoms (35).

Various lines of evidence suggest that depression in PD is an intrinsic part of the illness rather than a reaction to disability. Nonetheless, the psychosocial stressors that result from the illness often trigger or compound already existing depression. Depression in PD seldom reaches suicidal proportions except in cases with preexisting affective illness. On the other hand, even *subclinical or mild depression* can affect quality of life and impair cognition and motor function. There is no consensus on whether treating minor depression is warranted in PD, but if there is any doubt that the symptoms are interfering with quality of life, depression should be treated.

Management of bipolar illness in PD is complicated by the fact that dopamine agonists are capable of triggering a manic episode. These patients are best managed with mood stabilizers, appropriate antidepressants, and occasionally atypical antipsychotics. With these provisions, the judicious use of small doses of dopamine agonists may be possible in some cases. Among the mood stabilizers, lithium carbonate is poorly tolerated, as are large doses of valproic acid due to their potential to aggravate tremor and possibly other parkinsonian symptoms (24,27). Other potential mood stabilizers not formally tested in PD for which there are few data in PD include carbamazepine, lamotrigine, and topiramate.

Anxiety

Generalized anxiety disorders are also associated with PD. As in many other conditions, anxiety can appear in isolation or as an accompaniment to depression in PD (36). Unlike other conditions, in PD, anxiety can be due to an *akathesia equivalent* mediated by "dopamine hunger" (i.e., under-medication of motor symptoms) rather than dopamine blockade. This is compounded by the advent of motor fluctuation, which can precipitate panic attacks during the "off" periods (37,38). During the "off" periods associated anxiety is the most disabling to the patients. Patients describe a feeling of "doom" reminiscent of a drug withdrawal reaction. Anxiety increases as patients become demented, and it can be particularly severe in patients with LBD and delusions.

PSYCHOTIC SYMPTOMS

Hallucination and Delusions

The incidence of psychotic symptoms in PD varies greatly, ranging from 6 to 40%, depending on the age group of the population surveyed and the number of demented patients in the survey (39,40). Leading up to the first psychotic symptom, many patients exhibit behavioral changes, becoming erratic, temperamental, unreasonable, demanding, and seemingly self-centered, with apparent disregard for the needs of others. These personality changes can be multifactorial due to, for instance, emerging depression, conceptual disorganization due to emerging dementia, or mild delusional thinking due to drug-induced psychosis. The relation between the drugs, particularly dopamine agonists, and the psychotic symptoms is complex. In the absence of dementia, this behavior is typically drug-induced and equivalent to the BPSD psychosis mentioned above for demented patients.

Patients with LBD may experience all of the above even before being exposed to dopaminomimetic agents. For patients exhibiting the above mild and insidious nonpsychotic symptoms, the risk and the time course for developing psychotic symptoms remains unclear. When these symptoms are combined with sleep disturbances, the risk is significant.

Early drug-induced psychotic symptoms in PD are typified by formed visual hallucinations (usually people and animals) with retention of insight. The presence of auditory hallucinations suggests coexisting psychotic depression or dementia, or it may be a side effect of anticholinergic medications (41). In many instances, disturbing cognitive and psychiatric symptoms will cease with elimination of anticholinergics and amantadine. Although chronic dopaminomimetic therapy is associated with drug-induced hallucinations and possibly other psychotic symptoms, the mechanisms of this association are unclear. In one study acute elevation of plasma levodopa levels failed to trigger hallucinations in patients with a history of hallucinations, suggesting the effect is not simply a function of plasma levodopa levels or its pharmacokinetics (42). The phenomena of hallucinations depend on the chronic pharmacodynamic changes that take place downstream from the striatal dopamine receptor (43). In a clinicopathological study there was an association between the hallucinatory symptoms in demented PD patients and the presence of Lewy body (and presumably cholinergic) pathology in the amygdala and hippocampus (12). In a cerebral blood flow study, hallucinatory patients exhibited significantly lower blood flow in the left temporal regions than nonhallucinatory patients (44).

In hallucinating patients an attempt should be made to reduce the overall impact of the dopaminomimetic strategy. This is done in a systematic stepwise manner eliminating first the less effective drugs and, as necessary, eliminating longer-acting drugs before shorter-acting drugs before deciding on what to do with levodopa. Until the patient shows signs of improvement, sequentially eliminate selegiline, nocturnal doses of dopamine agonists or controlled release carbidopa-levodopa, reduce day-time doses of dopamine agonists, eliminate catechol-O-methyl transferase inhibitors, and finally reduce the dose of immediate release carbidopa-levodopa. If a significant reduction in antiparkinsonian therapy is required, the resulting aggravation of motor symptoms may be intolerable, requiring the introduction of selective atypical antipsychotics (41).

Delirium

Delirium refers to confusional states characterized by severe and fluctuating disturbances of arousal. In PD they are most often seen in patients with dementia and an intercurrent medical illness. These illnesses can be varied but commonly include infections, dehydration, metabolic disturbances, congestive heart failure, or analgesic use associated with chronic pain (45). Other common etiologies include use of anticholinergics, amantadine, selegiline, and dopamine agonists. Other agents include benzodiazepines, narcotic analgesics, and a host of drugs with anticholinergic side effects ranging from tricyclic antidepressants to bladder antispasmodics. Delirium may be due to underlying dementia. Before making this assumption it is important to first rule out the above medical causes, which are not only common, but equally likely to aggravate dementia-associated delirium and far easier to treat than the dementia itself. The treatment of dementia-induced delirium is far more complicated and may involve the use of dopamine antagonist doses higher than those used to treat hallucinations in PD, the introduction of acetyl-cholinesterase inhibitors, or a combination of both (46).

TREATMENT OF PSYCHIATRIC SYMPTOMS

Depression and Anxiety

Depression can be managed with drugs as well as changes in daily routine. Correcting abnormal sleep patterns, daily exercise, and behavioral approaches are recommended. Patients with depression may respond as well to conventional antidepressants [e.g., tricyclic antidepressants or selective serotonin reuptake inhibitors (SSRIs)]. Short-acting rather than long-acting SSRIs are preferred. Although all SSRIs are probably effective in PD, citalopram (10–30 mg/day), sertraline (50–150 mg/day), and paroxetine (10–30 mg/day) are particularly well tolerated (47). Buproprion (50–200 mg/day) and venlafaxin SR (37.5–150 mg/day) are less sedating. Concerns about the potential for hyperserotonergic reaction (delirium with myoclonus and hyperpyrexia) stemming from the combination of selegiline and SSRIs appear to be exaggerated (48). Finally, electroconvulsive therapy (ECT) is recommended for patients with PD who suffer from refractory or severe psychotic depression and are intolerant of oral antidepressants (49).

Antipsychotic Therapy

Given the pivotal role of dopaminomimetic agents in the genesis of psychotic symptoms in PD, in past years the treatment of motor symptoms was sacrificed in order to improve psychiatric symptoms. As was the case with "drug holidays," cognitive improvement was negated by the resulting worsening in motor symptoms. Since then, "drug holidays" have been largely abandoned due to their associated morbidity (50).

Conventional antipsychotics are poorly tolerated due to their associated tendency to aggravate parkinsonian symptoms in the elderly due to D_2 dopamine receptor blockade (51). The newer, selective, atypical antipsychotics have a lower incidence of extrapyramidal symptoms (e.g., parkinsonism) compared to conventional antipsychotics (52). This low tendency to generate extrapyramidal symptoms has been attributed to the high in vitro affinity for serotonin (5HT2a) receptors and the relatively low affinity for dopamine D_2 receptors of these compounds compared to typical antipsychotics. Not all atypical antipsychotics behave the same way. Using positron emission tomography, radioligand displacement studies have shown that the atypical antipsychotics clozapine and quetiapine tend to dissociate from striatal D_2 receptors faster (in less than 2 hours) than other atypicals (i.e., risperidone and olanzapine) and typical antipsychotics (53–55). This fast dissociation appears not to compromise the antipsychotic effect of these agents while reducing the risk of extrapyramidal symptoms. In other words, high affinity for and extended association with D_2 dopamine receptors is a better predictor of drug-induced parkinsonism than of antipsychotic response (56).

Clozapine has been shown to be highly effective in the treatment of drug-induced hallucinations in PD and may have additional beneficial effects on tremor, dystonia, and dyskinesias (57–60). Doses effective in the management of drug-induced hallucinations in non-demented PD patients are between 25–50 mg/day, typically administered at night before bedtime to help induce sleep and reduce the risk of early morning orthostatic hypotension. Higher doses may be needed to control behavioral symptoms in patients with LBD, PD/SDAT complex, or cases of dementia-associated delirium. Associated side effects include dizziness, orthostatic hypotension, sialorrhea, and confusion. Doses higher than 75–100 mg/day are not well tolerated in this population. It is widely accepted that the use of clozapine is tempered by the 1% risk of agranulocytosis, which requires frequent monitoring of the leukocyte count (61), and, more recently, by rare reported cases of myocarditis.

Quetiapine is now the first-line drug for the treatment of all psychotic symptoms in PD (62). It is not associated with serious toxicity and has a low incidence of drug-induced parkinsonism (63–67). In PD with drug-induced hallucinations, the median doses are 25–75 mg/day, with most of the dose administered at night. Daytime doses can be administered at noon or later. As with clozapine, the doses required to treat behavioral symptoms in LBD or dementia-associated delirium have not been well studied but may be higher. Side effects included sedation, orthostasis, dizziness, and, in demented patients, possible increased confusion. If the symptoms are not well controlled with quetiapine, the patient may be switched to clozapine (68).

Risperidone is the second oldest atypical antipsychotic. In small doses (0.25–1 mg/day) it is an effective antipsychotic in PD patients with drug-induced hallucinations. In some patients, a worsening of parkinsonian signs may occur (62). In fact in one study investigators failed to find a difference between the neurological effects of low-dose risperidone and haloperidol in PD patients being treated for psychotic symptoms (69). Olanzapine does not appear to be well tolerated by patients with PD (70–74).

Acetylcholinesterase Inhibitors

A novel strategy for the treatment of psychotic symptoms in LBD, and possibly PD, is the use of acetylcholinesterase inhibitors (22). In a 20-week, double-blind, placebo-controlled study, the acetylcholinesterase inhibitor rivastigmine in doses of 6–12 mg/day significantly improved hallucinations, delusions, anxiety, and apathy in patients with LBD (75). The improvement in psychotic symptoms was in the order of 30%, which is comparable to that typically obtained with the atypical antipsychotics. Patients did not experience increased tremor or a worsening of parkinsonian features, which had been previously reported with other acetylcholinesterase inhibitors (76,77). Similar findings were reported in patients with PD (with and without dementia) treated with donepezil for psychotic symptoms over the course of 6–26 weeks. In these small studies donepezil 5–10 mg/day produced a significant improvement in psychotic symptoms without worsening parkinsonian motor symptoms (78,79). Although the safety and efficacy of this approach needs further study, it may be worth considering in patients with PD and dementia who continue to experience apathy and delusions after an adequate trial of atypical antipsychotics.

SLEEP DISTURBANCES

General

Sleep disturbances are a common and underrecognized feature of PD (80). They can be part of a primary sleep disorder or be secondary to advancing PD or comorbid depression or dementia (81). Specific types of sleep disturbances in PD may even be linked to the pathophysiology of psychotic symptoms.

Sleep problems in PD range from delayed sleep onset and sleep fragmentation to periodic leg movements (PLMS), restless leg syndrome (RLS), and REM-related behavioral disorders (REM-BD). Recognizing these important elements of nonmotor dysfunction in PD is important due to the increasing evidence that they are critically linked to disability and emerging evidence that some sleep disorders may be linked to psychiatric symptomatology (2,82,83). Factors intrinsic to the illness or its treatment that may disrupt sleep include the dopaminergic pathology itself (84,85), the dopaminomimetic treatment strategies (86), and the diurnal fluctuations associated with the treatment. Nighttime reemergence of parkinsonian motor signs presents with reemergence of tremor, pain, and urinary urgency that forces the patient to get up (82). In addition, some patients experience sleep apnea, which may indirectly contribute to daytime somnolence and cognitive decline. Sleep apnea has been linked to cases of otherwise unexplained daytime fatigue (87). Untreated depression is also a major factor contributing to the high incidence of sleep disturbances in PD.

Drug-induced sleep disruption includes vivid dreams and hallucinations, as well as daytime somnolence with resulting nocturnal insomnia (83). When sleep abnormalities are successfully treated, improved daytime functional capability is realized ("sleep benefit") (88).

REM-Related Behavioral Disorder and a Possible Link to Psychotic Symptoms

REM-BD is yet another form of sleep disturbance that, although not specific to PD, may facilitate the development of psychotic symptoms (89,90). REM-BD is characterized by nocturnal vocalizations and bursts of motor activity during which the subject appears to be acting out his dreams (91). Polysomnographically, normal REM sleep appears during stages III and IV of sleep and is characterized by "awake-appearing" cortical desynchronization. REM sleep is normally accompanied by cardiorespiratory irregularities, muscle atonia, and dreaming, whereas REM-BD is associated with REM intrusions into stage I and II of sleep, sleep fragmentation, and motor and vocal phenomena (91). In addition to PD, REM-BD has been described in LBD, in multiple system atrophy (MSA), and in other conditions unrelated to PD (92).

A pathophysiological link between REM-BD and psychotic symptoms has been suggested by numerous observations and by a recent study in which 10 of 10 nondemented PD patients with hallucinations were found to have REM-BD (90). The finding is not specific since similar findings have been noted in LBD (92), and not all patients with REM-BD suffer from hallucinations (90). Nonetheless, daytime hallucinations coincident with REM intrusions during wakefulness were reported by all 10 and by none of the nonhallucinating patients, again suggesting a pathophysiological link between this phenomenon and the "dream-like state' of hallucinatory symptoms in PD (92).

Treatment of Sleep Disturbances

Treatment of sleep disorders in PD starts with the implementation of a sensible program of sleep hygiene (93). General principles include setting a regular time for rising and going to bed, providing bright lights during the daytime and darkness and a cool environment to sleep at night. Other suggestions include the use of satin sheets to facilitate moving in bed, avoiding liquids after supper, emptying the bladder before retiring for bed, and careful attention to bladder dysfunction. Parkinson-specific maneuvers include improving nocturnal akinesia and reemergence of tremor through the judicious use of controlled-release carbidopa/levodopa or dopamine agonists. Specific adjustments in other anti-PD medications include the discontinuation of the noon dose, or all doses of selegiline, which has a notable incidence of insomnia, or the use of nighttime doses of dopaminomimetics. In patients already experiencing hallucinations, this approach may lead to a worsening of psychotic symptoms, perhaps mediated by a "kindling effect" these drugs may have on psychiatric symptoms, particularly when administered at night (94). It is known that nighttime dopaminomimetics tend to block normal REM sleep, perhaps facilitating the REM shift from stages III and IV to stage I and II (95). Paradoxically, in patients with daytime sleepiness, the use of daytime stimulants like methylphenidate and modafinil may improve daytime arousal while improving nighttime sleep (96).

Other strategies to improve sleep in PD include ruling out or treating conditions like sleep apnea, PLMS and RLS. Trazadone or the judicious short-term use of hypnotics or benzodiazepines like clonazepam are viable alternatives. Other alternatives include the use of melatonin, small doses of tricyclic antidepressants like nortriptyline, or nighttime doses of a sedating antidepressant like mirtazapine. Treatment of REM-BD is more complex and may not work in all patients (97). The most effective treatment has been small doses of clonazepam (0.25–0.5 mg one hour before sleep). Dopamine agonists may help REM-BD but aggravate nightmares and possibly daytime psychotic symptoms (81). Atypical antipsychotics like clozapine and quetiapine have not been studied adequately. The effect of dopamine agonists is more variable, with some patients reporting improvement and others worsening. The reasons for this apparent heterogeneity to dopaminomimetic response is unknown but may have to do with clinical co-variants such as the presence of PLMS, RLS, and dementia.

ACKNOWLEDGMENTS

This work supported in part by Emory University's American Parkinson's Disease Association Center of Research Excellence in Parkinson's Disease (JLJ and RLW) and by NIH Grant 5RO1-AT006121-02AT(JLJ). Dr. Watts was also supported by the Lanier Family Foundation.

REFERENCES

1. Juncos J, DeLong M. Parkinson's disease and basal ganglia movement disorders. In: Wolinski J, ed. Scientific American Medicine. New York: Scientific American Publications, 1997.
2. Kuopio AM, Marttila RJ, Helenius H, et al. The quality of life in Parkinson's disease. Mov Disord 2000; 15(2):305–308.
3. Committee TGPsDSS. Factors impacting on quality of life in Parkinson's disease: results from an international survey. Mov Disord 2002; 17:60–67.
4. Goetz C, Stebbins G. Risk factors for nursing home placement in advanced Parkinson's disease. Neurology 1993; 43:2227–2229.
5. Aarsland D, Ballard C, Larsen JP, et al. A comparative study of psychiatric symptoms in dementia with Lewy bodies and Parkinson's disease with and without dementia. Int J Geriatr Psychiatry 2001; 16:528–536.
6. Catalan-Alonso MJ, Del Val J. Psicosis inducida por farmacos dopaminomimeticos en la enfermedad de Parkinson idiopatica:primer sintoma de deterioro cognitivo? Rev Neurol 2001; 32(11):1085–1087.
7. Kulisevsky J, Garcia-Sanchez C, Berthier ML, et al. Chronic effects of dopaminergic replacement on cognitive function in Parkinson's disease: a two-year follow-up study of previously untreated patients. Mov Disord 2000; 15(4):613–626.
8. Kulisevsky J. Role of dopamine in learning and memory: implications for the treatment of cognitive dysfunction in patients with Parkinson's disease. Drugs Aging 2000; 16(5):365–379.
9. Levy G, Schupf N, Tang M, et al. Combined effect of age and severity on the risk of dementia in Parkinson's disease. Ann Neurol 2002; 51(6):722–729.
10. Ditter S, Mirra S. Neuropathologic and clinical features of Parkinson's disease in Alzheimer's disease patients. Neurology 1987; 37:754–760.
11. Kotzbauer PT, Trojanowsk JQ, Lee VM. Lewy body pathology in Alzheimer's disease. J Mol Neurosci 2001; 17(2):225–232.
12. Churchyard A, Lees A. The relationship between dementia and direct involvement of the hippocampus and amygdala in Parkinson's disease. Neurology 1997; 49:1570–1576.
13. Galasko D, Katzman R, Salmon DP, et al. Clinical and neuropathological findings in Lewy body dementias. Brain Cognition 1996; 31(2):166–175.
14. Reisberg B, Borenstein J, Salob SP. Behavioral symptoms in Alzheimer's disease: phenomenology and treatment. J Clin Psychiatry 1987; 48(suppl):9–15.

15. Diagnostic and Statistical Manual of Mental Disorders. 4th ed. Washington, DC: American Psychiatric Association, 1994.
16. Kaufer DI, Catt KE, Lopez OL, et al. Dementia with Lewy bodies: response of delirium-like features to donepezil. Neurology 1998; 51:1512.
17. Monteiro IM, Auer SR, Blksay I, et al. New and promising modalities for assessment of behavioral and psychological symptoms of dementia. Int Psychogeriatr 2000; 12(suppl 1):175–178.
18. Morris SJ, Olichney JM, Corey-Bloom J. Psychosis in dementia with Lewy bodies. Semin Clin Neuropsychiatry 1998; 3(1).51–60.
19. Perry RH, McKeith IG, Perry EK. Dementia with Lewy Bodies: Clinical, Pathological, and Treatment Issues. New York: Cambridge University Press, 1996.
20. Ala TA, Yang KH, Sung JH, et al. Hallucinations and signs of parkinsonism help distinguish patients with dementia and cortical Lewy bodies from patients with Alzheimer's disease at presentation: a clinicopathological study. J Neurol Neurosurg Psych 1997; 62:16 21.
21. McKeith I, Del Ser T, Spano P, et al. Efficacy of rivastigmine in dementia with Lewy bodies: a randomized, double-blind, placebo-controlled international study. Lancet 2000; 356:2031–2036.
22. Cummings J. Cholinesterase inhibitors: expanding applications. Lancet 2000; 356:2024–2025.
23. Aarsland D, Cummings JL, Yenner G, et al. Relationship of aggressive behavior to other neuropsychiatric symptoms in patients with Alzheimer's disease. Am J Psychiatry 1996; 153:243–247.
24. Conforti D, Borgherini G, Fiorellini Bernardis L, et al. Extrapyramidal symptoms associated to a venlafaxine-valproic acid combination. Int Clin Psychopharmacol 1999; 14:197–198.
25. Porsteinsson AP, Tariot PN, Erb R, et al. Placebo-controlled study of divalproex sodium for agitation in dementia. Am J Geriatr Psychiatry 2000; 9(1):58–67.
26. Mellow AM, Solano-Lopez C, Davis S. Sodium valproate in the treatment of behavioral disturbance in dementia. J Geriatr Psychiatry Neurol 1993; 6(4):205–209.
27. Masmoudi K, Gras-Champel V, Bonnet I, et al. Dementia and extrapyramidal problems caused by long-term valproic acid. Therapie 2000; 55(5):629–634.
28. Cummings JL. Depression and Parkinson's disease: a review. Am J Psychiatry 1992; 149(4):443–454.
29. Allain H, Schuck S, Mauuit N. Depression in Parkinson's disease. BMJ 2000; 320(7245):1287–1288.
30. Tandberg E, Larsen JP, Aarsland D, et al. Risk factors for depression in Parkinson's disease. Arch Neurol 1997; 54(5):625–630.
31. Starkstein S, Mayberg, HS, Leiguarda, R, Preziosi, TJ, Robinson, RG. A prospective longitudinal study of depression, cognitive decline and physical impairments in patients with Parkinson's disease. J Neurol Neurosurg Psychiatry 1992; 55:377–382.

32. Kuhn W, Heye N, Muller T, et al. The motor performance test series in Parkinson's disease is influenced by depression. J Neural Transm 1996; 103(3):349–354.

33. Troster AI, Stalp LD, Paolo AM, et al. Neuropsychological impairment in Parkinson's disease with and without depression. Arch Neurol 1995; 52(12):1164–1169.

34. Norman S, Troster AI, Fields JA, et al. Effects of depression and Parkinson's disease on cognitive functioning. J Neuropsychiatry Clin Neurosci 2002; 14(1):31–36.

35. Okun M, McDonald WM, Hanfelt J, et al. Refractory nonmotor symptoms in male Parkinson patients due to testosterone deficiency: a common unrecognized comorbidity. Neurology 2002; 58(suppl 3):A284.

36. Menza MA, Sage J, Marshall E, et al. Mood changes and "on-off" phenomena in Parkinson's disease. Mov Disord 1990; 5(2):148–151.

37. Siemers ER, Shekhar A, Quaid K, et al. Anxiety and motor performance in Parkinson's disease. Mov Disord 1993; 8:501–506.

38. Stein MB, Heuser IJ, Juncos JL, et al. Anxiety disorders in patients with Parkinson's disease. Am J Psychiatry 1990; 147(2):217–220.

39. Cummings J. Behavioral complications of drug treatment of Parkinson's disease. J Am Geriatr Soc 1991; 39:708–716.

40. Factor SA, Molho ES, Podskalny GD, et al. Parkinson's disease: drug-induced psychiatric states. In: Weiner W, Lang A, eds. Behavioral Neurology of Movement Disorders. New York: Raven Press, 1995:115–138.

41. Juncos J. Management of psychotic aspects of Parkinson's disease. J Clin Psychiatry 1999; 60(58):42–53.

42. Goetz CG, Pappert EJ, Blasucci LM, et al. Intravenous levodopa in hallucinating Parkinson's disease patients: high dose challenge dose not precipitate hallucinations. Neurology 1998; 50:515–517.

43. Friedman JH. Intravenous levodopa in hallucinating PD patients. Neurology 1999; 52(1):219–220.

44. Okada K, Suyama N, Oguro H, et al. Medication-induced hallucination and cerebral blood flow in Parkinson's disease. J Neurol 1999; 246(5):365–368.

45. Samuels SC, Evers MM. Delirium: pragmatic guidance for managing a common, confounding, and sometimes lethal condition. Geriatrics 2002; 57:33–38.

46. Tune LE. The role of antipsychotics in treating delirium. Curr Psychiatry Rep 2002; 4:209–212.

47. Tom T, Cummimgs JL. Depression and Parkinson's disease. Drugs Aging 1998; 12(1):55–74.

48. Richard I, Maughn A, Kurlan R. Do serotonin reuptake inhibitor antidepressants worsen Parkinson's disease? A retrospective case series. Mov Disord 1999; 14(1):155–157.

49. Abrams R. ECT for Parkinson's disease. Am J Psychiatry 1989; 146:1391–1393.

50. Friedman J. Drug holidays in the treatment of Parkinson's disease: a brief review. Arch Intern Med 1985; 145:913–915.
51. Caligiuri MP, Lacro JP, Jeste DV. Incidence and predictors of drug-induced parkinsonism in older psychiatric patients treated with very low doses of neuroleptics. J Clin Psychopharmacol 1999; 19(4):322–328.
52. Jibson MD, Tandon R. New atypical antipsychotic medications. J Psychiatr Res 1998; 32:215–228.
53. Seeman P, Tallerico T. Antipsychotic drugs which elicit little or no parkinsonism bind more loosely than dopamine to brain D2 receptors, yet occupy high levels of these receptors [see comments]. Mol Psychiatry 1998; 3(2):123–134.
54. Seeman P, Tallerico T. Rapid release of antipsychotic drugs from dopamine D2 receptors: an explanation for low receptor occupancy and early clinical relapse upon withdrawal of clozapine or quetiapine. Am J Psychiatry 1999; 156(6):876–884.
55. Kapur S, Zipursky R, Coirey J, et al. A positron emission tomography study of quetiapine in schizophrenai: a preliminary finding of an antipsychotc effect with only transiently high dipamine D2 receptor occupancy. Arch Gen Psychiatry 2000; 57(6):553–559.
56. Kapur S, Seeman P. Does fast dissociation from the dopamine d(2) receptor explain the action of atypical antipsychotics?: A new hypothesis. Am J Psychiatry 2001; 158(3):360–369.
57. Friedman JH, Lannon MC, Factor S, et al. Low dose clozapine for the treatment of drug-induced psychosis in idiopathic Parkinson's disease: results of the double-blind, placebo-controlled trial. N Engl J Med 1999; 340(10):757–763.
58. Group FCPsS. Clozapine in drug-induced psychosis in parkinson's disease. Lancet 1999; 353:2041–2042.
59. Durif F, Vidailhet M, Assal F, et al. Low-dose clozapine improves dyskinesias in Parkinson's disease. Neurology 1997; 48:658–662.
60. Factor S, Friedman J. The emerging role of clozapine in the treatment of movement disorders. Mov Disord 1997; 12:483–496.
61. Honigfeld G, Arellano F, Sethi J, et al. Reducing clozapine-related morbidity and mortality: 5 years of experience with the Clozaril National Registry. J Clin Psychiatry 1998; 59:3–7.
62. Friedman JH, Factor SA. Atypical antipsychotics in the treatment of drug-induced psychosis in Parkinson's disease. Mov Disord 2000; 15(2):201–211.
63. Juncos J, Yeung P, Sweitzer D, et al. Quetiapine treatment of psychotic symptoms in Parkinson's disease: a one-year multicenter trial. Neurology 2000; 56:
64. Fernandez H, Friedman J, Jacques C, et al. Quietiapine for the treatment of drug-induced psychosis in Parkinson's disease. Mov Disord 1999; 14(3):484–487.

65. Juncos JL, Arvanitis L, Sweitzer D, et al. Quetiapine improves psychotic symptoms associated with Parkinson's disease. Neurology 1999; 52(suppl 2):262.

66. Samantha J, Stacey M. Quetiapine in the treatment of hallucinations in advanced Parkinson's disease. In: Fifth International Congress of Parkinson's disease and Movement Disorders, New York, 1998.

67. Targum SD, Abbott JL. Efficacy of quetiapine in Parkinson's patients with psychosis. J Clin Psychopharmacol 2000; 20(1):54–60.

68. Dewey RB, O'Suilleabhain PE. Treatment of drug-induced psychosis with quetiapine and clozapine in Parkinson's disease. Neurology 2000; 55:1753–1754.

69. Rosebush PI, Mazurek MF. Neurological side effects in neuroleptic-naive patients treated with haloperidol or risperidone. Neurology 1999; 52:782–785.

70. Jimenez-Jimenez FJ, Tallon-Barranco A, Orti-Pareja M, et al. Olanzapine can worsen parkinsonism. Neurology 1998; 50(2):1183–1184.

71. Molho E, Factor S. Worsening of motor features of Parkinson's disease with olanzapine. Mov Disord 1999; 14:1014–1016.

72. Goetz C, Blasucci L, Leurgans S, et al. Olanzapine and clozapine. Comparative effects on motor function in hallucinating PD patients. Neurology 2000; 55:789–794.

73. Gimenez-Roldan S, Mateo D, Navarro E, et al. Efficacy and safety of clozapine and olanzapine: an open-label study comparing tow groups of Parkinson's disease patients with dopaminergic-induced psychosis. Parkinsonism Relat Disord 2000; 7:121–127.

74. Marsh L, Lyketsos C, Reich SG. Olanzapine for the treatment of psychosis in patients with Parkinson's disease and dementia. Psychosomatics 2001; 42(6):477–481.

75. Del Ser T, McKeith I, Anand R, et al. Dementia with lewy bodies: findings from an international multicentre study. Int J Geriatr Psychiatry 2000; 15(11):1034–1045.

76. Hutchinson M, Fazzini E. Cholinesterase inhibition in Parkinson's disease [letter]. J Neurol Neurosurg Psychiatry 1996; 61(3):324–325.

77. Bourke D, Druckenbrod RW. Possible association between donepezil and worsening Parkinson's disease [letter]. Ann Pharmacother 1998; 32(5):610–611.

78. Bergman J, Lerner V. Successful use of donepezil for the treatment of psychotic symptoms in patients with Parkinson's disease. Clin Neuropharmacol 2002; 25(2):107–110.

79. Werber EA, Rabey JM. The beneficial effect of cholinesterase inhibitors on patients suffering from Parkinson's disease and dementia. J Neural Transmission – General Section 2001; 108(11):1319–1325.

80. Van Hilten B, Hoff JI, Middlekoop AM, et al. Sleep disruption in Parkinson's disease. Arch Neurol 1994; 51:922–928.

81. Olanow CW, Watts RL, Koller WC. An algorithm (decision tree) for the management of Parkinson's disease: treatment guidelines. Neurology 2001; 56(11 (suppl 5):S1–S88.

82. Bliwise DL, Watts RL, Watts N, et al. Disruptive nocturnal behavior in Parkinson's disease and Alzheimer's disease. J Geriatr Psychiatry Neurol 1995; 8:107–110.

83. Pappert E, Goetz C, Niederman F, et al. Hallucinations, sleep fragmentation, and altered dream phenomena in Parkinson's disease. Mov Disord 1999; 14(1):117 121.

84. Eisensehr I, Linke R, Noachtar S, et al. Reduced dopamine trasporters in idiopathis rapid eye movement sleep behavior disorders: comparison with Parkinson's disease and controls. Brain 2000; 123:1155–1160.

85. Rye DB, Jankovic J. Emerging view of dopamine in modulating sleep/wake state from an unlikely source: PD. Neurology 2002; 58:341–346.

86. Nausieda PA, Weiner WJ, Kaplan L, et al. Sleep disruption in the course of chronic levodopa therapy: an early feature of levodopa psychosis. Clin Neuropharmacol 1982; 5:183–194.

87. Hauser RA, Zesiewicz TA, Delgado HM, et al. Evaluation and treatment of fatigue in Parkinson's disease. Neurology 2002; 58(suppl 3):A433.

88. Factor SA, McAlarney T, Sanchez-Ramos JR, et al. Sleep disorders and sleep effect in Parkinson's disease. Mov Disord 1990; 5:280–285.

89. Schenk CS, Bundic SR, Patterson AL, et al. Rapid eye movement sleep behavior disorder. JAMA 1987; 257:1786–1789.

90. Arnulf I, Bonnet AM, Damier P, et al. Hallucinations, REM sleep, and Parkinson's disease: a medical hypothesis. Neurology 2000; 55(2):281–288.

91. Comella CL, Nardine TM, Diederich NJ, et al. Sleep-related violence, injury, and REM sleep behavior disorder in Parkinson's disease. Neurology 1998; 51(2):526–529.

92. Boeve BF, Silber MH, Ferman TJ, et al. REM sleep behavior disorder and degenerative dementia: an association likely reflecting Lewy body disease. Neurology 1998; 51(2):363–370.

93. Gillin JC, Byerley WF. Drug therapy: the diagnosis and management of insomnia. N Engl J Med 1990; 322:239–248.

94. Moskovitz C, Moses H, Klawans H. Levodopa-induced psychosis: a kindling phenomenon. Am J Psychiatry 1978; 135:669–675.

95. Gillin JC, Post RM, Wyatt RJ, et al. REM inhibitory effect of L-dopa infusion during human sleep. Electroenceph Clin Neurophysiol 1973; 35:181–186.

96. Ondo WG, Atassi F, Vuong KD, et al. Excessive daytime sleepines in Parkinson's disease: a double-blind, placebo-controlled, parallel design study of modafinil. Neurology 2002; 58(suppl 3):A433–434.

97. Ferini-Strambi L, Zucconi M. REM sleep behavior disorder. Clin Neurophysiol 2000; 111(suppl 2):S136–140.

8

Neuroimaging in Parkinson's Disease

Kenneth Marek, Danna Jennings, and John Seibyl
The Institute for Neurodegenerative Disorders, New Haven, Connecticut, U.S.A.

Neuroimaging has provided insight into the pathophysiology and natural history of Parkinson's disease (PD) and has emerged as a tool to monitor disease progression and to assess new potentially neuroprotective or neurorestorative therapies for PD. Diverse imaging methods have been successfully applied to neurological disorders. While technology like functional magnetic resonance imaging or magnetic resonance spectroscopy has been especially useful in assessing stroke, multiple sclerosis and epilepsy (1–3), in vivo neuroreceptor imaging using single photon emission tomography (SPECT) and positron emission tomogrpahy (PET) have so far been most valuable in assessing PD. SPECT and PET use specific radioactively labeled ligands to neurochemically tag or mark normal or abnormal brain chemistry. Recent advances in radiopharmaceutical development, imaging detector technologies, and image analysis software have expanded and accelerated the role of imaging in clinical research in PD, in general, and neurotherapeutics, in particular. In this overview we will focus on developments in neuroreceptor imaging in PD.

IMAGING TECHNOLOGY

Both PET, also called dual photon emission tomography, and SPECT are sensitive methods of measuring in vivo neurochemistry (4,5). The choice of imaging modality is ultimately determined by the specific study questions and study design. While, generally PET cameras have better resolution than SPECT cameras, SPECT studies may be technologically and clinically more feasible, particularly for large clinical studies and in clinical practice. PET studies may benefit from greater flexibility in the range of radiopharmaceuticals that can be tested, but SPECT studies have the advantage of longer half-life radiopharmaceuticals necessary for some studies.

The strengths and limitations of in vivo neuroreceptor imaging studies depend on the imaging technology utilized to measure brain neurochemistry and the ligand or biochemical marker used to tag a specific brain neurochemical system. The properties of the radiopharmaceutical are the most crucial issue in developing a useful imaging tool for PD. Some of the key steps in development of a potential radioligand include assessment of the brain penetration of the radioligand, the selectivity of the radioligand for the target site, the binding properties of the radioligand to the site, and the metabolic fate of the radioligand. These properties help to determine the signal-to-noise ratio of the ligand and the ease of quantitation of the imaging signal. While ligands targeting neuronal metabolism have been used successfully to study PD patients, this review will focus on dopaminergic ligands (6). Specific markers for the dopaminergic system including ^{18}F-DOPA (7–12), ^{11}C-VMAT2 (13–15), and dopamine transporter (DAT) ligands (16–22) (Fig. 1) have been widely used to evaluate patients with PD.

Dopamine ligands are useful to assess PD in so far as they reflect the ongoing dopaminergic degeneration in PD. In the study most directly correlating changes in dopamine neuronal numbers and imaging outcomes there is good correlation between dopamine neuron loss and ^{18}F-DOPA uptake, although conclusions are limited by a small sample size of five subjects (12). Numerous other studies have shown that the vesicular transporter and dopamine transporter are reduced in striatum in postmortem brain from PD patients (23–25). In turn numerous clinical imaging studies have shown reductions in ^{18}F-DOPA, ^{11}C-VMAT2, and DAT ligands uptake in PD patients and aging healthy subjects consistent with the expected pathology of PD and of normal aging. Specifically these imaging studies demonstrate asymmetric, putamen greater than caudate loss of dopaminergic uptake that is progressive (26–28) (Table 1). In addition both ^{11}C-VMAT2 and DAT ligands demonstrate reductions in activity with normal aging (13,29).

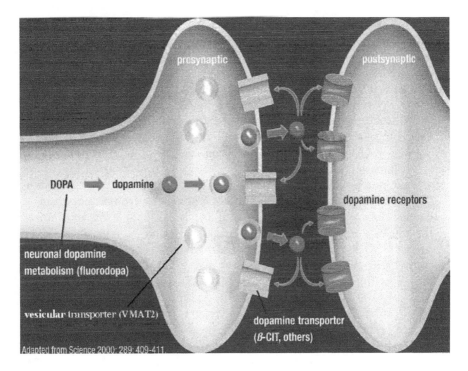

FIGURE 1   Idealized dopamine synapse showing targets for radiopharmaceutical in PD. (See color insert.)

TABLE 1   Comparison of Dopamine Presynaptic Ligands in PD Studies

	$[^{123}I]\beta$-CIT	^{11}C-VMAT2	^{18}F-DOPA
Target	DA transporter	Vesicular transporter	DA turnover
Bilateral reduction in hemi-PD	Yes	Yes	Yes
Correlates with UPDRS in cross section	Yes	Yes	Yes
Annual reduction change with aging (% loss from baseline)	0.8–1.4%	0.5%	No
Annual progression (% loss from baseline)	6–13%	10%	7–12%

Imaging with ^{18}F-DOPA, ^{11}C-VMAT2, and DAT ligands target different components of the presynaptic nigrostriatal neuron. The mechanism of each of these ligands has been elucidated in preclinical studies. Imaging with ^{18}F-DOPA depends on conversion of ^{18}F-DOPA by aromatic amino acid decarboxylase and uptake and trapping of ^{18}F-dopamine into synaptic vesicles. Studies in 1-methyl-4-Phenyl-1,2,3,6-tetrahydropyridine (MPTP)-treated monkeys have shown a correlation between the ^{18}F-DOPA uptake and both dopaminergic neuron number in the substantia nigra and dopamine levels in the striatum (30). The vesicular monoamine transporter acts to sequester newly synthesized or recovered monoamines (dopamine, serotonin, norepinephrine, and histamine) from the cytosol into the synaptic vesicles, thereby protecting the neurotransmitters from catabolism by cytosolic enzymes and packaging them for subsequent exocytotic release (31). VMAT2 ligand uptake is reduced in two commonly used rodent models of PD the 6-hydroxydopamine–treated rat and the MPTP-treated mouse (32,33). DAT, a protein on the nerve terminal, is responsible for reuptake of dopamine from the synaptic cleft. In MPTP-treated monkeys the loss of DAT paralleled that of dopamine in the striatum, and in MPTP monkeys treated with nigral implants recovery of behavioral function was correlated with changes in DAT imaging (34,35).

During the past decade, several DAT ligands have been developed and used to assess PD and related disorders. Table 2 provides a more detailed comparison of the properties of these ligands. This comparison both illustrates the increasing choice of radioligands available and underscores the distinction of those ligands that enable easy quantification of the imaging signal. DAT imaging agents are cocaine analogs with nanomolar affinity at the DAT (36–41). These ligands are chemically modified to alter

TABLE 2 Characteristics of SPECT Dopamine Transporter Radioligands

SPECT tracer	[123I]β-CIT	[123I]FP-CIT	^{99m}Tc-TRODAT	[123I]Altropane
Time to peak uptake	Protracted, 8–18 h	Rapid, 2–3 h	Rapid, 2–3 h	Rapid, 0.5–1 h
Washout phase	Prolonged	Prolonged	Intermediate	Rapid
DAT binding affinity	1.4 nM Ki	3.5 nM Ki	9.7 nm Ki	6.62 nM IC50
DAT:SERT selectivity	1.7:1	2.8:1	26:1	28:1
SPECT target:background tissue ratio	High	High	Low	Low

the rapid metabolism of cocaine at the ester linkage to provide more in vivo stability of the parent compound. Nonetheless, the kinetic properties of DAT radiotracers are quite different with regard to plasma protein binding, permeability across the blood-brain barrier, binding affinity, selectivity for the dopamine transporter, and elimination. These differences are crucial to the applications of the DAT ligand for imaging (42). For example, while a given DAT tracer may distinguish PD from healthy controls based on the qualitative appearance of striatal uptake, the ability to distinguish the longitudinal changes in severity of PD may be more difficult for tracers with relatively poorer signal-to-noise properties (lower specific to nonspecific brain uptake) (Table 2). The quantitative properties of the radiotracer must be well understood to assess disease progression. Specifically, does the imaging signal provide a measure that is related to Bmax, the density of DAT, and/or the integrity of dopamine neurons? For some tracers absolute quantitation of the DAT signal may require invasive methods involving full kinetic modeling, while other DAT tracers have a pharmacokinetic profile, which simplifies the methods for signal quantification. For example, the unusual binding kinetics of $[^{123}I]\beta$-CIT, with a protracted period of stable specific radiotracer uptake in the brain and extremely slow elimination from the DAT sites in striatum, permit reproducible quantitative determination of DAT density using a simple tissue ratio method (19,43). For DAT tracers with faster washout from specific binding sites, this simple ratio technique will overestimate the density of binding sites in healthy striatum relative to PD (44), although these tracers may permit better visual discrimination of diseased from control cases.

Of the DAT SPECT tracers in development, $[^{123}I]\beta$-CIT, $[^{123}I]FP$-CIT, $[^{123}I]$-altropane, and $[^{99m}Tc]$-TRODAT have been the most widely evaluated dopamine transporter agents for SPECT imaging (18,20,45) and ^{18}F-CFT (WIN 35,428) for PET (46,47). None of these tracers is commercially available as yet in North America, although one tropane derivative of cocaine (FP-CIT, DATSCAN®) is available as a $[^{123}I]$-labeled tracer in Europe.

PD DIAGNOSIS ACCURACY

The diagnosis of PD is currently based primarily on clinical judgment. However, the variability of disease presentation, progression, and response to medications often makes diagnosis uncertain. Prevalence studies of parkinsonism suggest a diagnostic accuracy of 80% after examination and application of clinical diagnostic criteria (48–50). Long-term clinicopathological studies evaluating the diagnostic accuracy of PD demonstrate that the diagnoses most commonly mistaken for PD are progressive supranuclear palsy (PSP) and multisystem atrophy (MSA) (51,52). However, early in the course of PD the diagnoses most commonly mistaken for PD include essential tremor, vascular parkinsonism, drug-induced parkinsonism, and Alzheimer's disease (53,54). It is estimated that diagnosis is incorrect in as many as 35% of those initially diagnosed as PD by generalists (55). In addition, symptoms of parkinsonism are relatively common in elderly subjects, making the diagnosis most challenging in this population. Subtle extrapyramidal signs on neurological evaluation are common in the elderly, with recorded prevalences of 32% (56) and 35% (57). Prevalence estimates for clinically evident parkinsonism in similarly aged subjects are much lower at around 3%. Neurologists with specialized training in parkinsonism are able to make the diagnosis of PD with higher accuracy than generalists as demonstrated by a follow-up study of the DATATOP cohort in which the diagnosis of PD was changed in only 8.1% of subjects at 6-year follow-up and by a study of movement disorder specialists in the United Kingdom demonstrating sensitivity of 91.1% for diagnosis of PD compared to the diagnosis based on pathology (58,59).

In vivo imaging holds the promise of improving diagnostic accuracy by providing an in vivo assessment of the nigrostriatal dopaminergic system early in disease. While comparison of imaging and pathology helps to confirm the validity of the imaging studies, it also highlights questions for which imaging studies may provide unique and otherwise unobtainable data. For example, in vivo imaging studies with either ^{18}F-DOPA/PET or [^{123}I]β-CIT/SPECT demonstrate a reduction in ligand uptake of approximately 50–70% in the putamen in PD subjects (20,60). The reduction in dopamine terminal function or DAT density and the pattern of striatal degeneration is consistent with the reduction in substantia nigra pars compacta neurons of greater than 80% and of putamenal dopamine content of 95% in PD brains (61–63). However, these imaging studies have shown at or near the threshold of diagnosis of PD a reduction in putamenal ^{18}F-DOPA or DAT activity of 40–60% rather than 80–90% as suggested by pathology studies (64–66). These imaging data acquired from early PD patients have clarified the natural history of disease, led to longitudinal studies on the rate of disease progression (as indicated below), and provide further impetus to develop therapies to protect the remaining 50% of dopaminergic neurons not yet affected at disease onset.

PD DIFFERENTIAL DIAGNOSIS AND SEVERITY

The first questions of an imaging ligand is whether it reliably distinguishes between subjects with and without known pathology (a marker for disease trait) and whether the changes in the imaging outcomes correlate with disease severity (a marker for disease state). In several studies both dopamine and vesicular transporter ligands and ^{18}F-DOPA discriminated between individuals with PD and healthy subjects with a sensitivity of >95% (11,13,20,67–69). These studies take advantage of the relatively greater dopaminergic loss in the putamen to enhance the discriminant function. Furthermore, the reduction in both dopamine and vesicular transporter and ^{18}F-DOPA imaging activity correlated with well-defined clinical rating scales of PD severity (16,20,28,70). Interestingly when specific PD symptoms are compared, the loss of dopaminergic activity measured by imaging correlated with bradykinesia but not with tremor (20,71). Cross-sectional studies show that severity of bradykinesia measured by clinical scales reflects the severity of the nigrostriatal dopamine neuron loss. Therefore, in vivo dopaminergic imaging provides a biomarker both for the presence of disease and for the severity of the pathological process.

In clinical practice, diagnosis is often difficult at the onset of symptoms. In studies focused on early PD patients, at the threshold of their illness, in vivo imaging demonstrated a 40–60% reduction in DAT or F-DOPA activity in the putamen contralateral to the symptomatic side. PD generally presents as a unilateral motor disorder and progresses during a variable period of 3–6 years to affect both sides although frequently remaining asymmetric (72). The unilateral motor presentation reflects the asymmetric dopaminergic pathology, which is in turn demonstrated by in vivo dopaminergic imaging (11,65,66).

Imaging may also be useful in special diagnostic situations such as psychogenic, drug-induced, traumatic, or vascular parkinsonism in distinguishing these syndromes without a presynaptic dopamine deficit from PD and other related disorders (73,74). A more difficult diagnostic problem is the distinction between the more specific diagnosis of PD and other related neurodegenerative disorders categorized as Parkinsonism or Parkinson's syndrome. The more common etiologies of Parkinson's syndrome are PSP, MSA, cortical basal ganglionic degeneration, and diffuse Lewy body disease, which may account for about 15–20% of patients with apparent PD. Parkinsonism is characterized by significant nigrostriatal neuronal loss, which is demonstrated by reduction in in vivo presynaptic dopaminergic imaging. While the severity of DAT or ^{18}F-DOPA loss does not discriminate between PD and other causes of Parkinson's syndrome, the pattern of loss in Parkinson's syndrome is less region specific (putamen and caudate equally affected) and more symmetric than PD. This strategy discriminates between PD and other causes of Parkinson's syndrome with a sensitivity of about 75–80% (75–77). In addition, the more widespread pathology associated with Parkinson's syndrome may be reflected in abnormalities in post-synaptic dopamine receptor imaging and in metabolic imaging which are not seen in PD. Therefore the pattern of presynaptic dopaminergic loss may be coupled with postsynaptic dopamine receptor imaging or metabolic imaging to distinguish PD from other related Parkinsonian syndromes (78,79).

PARKINSON'S DISEASE PROGRESSION

The rate of clinical progression of PD is highly variable and unpredictable (72). In clinical studies several clinical endpoints for progressive functional decline in PD have been used including Unified Parkinson's Disease Rating Scale (UPDRS) in the "defined off" state or after drug washout up to 2 weeks, time to need for dopaminergic therapy, or time to development of motor fluctuations (80–84). Clinical rating scales are extremely useful, but ratings may be investigator dependent and are frequently confounded by changes in symptomatic treatment. Pathological studies investigating rate of progression have been limited and rely entirely on cross-sectional data (62,63). These studies have in general considered patients with severe illness of long duration. In vivo imaging studies provide the opportunity to evaluate patients longitudinally from early to late disease using an objective biomarker for dopaminergic degeneration.

In several studies neuroreceptor imaging of the nigrostriatal dopaminergic system has been used as a research tool to monitor progressive dopaminergic neuron loss in PD. In longitudinal studies of PD progression both ^{18}F-DOPA and DAT imaging [β-CIT(2β-carboxymethoxy-3β(4-iodophenyl)tropane) and CFT] using both PET and SPECT have demonstrated an annualized rate of reduction in striatal ^{18}F-DOPA, ^{18}F-CFT, or [^{123}I]β-CIT uptake of about 6–13% in PD patients compared with 0–2.5% change in healthy controls (85–89). Similar findings have been reported for VMAT2 imaging (K. Frey, personal communication, 2002) (Fig. 2).

Evidence from studies of hemi-PD subjects provide further insight into the rate of progression of disease. In early hemi-PD there is a reduction in ^{18}F-DOPA and DAT uptake of about 50% in the affected putamen and of 25–30% in the unaffected putamen. Since most patients will progress clinically from unilateral to bilateral in 3–6 years, it is therefore likely that the loss of these in vivo imaging markers of dopaminergic degeneration in the previously unaffected putamen will progress at about 5–10% per annum (11,65).

Imaging has also been used to monitor progression of PD in patients receiving fetal substantia nigral transplants for PD. Several studies during the past several years show an increase in ^{18}F-DOPA uptake with follow-up of 6 months to 6 years posttransplant (90,91). The change in ^{18}F-DOPA

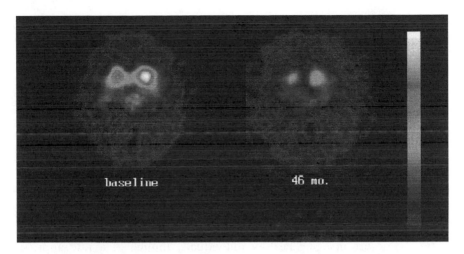

FIGURE 2   SPECT [^{123}I]β-CIT images from a patient with PD 2 years after diagnosis and 46 months later and from an age-matched healthy subject. Note the asymmetric reduction in [^{123}I]β-CIT uptake more marked in the putamen than caudate in the patient and the progressive loss of activity. Levels of SPECT activity are color-encoded from low (black) to high (yellow/white). (See color insert.)

uptake has been correlated with postmortem survival of grafted dopaminergic nigral cells (92).

The most important role of longitudinal imaging studies is to provide a tool to assess objectively potential neuroprotective and restorative therapies for PD. Imaging studies assessing progression of disease have provided data to estimate sample sizes required to detect slowing of disease progression due to study drug treatment. The sample size required depends on the effect of the disease-modifying drug and the duration of exposure to the drug. The effect of the drug is generally expressed as the percent reduction in rate of loss of the imaging marker in the group treated with the study drug versus a control group. More specifically, imaging studies have sought a reduction of between 25 and 50% in the rate of loss of ^{18}F-DOPA or [^{123}I]β-CIT uptake (i.e., a reduction from 10% to 5–7.5% per year). The sample size needed to detect a 25–50% reduction in the rate of loss of F-DOPA or β-CIT uptake during a 24-month interval ranges from approximately 30 to 120 research subjects in each study arm (85,93).

These data support the use of dopamine neuroreceptor imaging to assess the effects of potential neuroprotective drugs in PD, but there are several caveats in the study design and interpretation of these studies.

1. It must be acknowledged that imaging outcomes in studies of PD patients are biomarkers for brain activity, but are not true surrogates for drug effects in PD patients (94). These investigational drugs may have effects on dopamine neurons unrelated to slowed neuronal degeneration and may have effects outside the dopaminergic system.

2. The rate of change in imaging outcomes used to measure disease progression is slow, reflecting the slow clinical progression in PD and requiring the duration of these progression studies to be at least 18–24 months. In a recent study evaluating potential disease modifying effects of Neuroimmunophilin A, the study duration of 6 months resulted in an equivocal outcome necessitating a second, longer study to clarify the drug effects (95).

3. Progressive loss in brain dopaminergic imaging activity also occurs in aging healthy individuals, though at a rate approximately one-tenth that of PD patients (13,29).

4. The reliability of the imaging outcomes must be assessed. Recent test-retest studies using current technology and analyses methodology show good test-retest reproducibility of approximately 3–5% for ^{18}F-DOPA or VMAT2 studies and 5–7% for β-CIT SPECT (95–97).

5. Imaging outcomes of disease progression may be confounded by pharmacological effects of the study drug. In preclinical studies evaluation of the effect of dopamine agonists and antagonists and levodopa suggest possible regulation of both the DAT and dopamine turnover (32,98). The relevance of these studies to human imaging studies is questionable due to short duration of exposure to drugs, suprapharmacological dosing, and species differences. In another approach to assess regulation, in one of the few clinical studies comparing imaging ligands within subjects, 35 PD patients and 16 age-matched controls imaged with ^{11}C-methylphenidate (a dopamine transporter ligand), ^{18}F-DOPA and ^{11}C-dihydrotetrabenazine (a vesicular transporter ligand), demonstrated reduction in DAT which is greater than vesicular transporter which is greater than F-DOPA uptake. These data suggest that differential regulation of these imaging targets might occur in a progressively denervated striatum (14). These data were also consistent with the presumed upregulation of dopamine turnover in normal aging reflected in the lack of change in ^{18}F-DOPA imaging in aging healthy subjects (99). Other studies have more directly assessed the potential short-term regulation of imaging ligands by common PD medications. Available data does

not show regulation of DAT ligands or ^{18}F-DOPA uptake by levodopa or dopamine agonists. In the CALM-PD CIT study there was no significant change in β-CIT uptake after 10 weeks of treatment with either pramipexole (1.5–4.5 mg) or levodopa (300–600 mg) consistent with previous studies evaluating levodopa and selegiline effects after 6–12 weeks (100–102). In a similar study treatment with pergolide for 6 weeks also showed no significant changes in [^{123}I]β-CIT striatal, putamen, or caudate uptake, but an insignificant trend toward increased [^{123}I]β-CIT uptake (103). Data assessing RTI-32, another DAT ligand, demonstrated significant reductions from baseline in striatal DAT after 6 weeks of treatment with both levodopa and pramipexole, but also with placebo, and this pilot study could not detect differences between the treatment and placebo (104). There was no effect on ^{18}F-DOPA uptake in a study of five patients with restless legs syndrome who had been treated with levodopa (105). While these clinical studies do not demonstrate significant regulation of the DAT or ^{18}F-DOPA uptake, they do not exclude a significant short-term treatment-induced change in DAT, nor do they address the possibility that pharmacological effects may emerge in long-term studies.

Despite these caveats in interpretation of imaging results, neuroreceptor ligand biomarkers have become an increasingly useful method to assess the potential disease modifying effects of experimental drugs for PD. Several candidate drugs, including coenzyme Q10, a mitochondrial agent, neuroimmunophilin A, a potential growth factor, riluzole, a glutamatergic drug, CEP 1347 and CTCH 346, antiapoptotic agents, and pramipexole and ropinirole, dopamine agonists, have been or are in ongoing clinical studies of neuroprotection (80–82,84,106–108). Several other drugs are in preclinical testing as we seek the "holy grail" of neuroprotection.

Recently two similar studies compared the effect of initial treatment with a dopamine agonist [pramipexole (CALM-PD CIT) or ropinirole (REAL-PET)] or levodopa on the progression of PD as measured by [^{123}I]β-CIT or ^{18}F-DOPA imaging. These two clinical imaging studies targeting dopamine function with different imaging ligands and technology both demonstrate slowing in the rate of loss of [^{123}I]β-CIT or ^{18}F-DOPA uptake in early PD patients treated with dopamine agonists compared to levodopa. These studies evaluated two related, predominantly D2 dopamine receptor agonists, suggesting that the results may indicate a class effect. The relative reduction in the percent loss from baseline of [^{123}I]β-CIT uptake in the pramipexole versus the levodopa group was 47% at 22 months, 44% at 34 months, and 37% at 46 months after initiating treatment. The relative reduction of ^{18}F-DOPA uptake in the ropinirole group versus the levodopa group was 35% at 24 months. These data suggest that treatment with the dopamine agonists pramipexole and ropinirole and/or with levodopa may either slow or accelerate the dopaminergic degeneration of PD. Furthermore, these studies demonstrated that in vivo imaging can be used effectively to assess potential disease modifying drugs in well-controlled, blinded clinical studies (102,109)

In the CALM-PD CIT and REAL-PET studies there was no correlation between the percent change from baseline in the imaging outcome and the change from baseline in UPDRS at 22–24 months. There are several explanations for the lack of correlation between $[^{123}I]\beta$-CIT or ^{18}F-DOPA uptake and UPDRS in longitudinal studies. First, the UPDRS is confounded by the effects of the patient's anti-Parkinson medications both acutely after initiating therapy and with ongoing treatment. Even evaluation of the UPDRS in the "defined off" state or after prolonged washout does not eliminate the long-term symptomatic effects of these treatments (83,110). Second, in early PD the temporal patterns for rate of loss of DAT or ^{18}F-DOPA and the change in UPDRS may not be congruent. This is most evident in the preclinical period when the imaging outcomes are reduced by 40–60% prior to diagnosis. In the CALM-PD study the loss of striatal $[^{123}I]\beta$-CIT uptake from baseline was significantly correlated ($r = -0.40$; $p = 0.001$) with the change in UPDRS from baseline at 46-month evaluation, suggesting that the correlation between clinical and imaging outcomes begins to emerge with longer monitoring (102). These data suggest that particularly in early PD, clinical and imaging outcomes provide complementary data and that long-term follow-up will be required to correlate changes in clinical and imaging outcomes. Slowing the loss of imaging outcomes in PD is relevant only if these imaging changes ultimately result in meaningful, measurable, and persistent changes in clinical function in PD patients.

PRECLINICAL PARKINSON'S DISEASE

Neuroreceptor imaging studies provide a window into the preclinical period of PD, the time during which neurodegeneration has begun, but symptoms have not yet become manifest. Preclinical identification of affected subjects is particularly important if intervention exists that may prevent the progression of disease. The most extensive preclinical imaging data are from studies imaging patients with hemi-PD. In several imaging studies there is a significant reduction in putamen DAT or ^{18}F-DOPA uptake of about 25–30% in the "presymptomatic" striatum in these patients who are known to progress to bilateral disease (11,65,66).

Progression studies also elucidate the preclinical period of PD. For example, given the assumption that progression is linear, it is possible to back extrapolate from sequential imaging data and reported symptom duration to estimate the level of reduction in dopaminergic activity at symptom onset and the duration of the preclinical phase of PD (Fig. 3). Data from longitudinal imaging studies using both ^{18}F-DOPA and DAT imaging have been remarkably consistent with estimated disease onset at 70–75% of normal dopaminergic activity and a preclinical phase of 4–8 years (99,102). Interestingly these data are consistent with estimates of duration of the preclinical phase from pathology studies of 4.7 years derived from cross-sectional data (111). While the data available to calculate estimates of the preclinical phase must be viewed as preliminary, data acquired using different imaging methods measuring different components

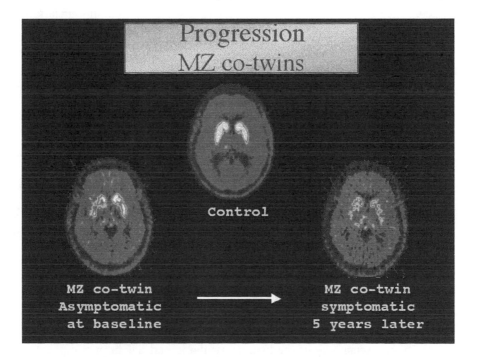

FIGURE 3   Presymptomatic loss of ^{18}F-DOPA in the asymptomatic co-twin of a PD patient. Note that the asymptomatic co-twin shows mild reduction in ^{18}F-DOPA at baseline that has worsened abnormality at 5-year follow-up associated with onset of symptoms. (Courtesy of D. Brooks, London, UK.) (See color insert.)

of the dopaminergic system and data from an independent pathology study suggest a relatively brief preclinical phase of less than a decade for PD. These data influence our understanding of disease etiology and development of strategies for disease screening and treatment. For example, if preclinical disease is relatively short, repetitive screening might be required to identify affected individuals in an at-risk population. Furthermore, as potential preventive or restorative therapies are developed, these treatments might be directed to the time period from onset of degeneration to onset of symptoms.

Other studies of the pre-clinical period have focused on potential at-risk individuals for PD such as family members or unaffected twins of PD patients. In studies of familial PD in several well-characterized kindreds 11 of 32 asymptomatic relatives were found to have reduced ^{18}F-DOPA uptake, and three of these subjects subsequently developed symptomatic PD (112). Several asymptomatic co-twins who also showed a reduction in ^{18}F-DOPA activity later developed symptoms of PD (Fig. 3), although the concordance rate for monozygotic and dyzygotic twins remains uncertain (113). Sporadic cases also have been reported of individuals imaged as presumed healthy subjects with mildly abnormal ^{18}F-DOPA uptake who later developed definite PD (114). Preclinical identification of subjects with PD forces us to reexamine our clinical definitions of disease. The recent identification of genes that confer the PD phenotype in familial PD will provide an opportunity to evaluate an at-risk population both clinically and with sequential imaging studies (115,116). As additional genetic markers are discovered, imaging will play an essential role in assessing neurodegeneration and possibly in redefining clinical disease onset.

FUTURE DIRECTIONS

Neuroimaging has provided key insights into the natural history of PD and has become a necessary if not sufficient test to assess potential new disease-modifying therapies for PD. While this review has focused on presynaptic dopamine ligands, several additional directions for imaging in PD have emerged or are under active study. Several postsynaptic dopamine imaging ligands have been used to study the postsynaptic dopaminergic receptors in PD (117–119), although quantitative information has been limited by relatively low sensitivity of the ligands available and has been complicated by uncertainty regarding endogenous dopamine binding to the receptor target. Postsynaptic dopamine receptor imaging studying dopamine release is a novel approach to using imaging to assess function particularly in studies involving cell-replacement therapy (120).

While dopamine degeneration is a crucial feature of PD, it is clear that there is widespread degeneration in the brain in PD and that many clinical manifestations of PD are likely not due to dopamine deficiency. Ligands for nondopaminergic targets have been and are being developed to investigate nondopaminergic manifestations of PD and to better understand the cause of PD and of dyskinesias. Some examples include recent data suggesting that uptake of a serotonin (5HT1A) receptor ligand 11C-Way100635 is reduced in the cortex of PD patients with associated depression, but not those without depression (121). Furthermore the reduction in 11C-Way100635 uptake correlates with tremor scores, suggesting that tremor may be related to serotonin deficiency. Ligands directed at the SP/neurokinin (NK1) receptor show reduction in thalamic uptake in dyskinetic but not in nondyskinetic PD patients, suggesting that this ligand may be a tool to help understand dyskinesias (122). In addition, imaging studies showed a reduction in acetylcholine activity in PD patients in cortex, and imaging of microglial activation has been demonstrated in cortex in Alzheimer's disease, and this approach may also be useful to understand the underlying pathology in PD (123).

The role of brain imaging in PD will continue to expand as new imaging targets emerge and additional disease-modifying drugs are developed. As simpler tools to identify preclinical at-risk individuals become available, neuroreceptor imaging will be widely used to establish and monitor the onset and progression of disease. As treatments become available that target the mechanisms that initiate and subsequently promote the course of disease progression, precise information about an individual's neurochemical status will be essential to optimize clinical management.

REFERENCES

1. OA Petroff, RH Mattson, DL Rothman. Proton MRS: GABA and glutamate. Adv Neurol 83:261–271, 2000.
2. F Fazekas, F Barkhof, M Filippi, R Grossman, D Li, W McDonald, H McFarland, D Paty, J Simon, J Wolinsky, D Miller. The contribution of magnetic resonance imaging to the diagnosis of multiple sclerosis. Neurology 53:448–456, 1999.
3. A Baird, S Warach. Imaging developing brain infarction. Curr Opin Neurol 12:65–71, 1999.
4. M Phelps. Positron emission tomography (PET). In: J Mazziota, S Gilman, eds. Clinical brain imaging: Principles and Applications. F.A. Davis: 1992, pp. 71–107.
5. N Lassen, S Holm. Single photon emission computerized tomography (SPECT). In: J Mazziota, S Gilman, eds. Clinical Brain Imaging: Principles and Applications. Philadelphia: F.A. Davis, 1992, pp 108–134.

6. D Eidelberg, C Edward. Functional brain imaging of movement disorders. Neurol Res 22:305–312, 2000.
7. K Leenders, A Antonini. PET 18F-fluorodopa (FD) uptake and disease progression in Parkinson's disease. Neurology 45:A220, 1995.
8. DJ Brooks. Advances in imaging Parkinson's disease. Curr Opin Neurol 10:327–331, 1997.
9. D Eidelberg, J Moeller, M Ishikawa, V Dhawan, P Spetsieris, T Chaly, A Belakhlef, F Mandel, S Przedborski, S Fahn. Early differential diagnosis of Parkinson's disease with 18F-fluorodeoxyglucose and positron emission tomography. Neurology 45:2005, 1995.
10. P Piccini, DJ Brooks. Etiology of Parkinson's disease: contributions from 18F-DOPA positron emission tomography. Adv Neurol 80:227–231, 1999.
11. G Sawle, E Playford, D Burn, V Cunnigham, D Brooks. Separating Parkinson's disease from normality: discriminant function analysis of [18F] dopa PET data. Arch Neurol 51:237–243, 1994.
12. B Snow, I Tooyama, E McGeer, D Calne. Human positron emission tomographic [18F] fluorodopa studies correlate with dopamine cell counts and levels. Ann Neurol 34:324–330, 1993.
13. KA Frey, RA Koeppe, MR Kilbourn, TM Vander Borght, RL Albin, S Gilman, DE Kuhl. Presynaptic monoaminergic vesicles in Parkinson's disease and normal aging. Ann Neurol 40:873–884, 1996.
14. CS Lee, A Samii, V Sossi, TJ Ruth, M Schulzer, JE Holden, J Wudel, PK Pal, R de la Fuente-Fernandez, DB Calne, AJ Stoessl. In vivo positron emission tomographic evidence for compensatory changes in presynaptic dopaminergic nerve terminals in Parkinson's disease. Ann Neurol 47:493–503, 2000.
15. K Frey, R Koeppe, M Kilbourn. Imaging the vesicular monoamine transporter. Adv Neurol 86:237–247, 2001.
16. S Asenbaum, T Brucke, W Pirker, I Podreka, P Angelberger, S Wenger, C Wober, C Muller, L Deecke. Imaging of dopamine transporters with iodine-123-B-CIT and SPECT in Parkinson's disease. J Nucl Med 38:1–6, 1997.
17. J Booij, G Tissingh, GJ Boer, JD Speelman, JC Stoof, AG Janssen, EC Wolters, EA van Royen. [^{123}I]FP-CIT SPECT shows a pronounced decline of striatal dopamine transporter labelling in early and advanced Parkinson's disease. J Neurol Neurosurg Psychiatry 62:133–140, 1997.
18. AJ Fischman, AA Bonab, JW Babich, EP Palmer, NM Alpert, DR Elmaleh, RJ Callahan, SA Barrow, W Graham, PC Meltzer, RN Hanson, BK Madras. Rapid detection of Parkinson's disease by SPECT with altropane: a selective ligand for dopamine transporters. Synapse 29:128–141, 1998.
19. RB Innis, JP Seibyl, BE Scanley, M Laruelle, A Abi-Dargham, E Wallace, RM Baldwin, Y Zea-Ponce, S Zoghbi, S Wang, et al. Single photon emission computed tomographic imaging demonstrates loss of striatal dopamine transporters in Parkinson disease. Proc Natl Acad Sci USA 90:11965–11969, 1993.
20. JP Seibyl, KL Marek, D Quinlan, K Sheff, S Zoghbi, Y Zea-Ponce, RM Baldwin, B Fussell, EO Smith, DS Charney, et al. Decreased single-photon

emission computed tomographic [123I]beta-CIT striatal uptake correlates with symptom severity in Parkinson's disease. Ann Neurol 38:589–598, 1995.

21. K Tatsch, J Schwarz, P Mosley, R Linker, O Poglarell, W Oertel, R Fieber, K Hahn, H Kung. Relationship between clinical features of Parkinson's disease and presynaptic dopamine transporter binding assessed with [123I]IPT and single-photon emission tomography. Eur J Nucl Med 24:415–421, 1997.

22. WS Huang, SZ Lin, JC Lin, SP Wey, G Ting, RS Liu. Evaluation of early-stage Parkinson's disease with 99mTc-TRODAT-1 imaging. J Nucl Med 42:1303–1308, 2001.

23. S Lehericy, JP Brandel, EC Hirsch, P Anglade, J Villares, D Scherman, C Duyckaerts, F Javoy-Agid, Y Agid. Monoamine vesicular uptake sites in patients with Parkinson's disease and Alzheimer's disease, as measured by tritiated dihydrotetrabenazine autoradiography. Brain Res 659:1–9, 1994.

24. M Kaufman, B Madras. Severe depletion of cocaine recognition sites associated with the dopamine transporter in Parkinson's diseased striatum. Synapse 9:43–49, 1991.

25. HB Niznik, EF Fogel, FF Fassos, P Seeman. The dopamine transporter is absent in Parkinsonian putamen and reduced in the caudate nucleus. J Neurochem 56:192–198, 1991.

26. K Marek. Dopaminergic dysfunction in parkinsonism: new lessons from imaging. Neuroscientist 5:333–339, 1999.

27. KA Frey, RA Koeppe, MR Kilbourn, Imaging the vesicular monoamine transporter. Adv Neurol 86:237–247, 2001.

28. DJ Brooks. Positron emission tomography studies in movement disorders. Neurosurg Clin North Am 9:263–282, 1998.

29. CH van Dyck, JP Seibyl, RT Malison, M Laruelle, SS Zoghbi, RM Baldwin, RB Innis. Age-related decline in dopamine transporters: analysis of striatal subregions, nonlinear effects, and hemispheric asymmetries. Am J Geriatric Psychiatry 10:36–43, 2002.

30. BD Pate, T Kawamata, T Yamada, EG McGeer, KA Hewitt, BJ Snow, TJ Ruth, DB Calne. Correlation of striatal fluorodopa uptake in the MPTP monkey with dopaminergic indices. Ann Neurol 34:331–338, 1993.

31. Y Liu, RH Edwards. The role of vesicular transport proteins in synaptic transmission and neural degeneration. Annu Rev Neurosci 20:125–156, 1997.

32. T Vander Borght, M Kilbourn, T Desmond, D Kuhl, K Frey. The vesicular monoamine transporter is not regulated by dopaminergic drug treatments. Eur J Pharmacol 294:577–583, 1995.

33. MR Kilbourn, K Kuszpit, P Sherman. Rapid and differential losses of in vivo dopamine transporter (DAT) and vesicular monoamine transporter (VMAT2) radioligand binding in MPTP-treated mice. Synapse 35:250–255, 2000.

34. E Bezard, S Dovero, C Prunier, P Ravenscroft, S Chalon, D Guilloteau, AR Crossman, B Bioulac, JM Brotchie, CE Gross. Relationship between the appearance of symptoms and the level of nigrostriatal degeneration in a progressive 1-methyl-4-phenyl-1,2,3,6 tetrahydropyridine-lesioned macaque model of Parkinson's disease. J Neurosci 21:6853–6861, 2001.

35. JD Elsworth, MS al-Tikriti, JR Sladek, JR Taylor, RB Innis, D. Redmond, RH Roth. Novel radioligands for the dopamine transporter demonstrate the presence of intrastriatal nigral grafts in the MPTP-treated monkey: correlation with improved behavioral function. Exp Neurol 126:300–304, 1994.

36. J Boja, A Patel, F Carroll, M Rahman, A Philip, A Lewin, T Kopajitic, M Kuhan. [125I]-RTI-55: a potent ligand for dopamine transporters. Eur J Pharmacol 194:133–194, 1991.

37. A Brouard, D Pelaprat, JW Boja, FI Carroll, M Vial, MJ Kuhar, W Rostene. Potent cocaine analogs inhibit [3H]dopamine uptake in rat mesencephalic cells in primary cultures: pharmacological selectivity of embryonic cocaine sites. Brain Res Dev Brain Res 75:13–17, 1993.

38. CL Coulter, HK Happe, DA Bergman, LC Murrin. Localization and quantification of the dopamine transporter: comparison of [3H]WIN 35,428 and [125I]RTI-55. Brain Res 690:217–224, 1995.

39. M Fujita, S Shimada, K Fukuchi, M Tohyama, T Nishimura. Distribution of cocaine recognition sites in rat brain: in vitro and ex vivo autoradiography with [125I]RTI-55. J Chem Neuroanat 7:13–23, 1994.

40. JK Staley, M Basile, DD Flynn, DC Mash. Visualizing dopamine and serotonin transporters in the human brain with the potent cocaine analogue [125I]RTI-55: in vitro binding and autoradiographic characterization. J Neurochem 62:549–556, 1994.

41. ND Volkow, SJ Gatley, JS Fowler, R Chen, J Logan, SL Dewey, YS Ding, N Pappas, P King, RR MacGregor, et al. Long-lasting inhibition of in vivo cocaine binding to dopamine transporters by 3 beta-(4-iodophenyl)tropane-2-carboxylic acid methyl ester: RTI-55 or beta CIT. Synapse 19:206–211, 1995.

42. A Abi-Dargham, MS Gandelman, GA DeErausquin, Y Zea-Ponce, SS Zoghbi, RM Baldwin, M Laruelle, DS Charney, PB Hoffer, JL Neumeyer, RB Innis. SPECT imaging of dopamine transporters in human brain with iodine-123-fluoroalkyl analogs of beta-CIT. J Nucl Med 37:1129–1133, 1996.

43. M Laruelle, E Wallace, JP Seibyl, RM Baldwin, Y Zea-Ponce, SS Zoghbi, JL Neumeyer, DS Charney, PB Hoffer, RB Innis. Graphical, kinetic, and equilibrium analyses of in vivo [123I] beta-CIT binding to dopamine transporters in healthy human subjects. J Cereb Blood Flow Metab 14:982–994, 1994.

44. J Seibyl, K Marek, K Sheff, R Innis. Within-subject comparison of [123IFP-CIT and [123I]B-CIT for SPECT imaging of dopamine transporters in Parkinson's disease. Neurology 46:A456, 1996.

45. MP Kung, DA Stevenson, K Plossl, SK Meegalla, A Beckwith, WD Essman, M Mu, I Lucki, HF Kung. [99mTc]TRODAT-1: a novel technetium-99m complex as a dopamine transporter imaging agent. Eur J Nucl Med 24:372–380, 1997.

46. JJ Frost, AJ Rosier, SG Reich, JS Smith, MD Ehlers, SH Snyder, HT Ravert, RF Dannals. Positron emission tomography imaging of the dopamine transporter with 11C WIN 35,428 reveals marked decline in mild Parkinson's disease. Ann Neurol 34:423–431, 1993.

47. JO Rinne, A Laihinen, K Nagren, H Ruottinen, U Ruotsalainen, UK Rinne. PET examination of the monoamine transporter with [11C]beta-CIT and [11C]beta-CFT in early Parkinson's disease. Synapse 21:97–103, 1995.

48. G Rosati, E Granieri, L Pinna, I Aiello, R Tola, P De Bastiani, A Pirisi, MC Devoto. The risk of Parkinson disease in Mediterranean people. Neurology 30:250–255, 1980.

49. R Maycux, K Marder, LJ Cote, J Denaro, N Hemenegildo, H Mejia, MX Tang, R Lantigua, D Wilder, B Gurland, et al. The frequency of idiopathic Parkinson's disease by age, ethnic group, and sex in northern Manhattan, 1988–1993. Am J Epidcmiol 142:820 827, 1995.

50. R Martilla, U Rinne, Epidemiology of Parkinson's disease in Finland. Acta Neurol Scand 43 (suppl 33):9–61, 1967.

51. A Rajput, B Rodzilsky, A Rajput. Accuracy of clinical diagnosis of Parkinsonism—a prospective study. Can J Neurol Sci 18:275–278, 1991.

52. AJ Hughes, SE Daniel, L Kilford, AJ Lees, Accuracy of clinical diagnosis of idiopathic Parkinson's disease: a clinico-pathological study of 100 cases. J Neurol Neurosurg Psychiatry 55:1142–1146, 1992.

53. N Quinn. Parkinsonism—recognition and differential diagnosis. Bmj 310:447–452, 1995.

54. J Meara, BK Bhowmick, P Hobson, Accuracy of diagnosis in patients with presumed Parkinson's disease. Age Ageing 28:99–102, 1999.

55. AJ Hughes, Y Ben-Shlomo, SE Daniel, AJ Lees. What features improve the accuracy of clinical diagnosis in Parkinson's disease: a clinicopathologic study. Neurology 42:1142–1146, 1992.

56. M Richards, Y Stern, R Mayeux. Subtle extrapyramidal signs can predict the development of dementia in elderly individuals. Neurology 43:2184–2188, 1993.

57. DA Bennett, LA Beckett, AM Murray, KM Shannon, CG Goetz, DM Pilgrim, DA Evans. Prevalence of parkinsonian signs and associated mortality in a community population of older people. N Engl J Med 334:71–76, 1996.

58. J Jankovic, AH Rajput, MP McDermott, DP Perl. The evolution of diagnosis in early Parkinson disease. Parkinson Study Group. Arch Neurol 57:369–372, 2000.

59. AJ Hughes, SE Daniel, Y Ben-Shlomo, AJ Lees. The accuracy of diagnosis of parkinsonian syndromes in a specialist movement disorder service. Brain 125:861–870, 2002.

60. DJ Brooks. Functional imaging in relation to parkinsonian syndromes. J Neurol Sci 115:1–17, 1993.

61. SJ Kish, K Shannak, O Hornykiewicz. Uneven pattern of dopamine loss in the striatum of patients with idiopathic Parkinson's disease. N Engl J Med 318:876–880, 1988.

62. PL McGeer, S Itagaki, H Akiyama, EG McGeer. Rate of cell death in parkinsonism indicates active neuropathological process. Ann Neurol 24.574–576, 1988.

63. J Fearnley, A Lees. Ageing and Parkinson's disease: substantia nigra regional selectivity. Brain 114:2283–2301, 1991.

64. P Morrish, G Sawlw, D Brooks, Clinical and [18F]dopa PET findings in early Parkinson's disease. J Neurol Neurosurg Psych 59:597–600, 1995.

65. K Marek, J Seibyl, B Scanley, M Laruelle, A Abi-Dargham, E Wallace, R Baldwin, Y Zea-Ponce, S Zoghbi, S Wang, G Y, J Neumeyer, D Charney, P Hoffer, R Innis. [I 123]CIT Spect imaging demonstrates bilateral loss of dopamine transporters in hemi Parkinson's disease. Neurology 46:231–237, 1996.

66. M Guttman, J Burkholder, S Kish, D Hussey, A Wilson, J DaSilva, S Houle. [11C]RTI-32 PET studies of the dopamine transporter in early dopa-naive Parkinson's disease. Neurology 48:1578–1583, 1997.

67. S Asenbaum, W Pirker, P Angelberger, G Bencsits, M Pruckmayer, T Brucke. [123I]beta-CIT and SPECT in essential tremor and Parkinson's disease. J Neural Transm 105:1213–1228, 1998.

68. TS Benamer, J Patterson, DG Grosset, J Booij, K de Bruin, E van Royen, JD Speelman, MH Horstink, HJ Sips, RA Dierckx, J Versijpt, D Decoo, C Van Der Linden, DM Hadley, M Doder, AJ Lees, DC Costa, S Gacinovic, WH Oertel, O Pogarell, H Hoeffken, K Joseph, K Tatsch, J Schwarz, V Ries. Accurate differentiation of parkinsonism and essential tremor using visual assessment of [123I]-FP-CIT SPECT imaging: the [123I]-FP CIT study group. Mov Disord 15:503–510, 2000.

69. Parkinson Study Group. A multicenter assessment of dopamine transporter imaging with Dopascan™/SPECT in parkinsonism. Neurology 55:1540–1547, 2000.

70. HT Benamer, J Patterson, DJ Wyper, DM Hadley, GJ Macphee, DG Grosset. Correlation of Parkinson's disease severity and duration with 123I-FP-CIT SPECT striatal uptake. Mov Disord 15:692–698, 2000.

71. FJ Vingerhoets, M Schulzer, DB Calne, BJ Snow. Which clinical sign of Parkinson's disease best reflects the nigrostriatal lesion? Ann Neurol 41:58–64, 1997.

72. MM Hoehn, MD Yahr. Parkinsonism: onset, progression and mortality. Neurology 17:427–442, 1967.

73. W Gerschlager, G Bencsits, W Pirker, BR Bloem, S Asenbaum, D Prayer, JC Zijlmans, M Hoffmann, T Brucke. [123I]beta-CIT SPECT distinguishes vascular parkinsonism from Parkinson's disease. Mov Disord 17:518–523, 2002.

74. S Goldstein, JH Friedman, R Innis, J Seibyl, K Marel. Hemi-parkinsonism due to a midbrain arteriovenous malformation: dopamine transporter imaging. Mov Disord 16:350–353, 2001.

75. T Brucke, S Asenbaum, W Pirker, S Djamshidian, S Wenger, C Wober, C Muller, I Podreka. Measurement of the dopaminergic degeneration in Parkinson's disease with [123I] beta-CIT and SPECT. Correlation with clinical findings and comparison with multiple system atrophy and progressive supranuclear palsy. J Neural Transm Suppl 50:9–24, 1997.

76. D Brooks, V Ibanez, G Sawle, E Playford, N Quinn, C Mathias, A Lees, C Marsden, R Bannister, R Frackowiak. Differing patterns of striatal 18F-DOPA uptake in Parkinson's disease, multiple system atrophy and progressive supranuclear palsy. Ann Neurol 28:547–555, 1990.

77. A Varrone, KL Marek, D Jennings, RB Innis, JP Seibyl. [(123)I]beta-CIT SPECT imaging demonstrates reduced density of striatal dopamine transporters in Parkinson's disease and multiple system atrophy. Mov Disord 16:1023–1032, 2001.

78. D Eidelberg, V Dhawan. Can imaging distinguish PSP from other neurodegenerative disorders? Neurology 58:997–998, 2002.

79. A Antonini, K Kazumata, A Feigin, F Mandel, V Dhawan, C Margouleff, D Eidelberg. Differential diagnosis of parkinsonism with [18F]fluorodeoxyglucose and PET. Mov Disord 13:268–274, 1998.

80. Parkinson Study Group. Effects of tocopherol and deprenyl on the progression of disability in early Parkinson's disease. N Engl J Med 328:176–183, 1993.

81. Parkinson Study Group. Pramipexole vs levodopa as initial therapy for Parkinson's disease. JAMA 284:1931–1938, 2000.

82. O Rascol, D Brooks, A Korczyn, P De Deyn, C Clarke, A Lang. A five-year study of the incidence of dyskinesia in patients with early Parkinson's disease who were treated with ropinirole or levodopa. N Engl J Med 342:1484–1491, 2000.

83. RA Hauser, WC Koller, JP Hubble, T Malapira, K Busenbark, CW Olanow. Time course of loss of clinical benefit following withdrawal of levodopa/carbidopa and bromocriptine in early Parkinson's disease. Mov Disord 15:485–489, 2000.

84. S Fahn. Parkinson disease, the effect of levodopa, and the ELLDOPA trial. Arch Neurol 56:529–535, 1999.

85. K Marek, R Innis, C van Dyck, B Fussell, M Early, S Eberly, D Oakes, J Seibyl. [123I]beta-CIT SPECT imaging assessment of the rate of Parkinson's disease progression. Neurology 57:2089–2094, 2001.

86. P Morrish, J Rakshi, D Bailey, G Sawle, D Brooks. Measuring the rate of progression and estimating the preclinical period of Parkinson's disease with [18F]dopa PET. J Neurol Neurosurg Psychiatry 64:314–319, 1998.

87. E Nurmi, H Ruottinen, V Kaasinen, J Bergman, M Haaparanta, O Solin, J Rinne. Progression in parkinson's disease: a positron emission tomography study with a dopamine transporter ligand [18F]CFT. Ann Neurol 47:804–808, 2000.

88. E Nurmi, H Ruottinen, J Bergman, M Haaparanta, O Solin, P Sonninen, J Rinne. Rate of progression in Parkinson's disease: A 6-[18F]fluoro-L-dopa PET study. Mov Disord 16:608–615, 2001.

89. W Pirker, S Djamshidian, S Asenbaum, W Gerschlager, G Tribl, M Hoffman, T Bruecke. Progression of dopaminergic degeneration in Parkinson's disease and atypical parkinsonism: a longitudinal β-CIT SPECT study. Mov Disord 17:45–53, 2002.

90. G Sawle, R Myers. The role of positron emission tomography in the asesment of human transplantation. Trends Neurosci 16:260–264, 1993.

91. T Nakamura, V Dhawan, T Chaly, M Fukuda, Y Ma, R Breeze, P Greene, S Fahn, C Freed, D Eidelberg. Blinded positron emission tomography study of dopamine cell implantation for Parkinson's disease. Ann Neurol 50:181–187, 2001.

92. CW Olanow, JH Kordower, TB Freeman. Fetal nigral transplantation as a therapy for Parkinson's disease. Trends Neurosci 19:102–109, 1996.

93. DJ Brooks. Monitoring neuroprotection and restorative therapies in Parkinson's disease with PET. J Neural Transm Suppl 60:125–137, 2000.

94. VG De Gruttola, P Clax, DL DeMets, GJ Downing, SS Ellenberg, L Friedman, MH Gail, R Prentice, J Wittes, SL Zeger. Considerations in the evaluation of surrogate endpoints in clinical trials. summary of a National Institutes of Health workshop. Control Clin Trials 22(5):485–502, 2001.

95. JP Seibyl, K Marek, D Jennings, L Powe, Nil-A Trial Group. 123 β-CIT SPECT imaging assessment of Parkinson disease patients treated for six months with a neuroimmunoplilin ligand, Nil A. Neurology 58(suppl3):A203, 2002

96. GL Chan, JE Holden, AJ Stoessl, A Samii, DJ Doudet, T Dobko, KS Morrison, M Adam, M Schulzer, DB Calne, TJ Ruth. Reproducibility studies with 11C-DTBZ, a monoamine vesicular transporter inhibitor in healthy human subjects. J Nucl Med 40:283–289, 1999.

97. R Ceravolo, P Piccini, DL Bailey, KM Jorga, H Bryson, DJ Brooks. 18F-Dopa PET evidence that tolcapone acts as a central COMT inhibitor in Parkinson's disease. Synapse 43:201–207, 2002.

98. MJ Zigmond, ED Abercrombie, TW Berger, AA Grace, EM Stricker. Compensations after lesions of central dopaminergic neurons: some clinical and basic implications. Trends Neurosci 13:290–296, 1990.

99. PK Morrish, GV Sawle, DJ Brooks. An [18F]Dopa-PET and clinical study of the rate of progression in Parkinson's disease. Brain 119 (Pt 2):585–591, 1996.

100. E Nurmi, J Bergman, O Eskola, O Solin, SM Hinkka, P Sonninen, and JO Rinne. Reproducibility and effect of levodopa on dopamine transporter function measurements: a [18F]CFT PET study. J Cereb Blood Flow Metab 20:1604–1609, 2000.

101. R Innis, K Marek, K Sheff, S Zogbi, J Castrnuovo, A Feigin, J Seibyl. Treatment with carbidopa/levodopa and selegiline on striatal transporter imaging with [123I]B-CIT. Mov Disord 14:436–443, 1999.

102. Parkinson Study Group. Dopamine transporter brain imaging to assess the effects of Pramipexole vs levodopa on Parkinson disease progression. JAMA 287:1653–1661, 2002.

103. JE Ahlskog, RJ Uitti, MK O'Connor, DM Maraganore, JY Matsumoto, KF Stark, MF Turk, OL Burnett. The effect of dopamine agonist therapy on dopamine transporter imaging in Parkinson's disease. Mov Disord 14:940–946, 1999.

104. M Guttman, D Stewart, D Hussey, A Wilson, S Houle, S Kish. Influence of L-dopa and pramipexole on striatal dopamine transporter in early PD. Neurology 56:1559–1564, 2001.
105. N Turjanski, AJ Lees, DJ Brooks. Striatal dopaminergic function in restless legs syndrome: 18F-dopa and 11C-raclopride PET studies. Neurology 52:932–937, 1999.
106. AC Maroney, JP Finn, D Bozyczko-Coyne, TM O'Kane, NT Neff, AM Tolkovsky, DS Park, CY Yan, CM Troy, LA Greene. CEP-1347 (KT7515), an inhibitor of JNK activation, rescues sympathetic neurons and neuronally differentiated PC12 cells from death evoked by three distinct insults. J Neurochem 73:1901–1912, 1999.
107. WG Tatton, RM Chalmers-Redman, WJ Ju, M Mammen, GW Carlile, AW Pong, NA Tatton. Propargylamines induce antiapoptotic new protein synthesis in serum- and nerve growth factor (NGF)-withdrawn, NGF-differentiated PC-12 cells. J Pharmacol Exp Ther 301:753–764, 2002.
108. CW Shults, AH Schapira. A cue to queue for CoQ? Neurology 57:375–376, 2001.
109. A Whone, P Remy, MR Davis, M Sabolek, C Nahmias, AJ Stoessl, RL Watts, DJ Brooks, The REAL-PET study: slower progression in early Parkinson's disease treated with ropinirole compared with L-Dopa. Neurology 58(suppl 3):A82–A83, 2002.
110. J Nutt, N Holford. The response of levodopa in Parkinson's disease: Imposing pharmacological law and order. Ann Neurol 39:561–573, 1996.
111. J Fearnley, A Lees. Striatonigral degeneration: a clinicopathological study. Brain 113:1823–1842, 1990.
112. P Piccini, PK Morrish, N Turjanski, GV Sawle, DJ Burn, RA Weeks, MH Mark, DM Maraganore, AJ Lees, DJ Brooks. Dopaminergic function in familial Parkinson's disease: a clinical and 18F-dopa positron emission tomography study. Ann Neurol 41:222–229, 1997.
113. DJ Burn, MH Mark, ED Playford, DM Maraganore, TR Zimmerman, Jr., RC Duvoisin, AE Harding, CD Marsden, DJ Brooks. Parkinson's disease in twins studied with 18F dopa and positron emission tomography. Neurology 42:1894–1900, 1992.
114. BJ Snow, RF Peppard, M Guttman, DB Calne. Positron emission tomographic scanning demonstrates a presynaptic dopaminergic lesion in Lytico-Bodig. Arch Neurol 47:870–874, 1990.
115. DJ Nicholl, JR Vaughan, NL Khan, SL Ho, DE Aldous, S Lincoln, M Farrer, JD Gayton, MB Davis, P Piccini, SE Daniel, GG Lennox, DJ Brooks, AC Williams, NW Wood. Two large British kindreds with familial Parkinson's disease: a clinico- pathological and genetic study. Brain 125:44–57, 2002.
116. R Kruger, W Kuhn, KL Leenders, R Sprengelmeyer, T Muller, D Woitalla, AT Portman, RP Maguire, L Veenma, U Schroder, L Schols, JT Epplen, O Riess, H Przuntek. Familial parkinsonism with synuclein pathology: clinical and PET studies of A30P mutation carriers. Neurology 56:1355–1362, 2001.

117. D Brooks, V Ibanez, G Sawle, E Playford, N Quinn, C Mathias, A Lees, C Marsden, R Bannister, R Frackowiak. Striatal D2 receptor status in patients with Parkinson's disease, striatonigral degeneration, and progressive supranuclear palsy, measured with 11C-raclopride and positron emission tomography. Ann Neurol 31:184–192, 1992.

118. A Antonini, J Schwarz, W Oertel, H Beer, U Madejo, K Leenders. [11C]Raclopride and positron emission tomography in previously untreated patients with Parkinson's disease: influence of L-dopa and lisuride therapy on striatal dopamine D2-receptors. Neurology 44:1325–1329, 1994.

119. K Tatsch, J Schwarz, W Oertel, C Kirsch. Dopamine D2 receptor imaging with I-123 IBZM SPECT to differentiate idiopathic from other parkinson syndromes (abstr). J Nucl Med 33:917–918, 1992.

120. P Piccini, DJ Brooks, A Bjorklund, RN Gunn, PM Grasby, O Rimoldi, P Brundin, P Hagell, S Rehncrona, H Widner, O Lindvall. Dopamine release from nigral transplants visualized in vivo in a Parkinson's patient. Nat Neurosci 2:1137–1140, 1999.

121. M Doder, E Rabiner, N Turjanski, A Lees, D Brooks. Imaging serotonin HT 1A binding in non-depressed and depressed Parkinson's disease patients with 11C Way100635 PET. Neurology 54:A112, 2000.

122. A Whone, E Rabiner, Y Arahata, S Luthra, R Hargreaves, D Brooks. Reduced substance P binding in Parkinson's disease complicated by dyskinesias: an 18F-L829165 PET study. Neurology 58(suppl 3):A488–489, 2002.

123. A Cagnin, DJ Brooks, AM Kennedy, RN Gunn, R Myers, FE Turkheimer, T Jones, RB Banati. In-vivo measurement of activated microglia in dementia. Lancet 358:461–467, 2001.

9

Neuropathology of Parkinsonism

Dennis W. Dickson
Mayo Clinic, Jacksonville, Florida, U.S.A.

INTRODUCTION

The common denominator of virtually all disorders associated with clinical parkinsonism is neuronal loss in the substantia nigra, particularly of dopaminergic neurons in the pars compacta that project to the striatum (Fig. 1). The ventrolateral tier of neurons appears to be the most vulnerable in many parkinsonian disorders, and these tend to project heavily to the putamen (1). The more medial groups of neurons send projections to forebrain and medial temporal lobe and are less affected. The dorsal tier of neurons may be most vulnerable to neuronal loss associated with aging (1).

PARKINSON'S DISEASE

The clinical features of Parkinson's disease (PD) include bradykinesia, rigidity, tremor, postural instability, autonomic dysfunction, and bradyphrenia. The most frequent pathological substrate for PD is Lewy body disease (LBD) (2). Some cases of otherwise clinically typical PD have other disorders, such as progressive supranuclear palsy (PSP), multiple system atrophy (MSA), or vascular disease, but these are uncommon, especially

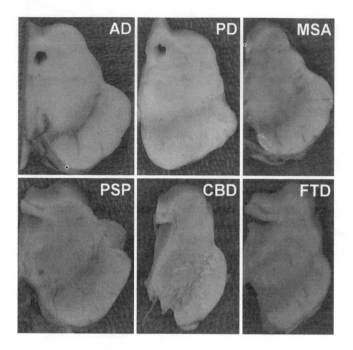

FIGURE 1 Midbrain sections from a variety of disorders associated with Parkinsonism, including Parkinson's disease (PD), multiple system atrophy (MSA), progressive supranuclear palsy (PSP), corticobasal degeneration (CBD), and frontotemporal dementia (FTD) and a disorder not associated with parkinsonism, Alzheimer's disease (AD). Note loss of pigment in the substantia nigra in all disorders except AD.

when the clinical diagnosis is made after several years of clinical follow-up (3,4). The diagnostic accuracy rate approached 90% in some recent series (5).

The brain is usually grossly normal when viewed from the outer surface. There may be mild frontal atrophy is some cases, but this is variable. The most obvious morphological change in PD is only visible after the brainstem is sectioned. The loss of neuromelanin pigmentation in the substantia nigra and locus ceruleus is usually grossly apparent and may be associated with a rust color in the pars reticulata, which correlates with increased iron deposition in the tissue. Histologically, there is neuronal loss in the substantia nigra pars compacta along with compensatory astrocytic and microglial proliferation. While biochemically there is loss of dopaminergic termini in the striatum, the striatum is histologically unremarkable. In the substantia nigra and locus ceruleus neuromelanin pigment may be found in the cytoplasm of macrophages. Less common are neurons undergoing neuronophagia (i.e., phagocytosis by macrophages). Hyaline cytoplasmic inclusions, so-called Lewy bodies (LBs), and less well-defined "pale bodies" are found in some of the residual neurons in the substantia nigra (Fig. 2). Similar pathology is found in the locus ceruleus, the dorsal motor nucleus of the vagus, as well as the basal forebrain (especially the basal nucleus of Meynert). The convexity neocortex usually does not have LBs, but the limbic cortex and the amygdala may be affected. Depending upon the age of the individual, varying degrees of Alzheimer type pathology may be detected, but if the person is not demented, this usually falls within the limits for that age. Some cases may have abundant senile plaques but few or no neurofibrillary tangles.

Lewy bodies are proteinaceous neuronal cytoplasmic inclusions (reviewed in Refs. 6 and 7). In some regions of the brain, such as the dorsal motor nucleus of the vagus, LBs tend to form within neuronal processes and are sometimes referred to as intraneuritic LBs. In most cases LBs are accompanied by a variable number of abnormal neuritic profiles, referred to as Lewy neurites. Lewy neurites were first described in the hippocampus (8), but they are also found in other regions of the brain, including the amygdala, cingulate gyrus, and temporal cortex. At the electron microscopic level, LBs are composed of densely aggregated

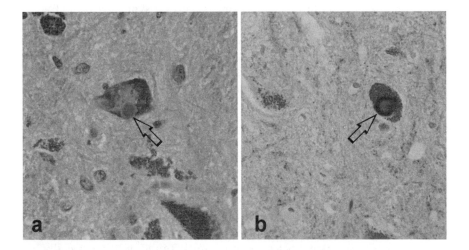

FIGURE 2   PD: Lewy bodies are hyaline inclusions visible with routine histological methods in pigmented neurons of the substantia nigra (arrow in a). They are immunostained with antibodies to synuclein (arrow in b).

filaments (9), and Lewy neurites also are filamentous, but they are usually not as densely packed (8).

Neurons that are most vulnerable to LBs include the monoaminergic neurons of the substantia nigra, locus ceruleus, and dorsal motor nucleus of the vagus, as well as cholinergic neurons in the basal forebrain. LBs are rarely detected in the basal ganglia or thalamus, but are common in the hypothalamus, especially the posterior and lateral hypothalamus, and the brainstem reticular formation. The oculomotor nuclear complex is also vulnerable. In the pons, the dorsal raphe and subpeduncular nuclei are often affected, but neurons of the pontine base are not. LBs have not been described in the cerebellar cortex. In the spinal cord, the neurons of the intermediolateral cell column are most vulnerable. LBs can be found in the autonomic ganglia, including submucosal ganglia of the esophagus.

While not usually numerous in typical PD, LBs can be found in cortical neurons, especially in the limbic lobe. Cortical LBs can be difficult to detect with routine histology, but they are visible with special staining techniques and are usually most numerous in small nonpyramidal neurons in lower cortical layers. Similar lesions in the substantia nigra are referred to as "pale bodies" or as "pre-Lewy bodies." Ultrastructural studies of cortical LBs demonstrate poorly organized filamentous structures similar to Lewy neurites.

The chemical composition of LBs has been inferred from immuno-histochemical studies. While antibodies to neurofilament were first shown to label LBs (10), ubiquitin (11) and more recently α-synuclein (12) (Fig. 2) antibodies are better markers for LBs, and α-synuclein appears to be the most specific marker currently available. Lewy neurites have the same immunoreactivity profile as LBs (13). Biochemical studies of purified LBs have not been accomplished, but evidence suggests that they may contain a mixture of proteins including neurofilament and α-synuclein (14–16).

DEMENTIA IN PD

Pathological findings considered to account for dementia in PD include severe pathology in monoaminergic and cholinergic nuclei that project to the cortex producing a "subcortical dementia" (39%), coexistent Alzhei-mer's disease (AD) (29%) and diffuse cortical LBs (26%) (17). The basal forebrain cholinergic system is the subcortical region most often implicated in dementia, and neurons in this region are damaged in both AD and LBD. Neuronal loss in the basal nucleus is consistently found in PD, especially PD with dementia (18). Cholinergic deficits are common in PD (19), and they may contribute to dementia in PD in those cases that do not have concurrent AD or cortical LBs.

While virtually all PD brains have a few cortical LBs (17), they are usually neither widespread nor numerous in PD patients who are not demented. Several recent studies have shown, however, that cortical LBs are numerous and widespread in PD with dementia (20–22) and that the density of cortical LBs and Lewy neurites, especially in the medial temporal lobe (23), correlates with the severity of dementia (24).

MULTIPLE SYSTEM ATROPHY

The term multiple system atrophy refers to a neurodegenerative disease characterized by parkinsonism, cerebellar ataxia, and autonomic dysfunction (25). The average age of onset is between 30 and 50 years, and the disease duration runs in the decades (25). There is no known genetic risk factor or genetic locus for MSA. The MSA brain shows varying degrees of atrophy of cerebellum, cerebellar peduncles, pons and medulla, as well as atrophy and discoloration of the posterolateral putamen and pigment loss in the substantia nigra. The histopathological findings include neuronal loss, gliosis, and microvacuolation, involving the putamen, substantia nigra, cerebellum, olivary nucleus, pontine base, and intermediolateral cell column of the spinal cord. White matter inevitably shows demyelination, with the brunt of the changes affecting white matter tracts in cerebellum and pons (Fig. 3).

Lantos and coworkers first described oligodendroglial inclusions in MSA and named them glial cytoplasmic inclusions (GCIs) (26). GCIs can be detected with silver stains, such as the Gallyas silver stain, but are best seen with antibodies to synuclein, where they appear as flame- or sickle-shaped inclusions in oligodendrocytes (Fig. 3). Like LBs, GCIs are also immunostained with antibodies to ubiquitin (26). At the ultrastructural level, GCIs are non–membrane-bound cytoplasmic inclusions composed of filaments (7–10 nm) and granular material that often coats the filaments, making precise measurements difficult (27). GCIs are specific for MSA and have not been found in other neurodegenerative diseases. In addition to GCIs, synuclein immunoreactive lesions are also detected in some neurons in MSA. Biochemical studies of synuclein in MSA have shown changes in its solubility (27).

NEUROPATHOLOGY OF PROGRESSIVE SUPRANUCLEAR PALSY

PSP, an atypical parkinsonian disorder associated with progressive axial rigidity, vertical gaze palsy, dysarthria, and dysphagia, was first described by Steele-Richardson-Olszewski (28). Frontal lobe syndrome and subcortical

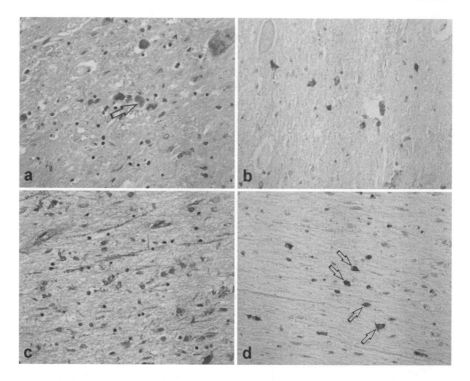

FIGURE 3   MSA: Substantia nigra neuronal loss in MSA is obvious in the cluster of pigment-laden macrophages (arrow in a), but neuronal inclusions are not present. Synuclein immunostaining of the substantia nigra shows many small inclusions in oligodendroglial cells (b). The white matter in the cerebellum shows marked myelin loss (Luxol fast blue stain for myelin) (c), and in the affected areas there are many synuclein-immunoreactive glial inclusions (arrows) (d).

dementia are present in some cases. In contrast to PD, gross examination of the brain often has distinctive features. Most cases have varying degrees of frontal atrophy that may involve the precentral gyrus. The midbrain, especially the midbrain tectum, and to a lesser extent the pons shows atrophy. The third ventricle and aqueduct of Sylvius may be dilated. The substantia nigra shows loss of pigment, while the locus ceruleus is often better preserved. The subthalamic nucleus is smaller than expected and may have a gray discoloration. The superior cerebellar peduncle and the hilus of the cerebellar dentate nucleus are usually atrophic and have a gray color due to myelinated fiber loss.

Microscopic findings include neuronal loss, gliosis, and neurofibrillary tangles (NFTs) affecting basal ganglia, diencephalon, and brainstem (Fig. 4). The nuclei most affected are the globus pallidus, subthalamic nucleus,

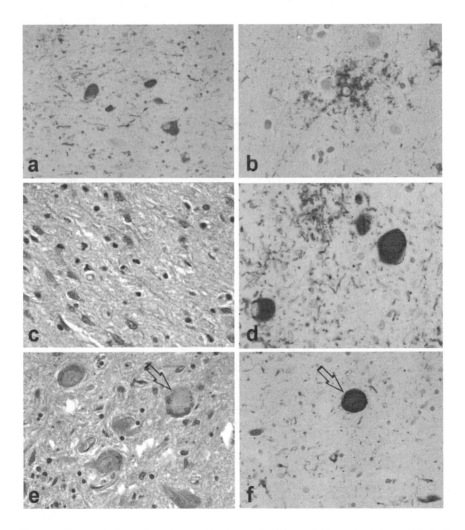

FIGURE 4   PSP: The basal ganglia have NFTs and threads (a) and tufted astrocytes (b) with tau immunostains. There is severe neuronal loss and gliosis in the subthalamic nucleus (c) and many NFT and glial lesions in the subthalamic nucleus (d). The substantia nigra has neuronal loss and NFTs in pigmented neurons (arrow) (e). The neurons in the substantia nigra have tau-immunoreactive NFTs (f).

and substantia nigra. The cerebral cortex is relatively spared, but lesions are common in the peri-Rolandic region. Recent studies suggest that cortical pathology may be more widespread in cases of PSP with atypical features, such as dementia (29). The limbic lobe is preserved in PSP.

The striatum and thalamus often have some degree of neuronal loss and gliosis, especially ventral anterior and lateral thalamic nuclei. The basal nucleus of Meynert usually has mild cell loss. The brainstem regions that are affected include the superior colliculus, periaqueductal gray matter, oculomotor nuclei, locus ceruleus, pontine nuclei, pontine tegmentum, vestibular nuclei, medullary tegmentum, and inferior olives. The cerebellar dentate nucleus is frequently affected and may show grumose degeneration, a type of neuronal degeneration associated with clusters of degenerating presynaptic terminals around dentate neurons. The dentatorubrothalamic pathway consistently shows fiber loss. The cerebellar cortex is preserved, but there may be mild Purkinje cell loss with scattered axonal torpedoes. The spinal cord is often affected, where neuronal inclusions can be found in anterior horn and intermediolateral cells.

Silver stains (e.g., Gallyas stain) or immunostaining for tau reveal NFTs in residual neurons in the basal ganglia, diencephalon, brainstem, and spinal cord. In addition to NFTs, special stains demonstrate argyrophilic, tau-positive inclusions in both astrocytes and oligodendrocytes. Tufted astrocytes are increasingly recognized as a characteristic feature of PSP and are commonly found in motor cortex and striatum (30) (Fig. 4). They are fibrillary lesions within astrocytes based upon double immunolabeling of tau and glial fibrillary acidic protein. Oligodendroglial lesions appear as argyrophilic and tau-positive perinuclear fibers, so-called coiled bodies, and they are often accompanied by thread-like processes in the white matter, especially in the diencephalon and cerebellar white matter.

NFTs in PSP are composed of 15 nm straight filaments (31). The abnormal filaments in glial cells in PSP also contain straight filaments. Biochemical studies also show differences between tau in AD and PSP. In AD the abnormal insoluble tau migrates as three major bands (68, 64, and 60 kDa) on Western blots, while in PSP it migrates as two bands (68 and 64 kDa) (32).

CORTICOBASAL DEGENERATION

Corticobasal degeneration (CBD) is only rarely mistaken for PD due to characteristic focal cortical signs that are the clinical hallmark of this disorder. Common clinical presentations include progressive asymmetrical rigidity and apraxia, progressive aphasia, and progressive frontal lobe dementia (33). Most cases also have some degree of parkinsonism, with bradykinesia, rigidity, and dystonia more common than tremor. Given the prominent cortical findings on clinical evaluations, it is not surprising that gross examination of the brain often reveals focal cortical atrophy. The atrophy may be severe and "knife-edge" in some cases or subtle and hardly noticeable in others. It may be asymmetrical. Atrophy is often most marked in the medial superior frontal gyrus, parasagittal pre- and postcentral gyri, and the superior parietal lobule. The temporal and occipital lobes are usually preserved. The brainstem does not have gross atrophy as in PSP, but pigment loss is common in the substantia nigra. In contrast to PSP, the superior cerebellar peduncle and the subthalamic nucleus are grossly normal.

The cerebral white matter in affected areas is often attenuated and may have a gray discoloration. The corpus callosum is sometimes thinned, and the frontal horn of the lateral ventricle is frequently dilated. The caudate head may have flattening. The thalamus may be smaller than usual.

Microscopic examination of atrophic cortical sections shows neuronal loss with superficial spongiosis, gliosis, and usually many achromatic or ballooned neurons. Ballooned neurons are swollen and vacuolated neurons found in the middle and lower cortical layers. They are variably positive with silver stains and tau immunohistochemistry, but intensely stained with immunohistochemistry for alpha-B-crystallin, a small heat shock protein, and for neurofilament (Fig. 5).

Cortical neurons in atrophic areas also have tau-immunoreactive lesions. In some neurons tau is densely packed into a small inclusion body, somewhat reminiscent of a Pick body or a small NFT. In other neurons, the filamentous inclusions are more dispersed and diffuse. As in PSP, neurofibrillary lesions in CBD are not detected well with most diagnostic silver stains and thioflavin fluorescent microscopy. Neurofibrillary lesions in brainstem monoaminergic nuclei, such as the locus ceruleus and substantia nigra, sometimes resemble globose NFT.

In addition to fibrillary lesions in perikarya of neurons, the neuropil of CBD invariably contains a large number of thread-like tau-immunoreactive processes. They are usually profuse in both gray and white matter, and this latter feature is an important attribute of CBD and a useful feature in differentiating it from other disorders (34).

The most characteristic tau-immunoreactive lesion in the cortex in CBD is an annular cluster of short, stubby processes with fuzzy outlines that may be highly suggestive of a neuritic plaque of AD (34) (Fig. 5). In contrast to AD plaques, they do not contain amyloid but rather tau-positive astrocytes and have been referred to as "astrocytic plaques." Astrocytic plaques differ from the tufted astrocytes seen in PSP, and the two lesions do

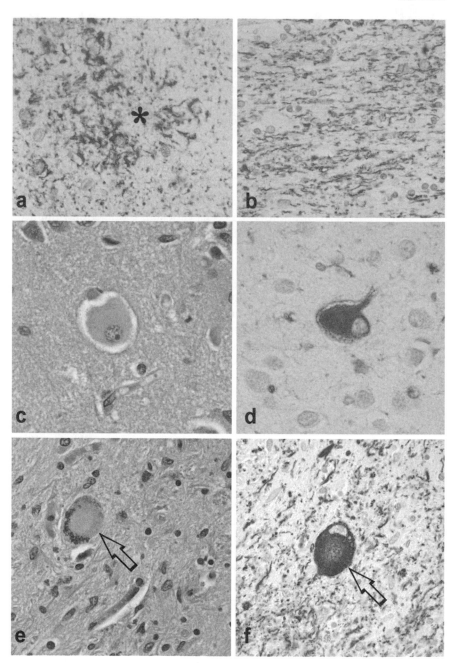

not coexist in the same brain (30). The astrocytic plaque may be the most specific histopathological lesion of CBD.

In addition to cortical pathology, deep gray matter is consistently affected in CBD. The globus pallidus and putamen show mild neuronal loss with gliosis. Thalamic nuclei may also be affected. In the basal ganglia, thread-like processes are often extensive, often in the pencil fibers of the striatum. Tau-positive neurons, but not NFT, are common in the striatum and globus pallidus. The internal capsule and thalamic fasciculus often have many thread-like processes. The subthalamic nucleus usually has a normal neuronal population, but neurons may have tau inclusions, and there may be many thread-like lesions in the nucleus. Fibrillary gliosis typical of PSP is not seen in the subthalamic nucleus in CBD.

The substantia nigra usually shows moderate to severe neuronal loss with extraneuronal neuromelanin and gliosis. Many of the remaining neurons contain NFT, which have also been termed "corticobasal bodies" (35) (Fig. 5). The locus ceruleus and raphe nuclei have similar inclusions. In contrast to PSP, where neurons in the pontine base almost always have at least a few NFT, the pontine base is largely free of NFTs in CBD. On the other hand, tau inclusions in glia and thread-like lesions are frequent in the pontine base. The cerebellum has mild Purkinje cell loss and axonal torpedoes. There is also mild neuronal loss in the dentate nucleus, but grumose degeneration is much less common than in PSP.

In CBD the filaments have a paired helical appearance at the electron microscopic level, but the diameter is wider and the periodicity is longer than the paired helical filaments of AD (34). These structures have been referred to as twisted ribbons. Similar to PSP, abnormal insoluble tau in CBD migrates as two prominent bands (68 and 64 kDa) on Western blots (32).

FIGURE 5   CBD: The hallmark lesion in CBD is the astrocytic plaque (asterisk), which is a cluster of irregular tau processes around a central astrocyte (a). The white matter and gray matter in CBD has numerous tau-immunoreactive thread-like processes (b). Cortical neurons have swelling characteristic of ballooning degeneration (c), and the ballooned neurons have intense immunoreactivity with the stress protein alpha-B-crystallin (d). Neurons in the substantia nigra have round inclusions called corticobasal bodies (arrow in e) that are positive for tau (arrow in f). Note also the many thread-like processes in (f).

POSTENCEPHALITIC PARKINSONISM

Parkinsonism following encephalitis lethargica during the influenza pandemic between 1916–1926 is known as postencephalitic parkinsonism (PEP). During the recovery phase of the acute viral encephalitis, parkinsonian rigidity developed with the most characteristic clinical features being oculogyric crises. The PEP brain has NFTs in cortex, basal ganglia, thalamus, hypothalamus, substantia nigra, brainstem tegmentum, and cerebellar dentate nucleus (36). The distribution of the pathology overlaps with PSP, and in recent studies it has not been possible to distinguish the two disorders by histopathological analysis alone (36). Biochemical studies of abnormal insoluble tau in PEP have features similar to AD with three major bands (68, 64, and 60 kDa) on Western blot studies, and electron microscopy shows paired helical filaments similar to those in AD (37).

GUAM PARKINSON-DEMENTIA COMPLEX

A characteristic parkinsonism with dementia (Parkinson dementia complex, PDC) with a number of features that overlap with PSP has been reported in the native Chamorro population of Guam since the 1950s (38). The frequency of PDC has declined in recent years for unknown reasons, and the etiology is unknown. The gross findings in PDC are notable for cortical atrophy affecting frontal and temporal lobes, as well as atrophy of the hippocampus and the tegmentum of the rostral brainstem (39). These areas typically have neuronal loss and gliosis with many NFTs in residual neurons. Extracellular NFTs are also numerous. In the cortex NFTs show a different laminar distribution from AD, with more NFTs in superficial cortical layers in Guam PDC and in lower cortical layers in AD (40). The hippocampus has numerous NFTs. The substantia nigra and locus ceruleus also have marked neuronal loss and many NFTs. The basal nucleus and large neurons in the striatum are also vulnerable to NFTs. Biochemically and morphologically, NFTs in Guam PDC are indistinguishable from those in AD (41).

DEMENTIA PUGILISTICA

An akinetic-rigid syndrome with dysarthria and dementia is sometimes a long-term outcome of repeated closed-head trauma, as seen in professional boxers. The pathology on gross examination, other than lesions that can be attributed to trauma, e.g., subdural membranes and cortical contusions, is nonspecific (42). The substantia nigra may also show pigment loss. Microscopically, there are NFTs similar to those in AD in brainstem monoaminergic nuclei, cortex, and hippocampus. At the electron microscopic level, they are composed of paired helical filaments and biochemically composed 68, 64, and 60 kDa forms (43).

FAMILIAL PARKINSONISM

While most parkinsonian disorders are sporadic, rare familial forms have been described and mutations have been found or genetic linkage analyses have suggested a strong genetic factor in their etiology (44). Perhaps the most common familial PD is autosomal recessive juvenile Parkinson's disease (ARJP). The clinical features are somewhat atypical in that dystonia is common in ARJP (45). The pathology of ARJP is based upon only a few autopsy reports. Initial studies emphasized severe neuronal loss in the substantia nigra with no LBs, but a more recent report of an individual who died prematurely in an automobile accident had LBs in the substantia nigra and other vulnerable regions (46). Even in sporadic PD there is an inverse relationship between the disease duration and the number of LBs in the substantia nigra. When the disease is very severe, there are very few residual neurons. Since LBs are intraneuronal inclusions that are phagocytosed after the neuron dies, it is not surprising that there are few LBs in cases of long duration.

Less common than ARJP are autosomal dominant forms of PD. The best characterized is the Contursi kindred, a familial PD due to a mutation in the α-synuclein gene (47). The pathology of the Contursi kindred is typical LB Parkinson's disease; however, given the young age of onset, by the time the individual dies, LB pathology is typically widespread in the brain. Lewy neurites are also prominent in many cortical areas.

Late-onset familial PD, such as Family C, has clinical characteristics and pathology that is virtually indistinguishable from sporadic PD (48). Some young-onset autosomal dominant PD kindred, such as the Iowa kindred, have atypical clinical presentations and include family members with dementia and psychosis. The pathology in at least some of these cases is associated with severe LB-related pathology in the cortex, hippocampus, and amygdala, in addition to the substantia nigra and other brainstem nuclei and in some cases glial inclusions similar to those in MSA are present (Fig. 6) (49).

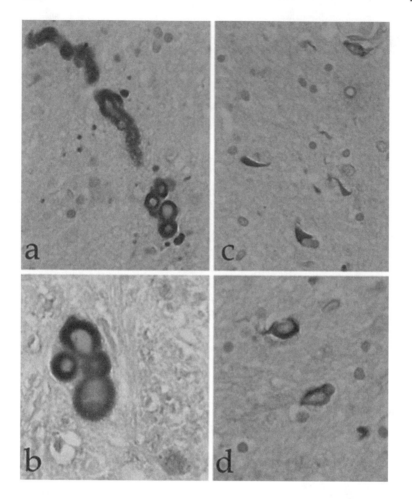

FIGURE 6 Familial PD: Many Lewy bodies are detected in early-onset familial cases, and some of the inclusions have unusual morphologies (a, b). Like MSA, synuclein-immunoreactive glial inclusions are also detected in some cases of familial early-onset PD.

ACKNOWLEDGMENTS

Supported by NIH AG16574, AG17216, AG14449, AG03949, NS40256, Mayo Foundation, State of Florida Alzheimer Disease Initiative, and the Society for Progressive Supranuclear Palsy.

REFERENCES

1. Gibb WR, Lees AJ. Anatomy, pigmentation, ventral and dorsal subpopulations of the substantia nigra, and differential cell death in Parkinson's disease. J Neurol Neurosurg Psychiatry 54:388–396, 1991.
2. Forno LS. Concentric hyaline intraneuronal inclusions of Lewy body type in the brains of elderly persons (50 incidental cases): relationship to parkinsonism. J Am Geriatr Soc 17:557–575, 1969.
3. Rajput AH, Rozdilsky B, Rajput A. Accuracy of clinical diagnosis in parkinsonism—a prospective study. Can J Neurol Sci 18:275–278, 1991.
4. Hughes AJ, Daniel SE, Kilford L, Lees AJ. Accuracy of clinical diagnosis of idiopathic Parkinson's disease: a clinico-pathological study of 100 cases. J Neurol Neurosurg Psychiatry 55:181–184, 1992.
5. Hughes AJ, Daniel SE, Lees AJ. Improved accuracy of clinical diagnosis of Lewy body Parkinson's disease. Neurology 57:1497–1499, 2001.
6. Pollanen MS, Dickson DW, Bergeron C. Pathology and biology of the Lewy body. J Neuropathol Exp Neurol 52:183–191, 1993.
7. Dickson DW. α-Synuclein and the Lewy body disorders. Curr Opin Neurol 14:423–432, 2001.
8. Dickson DW, Ruan D, Crystal H, Mark MH, Davies P, Kress Y, Yen S-H. Hippocampal degeneration differentiates diffuse Lewy body disease (DLBD) from Alzheimer's disease: light and electron microscopic immunocytochemistry of CA2-3 neurites specific to DLBD. Neurology 41:1402–1409, 1991.
9. Galloway PG, Mulvihill P, Perry G. Filaments of Lewy bodies contain insoluble cytoskeletal elements. Am J Pathol 140:809–815, 1992.
10. Goldman JE, Yen S-H, Chiu F-C, Peress NS. Lewy bodies of Parkinson's disease contain neurofilament antigens. Science 221:1082–1084, 1983.
11. Kuzuhara S, Mori H, Izumiyama N, Yoshimura M, Ihara Y. Lewy bodies are ubiquitinated: a light and electron microscopic immunocytochemical study. Acta Neuropathol 75:345–353, 1988.
12. Spillantini MG, Schmidt ML, Lee VM, Trojanowski JQ, Jakes R, Goedert M. Alpha-synuclein in Lewy bodies. Nature 388:839–840, 1997.
13. Irizarry MC, Growdon W, Gomez-Isla T, Newell K, George JM, Clayton DF, Hyman BT. Nigral and cortical Lewy bodies and dystrophic nigral neurites in Parkinson's disease and cortical Lewy body disease contain α-synuclein immunoreactivity. J Neuropathol Exp Neurol 57:334–337, 1998.
14. Pollanen MS, Bergeron C, Weyer L. Detergent-insoluble Lewy body fibrils share epitopes with neurofilament and tau. J Neurochem 58:1953–1956, 1992.
15. Iwatsubo T, Yamaguchi H, Fujimuro M, Yokosawa H, Ihara Y, Trojanowski JQ, Lee VM. Purification and characterization of Lewy bodies from the brains of patients with diffuse Lewy body disease. Am J Pathol 148:1517–1529, 1996.
16. Baba M, Nakajo S, Tu PH, Tomita T, Nakaya K, Lee VM, Trojanowski JQ, Iwatsubo T. Aggregation of alpha-synuclein in Lewy bodies of sporadic Parkinson's disease and dementia with Lewy bodies. Am J Pathol 152:879–884, 1998.

17. Hughes AJ, Daniel SE, Blankson S, Lees AJ. A clincopathologic study of 100 cases of Parkinson's disease. Arch Neurol 50:140–148, 1993.
18. Whitehouse PJ, Hedreen JC, White CL III, Price DL. Basal forebrain neurons in dementia of Parkinson disease. Ann Neurol 13:243–248, 1983.
19. Perry EK, McKeith I, Thompson P, Marshall E, Kerwin J, Jabeen S, Edwardson JA, Ince P, Blessed G, Irving D. Topography, extent, and clinical relevance of neurochemical deficits in dementia of Lewy body type, Parkinson's disease, and Alzheimer's disease. Ann NY Acad Sci 640:197–202, 1991.
20. Mattila PM, Roytta M, Torikka H, Dickson DW, Rinne JO. Cortical Lewy bodies and Alzheimer-type changes in patients with Parkinson's disease. Acta Neuropathol 95:576–582, 1998.
21. Hurtig HI, Trojanowski JQ, Galvin J, Ewbank D, Schmidt ML, Lee VM, Clark CM, Glosser G, Stern MB, Gollomp SM, Arnold SE. Alpha-synuclein cortical Lewy bodies correlate with dementia in Parkinson's disease. Neurology 54:1916–1921, 2000.
22. Apaydin H, Ahlskog JE, Parisi JE, Boeve BF, Dickson DW. Parkinson's disease neuropathology: later-developing dementia and loss of the levodopa response. Arch Neurol 59:102–112, 2002.
23. Churchyard A, Lees AJ. The relationship between dementia and direct involvement of the hippocampus and amygdala in Parkinson's disease. Neurology 49:1570–1576, 1997.
24. Lennox G, Lowe JS, Landon M, Byrne EJ, Mayer RJ, Godwin-Austen RB. Diffuse Lewy body disease: correlative neuropathology using anti-ubiquitin immunocytochemistry. J Neurol Neurosurg Psychiatry 52:1236–1247, 1989.
25. Wenning GK, Tison F, Ben Shlomo Y, Daniel SE, Quinn NP. Multiple system atrophy: a review of 203 pathologically proven cases. Mov Disord 12:133–147, 1997.
26. Lantos PL. The definition of multiple system atrophy: a review of recent developments. J Neuropathol Exp Neurol 57:1099–1111, 1998.
27. Dickson DW, Lin W, Liu WK, Yen SH. Multiple system atrophy: a sporadic synucleinopathy. Brain Pathol 9:721–732, 1999.
28. Steele JC, Richardson JC, Olszewski J. Progressive supranuclear palsy: a heterogenous degeneration involving the brainstem, basal ganglia and cerebellum with vertical gaze and pseudobulbar palsy, nuchal dystonia, and dementia. Arch Neurol 10:333–339, 1964.
29. Bigio EH, Brown DF, White CL 3rd. Progressive supranuclear palsy with dementia: cortical pathology. J Neuropathol Exp Neurol 58:359–364, 1999.
30. Komori T. Tau-positive glial inclusions in progressive supranuclear palsy, corticobasal degeneration and Pick's disease. Brain Pathol 9:663–679, 1999.
31. Tellez-Nagel I, Wisniewski HM. Ultrastructure of neurofibrillary tangles in Steele-Richardson-Olszewski syndrome. Arch Neurol 29:324–327, 1973.
32. Buee L, Delacourte A. Comparative biochemistry of tau in progressive supranuclear palsy, corticobasal degeneration, FTDP-17 and Pick's disease. Brain Pathol 9:681–693, 1999.

33. Litvan I, Grimes DA, Lang AE, Jankovic J, McKee A, Verny M, Jellinger K, Chaudhuri KR, Pearce RK, Clinical features differentiating patients with postmortem confirmed progressive supranuclear palsy and corticobasal degeneration. J Neurol 246(suppl 2):1–5, 1999.
34. Dickson DW, Liu W-K, Ksiezak-Reding H, Yen S-H. Neuropathologic and molecular considerations. In: Litvan I, Goetz CG, Lang AE, eds. Corticobasal Degeneration and Related Disorders. Advances in Neurology, Vol. 82. New York: Lippincott-Raven, 2000, pp 9–27.
35. Gibb WRG, Luthert PJ, Marsden CD. Corticobasal degeneration. Brain 112:1171–1192, 1989.
36. Geddes JF, Hughes AJ, Lees AJ, Daniel SE. Pathological overlap in cases of parkinsonism associated with neurofibrillary tangles. A study of recent cases of postencephalitic parkinsonism and comparison with progressive supranuclear palsy and Guamanian parkinsonism-dementia complex. Brain 116:281–302, 1993.
37. Buée-Scherer V, Buée L, Leveugle B, Perl DP, Vermersch P, Hof PR, Delacourte A. Pathological tau proteins in postencephalitic parkinsonism: comparison with Alzheimer's disease and other neurodegenerative disorders. Ann Neurol 42:356–359, 1997.
38. Hirano A, Malamud N, Kurland LT. Parkinsonism—dementia complex is an endemic disease on the island of Guam. II. Pathological features. Brain 84:662–679, 1961.
39. Oyanagi K, Makifuchi T, Ohtoh T, Chen KM, van der Schaaf T, Gajdusek DC, Chase TN, Ikuta F. Amyotrophic lateral sclerosis of Guam: the nature of the neuropathological findings. Acta Neuropathol 88:405–412, 1994.
40. Hof PR, Perl DP, Loerzel AJ, Morrison JH. Neurofibrillary tangle distribution in the cerebral cortex of parkinsonism-dementia cases from Guam: differences with Alzheimer's disease. Brain Res 564:306–313, 1991.
41. Buee-Scherrer V, Buee L, Hof PR, Leveugle B, Gilles C, Loerzel AJ, Perl DP, Delacourte A. Neurofibrillary degeneration in amyotrophic lateral sclerosis/parkinsonism-dementia complex of Guam. Immunochemical characterization of tau proteins. Am J Pathol 146:924–932, 1995.
42. Graham DI, Gennarelli TA. Trauma. In: Graham DI, Lantos PL, eds. Greenfield's Neuropathology, 6th ed. London: Arnold, 1997, pp 197–263.
43. Schmidt ML, Zhukareva V, Newell KL, Lee VM, Trojanowski JQ. Tau isoform profile and phosphorylation state in dementia pugilistica recapitulate Alzheimer's disease. Acta Neuropathol 101:518–524, 2001.
44. Gasser T. Genetics of Parkinson's disease. J Neurol 248:833–840, 2001.
45. Hattori N, Shimura H, Kubo S, Kitada T, Wang M, Asakawa S, Minashima S, Shimizu N, Suzuki T, Tanaka K, Mizuno Y. Autosomal recessive juvenile parkinsonism: a key to understanding nigral degeneration in sporadic Parkinson's disease. Neuropathology 20(suppl):S85–S90, 2000.
46. Farrer M, Chan P, Chen R, Tan L, Lincoln S, Hernandez D, Forno L, Gwinn-Hardy K, Petrucelli L, Hussey J, Singleton A, Tanner C, Hardy J, Langston

JW. Lewy bodies and parkinsonism in families with parkin mutations. Ann Neurol 50:293–300, 2001.

47. Polymeropoulos MHC, Lavedan C, Leroy E, Ide SE, Dehejia A, Dutra A, Pike B, Root H, Rubenstein J, Boyer R, Stenroos ES, Chandrasekharappa S, Athanassiadou A, Papapetropoulos T, Johnson WG, Lazzarini AM, Duvoisin RC, Di Iorio G, Golbe LI, Nussbaum RL. Mutation in the alpha-synuclein gene identified in families with Parkinson's disease. Science 276:2045–2047, 1997.

48. Wszolek ZK, Gwinn-Hardy K, Wszolek EK, Muenter MD, Pfeiffer RF, Rodnitzky RL, Uitti RJ, McComb RD, Gasser T, Dickson DW. Neuropathology of two members of a German-American kindred (Family C) with late onset parkinsonism. Acta Neuropathol 103:344–350, 2002.

49. Gwinn-Hardy K, Mehta ND, Farrer M, Maraganore D, Muenter M, Yen SH, Hardy J, Dickson DW. Distinctive neuropathology revealed by alpha-synuclein antibodies in hereditary parkinsonism and dementia linked to chromosome 4p. Acta Neuropathol 99:663–672, 2000.

10

Neurochemistry of Nigral Degeneration

Jayaraman Rao
Louisiana State University Health Sciences Center,
New Orleans, Louisiana, U.S.A.

INTRODUCTION

Progressive degeneration of the dopaminergic neurons of the substantia nigra is the pathological hallmark of idiopathic Parkinson's disease (PD). Based on cytoarchitectonics and melanization, Hassler divided the human substantia nigra into many subsections and demonstrated that the ventral and lateral regions of the substantia nigra may be preferentially involved in early stages of the disease (1,2) (Fig. 1), an observation that was later confirmed in human PD (3,4). The etiology of the progressive degeneration of the substantia nigra pars compacta cells is unknown. It has been proposed that the clinical signs and symptoms of PD emerge only after a loss of 75% of the nigral neurons. Positron emission tomography (PET) and single photon emission computed tomography (SPECT) studies also indicate that the rate of loss of dopaminergic neurons is about 6–13% in patients with PD compared to 0–2.5% in healthy controls (5). These facts suggest that the process of degeneration of nigral neurons is initiated several years ahead of the onset of the clinical expression of the disease.

Epidemiological evidence emphasizes the role of environmental toxins in the development of PD. Discoveries of gene mutations responsible for

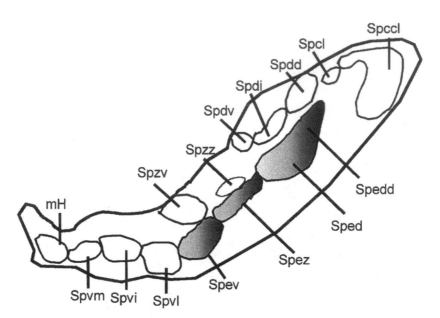

FIGURE 1   A diagrammatic representation of the subdivisions of human substantia nigra as defined by Hassler. The shaded subnuclei in the ventral and lateral regions degenerate selectively in the early stages of PD. (Adapted from Refs. 1, 2.)

inherited forms of PD have increased interest in the role of genetics in the etiology of PD. Modern molecular biological approaches are pointing to the possibility that dysfunction of a variety of cellular mechanisms may result in an insidious and a slowly progressive levodopa-responsive parkinsonism that is indistinguishable from PD. These observations raise the issue of whether there may be multiple etiologies for PD. In this chapter, some of the neurochemical changes noted in the degenerating dopaminergic neurons of the substantia nigra in experimental models of PD, inherited forms of PD, and idiopathic PD will be summarized.

GROWTH FACTORS AND THE SUBSTANTIA NIGRA

Neurons and glia need a very small concentration of trophic or growth factor(s) for their continued existence, maintenance of a normal connectivity and physiological state, as well as recovery from chemical and physical injury (6). If these growth factors are withdrawn or if their continuing influence is affected both neurons and glia may fail to differentiate and die during embryogenesis. As adult neurons, they may lose their efficiency or become vulnerable to toxic factors and ultimately die. Under stressful circumstances, neurons and glia upregulate the expression of growth factors and their specific receptors or acquire them from their target neurons and the surrounding glial cells and recover from the injury. Age-dependent decline and withdrawal of neurotrophins and their receptors (7,8) are thought to play an important role in the pathogenesis of Alzheimer's disease. The dopaminergic neurons of the substantia nigra are dependant on several such trophic and growth factors for normal ontogenesis and survival as fully differentiated mature adult neurons. In experimental models of PD and in idiopathic PD, the dopamine neurons of the substantia nigra show a deficiency of expression of several growth factors. It is possible that withdrawal of these growth factors in the dopaminergic neurons of the substantia nigra may contribute to the pathogenesis of idiopathic PD.

Trophic Factors and Ontogenesis of Dopaminergic Neurons of the Substantia Nigra

The normal development of dopaminergic neurons in ventral mesencephalon depends on the influence of many trophic factors. Between embryonic days E9.5 and E16, several trophic factors play important roles in the induction, differentiation, as well as complete maturation of dopamine synthesis, release, and reuptake machinery of ventral mesencephalic dopamine neurons (Fig. 2). Around the embryonic day of E 9.5, two such factors, namely sonic hedgehog (SHH) (9) and fibroblast growth factor 8 (FGF8), define the site of induction of dopamine neurons in the ventral mesencephalon. SHH is a member of the hedgehog family of signaling protein that plays a major role in the differentiation of diverse groups of neurons in the ventral half of the neural tube, including dopamine and serotoninergic neurons (10). SHH may even play an important role in maintenance of adult dopamine neurons since intrastriatal injection of SHH diminishes the motor behavioral defects of 6-hydroxydopamine (6-OHDA) models of PD (11).

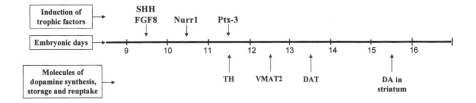

FIGURE 2 The ontogenesis of dopaminergic neurons of substantia nigra in rats and mice. (Adapted from Refs. 9, 12, 26, 27, 28.)

Around embryonic day E10.5, Nurrl is expressed in a group of cells in the ventral mesencephalic region (12). Nurrl is a member of the "orphan receptors" transcription factors and is expressed in several areas of the brain, but it is expressed intensely and selectively in the dopaminergic neurons of the ventral mesencephalon (12,13). Nurrl knockout results in the complete lack of development of dopaminergic neurons in the midbrain (14,15) with almost 98% reduction of dopamine in the striatum (16). Nurrl and tyrosine hydroxylase (TH) are coexpressed, with the maximum intensity in the midbrain substantia nigra neurons (17–19). The expression of dopamine transporter molecule may also be dependant on the Nurrl gene (20). Nurrl is expressed even in adult neurons, suggesting a role for a continuing influence on TH expression and survival of adult nigral dopamine neurons (21). Nurrl-deficient animals are more susceptible to 1-methyl-4-phenyl-1,2,3,6-tetrahydropyridine (MPTP) treatment (22), and Nurrl polymorphism may be associated with familial and idiopathic PD (23).

One day after expression of Nurrl, on E11.5, another factor, Pentraxin 3 (Ptx3), is expressed solely in the dopaminergic neurons of the ventral tegmental area and the substantia nigra (24). Ptx3 is reduced in the 6-OHDA model of PD as well as in idiopathic PD (24). The expression of Ptx3 in these neurons coincides with the expression of the TH gene in the same neurons (25). The appearance of Nurrl and Ptx3 early in the ontogenesis of dopaminergic neurons suggests that these factors are responsible for differentiation and maturation of ventral mesencephalic dopamine neurons rather than establishment of connectivity to the striatum. The expression and maturation of other components of dopamine release, reuptake, and storage are completed by the embryonic day E16, and the release of dopamine in the striatum is first noted around E17 (26–28).

Besides SHH, Nurr-1, and Ptx-3, NFIAb (29), LMX1b (30), heparin-binding epidermal growth factor-like growth factor (HB-EGF) (31), En-1, and En-2 of the engrailed gene family (32) have roles in the survival of the midbrain dopaminergic system during ontogenesis. En-1 and En-2 also appear to regulate the expression of α-synuclein, the major constituent of Lewy bodies in PD (32).

Growth Factors and Nigral Injury

Besides these trophic factors that play important roles in the ontogenesis of nigral dopamine neurons as well as maintaining the survival of differentiated adult dopamine neurons in the nigra, several other neurotrophic factors may play a neuroprotective role in many models of injury to the dopaminergic neurons of the substantia nigra (8,33). These neurotrophic factors have significant structural and functional similarities and are classified into the nerve-growth factor (NGF) superfamily, the glial-derived neurotrophic factor (GDNF) family, the neurokine family, and the nonneuronal growth factors.

The superfamily of neurotrophins includes the NGF, brain-derived neurotrophic factor (BDNF), and neurotrophins (NT) 3, 4/5, and 6. All members of the neurotrophin family interact with two structurally unrelated receptors, namely the tyrosine kinases (*trk*A, *trk*B, and *trk*C) and the low-affinity binding neurotrophin receptor p75^{NTR} (34,35). Recent studies have shown that the *trk* and p75^{NTR} are coexpressed in the same cell and that the molecular signaling pathways of these two receptors may be stimulated independently or coactivated (36,37). Even though stimulation of these two pathways may interact with each other, they may have opposite effects. Stimulation of the *trk* receptors subserves a neuroprotective effect by inactivating several factors that are apoptotic (35). The p75^{NTR} is structurally unlike the *trk* receptors. It belongs to the tumor necrosis factor (TNF) receptor family and contains the "death domain" (35,38). Stimulation of p75^{NTR} has been shown to induce several molecules that can initiate apoptosis, but under other conditions p75^{NTR} stimulation can be antiapoptotic (34,35).

The dopaminergic neurons of the substantia nigra in humans immunostain for proteins of FGF, BDNF, and NT3 as well as *trk*A, *trk*B, and *trk*C. The immunoreactivity is noted more intensely in the medial areas of the nigra than the lateral areas (39), providing one piece of evidence for selective loss of neurons in the lateral regions. BDNF, when injected into the striatum, is transported only to the soma of dopaminergic neurons of the substantia nigra. These findings suggest that BDNF found in nigral neurons may be synthesized locally within the neurons or can be acquired by retrograde transport from the striatal neurons (40). The melanized dopamine-containing neurons of the substantia nigra show a greater loss of BDNF than the nonmelanized cells (41,42). BDNF prevents nigral degeneration induced in MPTP models of PD (43).

GDNF, a neurotrophic factor belonging to the TGF-β superfamily, and its receptors, Ret and GDNF-α1, are expressed highly in the dopaminergic neurons of the substantia nigra (8,33). GDNF concentrations are decreased in the nigral neurons in PD (44). When injected in the striatum, GDNF is selectively transported retrogradely to nigral dopaminergic neurons (40). GDNF, like BDNF, protects mesencephalic dopamine neurons from 6-OHDA and MPTP toxicity and improves motor functions in these models of PD (45,46). However, the molecular pathways that mediate neuroprotective effects of these two neurotrophic factors may be different (47).

Neurokines are neuropoietic cytokines. Among the neurokines, an increased level of interleukin-6 (IL-6) has been demonstrated in the striatum. Many cytokines, which are traditionally recognized to play anti-inflammatory roles outside the brain, have now been recognized to be expressed in the brain (48) in response to tissue injury or inflammation (e.g., multiple sclerosis) (49). Some of these cytokines may be neuroprotective and others apoptotic. In this regard, levels of TNF-α, TGF-α, TGF-β, IL-1β, IL-4, and IL-6 are elevated in the striatum in PD. This has led to the hypothesis that the pathogenesis of PD may be the result of an imbalance between the actions of the antiapoptotic neurotrophic factors and the proapoptotic factors (50,51).

Several neurotrophic factors have been recognized to be expressed by nonneural cells. Among these, basic fibroblast growth factor (bFGF or FGF2) has been demonstrated to be expressed in the substantia nigra (52), and a profound depletion of bFGF was noted in the nigral neurons in PD (53,54). Acute and intermittent injections of nicotine increase FGF2 expression and mediate neuroprotective effects in several models of neuronal injury (55,56) including 6-OHDA and MPTP models of PD (57–59).

Summary

It is important to point out that it is unclear whether the reduction of the neurotrophic factors noted in the nigral neurons of PD is the cause or a consequence of nigral degeneration. While in animal models of acute injury the striatum and the dopaminergic neurons of the substantia nigra may be protected by these neurotrophic factors, the role played by these factors in PD remains to be established. Even if the observed decrease in neurotrophic factors and their receptors is a consequence of the disease itself and not the cause, reintroduction of these trophic factors using viral vectors or drugs that will inhibit or activate the different molecules involved in the pro- and antiapoptotic pathways, respectively, will be an important mode of therapy for PD, Alzheimer's disease, and other neurodegenerative disorders in the future. Among these neurotrophic factors, at the present time BDNF, GDNF, and FGF2 appear to show the greatest promise.

DYSREGULATION OF PROTEIN METABOLISM

The identification of gene mutations that are responsible for causing inherited forms of PD has expanded our focus from environmental causes of PD to the possible role of genetics in the etiology of PD. Several studies demonstrate that mutations of genes result in mutant proteins that are inefficiently catabolized by the protein removal system, the ubiquitin-proteasome pathway. A defective ubiquitin-proteasome pathway can also be the result of gene defects. Failure of the ubiquitin-proteasome system to degrade a protein because it is unable to recognize the mutant protein or due to an inefficiency of the ubiquitin-proteasome system itself will result in aggregation of the mutant proteins within nigral cells and cause neurotoxicity. Evidence for both types of abnormalities has been observed in inherited forms of PD. Dysfunction of the ubiquitin-proteasome system could potentially be an important factor in the pathogenesis of PD.

Mutant Proteins and Inherited Forms of PD

An alanine-to-threonine substitution at codon 53 (A53T) of the gene for α-synuclein has been identified in several families with Italian-Greek pedigree (60). A substitution of proline for alanine at codon 30 (A30P) of the α-synuclein gene was also described in a family of German pedigree (61). The mRNA of α-synuclein is expressed throughout the brain, but expressed at a very low intensity in the substantia nigra, and the level of expression of mRNA for α-synuclein is much lower than normal in the nigral neurons of PD brains (62). The protein of α-synuclein localizes to both the nucleus and the synapse, but its function is predominantly presynaptic (63). α-Synuclein has structural similarities to the chaperone protein 14-3-3 (64), and together, α-synuclein and 14-3-3 regulate the expression of TH (65).

Recognition that mutations of the Parkin gene are responsible for autosomal recessive-juvenile parkinsonism (AR-JP) is a major breakthrough in our understanding of the pathogenesis of PD (66). The Parkin gene maps to chromosome 6q25.2-q27 and has 12 exons coding for a 465-amino-acid protein. Mutations of the Parkin gene are the most common type noted in autosomal recessive PD (66). Parkin is an E3 ubiquitin ligase (67), an enzyme that plays an important role in the ubiquitin-proteasome protein degradation pathway. The E3 ubiquitin ligase family consists of a large number of members and among these, Parkin is the type that contains, within the same molecule, a ring finger domain that binds to ubiquitin as well as a site that recognizes and binds to the substrate (68).

α-Synuclein (66), alphaSp22, which is a glycosylated isoform of α-synuclein (69), CDCrel-1 (67), a synaptic vesicle–associated protein, synphilin-1 (70), Pael receptor (Parkin-associated endothelin receptor-like receptor) (71), and a G-protein–coupled transmembrane polypeptide that is expressed most intensely in the TH-positive neurons of the nigra (72) are some of the substrates that interact with Parkin.

A mutation of the gene that codes for ubiquitin carboxy-terminal hydrolase (UCH-L1) has been recognized in one family with an inherited form of PD (73). Ubiquitin hydrolases are deubiquitinating enzymes that play a pivotal role in maintaining a steady-state level of ubiquitin by generating and recycling ubiquitin (68). A mutation of the human neurofilament M gene has also been reported in a patient with young-onset PD with a French-Canadian pedigree (74).

Ubiquitin-Proteasome Protein Degradation Pathway and PD

Ubiquitin-proteasome–mediated protein catabolic pathway plays a major role in maintaining a viable and normal functioning cell. Dysfunction of the ubiquitin-proteasome pathway has been proposed to be involved in many neurodegenerative disorders, including Alzheimer's disease, frontotemporal dementia, Huntington's disease, and several types of malignancies (68,75). The two basic mechanisms that are involved in the catabolism of proteins by the ubiquitin-proteasome pathway are (1) the protein that needs to be degraded is tagged with ubiquitin and (2) the tagged protein is then transferred to a protease, 26S proteasome, which degrades the tagged protein into small peptides. The initial step for ubiquitination of the substrate consists of activation of the inactive form of ubiquitin by the ubiquitin-activating enzyme E1. The activated ubiquitin is then transferred to the ubiquitin carrier protein family of enzymes (ubiquitin conjugating enzyme or Ubc) E2. Among the 13 subtypes of E2, UbcH7 and UbcH8 appear to play a more prominent role in interacting with the subtype of E3 ubiquitin ligase implicated in AR-JP (66). E3 (ubiquitin ligase), consisting of a large family of ligases, is responsible for recognizing the substrate protein that is to be degraded and facilitating the transfer of activated ubiquitin from E2 so that the substrate can be tagged with ubiquitin and subsequently recognized by the proteasome. This substrate-ubiquitin complex is further polyubiquitinated by a polyubiquitinating enzyme E4 and presented to the 26S proteasome. The proteasome then degrades the tagged protein to small polypeptides, and peptidases further degrade the peptides into amino acids. Ubiquitin is released for further use by one of several deubiquitinating enzymes. The deubiquitinating enzymes play the important role of regulating the amount of ubiquitin available (Fig. 3).

Gene defects resulting in dysfunction of many of the different molecules involved in the ubiquitin-proteasome pathway have been shown to induce PD. These mutations of the genes may result in (1) mutant forms of ubiquitin-domain proteins (UDPs), which will decrease the availability of free UDPs; (2) mutant ubiquitin ligase (E3), which will result in a failure of E3 to recognize the substrate; (3) mutations of the protein substrate; or (4) a failure to deubiquitinate, which will result in a decreased supply of free ubiquitin to inadequate recycling of ubiquitin. The N-terminal region of the

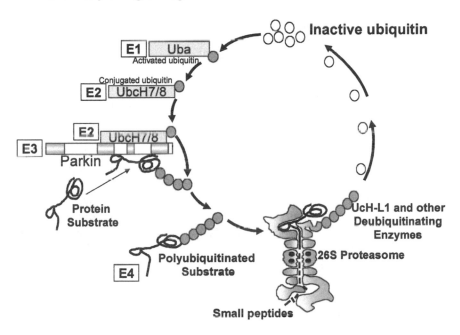

FIGURE 3 Diagrammatic representation of the Parkin-Ubiquitin proteasome pathway. See text for details. (Adapted from Refs. 66, 67, 68, 72.)

Parkin protein codes for an ubiquitin-domain protein (UDP). The UDPs have structural similarities to ubiquitin and function as proteasome adapters (76). A mutation of the ubiquitin-like domain coding regions of exons 2 and 3 of the Parkin gene alone has been observed in AR-JP (66). Deletion, duplication, and mutations of several regions of the Parkin gene have been recognized to cause AR-JP. Among these, mutations in the regions coding for ring fingers appear to be quite frequent among AR-JP patients (66). Mutation of α-synuclein may result in failure of the ubiquitinating system to recognize the substrate. Even though only two members of the family were reported to have mutations of the gene of UCH-L1, resulting in only a partial suppression of the deubiquitinating enzyme UCH-L2, these two patients reinforce the concept that disturbances of the protein degradation system will lead to aggregation of protein within the neuron. Proteasomal dysfunctions have also been observed in PD (77).

Neurochemistry of the Lewy Body

Mutated and misfolded proteins tend to aggregate. During aggregation, as commonly seen in polyglutamine repeat diseases, these fibrillary proteins may also sequester other proteins, including chaperone proteins and ubiquitin-conjugating enzymes, and further contribute to prevention of catabolism of these mutant proteins (78). The presence of the Lewy body, an example of such protein aggregation, in the substantia nigra is considered pathognomonic of PD. Electron microscopically, the Lewy body consists of a dense circular central core surrounded by neurofilaments located in the pale halo at the periphery (79). Aggregated α-synuclein is a major constituent of Lewy bodies in PD. The central core as well as the peripheral halo immunostain very strongly for the full length of α-synuclein (80). β or γ-Synuclein appears to aggregate in the axon terminals of hippocampal neurons of PD and diffuse Lewy body brains (81).

An overexpression of α-synuclein, as demonstrated in *Drosophila* models of PD (82), is neurotoxic to nigral neurons, but this toxicity can be reversed by overexpression of two other chaperone proteins, namely HSP70 and HSP40 (83). In the presence of iron, which accumulates in the ventral mesencephalon in PD, or of aluminum, copper, or manganese ions, α-synuclein appears to be insoluble (84). Increased oxidative stress can be an early step for aggregation of α-synuclein (85), and in turn, aggregation of α-synuclein can promote further mitochondrial dysfunction and oxidative stress (86). α-Synuclein accumulation can decrease the effectiveness of proteasomal function and contribute to the accumulation of other proteins that are substrates for proteasomal degradation. Understanding the mechanisms of insolubility of α-synuclein is crucial to creating new modes of therapy for PD and other synucleinopathies.

Besides α-synuclein, Lewy bodies also contain several other proteins. These proteins can be broadly grouped into several types, namely (1) proteins that have presynaptic functions, (2) neurofilaments and related proteins, (3) markers of oxidative stress, (4) pro- and antiapoptotic proteins, (5) molecular chaperones, and (6) members of the ubiquitin-proteasome system (Fig. 4).

Summary

The discovery that mutations of the α-synuclein and Parkin genes cause a parkinsonian syndrome has led to a better understanding of the mechanisms with which the dopaminergic neurons of the substantia nigra handle protein degradation. The evidence indicates that in PD, as in several other synucleinopathies, the aggregation of α-synuclein and ubiquitin in Lewy bodies is the result of ineffective removal of proteins by the ubiquitin-proteasomal system of the dopaminergic neurons of the substantia nigra.

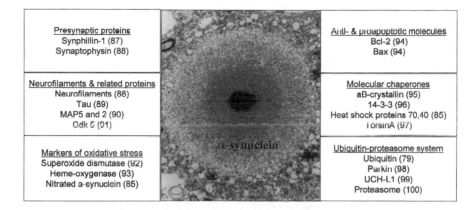

Presynaptic proteins		Anti- & proapoptotic molecules
Synphillin-1 (87)		Bcl-2 (94)
Synaptophysin (88)		Bax (94)
Neurofilaments & related proteins		**Molecular chaperones**
Neurofilaments (88)		aB-crystallin (95)
Tau (89)		14-3-3 (96)
MAP5 and 2 (90)		Heat shock proteins 70,40 (85)
Cdk 5 (91)	α-synuclein	TorsinA (97)
Markers of oxidative stress		**Ubiquitin-proteasome system**
Superoxide dismutase (92)		Ubiquitin (79)
Heme-oxygenase (93)		Parkin (98)
Nitrated a-synuclein (85)		UCH-L1 (99)
		Proteasome (100)

FIGURE 4 Diagrammatic representation of a Lewy body. The different proteins that are associated with Lewy bodies in PD are listed in boxes.

MITOCHONDRIAL DAMAGE AND THE SUBSTANTIA NIGRA

The concept that mitochondrial dysfunction can cause a parkinsonian syndrome came into focus with the observation that MPTP induced PD in "frozen" addicts (101–103). Mitochondrion is the major source of cellular energy. Each cell has thousands of mitochondria throughout the cytoplasm. In addition to generating most of the energy in the form of adenosine triphosphate (ATP) required by the cell through the oxidative phosphorylation system (OXPHOS), mitochondria also generate and remove free radicals and play the central role in initiating many of the key steps for apoptosis (104). Mitochondrial dysfunctions are now recognized to be the major cause of nigral degeneration in experimental models of PD (105,106) and possibly even in idiopathic PD.

Electron Transfer Chain Dysfunction

The electron transfer chain (ETC) is an important component of the OXPHOS system. The respiratory complexes I, II, III, IV, and V are located within the inner membrane of the mitochondria and play a critical role in transferring electrons from different sources within the mitochondria. Dysfunction of these respiratory complexes will lead to significant loss in the generation of stored energy in the form of ATP as well as increased oxidative damage due to accumulation of reactive oxygen species.

The MPTP model of PD clearly suggests that inhibition of the ETC, especially at the Complex I level, is toxic to nigral neurons (107). There is a significant decrease in the levels of complex I in the nigral neurons of PD (108,109). Among the different diseases of the basal ganglia, the deficiency of Complex I in the nigra may be specific to PD (110). Complex I deficiency is not restricted to the brain, but is also found in the skeletal muscle, platelets, fibroblasts, and lymphocytes (111) in PD. It is important to recognize that in the two most commonly used animal models of PD, 6-OHDA– and MPTP-induced models, the toxins decrease the efficiency of Complex I (105,106).

Chronic injections of a commonly used pesticide, rotenone, cause selective degeneration of the nigrostriatal system and result in aggregation of ubiquitin and α-synuclein (112). This is important in understanding the etiology of PD. Rotenone, a toxin that is used to kill fish in ponds, is a mitochondrial toxin, which easily crosses the blood-brain barrier and inhibits Complex I. The clinical syndrome that results with chronic rotenone administration has significant similarities to human PD, including hypokinesia, stooped posture, and tremor. A dysfunction of Complex III has also been suggested to occur in PD (113). Recent studies suggest that nitric oxide (NO) can inhibit Complex IV, and this inhibition may accentuate the toxic effects of methyl-4-phenylpyridium(MPP+) on Complex I (114).

Free Radicals and Mitochondrial Toxicity

Mitochondria are the major source of energy production for the cell and the major site of utilization of cellular oxygen. During the synthesis of stored energy in the form of ATP, mitochondria produce several reactive oxygen species (ROS). It is estimated that 2–4% of the utilized oxygen is converted into ROS. ROS consists of superoxide anions, hydroxyl radicals, and hydrogen peroxide. The majority of the ROS produced in a cell is derived from the mitochondria. ROS are produced at Complex I and Complex III of the ETC system (115).

ROS are toxic to neurons. An increased level of ROS within the mitochondria can decrease the efficiency of Complex I and the ETC system. This will decrease energy production and cause further accumulation of free radicals, mtDNA damage, and production of additional free radicals through Fenton reaction. All of these events may induce aging of the cell and mitochondria-mediated apoptotic mechanisms of cell death (115). An increased accumulation of ROS can occur either due to increased synthesis of ROS or because of failure or a decreased level of removal by the glutathione system. Evidence for both increased production as well as decreased clearance of these free radicals has been observed in PD.

The different metabolic breakdown pathways of levodopa may be an important source of an increased production of free radicals. There is controversy regarding the neurotoxic vs. neuroprotective role of levodopa in PD (116–118). There is extensive literature to suggest that, at least in experimental conditions, especially in conditions using cell culture techniques, levodopa can produce free radicals and can destroy the cells in culture. In the presence of iron, there is an even greater increase in the levels of free radicals synthesized (119,120). Extensive review of this issue suggests that the evidence supporting the neurotoxic role of levodopa is insufficient in patients with PD (118). In fact, the cytotoxic effects of dopamine may be an artifact of cell culture technique (121), and the neurotoxic effects of accumulated iron may be due to its ability to promote aggregation of α-synuclein (84) and may contribute to Lewy body pathology.

An increased level of free radicals may be from sources other than the mitochondria. NO may be one such source of free radicals (122). An increased production of nitric oxide synthase, as noted in MPTP models of PD (123), can lead to increased levels of NO, which in turn results in an increased synthesis and accumulation of free radicals within the nigral cells. NO may play an important role in inducing nigral degeneration in amphetamine and MPTP-induced PD. Increased NO levels can lead to increased formation of peroxynitrite, a potent oxidant, and peroxynitrite may interact with dopamine autooxidant products and neuromelanin (124,125) and can cause free radical mediated nigral neurotoxicity.

The presence of a defective free radical removal system has been established in PD. ROS is removed by superoxide dismutase (SOD), catalase, and glutathione peroxidase. SOD facilitates the conversion of superoxide to hydrogen peroxide, and catalase and glutathione peroxidase convert hydrogen peroxide to water (115). Decreased levels of glutathione, glutathione peroxidase, and catalase have been observed in PD (126,127). In fact, glutathione depletion may be one of the earliest events in the evolution of mitochondrial dysfunctions in PD (128). Decreased glutathione may actually cause a selective inhibition of Complex I and result in an inefficient ETC system (129,130).

mtDNA Defects

Mitochondria's own genome (mtDNA) is localized in the matrix compartment. mtDNA consists of a 16.5 kb molecule coding for a total of 37 genes, 13 of which code for the oxidative phosphorylation system (OXPHOS), 2 for ribosomal RNAs (12S and 16S rRNA), and 22 for transfer RNAs (tRNA), molecules that are necessary for the translation of mtDNA structural genes (104,131). Mutations of mtDNA increase with age. Cybrid studies have suggested that the Complex I deficiency noted in idiopathic PD may be due to mtDNA aberrations. Transmitochondridal cybrid lines, using mitochondria of platelets from PD patients, show several features of oxidative stress, increased vulnerability to MPP+, and an increased expression of apoptotic molecules (132,133). More recently, the presence of tRNA mutations have been observed in histologically confirmed PD patients (134).

Summary

This evidence suggests that toxins in the environment and toxins generated intrinsically can result in dysfunction of nigral mitochondria and lead to nigral degeneration and the induction of a slowly progressive syndrome similar to PD.

NIGRA AND APOPTOSIS

There is a significant controversy about whether apoptotic mechanisms play a role in the death of substantia nigra neurons in PD (135,136). However, experimental evidence of several well-recognized markers of apoptosis has been demonstrated in the nigral cells of both experimental models of PD and human PD (137).

Apoptosis, an established mechanism of cell death during embryogenesis and brain maturation, is characterized by a well-defined stereotypical pattern of neurochemical and morphological changes (138,139). The process involves caspase-induced cleaving of DNA and numerous other intracellular polypeptides, which ultimately leads to cellular death. Activation of caspases is a key triggering event for apoptosis. Caspases may be activated by at least by two different mechanisms: an extrinsic system which involves stimulation of death receptors by extracellular "death ligands" (139) or an intrinsic pathway, which requires the activation of the mitochondrial pathway. Death ligands bind to members of TNF receptor gene superfamily of death receptors, namely Fas, TNFR1, DR3, DR4, and DR5 (38), and cause apoptosis. Once stimulated, the death receptors activate the initiator caspase 9, and this in turn activates effector caspases 3 and 6 and executes apoptosis.

Mitochondrial Apoptotic Pathways and the Substantia Nigra

Many apoptotic and antiapoptotic factors converge upon the mitochondria. The expression of many of these factors is dependant on the activation of

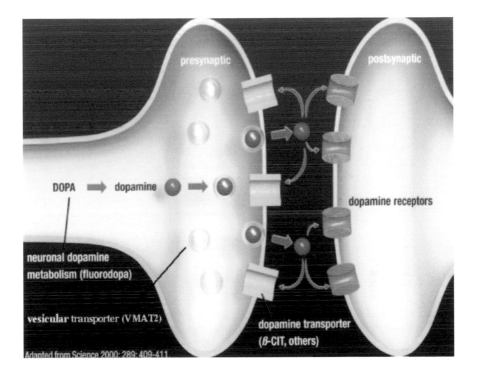

FIGURE 8.1 Idealized dopamine synapse showing targets for radiopharmaceutical in PD.

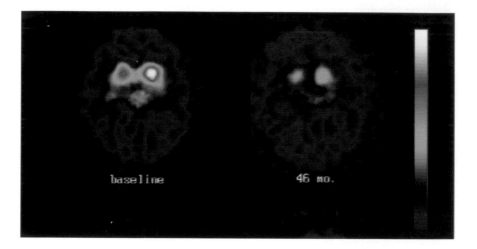

FIGURE 8.2 SPECT [^{123}I]β-CIT images from a patient with PD 2 years after diagnosis and 46 months later and from an age-matched healthy subject. Note the asymmetric reduction in [^{123}I]β-CIT uptake more marked in the putamen than caudate in the patient and the progressive loss of activity. Levels of SPECT activity are color-encoded from low (black) to high (yellow/white).

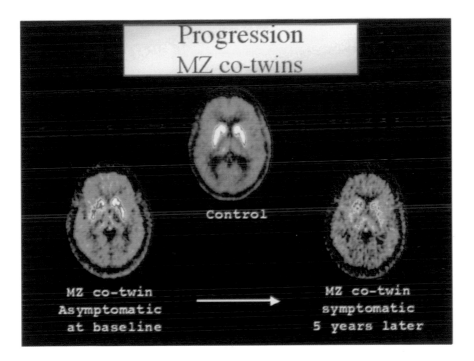

FIGURE 8.3 Presymptomatic loss of ^{18}F-DOPA in the asymptomatic co-twin of a PD patient. Note that the asymptomatic co-twin shows mild reduction in ^{18}F-DOPA at baseline that has worsened abnormality at 5-year follow-up associated with onset of symptoms. (Courtesy of D. Brooks, London, UK.)

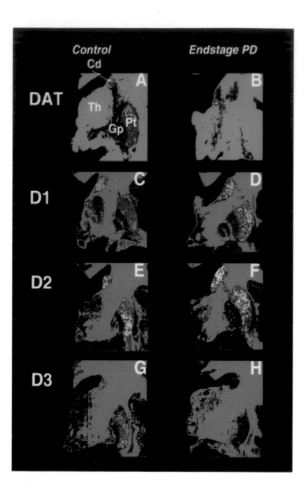

FIGURE 13.1 Autoradiographic localization of the distribution of D1, D2, and D3 receptors in representative coronal half-hemisphere sections of the human brain. Brain autoradiograms are shown in pseudocolor codes corresponding to a rainbow scale (red = high densities; green = intermediate densities; purple = low densities) for a control subject (male, age 72 yrs) and a patient with Parkinson's disease (male, age 67 yrs). The dopamine transporter was labeled with [3H]WIN 35, 428 (panels A and E) and shows the severity of the loss of dopamine terminals in endstage Parkinson's disease. Panels B and F illustrate the distribution of D1 receptors with 1 nM [^{3}H]SCH 23390 in the presence of 10 nM mianserin to occlude labeling of the 5-HT$_2$ receptor. Panels C and G show the distribution of D2 receptors labeled with 2 nM [^{3}H] raclopride. Panels D and H illustrate the distribution of D3 receptors labeled with [^{3}H]7OH DPAT. Panels C and F show the distribution of D3 receptors labeled with [3H]7OH-DPAT (for method see Ref. 68). Cd, caudate; Gp, globus pallidus; Pt, putamen; Th, thalamus.

neurotrophin and *trk*-mediated antiapoptotic or the p75^{NTR}-mediated apoptotic molecular cascades (Fig. 5). The members of the Bcl-2 family, namely Bcl-2, Bcl-xl, and Bcl-w, are antiapoptotic. Bax, Bak, and another group of polypeptides that includes Bid, Bad, Bim, and Bik are proapoptotic (139) (Figs. 4 and 5). Activation of caspases through the mitochondrial pathway is mediated by proapoptotic molecules facilitating the release of cytochrome *c* from the mitochondria as well as apoptotic-inducing factor (AIF) and endonuclease G, two other molecules released from the mitochondria that participate in apoptosis. Release of cytochrome *c* into the cytoplasm triggers activation of initiator caspase 9, formation of apoptosome, and subsequent activation of the effector caspases 3 and 6 and results in the destruction of the cytoplasm. The AIF translocates to the nucleus and contributes to DNA fragmentation and chromatin destruction and ultimately to cell death (139).

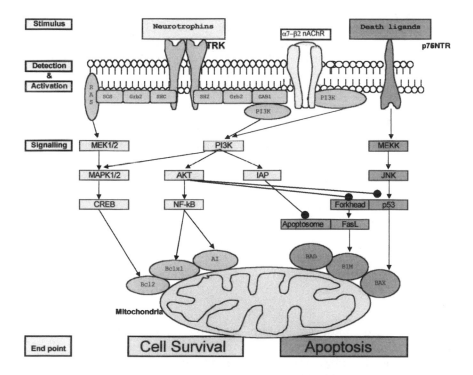

FIGURE 5 The neurotrophin-mediated pathways influencing the expression of different proapoptotic and antiapoptotic molecules on the mitochondria. (Adapted from Refs. 35,139,158.)

Bax, the proapoptotic protein, is expressed ubiquitously in normal and degenerating neurons of human nigra, but the numbers of Bax-positive neurons are significantly higher among the melanized degenerating nigral neurons in PD (140,141). p53-deficient mice were resistant to MPP+-induced neurotoxicity of dopaminergic neurons of nigra (142). Bax ablation prevents the MPTP-induced mouse model of PD (143). Overexpression of Bcl-2 protects catecholaminergic neurons from MPP+ and 6-OHDA toxicity of PC12 cells and neurons (144,145).

The effector caspase, caspase 3, is activated in 6-OHDA models of PD (146–149). Similarly, MPTP-induced nigral neurotoxicity has also been shown to be apoptotic. MPP+ also induces significant elevations of levels of caspase 3, caspase 8, and caspase 1 in the nigral neurons of mice, and inhibition of caspase activity prevents MPP+ neurotoxicity (150). Caspase 1 and 3 activities are increased in human nigral dopaminergic neurons of PD (151–153).

TUNEL-positive cells, an indicator of DNA fragmentation from apoptosis, have been noted in the MPTP-induced degeneration of nigral neurons and in melanized dopaminergic neurons of human nigra in PD (154–156). These and other studies strongly suggest that activation of the molecular cascades of proapoptotic pathways plays an important role in the death of substantia nigra neurons in PD.

Death Receptors and the Substantia Nigra

Apoptosis can also be induced by activation of several receptors of the TNF receptor gene superfamily. When "death ligands" bind to the receptors, the cells trigger several molecules that instruct the cells to self-destruct. So far, the ligands that directly activate the death receptors in PD have not been identified. TNF-receptor1, a receptor that contains the "death domain," is expressed in the nigral dopaminergic neurons and the glial cells that express this receptor. These are higher in the substantia nigra of PD than in controls (157).

Summary

The evidence for mitochondrial apoptotic pathways playing an important role in the death of dopaminergic neurons in PD is being established. The possible role of the receptors with death domain in the pathogenesis of PD and the role of increased levels of cytokines that have the potential to stimulate these death receptors is just beginning to be explored.

CONCLUSION

From the evidence discussed above, it is clear that both environmental and genetic factors can cause a parkinsonian syndrome that is similar to idiopathic PD. Environmental toxins induced mitochondrial dysfunction might be the most common cause of PD. In this regard, the observation that chronic administration of rotenone, a common toxin, can lead to a neurochemical and clinical syndrome that has significant similarities to that of idiopathic PD is a seminal one. This study certainly reinforces the prevailing epidemiological evidence that environmental toxins may cause PD.

However, based on the pathogenesis of familial PD, it is also recognized that dysfunction of the ubiquitin-proteasome system can lead to protein aggregation and resultant toxicity to nigral neurons. Accumulation and aggregation of proteins because of abnormal folding of proteins or inefficiency of molecular chaperones or proteasomal functions may occur even in the absence of any gene defects or toxins. Such mechanisms may play a role in aggregation of proteins in non-familial forms of Alzheimer's, prion and motor neuron diseases (68,75,78).

The survival of a neuron may also be dependant on a delicate balance between the neurotrophin and *trk* receptor–mediated antiapoptotic pathway and the proapoptotic pathway mediated by p75^{NTR} and other death receptors (139,158). As of yet, there is no direct evidence to support the hypothesis that withdrawal of growth factors or stimulation of the death receptors and accessing the direct pathway to apoptosis exists in PD. However, the role of a decreased level of growth factors as well as increased levels of cytokines observed in the dopaminergic neurons of the substantia nigra in PD remains to be explored.

As the understanding of the trophic factors that influence normal differentiation and maturation of nigral dopaminergic neurons is expanding, the possibility that lack of or reduced influence of these ontogenic trophic factors may somehow result in either a decreased number or defective dopamine neurons in adulthood exists. Such a decrease in the number or efficiency of dopamine neurons may be a risk factor for developing PD later in life.

While many of these concepts about multiple etiologies for PD are nothing more than hypothetical at present, the knowledge derived from modern experimental approaches will certainly allow us to enter into a new and exciting phase of diagnosing these patients early in the course of the disease and treat them with molecules that will either slow the progression of PD or, hopefully, even stop the progression of the disease.

ACKNOWLEDGMENTS

Supported by the Carl Baldridge Parkinson's Disease Research Fund. Dedicated to my mentors Drs. B. Ramamurthi, T. Umeshraya Pai, C. H. Narayanan, Malcolm Carpenter, Stanley Fahn, Joseph Chusid, Hyman Donnenfeld, and George Uhl.

REFERENCES

1. R Hassler. Zur Normalantomie de Substantia nigra. J Psychol Neurol 48:1–55, 1937.
2. R. Hassler. Zur Pathologie der Paralysis agitans und des postencephalitischen Parkinsonismus. J. psychol. Neurology 48:387–455, 1938.
3. JM Fearnley, AJ Lees. Ageing and Parkinson's disease: substantia nigra regional selectivity. Brain 114:2283–2301, 1991.
4. WR Gibb, AJ Lees. Anatomy, pigmentation, ventral and dorsal subpopulations of the substantia nigra, and differential cell death in Parkinson's disease. J Neurol Neurosurg Psychiatry 54:388–396, 1991.
5. Parkinson Study Group. Dopamine transporter brain imaging to assess the effects of pramipexole vs levodopa on Parkinson disease progression. JAMA 287:1653–1661,2002.
6. YA Barde. Trophic factors and neuronal survival. Neuron 2:1525–1534,1989.
7. MV Sofroniew, CL Howe, WC Mobley. Nerve growth factor signaling, neuroprotection, and neural repair. Annu Rev Neurosci 24:1217–1281, 2001.
8. B Connor, M Dragunow. The role of neuronal growth factors in neurodegenerative disorders of the human brain. Brain Res Brain Res Rev 27:1–39, 1998.
9. M Hynes, JA Porter, C Chiang, D Chang, M Tessier-Lavigne, PA Beachy, A Rosenthal. Induction of midbrain dopaminergic neurons by sonic hedgehog. Neuron 15:35–44, 1995.
10. J Briscoe, J Erickson. Specification of neuronal fates in the ventral neural tube. Curr Opin Neurobiol 11:43–49, 2001.
11. K Tsuboi, CW Shults. Intrastriatal injection of sonic hedgehog reduces behavioral impairment in a rat model of Parkinson's disease. Exp Neurol 173:95–104, 2002.
12. O Saucedo-Cardenas, JD Quintana-Hau, WD Le, MP Smidt, JJ Cox, F De Mayo, JP Burbach, OM Conneely. Nurrl is essential for the induction of the dopaminergic phenotype and the survival of ventral mesencephalic late dopaminergic precursor neurons. Proc Natl Acad Sci USA 95:4013–4018, 1998.
13. C Backman, T Perlmann, A Wallen, BJ Hoffer, M Morales. A selective group of dopaminergic neurons express Nurrl in the adult mouse brain. Brain Res 851:125–132, 1999.
14. RH Zetterstrom, L Solomin, L Jansson, BJ Hoffer, L Olson, T Perlmann. Dopamine neuron agenesis in Nurrl-deficient mice. Science 276:248–250, 1997.

15. SO Castillo, JS Baffi, M Palkovits, DS Goldstein, IJ Kopin, J Witta, MA Magnuson, VM Nikodem. Dopamine biosynthesis is selectively abolished in substantia nigra/ventral tegmental area but not in hypothalamic neurons in mice with targeted disruption of the Nurrl gene. Mol Cell Neurosci 11:36–46, 1998.

16. W Le, OM Conneely, L Zou, Y He, O Saucedo-Cardenas, J Jankovic, DR Mosier, SH Appel. Selective agenesis of mesencephalic dopaminergic neurons in Nurrl-deficient mice. Exp Neurol 159:451–458, 1999.

17. K Sakurada, M Ohshima-Sakurada, TD Palmer, FH Gage. Nurrl, an orphan nuclear receptor, is a transcriptional activator of endogenous tyrosine hydroxylase in neural progenitor cells derived from the adult brain. Development 126:4017–4026, 1999.

18. JS Baffi, M Palkovits, SO Castillo, E Mezey, VM Nikodem. Differential expression of tyrosine hydroxylase in catecholaminergic neurons of neonatal wild-type and Nurrl-deficient mice. Neuroscience 93:631–642, 1999.

19. T Iwawaki, K Kohno, K Kobayashi. Identification of a potential nurrl response element that activates the tyrosine hydroxylase gene promoter in cultured cells. Biochem Biophys Res Commun 274:590–595, 2000.

20. P Sacchetti, TR Mitchell, JG Granneman, MJ Bannon. Nurrl enhances transcription of the human dopamine transporter gene through a novel mechanism. J Neurochem 76:1565–1572, 2001.

21. RH Zetterstrom, R Williams, T Perlmann, L Olson. Cellular expression of the immediate early transcription factors Nurrl and NGFI-B suggests a gene regulatory role in several brain regions including the nigrostriatal dopamine system. Brain Res Mol Brain Res 41:111–120, 1996.

22. W Le, OM Conneely, Y He, J Jankovic, SH Appel. Reduced Nurrl expression increases the vulnerability of mesencephalic dopamine neurons to MPTP-induced injury. J Neurochem 73:2218–2221, 1999.

23. PY Xu, R Liang, J Jankovic, C Hunter, YX Zeng, T Ashizawa, D Lai, WD Le. Association of homozygous 7048G7049 variant in the intron six of Nurrl gene with Parkinson's disease. Neurology 58:881–884, 2002.

24. MP Smidt, HS van Schaick, C Lanctot, JJ Tremblay, JJ Cox, AA van der Kleij, G Wolterink, J Drouin, JP Burbach. A homeodomain gene Ptx3 has highly restricted brain expression in mesencephalic dopaminergic neurons. Proc Natl Acad Sci USA 94:13305–13310, 1997.

25. M Lebel, Y Gauthier, A Moreau, J Drouin. Pitx3 activates mouse tyrosine hydroxylase promoter via a high-affinity binding site. J Neurochem 77:558–567, 2001.

26. M Fujita, S Shimada, T Nishimura, GR Uhl, M Tohyama. Ontogeny of dopamine transporter mRNA expression in the rat brain. Brain Res Mol Brain Res 19:222–226, 1993.

27. SR Hansson, BJ Hoffman, E Mezey. Ontogeny of vesicular monoamine transporter mRNAs VMAT1 and VMAT2. I. The developing rat central nervous system. Brain Res Dev Brain Res 110:135–158, 1998.

28. C Perrone-Capano, P Da Pozzo, U di Porzio. Epigenetic cues in midbrain dopaminergic neuron development. Neurosci Biobehav Rev 24:119–124, 2000.
29. DB Ramsden, RB Parsons, SL Ho, RH Waring. The aetiology of idiopathic Parkinson's disease. Mol Pathol 54:369–380, 2001.
30. MP Smidt, CH Asbreuk, JJ Cox, H Chen, RL Johnson, JP Burbach. A second independent pathway for development of mesencephalic dopaminergic neurons requires Lmxlb. Nat Neurosci 3:337–341, 2000.
31. LM Farkas, K Krieglstein. Heparin-binding epidermal growth factor-like growth factor (HB-EGF) regulates survival of midbrain dopaminergic neurons. J Neural Transm 109:267–277, 2002.
32. HH Simon, H Saueressig, W Wurst, MD Goulding, DD O'Leary. Fate of midbrain dopaminergic neurons controlled by the engrailed genes. J Neurosci 21:3126–3134, 2001.
33. GJ Siegel, NB Chauhan. Neurotrophic factors in Alzheimer's and Parkinson's disease brain. Brain Res Brain Res Rev 33:199–227, 2000.
34. DR Kaplan, FD Miller. Signal transduction by the neurotrophin receptors. Curr Opin Cell Biol 9:213–221, 1997.
35. DR Kaplan, FD Miller. Neurotrophin signal transduction in the nervous system. Curr Opin Neurobiol 10:381–391, 2000.
36. Bibel, E Hoppe, YA Barde. Biochemical and functional interactions between the neurotrophin receptors trk and p75NTR. Embo J 18:616–622, 1999.
37. G Dechant. Molecular interactions between neurotrophin receptors. Cell Tissue Res 305:229–238, 2001.
38. A Ashkenazi, VM Dixit. Death receptors: signaling and modulation. Science 281:1305–1308, 1998.
39. T Nishio, S Furukawa, I Akiguchi, N Sunohara. Medial nigral dopamine neurons have rich neurotrophin support in humans. Neuroreport 9:2847–2851, 1998.
40. EJ Mufson, JS Kroin, TJ Sendera, T Sobreviela. Distribution and retrograde transport of trophic factors in the central nervous system: functional implications for the treatment of neurodegenerative diseases. Prog Neurobiol 57:451–484, 1999.
41. M Mogi, A Togari, T Kondo, Y Mizuno, O Komure, S Kuno, H Ichinose, T Nagatsu. Brain-derived growth factor and nerve growth factor concentrations are decreased in the substantia nigra in Parkinson's disease. Neurosci Lett 270:45–48, 1999.
42. K Parain, MG Murer, Q Yan, B Faucheux, Y Agid, E Hirsch, R Raisman-Vozari. Reduced expression of brain-derived neurotrophic factor protein in Parkinson's disease substantia nigra. Neuroreport 10:557–561, 1999.
43. DM Frim, TA Uhler, WR Galpern, MF Beal, XO Breakefield, O Isacson. Implanted fibroblasts genetically engineered to produce brain-derived neurotrophic factor prevent 1-methyl-4-phenylpyridinium toxicity to dopaminergic neurons in the rat. Proc Natl Acad Sci USA 91:5104–5108, 1994.

44. NB Chauhan, GJ Siegel, JM Lee. Depletion of glial cell line-derived neurotrophic factor in substantia nigra neurons of Parkinson's disease brain. J Chem Neuroanat 21:277–288, 2001.

45. CW Shults, T Kimber, D Martin. Intrastriatal injection of GDNF attenuates the effects of 6-hydroxydopamine. Neuroreport 7:627–631, 1996.

46. JH Kordower, ME Emborg, J Bloch, SY Ma, Y Chu, L Leventhal, J McBride, EY Chen, S Palfi, BZ Roitberg, WD Brown, JE Holden, R Pyzalski, MD Taylor, P Carvey, Z Ling, D Trono, P Hantraye, N Deglon, P Aebischer. Neurodegeneration prevented by lentiviral vector delivery of GDNF in primate models of Parkinson's disease. Science 290:767–773, 2000.

47. L Feng, CY Wang, H Jiang, C Oho, M Dugich-Djordjevic, L Mei, B Lu. Differential signaling of glial cell line-derived neurothrophic factor and brain-derived neurotrophic factor in cultured ventral mesencephalic neurons. Neuroscience 93:265–273, 1999.

48. NJ Rothwell. Annual review prize lecture cytokines—killers in the brain? J Physiol 514:3–17, 1999.

49. R Martin, CS Sturzebecher, HF McFarland. Immunotherapy of multiple sclerosis: Where are we? Where should we go? Nat Immunol 2:785–788, 2001.

50. M Mogi, M Harada, T Kondo, P Riederer, H Inagaki, M Minami, T Nagatsu. Interleukin-1 beta, interleukin-6, epidermal growth factor and transforming growth factor-alpha are elevated in the brain from parkinsonian patients. Neurosci Lett 180:147–150, 1994.

51. T Nagatsu, M Mogi, H Ichinose, A Togari. Cytokines in Parkinson's disease. J Neural Transm (suppl)58:143–151, 2000.

52. A Cintra, YH Cao, C Oellig, B Tinner, F Bortolotti, M Goldstein, RF Pettersson, K Fuxe. Basic FGF is present in dopaminergic neurons of the ventral midbrain of the rat. Neuroreport 2:597–600, 1991.

53. I Tooyama, T Kawamata, D Walker, T Yamada, K Hanai, H Kimura, M Iwane, K Igarashi, EG McGeer, PL McGeer. Loss of basic fibroblast growth factor in substantia nigra neurons in Parkinson's disease. Neurology 43:372–376, 1993.

54. I Tooyama, EG McGeer, T Kawamata, H Kimura, PL McGeer. Retention of basic fibroblast growth factor immunoreactivity in dopaminergic neurons of the substantia nigra during normal aging in humans contrasts with loss in Parkinson's disease. Brain Res 656:165–168, 1994.

55. T Kihara, S Shimohama, H Sawada, K Honda, T Nakamizo, H Shibasaki, T Kume, A Akaike. alpha 7 nicotinic receptor transduces signals to phosphatidylinositol 3-kinase to block A beta-amyloid-induced neurotoxicity. J Biol Chem 276:13541–13546, 2001.

56. P Marin, M Maus, S Desagher, J Glowinski, J Premont. Nicotine protects cultured striatal neurones against N-methyl-D-aspartate receptor-mediated neurotoxicity. Neuroreport 5:1977–1980, 1994.

57. R Maggio, M Riva, F Vaglini, F Fornai, R Molteni, M Armogida, G Racagni, GU Corsini. Nicotine prevents experimental parkinsonism in rodents and

induces striatal increase of neurotrophic factors. J Neurochem 71:2439–2446, 1998.

58. RE Ryan, SA Ross, J Drago, RE Loiacono. Dose-related neuroprotective effects of chronic nicotine in 6-hydroxydopamine treated rats, and loss of neuroprotection in alpha4 nicotinic receptor subunit knockout mice. Br J Pharmacol 132:1650–1656, 2001.

59. M Quik, DA Di Monte. Nicotine administration reduces striatal MPP+levels in mice. Brain Res 917:219–224, 2001.

60. MH Polymeropoulos, C Lavedan, E Leroy, SE Ide, A Dehejia, A Dutra, B Pike, H Root, J Rubenstein, R Boyer, ES Stenroos, S Chandrasekharappa, A Athanassiadou, T Papapetropoulos, WG Johnson, AM Lazzarini, RC Duvoisin, G Di Iorio, LI Golbe, RL Nussbaum. Mutation in the alpha-synuclein gene identified in families with Parkinson's disease. Science 276:2045–2047, 1997

61. R Kruger, W Kuhn, T Muller, D Woitalla, M Graeber, S Kosel, H Przuntek, JT Epplen, L Schols, O Riess. Ala30Pro mutation in the gene encoding alpha-synuclein in Parkinson's disease. Nat Genet 18:106–108, 1998.

62. M Neystat, T Lynch, S Przedborski, N Kholodilov, M Rzhetskaya, RE Burke. Alpha-synuclein expression in substantia nigra and cortex in Parkinson's disease. Mov Disord 14:417–422, 1999.

63. NB Cole, DD Murphy. The cell biology of alpha-synuclein: a sticky problem? Neuromolecular Med 1:95–109, 2002. LA Hansen, M Mallory, JQ Trojanowski, D Galasko, E Masliah. Altered expression of the synuclein family mRNA in Lewy body and Alzheimer's disease. Brain Res 914:48–56, 2001.

64. N Ostrerova, L Petrucelli, M Farrer, N Mehta, P Choi, J Hardy, B Wolozin. Alpha-synuclein shares physical and functional homology with 14-3-3 proteins. J Neurosci 19:5782–5791, 1999.

65. RG Perez, JC Waymire, E Lin, JJ Liu, F Guo, MJ Zigmond. A role for alpha-synuclein in the regulation of dopamine biosynthesis. J Neurosci 22:3090–3099, 2002.

66. K Tanaka, T Suzuki, T Chiba, H Shimura, N Hattori, Y Mizuno. Parkin is linked to the ubiquitin pathway. J Mol Med 79:482–494, 2001.

67. Y Zhang, J Gao, KK Chung, H Huang, VL Dawson, TM Dawson. Parkin functions as an E2-dependent ubiquitin- protein ligase and promotes the degradation of the synaptic vesicle-associated protein, CDCrel-1. Proc Natl Acad Sci USA 97:13354–13359, 2000.

68. MH Glickman, A Ciechanover. The ubiquitin-proteasome proteolytic pathway: destruction for the sake of construction. Physiol Rev 82:373–428, 2002.

69. H Shimura, MG Schlossmacher, N Hattori, MP Frosch, A Trockenbacher, R Schneider, Y Mizuno, KS Kosik, DJ Selkoe. Ubiquitination of a new form of alpha-synuclein by parkin from human brain: implications for Parkinson's disease. Science 293:263–269, 2001.

70. KK Chung, Y Zhang, KL Lim, Y Tanaka, H Huang, J Gao, CA Ross, VL Dawson, TM Dawson. Parkin ubiquitinates the alpha-synuclein-interacting

protein, synphilin-1: implications for Lewy-body formation in Parkinson disease. Nat Med 7:1144–1150, 2001.

71. Y Imai, M Soda, H Inoue, N Hattori, Y Mizuno, R Takahashi. An unfolded putative transmembrane polypeptide, which can lead to endoplasmic reticulum stress, is a substrate of Parkin. Cell 105:891–902, 2001.

72. BI Giasson, VM Lee. Parkin and the molecular pathways of Parkinson's disease. Neuron 31:885–888, 2001.

73. E Leroy, R Boyer, G Auburger, B Leube, G Ulm, E Mezey, G Harta, MJ Brownstein, S Jonnalagada, T Chernova, A Dehejia, C Lavedan, T Gasser, PJ Steinbach, KD Wilkinson, MH Polymeropoulos. The ubiquitin pathway in Parkinson's disease. Nature 395:451–452, 1998.

74. C Lavedan, S Buchholtz, RL Nussbaum, RL Albin, MH Polymeropoulos. A mutation in the human neurofilament M gene in Parkinson's disease that suggests a role for the cytoskeleton in neuronal degeneration. Neurosci Lett 322:57–61, 2002.

75. R Layfield, A Alban, RJ Mayer, J Lowe. The ubiquitin protein catabolic disorders. Neuropathol Appl Neurobiol 27:171–179, 2001.

76. S Jentsch, G Pyrowolakis. Ubiquitin and its kin: How close are the family ties? Trends Cell Biol 10:335–342, 2000.

77. KS McNaught, P Jenner. Proteasomal function is impaired in substantia nigra in Parkinson's disease. Neurosci Lett 297:191–194, 2001.

78. MD Kaytor, ST Warren. Aberrant protein deposition and neurological disease. J Biol Chem 274:37507–37510, 1999.

79. H Takahashi, K Wakabayashi. The cellular pathology of Parkinson's disease. Neuropathology 21:315–322, 2001.

80. MG Spillantini, RA Crowther, R Jakes, M Hasegawa, M Goedert. alpha-synuclein in filamentous inclusions of Lewy bodies from Parkinson's disease and dementia with lewy bodies. Proc Natl Acad Sci USA 95:6469–6473, 1998.

81. JE Galvin, K Uryu, VM Lee, JQ Trojanowski. Axon pathology in Parkinson's disease and Lewy body dementia hippocampus contains alpha-, beta-, and gamma-synuclein. Proc Natl Acad Sci USA 96:13450–13455, 1999.

82. MB Feany and WW Bender. A Drosophila model of Parkinson's disease. Nature 404:394–398, 2000.

83. PK Auluck, HY Chan, JQ Trojanowski, VM Lee, NM Bonini. Chaperone suppression of alpha-synuclein toxicity in a Drosophila model for Parkinson's disease. Science 295:865–868, 2002.

84. VN Uversky, J Li, AL Fink. Metal-triggered structural transformations, aggregation, and fibrillation of human alpha-synuclein. A possible molecular NK between Parkinson's disease and heavy metal exposure. J Biol Chem 276:44284–44296, 2001.

85. BI Giasson, JE Duda, IV Murray, Q Chen, JM Souza, HI Hurtig, H Ischiropoulos, JQ Trojanowski, VM Lee. Oxidative damage linked to neurodegeneration by selective alpha-synuclein nitration in synucleinopathy lesions. Science 290:985–989, 2000.

86. LJ Hsu, Y Sagara, A Arroyo, E Rockenstein, A Sisk, M Mallory, J Wong, T Takenouchi, M Hashimoto, E Masliah. alpha-synuclein promotes mitochondrial deficit and oxidative stress. Am J Pathol 157:401–410, 2000.

87. S Engelender, Z Kaminsky, X Guo, AH Sharp, RK Amaravi, JJ Kleiderlein, RL Margolis, JC Troncoso, AA Lanahan, PF Worley, VL Dawson, TM Dawson, CA Ross. Synphilin-1 associates with alpha-synuclein and promotes the formation of cytosolic inclusions. Nat Genet 22:110–114, 1999.

88. A Takeda, M Mallory, M Sundsmo, W Honer, L Hansen, E Masliah. Abnormal accumulation of NACP/alpha-synuclein in neurodegenerative disorders. Am J Pathol 152:367–372, 1998.

89. K Arima, S Hirai, N Sunohara, K Aoto, Y Izumiyama, K Ueda, K Ikeda, M Kawai. Cellular co-localization of phosphorylated tau- and NACP/alpha-synuclein-epitopes in lewy bodies in sporadic Parkinson's disease and in dementia with Lewy bodies. Brain Res 843:53–61, 1999.

90. WP Gai, PC Blumbergs and WW Blessing. Microtubule-associated protein 5 is a component of Lewy bodies and Lewy neurites in the brainstem and forebrain regions affected in Parkinson's disease. Acta Neuropathol (Berl) 91:78–81, 1996.

91. S Nakamura, Y Kawamoto, S Nakano, I Akiguchi and J Kimura. p35nck5a and cyclin-dependent kinase 5 colocalize in Lewy bodies of brains with Parkinson's disease. Acta Neuropathol (Berl) 94:153–157, 1997.

92. K Nishiyama, S Murayama, J Shimizu, Y Ohya, S Kwak, K Asayama, I Kanazawa. Cu/Zn superoxide dismutase-like immunoreactivity is present in Lewy bodies from Parkinson disease: a light and electron microscopic immunocytochemical study. Acta Neuropathol (Berl) 89:471–474, 1995.

93. HM Schipper, A Liberman, EG Stopa. Neural heme oxygenase-1 expression in idiopathic Parkinson's disease. Exp Neurol 150:60–68, 1998.

94. A Tortosa, E Lopez, I Ferrer. Bcl-2 and Bax proteins in Lewy bodies from patients with Parkinson's disease and diffuse Lewy body disease. Neurosci Lett 238:78–80, 1997.

95. J Lowe, H McDermott, I Pike, I Spendlove, M Landon, RJ Mayer. alpha B crystallin expression in non-lenticular tissues and selective presence in ubiquitinated inclusion bodies in human disease. J Pathol 166:61–68, 1992.

96. Y Kawamoto, I Akiguchi, S Nakamura, Y Honjyo, H Shibasaki, H Budka. 14-3-3 proteins in Lewy bodies in Parkinson disease and diffuse Lewy body disease brains. J Neuropathol Exp Neurol 61:245–253, 2002.

97. P Shashidharan, PF Good, A Hsu, DP Perl, MF Brin, CW Olanow. TorsinA accumulation in Lewy bodies in sporadic Parkinson's disease. Brain Res 877:379–381, 2000.

98. MG Schlossmacher, MP Frosch, WP Gai, M Medina, N Sharma, L Forno, T Ochiishi, H Shimura, R Sharon, N Hattori, JW Langston, Y Mizuno, BT Hyman, DJ Selkoe, KS Kosik. Parkin localizes to the Lewy bodies of Parkinson disease and dementia with Lewy bodies. Am J Pathol 160:1655–1667, 2002.

99. J Lowe, H McDermott, M Landon, RJ Mayer, KD Wilkinson. Ubiquitin carboxyl-terminal hydrolase (PGP 9.5) is selectively present in ubiquitinated inclusion bodies characteristic of human neurodegenerative diseases. J Pathol 161:153–160, 1990.

100. K Ii, H Ito, K Tanaka and A Hirano. Immunocytochemical co-localization of the proteasome in ubiquitinated structures in neurodegenerative diseases and the elderly. J Neuropathol Exp Neurol 56:125–131, 1997.

101. GC Davis, AC Williams, SP Markey, MH Ebert, ED Caine, CM Reichert, IJ Kopin. Chronic Parkinsonism secondary to intravenous injection of meperidine analogues. Psychiatry Res 1:249–254, 1979.

102. JW Langston, P Ballard, JW Tetrud, I Irwin. Chronic Parkinsonism in humans due to a product of meperidine-analog synthesis. Science 219:979–980, 1983.

103. JW Langston. The Case of the Frozen Addicts. Santa Rosa, CA: Vintage Publications, 1996.

104. DC Wallace. Mitochondrial diseases in man and mouse. Science 283:1482–1488, 1999.

105. HS Chun, GE Gibson, LA DeGiorgio, H Zhang, VJ Kidd, JH Son. Dopaminergic cell death induced by MPP(+), oxidant and specific neurotoxicants shares the common molecular mechanism. J Neurochem 76:1010–1021, 2001.

106. R Betarbet, TB Sherer, JT Greenamyre. Animal models of Parkinson's disease. Bioessays 24:308–318, 2002.

107. I Vyas, RE Heikkila, WJ Nicklas. Studies on the neurotoxicity of 1-methyl-4-phenyl-1,2,3,6-tetrahydropyridine: inhibition of NAD-linked substrate oxidation by its metabolite, 1-methyl-4-phenylpyridinium. J Neurochem 46:1501–1507, 1986.

108. Y Mizuno, S Ohta, M Tanaka, S Takamiya, K Suzuki, T Sato, H Oya, T Ozawa, Y Kagawa. Deficiencies in complex I subunits of the respiratory chain in Parkinson's disease. Biochem Biophys Res Commun 163:1450–1455, 1989.

109. AHV Schapira, JM Cooper, D Dexter, P Jenner, JB Clark, CD Marsden. Mitochondrial complex I deficiency in Parkinson's disease. Lancet 1:1269, 1989.

110. AHV Schapira, VM Mann, JM Cooper, D Dexter, SE Daniel, P Jenner, JB Clark, CD Marsden. Anatomic and disease specificity of NADH CoQ1 reductase (complex I) deficiency in Parkinson's disease. J Neurochem 55:2142–2145, 1990.

111. M Orth, AH Schapira. Mitochondrial involvement in Parkinson's disease. Neurochem Int 40:533–541, 2002.

112. R Betarbet, TB Sherer, G MacKenzie, M Garcia-Osuna, AV Panov, JT Greenamyre. Chronic systemic pesticide exposure reproduces features of Parkinson's disease. Nat Neurosci 3:1301–1306, 2000.

113. Y Mizuno, K Suzuki, S Ohta. Postmortem changes in mitochondrial respiratory enzymes in brain and a preliminary observation in Parkinson's disease. J Neurol Sci 96:49–57, 1990.

114. MW Cleeter, JM Cooper, AH Schapira. Nitric oxide enhances MPP(+) inhibition of complex I. FEBS Lett 504:50–52, 2001.

115. T Finkel, NJ Holbrook. Oxidants, oxidative stress and the biology of ageing. Nature 408:239–247, 2000.

116. Y Agid. Levodopa: is toxicity a myth? Neurology 50:858–863, 1998.

117. Y Agid. Levodopa. Is toxicity a myth? 1998. Neurology 57:S46–51, 2001.

118. J Jankovic. Levodopa strengths and weaknesses. Neurology 58:S19–32, 2002.

119. D Berg, M Gerlach, MB Youdim, KL Double, L. Zecca, P Riederer, G Becker. Brain iron pathways and their relevance to Parkinson's disease. J Neurochem 79:225–236, 2001.

120. M Gu, AD Owen, SE Toffa, JM Cooper, DT Dexter, P Jenner, CD Marsden, AH Schapira. Mitochondrial function, GSH and iron in neurodegeneration and Lewy body diseases. J Neurol Sci 158:24–29, 1998.

121. MV Clement, LH Long, J Ramalingam, B Halliwell. The cytotoxicity of dopamine may be an artefact of cell culture. J Neurochem 81:414–421, 2002.

122. M Gerlach, D Blum-Degen, J Lan, P Riederer. Nitric oxide in the pathogenesis of Parkinson's disease. Adv Neurol 80:239–245, 1999.

123. GT Liberatore, V Jackson-Lewis, S Vukosavic, AS Mandir, M Vila, WG McAuliffe, VL Dawson, TM Dawson, S Przedborski. Inducible nitric oxide synthase stimulates dopaminergic neurodegeneration in the MPTP model of Parkinson disease. Nat Med 5:1403–1409, 1999.

124. MJ LaVoie, TG Hastings. Peroxynitrite- and nitrite-induced oxidation of dopamine: implications for nitric oxide in dopaminergic cell loss. J Neurochem 73:2546–2554, 1999.

125. AJ Nappi, E Vass. The effects of nitric oxide on the oxidations of l-dopa and dopamine mediated by tyrosinase and peroxidase. J Biol Chem 276:11214–11222, 2001.

126. TL Perry, DV Godin, S Hansen. Parkinson's disease: a disorder due to nigral glutathione deficiency? Neurosci Lett 33:305–310, 1982.

127. SJ Kish, C Morito, O Hornykiewicz. Glutathione peroxidase activity in Parkinson's disease brain. Neurosci Lett 58:343–346, 1985.

128. P Jenner. Presymptomatic detection of Parkinson's disease. J Neural Transm Suppl 40:23–36, 1993.

129. M Merad-Boudia, A Nicole, D Santiard-Baron, C Saille, I Ceballos-Picot. Mitochondrial impairment as an early event in the process of apoptosis induced by glutathione depletion in neuronal cells: relevance to Parkinson's disease. Biochem Pharmacol 56:645–655, 1998.

130. N Jha, O Jurma, G Lalli, Y Liu, EH Pettus, JT Greenamyre, RM Liu, HJ Forman, JK Andersen. Glutathione depletion in PC12 results in selective inhibition of mitochondrial complex I activity. Implications for Parkinson's disease. J Biol Chem 275:26096–26101, 2000.

131. RH Swerdlow. Mitochondrial DNA–related mitochondrial dysfunction in neurodegenerative diseases. Arch Pathol Lab Med 126:271–280, 2002.

132. RH Swerdlow, JK Parks, JN Davis, 2nd, DS Cassarino, PA Trimmer, LJ Currie, J Dougherty, WS Bridges, JP Bennett, Jr., GF Wooten, WD Parker.

Matrilineal inheritance of complex I dysfunction in a multigenerational Parkinson's disease family. Ann Neurol 44:873–881, 1998.

133. M Gu, JM Cooper, JW Taanman, AH Schapira. Mitochondrial DNA transmission of the mitochondrial defect in Parkinson's disease. Ann Neurol 44:177–186, 1998.

134. EM Grasbon-Frodl, S Kosel, M Sprinzl, U von Eitzen, P Mehraein, MB Graeber. Two novel point mutations of mitochondrial tRNA genes in histologically confirmed Parkinson disease. Neurogenetics 2:121–127, 1999.

135. RE Burke and NG Kholodilov. Programmed cell death: does it play a role in Parkinson's disease? Ann Neurol 44:S126–133, 1998.

136. EC Hirsch, S Hunot, B Faucheux, Y Agid, Y Mizuno, H Mochizuki, WG Tatton, N Tatton, WC Olanow. Dopaminergic neurons degenerate by apoptosis in Parkinson's disease. Mov Disord 14:383–385, 1999.

137. D Blum, S Torch, N Lambeng, M Nissou, AL Benabid, R Sadoul, JM Verna. Molecular pathways involved in the neurotoxicity of 6-OHDA, dopamine and MPTP: contribution to the apoptotic theory in Parkinson's disease. Prog Neurobiol 65:135–172, 2001.

138. DL Vaux, A Strasser. The molecular biology of apoptosis. Proc Natl Acad Sci USA 93:2239–2244, 1996.

139. SH Kaufmann, MO Hengartner. Programmed cell death: alive and well in the new millennium. Trends Cell Biol 11:526–534, 2001.

140. NA Tatton. Increased caspase 3 and Bax immunoreactivity accompany nuclear GAPDH translocation and neuronal apoptosis in Parkinson's disease. Exp Neurol 166:29–43, 2000.

141. A Hartmann, PP Michel, JD Troadec, A Mouatt-Prigent, BA Faucheux, M Ruberg, Y Agid, EC Hirsch. Is Bax a mitochondrial mediator in apoptotic death of dopaminergic neurons in Parkinson's disease? J Neurochem 76:1785–1793, 2001.

142. PA Trimmer, TS Smith, AB Jung, JP Bennett, Jr. Dopamine neurons from transgenic mice with a knockout of the p53 gene resist MPTP neurotoxicity. Neurodegeneration 5:233–239, 1996.

143. M Vila, V Jackson-Lewis, S Vukosavic, R Djaldetti, G Liberatore, D Offen, SJ Korsmeyer, S Przedborski. Bax ablation prevents dopaminergic neurodegeneration in the 1-methyl-4-phenyl-1,2,3,6-tetrahydropyridine mouse model of Parkinson's disease. Proc Natl Acad Sci USA 98:2837–2842, 2001.

144. D Offen, PM Beart, NS Cheung, CJ Pascoe, A Hochman, S Gorodin, E Melamed, R Bernard, O Bernard. Transgenic mice expressing human Bcl-2 in their neurons are resistant to 6-hydroxydopamine and 1-methyl-4-phenyl-1,2,3,6-tetrahydropyridine neurotoxicity. Proc Natl Acad Sci USA 95:5789–5794, 1998.

145. L Yang, RT Matthews, JB Schulz, T Klockgether, AW Liao, JC Martinou, JB Penney, Jr., BT Hyman, MF Beal. 1-Methyl-4-phenyl-1,2,3,6-tetrahydropyride neurotoxicity is attenuated in mice overexpressing Bcl-2. J Neurosci 18:8145–8152, 1998.

146. B Cutillas, M Espejo, J Gil, I Ferrer, S Ambrosio. Caspase inhibition protects nigral neurons against 6-OHDA-induced retrograde degeneration. Neuroreport 10:2605–2608, 1999.

147. BS Jeon, NG Kholodilov, TF Oo, SY Kim, KJ Tomaselli, A Srinivasan, L Stefanis, RE Burke. Activation of caspase-3 in developmental models of programmed cell death in neurons of the substantia nigra. J Neurochem 73:322–333, 1999.

148. N Takai, H Nakanishi, K Tanabe, T Nishioku, T Sugiyama, M Fujiwara, K Yamamoto. Involvement of caspase-like proteinases in apoptosis of neuronal PC12 cells and primary cultured microglia induced by 6-hydroxydopamine. J Neurosci Res 54:214–222, 1998.

149. RC Dodel, Y Du, KR Bales, Z Ling, PM Carvey, SM Paul. Caspase-3-like proteases and 6-hydroxydopamine induced neuronal cell death. Brain Res Mol Brain Res 64:141–148, 1999.

150. H Turmel, A Hartmann, K Parain, A Douhou, A Srinivasan, Y Agid, EC Hirsch. Caspase-3 activation in 1-methyl-4-phenyl-1,2,3,6-tetrahydropyridine (MPTP)-treated mice. Mov Disord 16:185–189, 2001.

151. M Mogi, A Togari, T Kondo, Y Mizuno, O Komure, S Kuno, H Ichinose, T Nagatsu. Caspase activities and tumor necrosis factor receptor R1 (p55) level are elevated in the substantia nigra from parkinsonian brain. J Neural Transm 107:335–341, 2000.

152. A Hartmann, S Hunot, PP Michel, MP Muriel, S Vyas, BA Faucheux, A Mouatt-Prigent, H Turmel, A Srinivasan, M Ruberg, GI Evan, Y Agid, EC Hirsch. Caspase-3: a vulnerability factor and final effector in apoptotic death of dopaminergic neurons in Parkinson's disease. Proc Natl Acad Sci USA 97:2875–2880, 2000.

153. A Hartmann, JD Troadec, S Hunot, K Kikly, BA Faucheux, A Mouatt-Prigent, M Ruberg, Y Agid, EC Hirsch. Caspase-8 is an effector in apoptotic death of dopaminergic neurons in Parkinson's disease, but pathway inhibition results in neuronal necrosis. J Neurosci 21:2247–2255, 2001.

154. P Anglade, S Vyas, F Javoy-Agid, MT Herrero, PP Michel, J Marquez, A Mouatt-Prigent, M Ruberg, EC Hirsch, Y Agid. Apoptosis and autophagy in nigral neurons of patients with Parkinson's disease. Histol Histopathol 12:25–31, 1997.

155. H Mochizuki, K Goto, H Mori, Y Mizuno. Histochemical detection of apoptosis in Parkinson's disease. J Neurol Sci 137:120–123, 1996.

156. H Mochizuki, H Mori, Y Mizuno. Apoptosis in neurodegenerative disorders. J Neural Transm Suppl 50:125–140, 1997.

157. A Hartmann, A Mouatt-Prigent, BA Faucheux, Y Agid, EC Hirsch. FADD: a link between TNF family receptors and caspases in Parkinson's disease. Neurology 58:308–310, 2002.

158. SR Datta, A Brunet, ME Greenberg. Cellular survival: a play in three Akts. Genes Dev 13:2905–2927, 1999.

11

Neurophysiology/Circuitry

Erwin B. Montgomery, Jr.
Cleveland Clinic Foundation, Cleveland, Ohio, U.S.A.

INTRODUCTION

Theories of the role of the basal ganglia within the functional circuitry of the basal ganglia-thalamic-cortical system are entering a state of flux. Current theories, while of heuristic value in explaining many observations, are now inconsistent with an expanding body of knowledge. Most likely, observations supportive of the current theories and their associated circumstances will be found to be special cases of a larger new theory. There is no new general theory yet proposed that is a clear successor. Consequently, there is considerable value in analyzing the epistemic basis of current theories, if for no other reason than avoiding the types of inferences that, in retrospect, are erroneous. Also, such an exercise may help to form a framework by which new theories can develop and be judged. As Charcot said, "we see only what we are ready to see" (1). Typically this statement is made in retrospect to explain why observations and insights are missed or late in being made. A better use would be to prepare prospectively to facilitate new observations and insights. Such preparation must necessarily be theoretical and, to some extent, philosophical because such discussions precede recognition of data.

Understanding the functional circuitry of the basal ganglia-thalamus-cortex in terms of neuronal activities and interrelationships within a large-scale dynamical system is important now and will become increasingly important in the future. The resurgence of functional stereotactic surgery, both ablative and utilizing deep brain stimulation (DBS), has been fueled by improvement in surgical techniques such as image-based and microelectrode navigation, a realization of the limitations of pharmacological therapy, as well as a justifying rationale based on better understanding of neuronal pathophysiology. Systems physiology and pathophysiology will play an ever-increasing role in developing new electrophysiologically based techniques such as DBS.

Systems physiology and pathophysiology also will play a large role in the further development of neurotransplantation of both fetal dopamine and stem cells. The occurrence of "runaway" dyskinesia in patients who underwent neurotransplantation with fetal cells emphasizes the importance of physiological controls on the implanted cells (2). Considerable research is underway to develop methods to dynamically control transplanted neurons, as well as a greater understanding of the importance of the physiological context or environment. For example, fetal dopamine neurons extracted from the region of the substantia nigra pars compacta (SNpc) have been transplanted into the striatum. However, this is not the normal location for these neurons, and the usual efferents to SNpc that control dopamine neuron function are not located in the striatum.

ANATOMY: THE BASICS FOR CIRCUITRY

This section reviews the basic anatomical interconnections between neurons that make up the basal ganglia-thalamic-cortical circuits. The anatomy is discussed only to a level of detail necessary for conceptual understanding of current models of function and dysfunction and for possible future theories. This section will not cover a fine-grained analysis of interconnections nor the histology (3,4).

Traditional approaches to the anatomy of the basal ganglia have divided it into input and output stages. This approach will be avoided here because such a description implies a sequential and hierarchical organization, which probably is misleading from a physiological perspective. Just as it is hard to say where a circle starts and an arbitrary starting point must be selected, this description will begin with the striatum. The caudate nucleus and putamen (Pt) make up the striatum.

The major sources of input to the striatum come from the cerebral cortex and thalamus. Virtually the entire cortex projects to the striatum in a topographic fashion. Frontal cortex projects to the head of the caudate and anterior putamen while motor and somatosensory cortex project to the postcommissural Pt and temporal cortex projects to the tail of the caudate.

Inputs from the thalamus include projections from the centromedian (CM) and parafasciculus (PF) nuclei of the thalamus. The striatum projects to the globus pallidus external segment (GPe), globus pallidus internal segment (GPi), and substantia nigra pars reticulata (SNr). There appears to be two separate groups of striatal neurons based on projection targets and neurotransmitters. All outputs from the striatum utilize gamma aminobutyric acid (GABA) but differ in the polypeptide cotransmitter. Striatal neurons projecting to the GPe express enkephalin and have predominantly D_2 receptors. Striatal neurons projecting to GPi express substance P and dynorphin and have predominantly D_1 receptors (5).

The GPe has inhibitory GABAergic projections to the subthalamic nucleus (STN) and GPi. The STN has excitatory glutamatergic projections to the GPi and SNr and back to GPe. GPi has GABAergic outputs to the ventrolateral (VL) and ventroanterior (VA) nuclei of the thalamus, which then has extensive projections back to the cerebral cortex. In addition, GPi projects to the pedunculopontine nucleus (PPN) in the brainstem. The PPN has received considerable attention recently. Injections of bicucullin, a GABA antagonist, alleviate symptoms of experimental parkinsonism induced by administration of n-methyl-4 phenyl-1,2,3,6-tetrahydropyridine (MPTP) in nonhuman primates (6). The SNr projects to the superior colliculi and are conceived to be involved in eye movements.

CURRENT CONCEPTS OF PARKINSON'S DISEASE PATHOPHYSIOLOGY

These anatomical/neurochemical circuits have been conceptualized by current theories of physiology and pathophysiology into direct and indirect pathways (7,8). The direct pathway includes the striatum to the GPi to the VL thalamus, finally to motor cortex (MC) and supplementary motor area (SMA). The indirect pathway includes the striatum to GPe to STN to GPi to VL thalamus and then to MC and SMA. SNpc dopamine neurons are excitatory of striatal neurons participating in the indirect pathway and inhibitory of striatal neurons participating in the direct pathway. Consequently, the result of loss of SNpc dopamine neurons can be hypothesized to cause decreased activity in the striatal neurons of the direct pathway. This would result in a reduction of inhibition of GPi neurons, which in turn would result in increased inhibition of the VL thalamus and a reduction of excitation of the MC and SMA, thus providing an explanation for loss and slowing of movements (Fig. 1).

Loss of SNpc dopaminergic drive to striatal neurons of the indirect pathway would result in decreased inhibition of these striatal neurons, which in turn would increase the inhibition of the GPe. Consequent

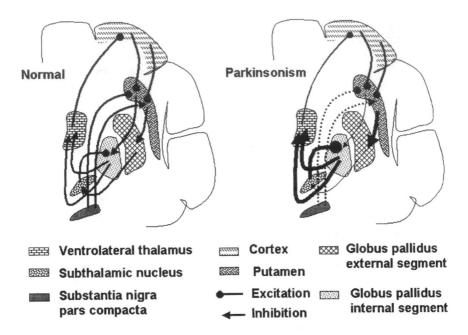

Normal   **Parkinsonism**

▦ **Ventrolateral thalamus**	▨ **Cortex**	▧ **Globus pallidus**
▨ **Subthalamic nucleus**	▨ **Putamen**	**external segment**
▬ **Substantia nigra**	●— **Excitation**	▨ **Globus pallidus**
pars compacta	◄— **Inhibition**	**internal segment**

FIGURE 1 Schematic representation of the basal ganglia-thalamic-cortical circuits. There are two general pathways, termed the direct and indirect pathways. The direct pathway goes from putamen directly to globus pallidus internal segment, while the indirect pathway goes through, the globus pallidus external segment and subthalamic nucleus before reaching the globus pallidus internal segment. These two pathways also differ in the effect of dopaminergic inputs from the substantia nigra pars compacta. The dopaminergic input is inhibitory of putamen neurons participating in the indirect pathway and excitatory of those putamen neurons participating in the direct pathway. The figure on the left shows the normal circumstance, while the figure on the right shows the consequence of dopamine depletion (represented by the broken arrows) such as occurs in Parkinson's disease. The net result is reduction of inhibition, represented by the thinner arrows, and an increase in excitatory input, represented by the thicker arrow, onto the globus pallidus internal segment with increased inhibition of the ventrolateral thalamus.

decreased activity in GPe would result in reduced inhibition of and increased activity in STN. The increased activity of STN then causes further increased activity in GPi (Fig. 1).

There is considerable empirical evidence in support of this model. However, most of that evidence is indirect. Direct evidence comes from microelectrode recordings in non-human primates before and after the induction of experimental parkinsonism by the administration of MPTP, which selectively degenerates dopaminergic neurons (9). Some studies have demonstrated the predicted increases in GPi and STN neuronal activities following experimental parkinsonism. Microelectrode recordings in the STN of PD patients also have higher discharge rates than in epilepsy patients undergoing DBS (10). However, STN neurons in PD patients also were more irregular in their firing patterns.

The observations of increased neuronal activity in the STN and GPi and reduced activity in the GPe cannot escape the possibility of being epiphenomenal rather than causally related to the symptoms of PD. These observations could be a special case more related to the severity of dopamine loss than two causal mechanisms. Others have shown no significant changes in baseline neuronal activity of either the striatum, GPe, VL thalamus, or MC following MPTP and animals clearly parkinsonian as evidenced by bradykinesia and changes in regional 2-deoxyglucose utilization typical of parkinsonian nonhuman primates (11). Filion and Tremblay (12) demonstrated that GPi neurons increased activity after MPTP, but the level of neuronal activity returned to baseline within a few weeks. Thus, dopamine depletion to the degree of producing changes in baseline neuronal activity is not a necessary condition for the production of parkinsonism.

Additional evidence offered in support of the current model is the clinical efficacy of pallidotomy. Destruction of the GPi would certainly remove abnormal increased GPi activity and thereby lessen inhibitory inputs onto VL thalamic neurons. However, it is also likely that pallidotomy would eliminate abnormal neuronal firing patterns. Additional supportive evidence of the current models is that dopaminergic replacement reduces neuronal activity in the GPi and STN of human parkinsonian patients.

The current model has been criticized on a number of grounds, primarily anatomical and clinical (13,14). Perhaps the strongest evidence against the current model is the remarkable efficacy of DBS (15). While there remains some controversy regarding the mechanisms of action of DBS, there is increasing evidence in direct microelectrodes in both humans and nonprimates that DBS increases the output of the stimulated structures rather than inhibiting or reducing activity within the stimulated structure. Thus, high-frequency DBS in the STN and GPi drives the output of the GPi at frequencies higher than in PD. Clearly, overactivity of this structure cannot be causally related to the mechanisms of PD.

NEURONAL MECHANISMS OF STN DBS

Preliminary results are reported from microelectrode recordings of GPi neuronal activities during stimulation in the vicinity of the STN in a nonhuman primate. A DBS lead one-quarter scale relative to the human DBS lead was used to approximate DBS in humans. This type of stimulation is not specific to any single structure, whether it is the STN, axons of cortical projections to the STN, or pallidal-fugal fibers, but it does reflect how DBS leads are used in humans. The anatomical localization of the DBS lead and recording sites within the GPi were histologically confirmed.

DBS stimulation utilized the most ventral contact as the cathode (initial phase) and the most dorsal contact as the anode (initial phase). This reflects the most common active electrode arrangements we use clinically. Stimulation utilized biphasic current balanced stimulation with each phase 90 μs in duration. The current passed was made 80% of the threshold for stimulation to induce a muscle contraction of the contralateral body. This was determined to be 3.9 microcoulombs/cm^2/phase, well below the threshold for tissue injury. Neuronal activity was recorded for 30 seconds before, 30 seconds during, and 30 seconds after stimulation. Three to four trials of each of stimulation were obtained.

Computer software was developed that allowed removal of stimulus-induced artifact such that neuronal activity could be directly studied during stimulation. Previous studies analyzed activity immediately after cessation of stimulation because they were unable to analyze activity during stimulation (16). They inferred that this represented activity during stimulation, which will be shown to be false.

Average neuronal discharge frequencies were determined for prestimulation, during stimulation, and poststimulation for each set of trials associated with each frequency of stimulation. The percent change in the average GPi neuronal discharge frequency during stimulation was compared to the prestimulation period. Cross-correlograms were constructed of GPi neuronal activity referenced to the time of occurrence of the stimulation pulses.

Figure 2 shows a representative recording in GPi. The tracing shows the raw data after stimulus artifact removal. There is greater activity in the GPi segment during stimulation compared to before. Also, the activity following stimulation is less than before stimulation. This is evidence that one cannot infer that the neuronal activity immediately following cessation of stimulation reflects what occurs during stimulation.

One hundred and eleven neurons were recorded before, during, and after stimulation at 130-pulses per second (pps) in the GPi. Sixty-one (55%) neurons increased their discharge frequency associated with stimulation, while 50 (45%) decreased. Cross-correlograms are a method of relating the occurrence of a neuronal discharge to the stimulation pulse (Fig. 3). They are constructed by measuring the time of each neuronal discharge within a

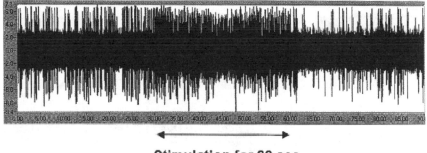

Stimulation for 30 sec

FIGURE 2 Microelectrode recording of the extracellular action potentials of a globus pallidus internal segment neuron in response to DBS in the vicinity of the subthalamic nucleus. There is a 30-second baseline recording followed by 30 seconds of stimulation and then recording for an additional 30 seconds.

defined time period following each stimulation pulse. Thus, the cross-correlogram can be interpreted as the relative probability that the neuron will discharge at a defined time period following delivery of a stimulation pulse. Representative cross-correlograms of GPi neuronal activity indexed to the occurrence of the stimulation pulses are shown Fig. 4, in which several

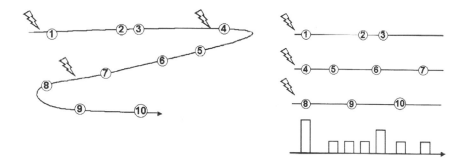

FIGURE 3 Schematic explanation of the cross- correlogram of neuronal activity reference to the stimulation pulses (lightning bolts). The time of each neuronal extracellular action potential are represented by the numbered circle. The figure on the left represents a recording during which three stimuli are delivered. The figure on the right separates the recording into three segments at the time of each stimulus. The times of neuronal discharge relative to the stimuli are then summed across trials to generate a histogram that is the cross-correlogram. The height of each interval in the histogram indicates the relative probability of a spike occurring in a time locked fashion in response to the stimuli.

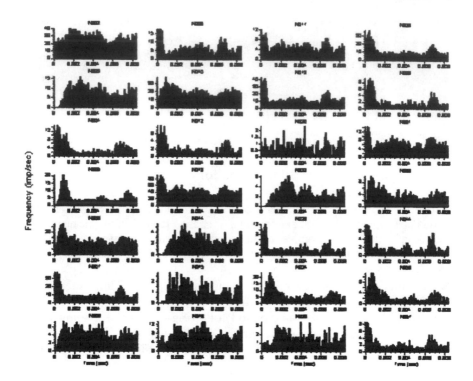

FIGURE 4 Cross-correlogram of activity of globus pallidus internal segment neurons to DBS in the vicinity of the subthalamic nucleus. The activities are reference to a stimulus pulse delivered at 130 pulses per second. The time line for each correlogram is 8 ms and the bin width is 0.1 ms. See text for description.

peaks are seen at different times. An early and narrow peak at approximately 1 msec is most consistent with, although not proof of, antidromic activation of the GPi neuron by stimulation of pallidal-fugal fibers traveling in the lenticular fasciculis and ansa lenticularis near the STN.

Later and border peaks are consistent with mono- and polysynaptic orthodromic activation, perhaps due to stimulation of the STN axons projecting to the GPi. Cross-correlograms of neurons, which, on average, decreased activity with stimulation, also showed activity correlated with stimulation but associated with a reduction of activity. Even neurons that reduced average activity with stimulation had at least a transient increase in neuronal activity with each stimulation pulse. Hasmimoto et al. (17) also demonstrated increased activity in GPi with STN DBS. Anderson (18) demonstrated reduced activity in VL thalamus consistent with increased GPi output with GPi DBS.

Dostrovsky et al. (19) reported reduced GPi neuronal activity with microelectrode stimulation of the GPi using pairs of microelectrodes to simultaneously stimulate and record. They attributed these findings to increased release of presynaptic inhibitory neurotransmitters onto GPi neurons. However, DBS effects on GPi neuronal cell bodies as would be recorded with microelectrodes may be dissociated from effects on the axon hillocks (initial segments) or first internodes between myelin segments. Thus, stimulation could lead to decreased discharge of the neuronal cell body but increased output due to excited axon hillocks or first internotes as supported by computer modeling of thalamic neurons based on membrane properties, neuronal geometries, and conductance channels (20). STN DBS effects on electromyographic (EMG) activity (21), STN DBS-evoked scalp potentials (22), and clinical efficacy related to chronaxie (23) are consistent with axonal mechanisms.

Preliminary data described here strongly support the notion that DBS drives output. The mechanisms are complex and varied, including antidromic and mono- and polysynaptic orthodromic activation. This is probably related to the many different structures in the region of the STN DBS leads. Consequently, high-frequency therapeutic DBS drives GPi neurons at frequencies higher than in the normal and in the MPTP-parkinsonian nonhuman primate. It is reasonable to conclude that high-frequency DBS also drives human GPi well above the abnormal baseline frequencies associated with PD. Therefore, it cannot be that the pathophysiology of PD is due to overactivity of the GPi, or else high-frequency DBS would make PD symptoms worse instead of better. Rather, these changes in baseline activity most likely represent epiphenomena. The current theory needs restructuring or to be discarded altogether.

ALTERNATIVE HYPOTHESES

The question arises as to what theories will replace the current ones. There are some observations that suggest where to begin. First, pallidotomy and GPi DBS are very effective for levodopa-induced dyskinesia (24), dystonia (25), and hemiballismus (25). In contrast to the overactivity of the GPi in PD, GPi neuronal activity in these other conditions is lower than what is thought normal. However, common to all these conditions is the fact that the pathological neuronal activity is more irregular. Perhaps the therapeutic mechanism of DBS is more related to the irregular activity than changes in average neuronal activity. The question then is how an irregular pattern of activity leads to the symptoms of these disorders.

Information Processing and Misinformation

Information is encoded in the patterns of neuronal activity. Abnormal patterns of activity translate into misinformation. In addition, irregular neuronal activity can have an abnormal effect on downstream information processing through a mechanism of stochastic resonance. This phenomenon is the increase in the signal-to-noise ratio when noise is added. Computer modeling of information transfer and processing demonstrates that stochastic resonance effect is greatest with low-frequency regular and irregular activity (26). The stochastic resonance effect is the least with high-frequency regular activity.

The computer model used two neurons (X and Y) synapsing on a third neuron (Z) (Fig. 5). The effects of activity in neuron Y, either spontaneous or in response to DBS, on information transfer between neurons X and Z were analyzed. The information was represented by an idealized waveform to which Gaussian noise was added and then converted to neuronal like activity. Neuron Z simply added the inputs from neurons X and Y. The gain

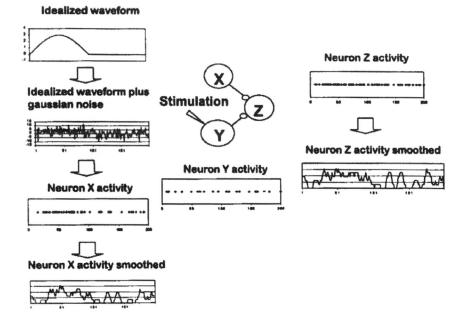

FIGURE 5   Schematic representation of the modeling of information processing: the effects of activity in neuron Y, either spontaneous or in response to DBS, on information transfer from neuron X to neuron Z. See text for description. (From Ref. 26.)

of information between neuron X and Z was determined where a positive difference represents information gain and a negative difference represents information loss. High-frequency irregular activity nearly always results in a loss of signal-to-noise ratio. Low-frequency regular or irregular activity also results in instances of loss of signal-to-noise ratio but occasionally results in abnormal gain. The high frequency and regular activity pattern had the least impact (Fig. 6).

PD results in overall loss of function because of the higher and more irregular GPI activity. The slow and irregular GPI neuronal activity in levodopa-induced dyskinesia, dystonia, and Huntington disease results in

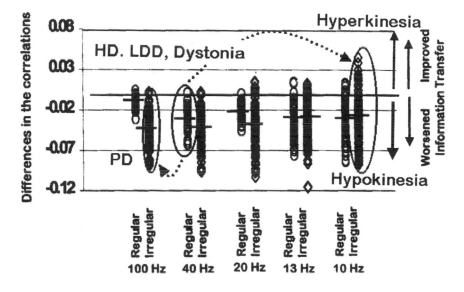

FIGURE 6 Results of computational modeling of the effects of neuron Y on information transfer from neuron X to neuron Z. A difference in correlation below zero represents loss of information, while differences in correlations above zero represent a gain in information. The effects of pathology of the basal ganglia are represented. Normal activity of the globus pallidus internal segment is represented by the circle for 40 Hz regular activity in neuron Y. In Parkinson's disease (PD) there is an increase in neuronal activity that becomes more irregularly represented. In contrast, Huntington's disease (HD), levodopa induced dyskinesia (LDD), and dystonia result in information transfer that loses information as well as instances of abnormal gain of information. The former may account for many of the negative symptoms associated with Huntington's disease, levodopa-induced dyskinesia, and dystonia, while the episodes of abnormal gain of information may account for the hypherkinesias or involuntary movement. (Modified from Ref. 26.)

both a loss of function and episodes of abnormal gain of function that could explain the involuntary movements of these disorders. Driving GPi to high frequency and regular activity minimizes the misinformation and abnormal loss or gain in the signal-to-noise ratio or information content (Fig. 7).

Preliminary studies described above support the hypothesis of more regular activity in GPi with STN DBS. Figure 8 is a schematic explanation of the autocorrelogram, which is similar to a cross-correlogram. The autocorrelogram indicates the relative probability that one neuronal discharge will be associated with another discharge occurring at some defined time earlier or later. Peaks in the autocorrelogram indicate organization in the spike train such as oscillatory or regular behavior. There is better organization of GPi neuronal activities during stimulation at 130 pps as evidenced by peaks in the autocorrelogram during stimulation compared to before stimulation (Fig. 9). This is particularly evident in the autocorrelogram of the population of GPi neurons. Thus, GPi neuronal

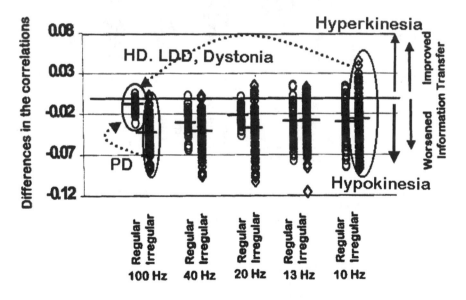

FIGURE 7 Schematic representation of the possible effects of high-frequency DBS. In Parkinson's disease (PD), Huntington's disease (HD), levodopa-induced dyskinesia (LDD), and dystonia, high-frequency DBS drives the activity of the globus pallidus internal segment to high and regular frequencies, thereby minimizing the effects on information processing downstream and mitigating disease symptoms, both positive and negative. (Modified from Ref. 26.)

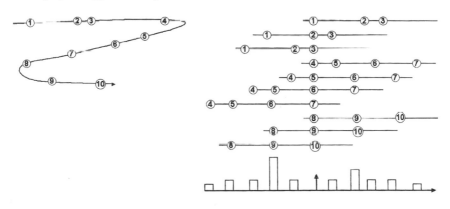

FIGURE 8 Schematic explanation of the autocorrelogram. The figure on the left shows the time course of a recording of neuronal activity. The figure on the right shows the time course broken into segments. Segments are duplicated and organized so that each neuron discharge becomes centered on the upward arrow. The times of neuronal discharge are then collapsed across trials and summed in the resulting histogram. The height of each interval in the histogram indicates the relative probability of a neuronal discharge occurring at a specific time before and after the occurrence of an individual discharge. Peaks in the autocorrelogram indicate organized activity that may be oscillatory.

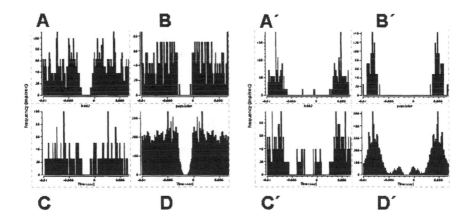

FIGURE 9 Autocorrelograms of three individual neurons (A and A', B and B', and C and C') and the ensemble population of eleven neurons (D and D') recorded at a single site in the globus pallidus internal segment. Autocorrelograms A, B, C, and D were from recording 30 s before DBS in the vicinity of the subthalamic nucleus at a regular 130 pulses per second. Autocorrelograms A', B', C', and D' were from recordings during 30 s of stimulation. The time line for each correlogram is 10 ms and the bin width is 0.1 ms.

activity is more regular during STN DBS, which then removes information content (27).

The hypothesis follows that the abnormal patterns of GPi neuronal activity result in misinformation and that DBS changes misinformation to essentially no information. Ablation eliminates the source of the mis-information. This may explain the similarity of the clinical efficacy of pallidotomy and DBS.

DBS Effects on "Systems"

The effects of DBS are not limited to the STN or GPi but rather influence multiple components of the basal ganglia-thalamic-cortical circuits or systems. It is possible that the therapeutic mechanisms of DBS are due to these effects and, if so, that concepts of PD pathophysiology need to be extended to these systems.

Preliminary studies in a nonhuman primate, as described above, included analysis of responses of neurons in the MC and Pt (Fig. 10). The responses to STN DBS included very short duration narrow responses, suggesting antidromic activation of neurons in the motor cortex and longer latency and broader peak responses, suggestive of polysynaptic orthodromic activation in both the MC and Pt. It is interesting to note the temporal relationships between the peaks of the increased polysynaptic activity in the Pt and GPi. Increased activity within the Pt was followed by decreased activity in the GPi with a lag time of approximately 1.6 msec, which is consistent with the monosynaptic connections between Pt and GPi (Fig. 10). This is analyzed further in Fig. 11. The top tracing shows the cross-correlogram of 12 Pt neurons that are normalized to the maximum value in each correlogram. The tracings of each cross-correlogram are superimposed. A similar analysis for GPi neurons is shown in the middle tracing of Fig. 11. The bottom tracing shows the average of the individual tracings for the Pt and GPi superimposed. A phase relationship with a lag time of approximately 1.6 msec can be seen. There is a suggestion of a similar relationship between cortical and Pt activity. High-frequency DBS in the vicinity of the STN generates oscillations within the basal ganglia-thalamic-cortical circuits as evidenced by STN DBS evoked potentials found over the scalp and in the contralateral STN (22).

How activation of oscillations within this circuit is causally related to the therapeutic mechanisms of action of high-frequency DBS is unclear. One possibility might be reinforcement of a resonance frequency within the basal ganglia-thalamic-cortical circuit. If one assumes a four-segment circuit reflecting the direct pathway and further assumes a 1.6 ms time lag (seen in the cross-correlograms of Fig. 10 and the modified cross-correlogram of Fig.

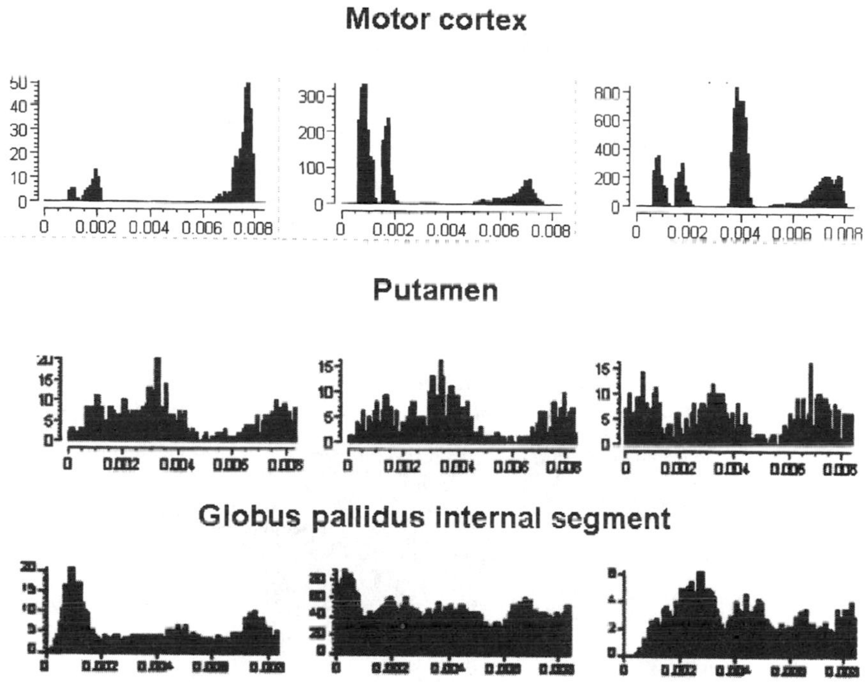

Motor cortex

Putamen

Globus pallidus internal segment

FIGURE 10 Representative cross-correlogram of activity of globus pallidus internal segment, motor cortex, and putamen neurons to DBS in the vicinity of the subthalamic nucleus. The activities are reference to a stimulus pulse delivered at 130 pulses per second. The time line for each correlogram is 8 ms and the bin width is 0.1 ms. See text for description.

11) between activities within the circuits, then information could circulate the circuit in approximately 6.4 ms. This would correspond to a frequency of 156 Hz. Information could traverse the indirect pathway, made up of five segments, with a frequency of 125 Hz. These frequencies are in the range of those found therapeutic for DBS. Stimulation at the resonance frequency could reinforce normal information processing within the basal ganglia-thalamic-cortical circuit and, therefore, improve motor function.

"Systems" and "Theoretical" Approach

The critical question now becomes: What will be the basis for a future model of basal ganglia physiology and pathophysiology? The current model is a model of anatomy and neurochemistry rather than physiology. Most of the

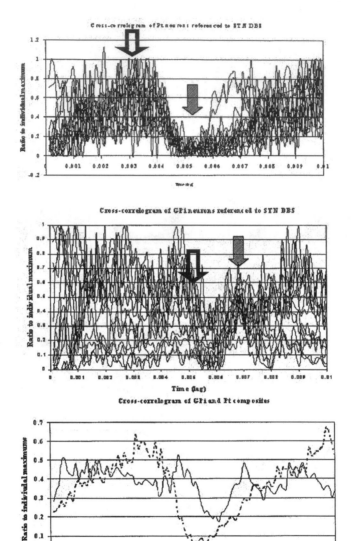

FIGURE 11 Normalized tracings from the cross- correlograms of Pt and GPi neurons. The upper tracings are from Pt neurons and the middle tracings from GPi neurons. The bottom tracing shows the average of the individual tracings, solid line for Pt and broken line for GPi. The peak of neuronal activity in Pt is followed by a reduction in GPi activity (open arrows), while a reduction in Pt activity is followed by an increase in GPi activity (gray-filled arrows).

physiological assertions are inferences from the anatomy and neurochemistry. As will be discussed, these inferences do not explain the temporal dynamics of complex systems.

The current model uses single neurons substituted for whole structures. This is referred to as the "macro-neuronal" approach. For example, single neurons represent the cortex, Pt, of the indirect pathway, Pt of the direct pathway, GPe, GPi, STN, SNpc, SNr and VL thalamus. These "macro-neurons" are linked by inhibitory or excitatory neurotransmitters. The dynamics of this model are one-dimensional "push-pull" interactions (Fig. 1). The predicted findings of this model have been supported for changes in baseline, steady-state, or resting activity of the different basal ganglia structures. However, these changes may be epiphenomenal as described above.

The temporal dynamics of the circuits relative to the behaviors they are thought to mediate is critically important. For example, Fig. 12 shows the time course of neuronal activity in the motor cortex associated with a

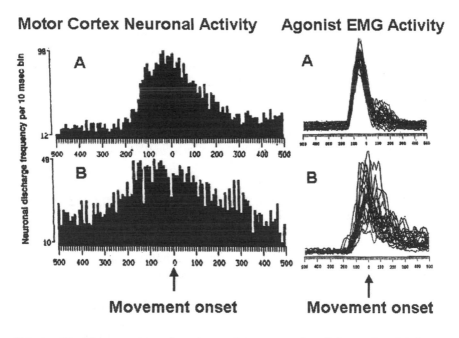

FIGURE 12 Time course of motor cortex neuronal activity and wrist flexor electromyographic (EMG) activity associated with a wrist flexion task in a nonhuman primate before (A) and after (B) induction of parkinsonism using *n*-methyl-4-phenyl-1,2,3,6-tetrahydropyridine (MPTP). Recordings are made from 500 ms before to 500 ms after movement onset over multiple trials. (From Ref. 28.)

wrist flexion task (28). Changes in neuronal activity in the normal condition begin approximately 200 ms before movement onset and reach a new baseline or steady state approximately 300 ms after movement onset. Information can traverse the basal ganglia-thalamic-motor cortex within 6.4–8 ms. It is possible for information to have traversed the circuits 63–78 times during the course of a 500-ms-long behavior. Thus, the sequential nature of the one-dimensional "push-pull" dynamics of the current model cannot begin to account for such a complex reentrant system. Rather, the function or dysfunction associated with disorders of the basal ganglia must be reconceptualized into a distributed and parallel system of re-entrant oscillating circuits. The basic units of function and therefore the subject of analyses are no longer the individual structures of the cortex, basal ganglia, and thalamus but rather the basal ganglia-thalamic-cortical circuit as a whole.

Evidence in support of a parallel and distributed system within the time frame of behavior is seen in recordings of MC and Pt neuronal activity during the course of a wrist flexion and extension task (29). Utilizing a method that relates changes in neuronal activity to behavioral events (30), it was possible to determine which behavioral event was best related to the change in neuronal activities. Thus, neurons in MC and Pt were identified that were preferentially related to the appearance of the go signal or movement onset. Neurons responding to the go signal typically became active before those related to movement onset (Fig. 13). However, go signal–related neurons in the Pt became active at nearly the same time as those in the MC. Similarly movement onset–related Pt neurons became active at the same time as movement onset–related neurons in MC.

EPISTEMOLOGY OF CURRENT MODELS OF PHYSIOLOGY AND PATHOPHYSIOLOGY

Scientists and philosophers repeatedly warn that attention to how something is known often is as important as what is known. Numerous aphorisms have been coined for such warnings, such as "we see what we are prepared to see" or "when all you have is a hammer, everything becomes a nail." Unfortunately, epistemic discussions in neurophysiology are rare. What follows is such a discussion of our current conceptual approaches to systems neurophysiology that may help to understand why specific questions have been asked rather than others and the origins of the assumptions that underlie those questions. This effort will be very important in creating the new theories of basal ganglia physiology and pathophysiology.

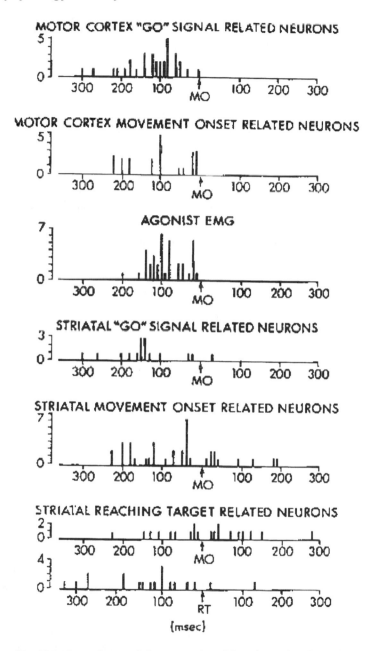

FIGURE 13 The time of onset of neuronal activity of go-signal– and movement onset–related neurons in motor cortex and putamen demonstrating nearly virtually simultaneous onset of activity change. (From Ref. 29.)

Reasoning by Anatomy

The proposition is offered that in conceptual approaches to systems neurophysiology are the results of anatomical studies to the greatest degree followed by clinical observations of disease states. The actual incremental increases in our understanding offered by direct recordings of neuronal activities during the course of behavior have contributed relatively little in comparison. Indeed, there have been circumstances where recordings of neuronal activity would appear contradictory to the inferences drawn from the anatomy (11,26). These contradictory findings have received scant attention.

This is not to discount the importance of anatomical understanding or research. In fact, anatomical data provide a critical reality check because any theory of systems neurophysiology cannot contradict validated anatomical fact. However, the anatomy can only provide information in the widest sense in that its limits are only the maximum possibilities and the physiological realities are likely to be only a subset of the anatomical possibilities (31). Further, as the complexities of anatomical organization and interconnections increase, it will become increasingly difficult to predict function from the structure. This is particularly true if, as is likely, the interactions are highly nonlinear. Any new model would require as its basis the same anatomical facts that underlie the current anatomical model. However, as will be seen, there may be emergent properties of the new dynamical models that are not intuitive from the current anatomical model and, therefore, represent such a quantitative change as to be qualitatively different.

Hierarchical Processing

The macro-neuron approach leads to structures that are then linked with a very specific directional aspect, for example, the cortex projects to Pt, which in turn projects to GPi, which projects to the VL thalamus. Consequently, the presumption has been that information is processed within the cortex, which is relayed to Pt for processing. When completed, the information is then relayed to GPi and so on. This has led to attempts to identify specific functions unique to each structure and to demonstrate timing differences of changes in neuronal activities associated with behavior. For example, experiments attempted to demonstrate that the GPi or Pt nucleus became active before the MC. The results of these experiments were either inconclusive or failed to demonstrate the anticipated timing differences (8,32–34).

The anatomically derived hierarchical conceptual approach fails to distinguish anatomical proximity form physiological proximity. The presumption is that neurons in close proximity to each other (such as being within the same nuclei or restricted region of cortex) interact to carry out specific physiological functions. However, it is quite possible, indeed probable in the case of the basal ganglia, that neurons in different and separate structures are more directly linked physiologically than adjacent neurons in the same structure. For example, the majority of neuronal recording studies of simultaneously recorded putamen neurons in close proximity are not cross-correlated, demonstrating very little if any physiological interactions. Yet, there is a very precise and robust physiological interaction between cortex and Pt neurons. Physiologically, it may make better sense to consider neurons tightly linked in the cortical-basal ganglia-thalamic circuit as being the more fundamental physiological working unit, rather than any of the separate nuclei or cortical structures.

The degree of independence between these circuits has been discussed at length (35–37). Evidence for separate basal ganglia-thalamic-cortical loops comes from anatomical studies. Studies using viruses to trace anatomical projections across synapses suggest that there is little or no anatomical overlap between those circuits serving cognitive, limbic, or motor functions (36). However, these studies were not done at the levels of resolution of neuronal populations related to individual extremities or muscles. Recent functional magnetic resonance imaging (fMRI) studies have suggested overlap in areas of the Pt representing the face, fingers, and toes (38). Electrophysiological studies can estimate the degree that electrical activities in individual neurons are coupled using cross-correlation techniques. Little evidence of coupling is found for pallidal neurons, although more couplings have been found for tonically acting striatal neurons, which are probably cholinergic interneurons (35).

An alternative to the anatomically based hierarchical conceptual approach posits that physiological function, such as responding to a go signal, initiating a movement, or completing a movement, is represented in separate basal ganglia-thalamic-cortical circuits. Processing within the circuit is virtually simultaneous within the components of the circuit. There is a hierarchical structure, but it is in physiological terms not anatomical. Thus, during behaviors such as making a movement to a target in response to a go signal, the basal ganglia-thalamic-cortical circuit related to responding to the go signal is hierarchical to the basal ganglia-thalamic-cortical circuit that is associated with movement initiation. This, in turn, is hierarchical to the circuit whose activity changes are preferentially related to reaching the target. This hierarchical organization of function is paralleled by differences in the timing of activity changes in these circuits.

The macro-neuron approach also leads to the inference that physiological functions are specific to the nucleus or subdivision of the nucleus or to a specific region of the cortex. Evidence against the hierarchical arrangement suggested by the macro-neuron model lies in the fact that diseases affecting different structures may produce very similar if not indistinguishable symptoms. For example, lesions of the GPi, SNpc, and the SMA (39–43) all produce parkinsonian akinesia and bradykinesia. As described above, Huntington's disease patients have prolonged reaction times and slowed movement (44). Consequently, physiological function is not likely separately represented in specific and unique structures, otherwise lesions of each specific and unique nucleus would result in specific and distinct dysfunction.

THE NEED FOR MATHEMATICALTHEORETICAL NEUROPHYSIOLOGY

The relative lack of knowledge and understanding in systems physiology and pathophysiology is not for want of talent or effort. More likely it is related to the incredible difficulties encountered and the type of explanation required. The complexities of any interacting system increase enormously as the number of agents and mechanisms of interaction increases. Systems physiology of necessity requires study of large numbers of agents and interactions. One approach to managing complexity is to use statistical descriptions of empirical descriptions gleaned from populations and to use correlations as surrogate markers for causal interactions. However, this is not the level that will provide mechanistic insights that will power development of future research.

Given the daunting challenge, what will it take to reach a full understanding of how complex interconnected neurons organize and interact to create the human experience? Note that the aim is an understanding and not knowledge as in a complete specification of every element. Indeed, it is likely that such a complete specification at the most fundamental level will be so improbable as to be impossible. The question then arises whether there is a level of understanding that has sufficient resolution as to be useful. There are at least two responses. The first is the concept of emergent properties. The second is the use of metaphors of sufficient complexity and realism and whose validation will be in the ability of the metaphors to generate succeeding generations of biologically testable hypotheses.

Emergent properties are reflected in regularities of observed or macroscopic behavior that are not readily apparent from microscopic observation of its constituent agents. For example, it is not possible to observe the activity of individual neurons in the brain and precisely predict any behavior. However, the notion of emergent properties is not hostile to reductionism. Ultimately, behavior must be the result of activities of individual neurons. But knowledge at the level of the individual neuron is not a necessary, or perhaps even possible, requirement for understanding of behavior as evidenced by the remarkable successes of cognitive neuroscience. For the systems neurophysiologist, the issue becomes whether there are emergent properties at tractable levels of analysis that can be useful.

What alternatives exist to metaphorical knowledge to provide understanding? No alternatives loom on the horizon. Consequently, how can metaphors be made to be useful as surrogate knowledge of brain function? There are two critical pitfalls using metaphors. These are the fallacy of induction and the related logical error of confirming the consequence. The fallacy of induction translates that just because one metaphor may explain a biological phenomena, it is not possible to exclude the possibility that an alternative exists. The only options then are to insist that the biological phenomena be of sufficient richness as to make it hard for a large number of possible alternatives to exist and that an appropriate level of analysis (i.e., emergent properties) is used to determine whether alternatives are truly different.

The second derivative problem is the penchant of experimenters to fall victim to the logical error of confirming the antecedent. This error is of the form (1) if "a" then "b"; (2) "b" is true; therefore (3) "a" is true. In relevant terms, an error backpropagation neural network model can solve a biological problem, such as distinguishing phonemes in speech, biological systems can distinguish phonemes, therefore, biological systems use backpropagation and the search is on to find backpropagation in individual neurons. These logical errors do not necessarily mean that backpropagation could or would not be demonstrable, but if they are, it is not from logical deduction. These difficulties are probably largely responsible for the hostility that biologists have for model-based explanations. However, at an emergent level there is validity to a backpropagation notion because organisms do learn from their mistakes.

Clearly, the systems neurophysiologist will have to operate at the level of metaphor if there is any chance of formulating an interesting and useful biological testable hypothesis that will drive future empirical research. The issue is what has driven the development of metaphors to date, and what the survival value of continuing that line of development is. The use of metaphors can be liberating or confining. It will be argued that the current basis for metaphor development in the area of basal ganglia physiology and pathophysiology has been anatomical and therefore static. The anatomically based metaphor has resulted in simplistic expectations that, unfortunately, have been found to be epiphenomenonally true and has created false local minimas in the ignorance of basal ganglia physiology and pathophysiology. So pervasive and seductive has the anatomical metaphor been that it has defied physiological common sense—hence, the false local minimas.

There may be an inclination to avoid constructing any models in the hope that sufficient empirical data could be obtained to provide a sufficient intuitive or self-evident explanation. However, the odds of this are extremely small. Clearly, models of vastly increased complexity, one day possibly approaching the degree of complexity inherent in biological systems, are necessary. Validating such complex models requires developing experimental, analytical, and conceptual methods to understand biological activity of a corresponding degree of complexity. Rapid advances in computer technology and multiple microelectrode arrays will provide vast amounts of empirical data. But there is the danger that the magnitude of the empirical data will overwhelm the ability to make sense of the data. Therefore, conceptual methods of data reduction, particularly nonlinear methods such as chaos and fractal analyses, will become increasingly important. Models will have to be constructed to act as metaphors by which to understand the empirical data. While this approach risks circularity, there seems little alternative.

REFERENCES

1. Strauss MB, ed. Familiar Medical Quotations. Boston: Little Brown, 1968, p 335.
2. Hagell P, Piccini P, Bjorklund A, Brundin P, Rehncrona S, Widner H, Crabb L, Pavese N, Oertel W, Quinn N, Brooks DJ, Lindvall O. Dyskinesias following neural transplantation in Parkinson's disease. Nat Neurosci 5:627–628, 2002.
3. Parent A, Hazarati L-N. Functional anatomy of the basal ganglia. I. The cortico-basal ganglia-thalamo-cortical loop. Brain Res Rev 20:91–127, 1995.
4. Parent A, Hazarati L-N. Functional anatomy of the basal ganglia. II. The place of subthalamic nucleus and external pallidum in basal ganglia circuitry. Brain Res Rev 20:127–154, 1995.
5. Smith Y, Shink E, Sidibé M, Neuronal circuitry and synaptic connectivity of the basal ganglia. Neurosurg Clin North Am 9:203–222, 1998.
6. Nandi D, Aziz TZ, Liu X, Stein JF, Brainstem motor loops in the control of movement. Mov Disord 17:S22–S27, 2002.
7. Penny JB, Young AB. Striatal inhomogeneities and basal ganglia function. Mov Disord 1:3–15, 1983.
8. DeLong MR. Activity of the basal ganglia neurons during movement. Brain Res 40:127–135, 1972.

9. Wichmann T, Bergman H, Starr PA, Subramanian T, Watts R, DeLong MR, Comparison of MPTP-induced changes in spontaneous neuronal discharge in the internal pallidal segment and in the substantia nigra pars reticulata in primate. Exp Brain Res 125:397–409, 1999.

10. Montgomery Jr. EB, Baker KB, Rezai A, Bingaman W, Barnett G. Lüders HO. Subthalamic neuronal resting activities in humans with and without Parkinson's disease. The Movement Disorder Society's 7th International Congress of Parkinson's Disease and Movement Disorders, November 10–14, 2002.

11. Montgomery Jr EB, Buchholz SR, Delitto A, Collins RC. Alterations in basal ganglia physiology following MPTP in monkeys. In: Markey SP, Castagnoli N, Trevor AJ, Kopin IJ, eds, A Neurotoxin Producing a Parkinsonian Syndrome. Academic Press, Inc., 1986, pp 679–682.

12. Filion M, Tremblay L. Abnormal spontaneous activity of globus pallidus neurons in monkeys with MPTP-induced parkinsonism. Brain Res 547:142–151, 1991.

13. Parent A, Sato F, Wu Y, Gauthier J, Levesque M, Parent M. Organization of the basal ganglia: the importance of axonal collateralization. Trends Neurosci 23:S20–S27, 2000.

14. Obeso JA, Rodriguez-Oroz MC, Rodriguez M, Lanciego JL, Artieda J, Gonzalo N, Olanow W. The physiology of the basal ganglia in Parkinson's disease. TINS 23 (suppl):S8–S19, 2000.

15. Deep-Brain Stimulation for Parkinson's Disease Study Group. Deep-brain stimulation of the subthalamic nucleus or the pars interna of the globus pallidus in Parkinson's disease. N Engl J Med 345:956–963, 2001.

16. Bennazzouz A, Piallat B, Pollak P, Benabid AL. Responses of substantia nigra pars reticulata and globus pallidus complex to high frequency stimulation on the subthalamic nucleus in rats: electrophysiological data. Neurosci Lett 189:77–80, 1995.

17. Hasmimoto T, Elder CM, DeLong MR, Viteck JL. Responses of pallidal neurons to electrical stimulation of the subthalamic nucleus in experimental parkinsonism. Soc Neurosci abst. #750.0, 2001.

18. M. Anderson, personal communication, 2001.

19. Dostrovsky JO, Levy R, Wu JP, Hutchison WD, Tasker RR, Lozano AM. Microstimulaiton-induced inhibition of neuronal firing in human globus pallidus. J Neurophysiol 84:570–574, 2000.

20. McIntyre CC, Grill WM. Excitation of central nervous system neurons by nonuniform electric fields. Biophys J 76:878–888, 1999.

21. Ashby P, Kim YJ, Kumar R, Lang AE, Lozano AM, Neruophysiological effects of stimulation through electrodes in the human subthalamic nucleus. Brain 122:1919–1931, 1999.

22. Baker KB, Montgomery Jr, EB, Rezai A, Burgess B, Lüders HO. Subthalamic nucleus DBS evoked potentials: physiology and therapeutic implications. Mov Disord 17:969–983, 2002.

23. Rizzone M, Lanotte M, Bergamasco B, Tavella A, Torre E, Faccani G, Melcarne A, Lopiano L. Deep brain stimulation of the subthalamic nucleus in Parkinson's disease: effects of variation in stimulation parameters. J Neurol Neurosurg Psychiatry 71:215–219, 2001.

24. Papa SM, Desimone R, Fiorani M, Oldfield EH. Internal globus pallidus discharge is nearly suppressed during levodopa-induced dyskinesia. Ann Neurol 46:732–738, 1999.

25. Vitek JL, Chockkan V, Zhang J-Y, Kaneoke Y, Evatt M, DeLong MR, Triche S, Mewes K, Hashimoto T, Bakay RAE. Neuronal activity in the basal ganglia in patients with generalized dystonia and hemiballismus. Ann Neurol 46:22–35, 1999.

26. Montgomery Jr EB, Baker KB. Mechanisms of deep brain stimulation and future technical developments. Neurol Res 22:259–266, 2000.

27. Shannon CE, Weaver W. The Mathematical Theory of Communication. University of Illinois Press, 1998.

28. Mandir AS, Watts RL, Buchholz SR, Montgomery EB Jr. Changes in motor cortex neuronal activity associated with increased reaction time in MPTP parkinsonism. Soc Neurosci Abst 15:787, 1989.

29. Montgomery Jr EB, Buchholz SR. The striatum and motor cortex in motor initiation and execution. Brain Res 549:222–229, 1991.

30. Montgomery EB, Jr. A new method for relating behavior to neural activity in performing monkeys. J Neurosci Methods 28:197–204, 1989.

31. Montgomery EB Jr, Clare MH, Sahrman S, Buchholz SR, Hibbard LS, Landau WM. Neuronal multipotentiality: evidence for network representation of physiological function. Brain Res 580:49–61, 1992.

32. Crutcher MD, DeLong MR. Single cell studies of the primate putamen. II. Relations to direction of movement and pattern of muscular activity. Exp Brain Res 53:244–258, 1984.

33. Liles SL, Updyke BV. Projection of the digit and wrist area of precentral gyrus to the putamen: relation between topography and physiological properties of neurons in the putamen. Brain Res 339:245–255, 1985.

34. Anderson ME, Horak FB. Influence of the globus pallidus on arm movements in monkeys. III. Timing of movement- related information. J Neurophysiol 54:433–448, 1985.

35. Bergman H, Feingold A, Nini A, Raz A, Slovin H, Abeles M, Vaadia E. Physiological aspects of information processing in the basal ganglia of normal and parkinsonian primates. Trends Neurosci 21:32–38, 1998.

36. Middleton FA, Strick PL. Basal ganglia and cerebellar loops: motor and cognitive circuits. Brain Res Rev 31:236–250, 2000.

37. Bolam JP, Hanley JJ, Booth PAC, Bevan MD. Synaptic organization of the basal ganglia. J Anat 196:527–542, 2000.

38. Maillard L, Ishii K, Bushara K, Waldvogel D, Schulman AE, Hallet M. Mapping the basal ganglia: fMRI evidence for somatotopic representation of face, hand, and foot. Neurology 55:377–383, 2000.

39. Laplane D, Talairach J, Meinger V, Bancaud J, Orgogozw JM. Clinical consequences of corticectomies involvinb the supplementary motor area in man. J Neurol Sci 34:301–314, 1977.
40. Gelmers HJ. Non-paralytic motor disturbances and speech disorders: the role of the supplementary motor area. J Neurol Neurosurg and Psych 46:1052–1054, 1983.
41. Peled R, Harnes B, Borovich B, Sharf B. Speech arrest and supplementary motor area seizures. Neurology 34:110–111, 1984.
42. Dick JP, Benecke R, Rothwell JC, Bay BL, Marsden CD. Simple and complex movements in a patient with infarction of the right supplementary motor area. Mov Disord 1:255–266, 1986.
43. Watson RT, Fleet WS, Gonzalez Rothi L, Heilman KM. Apraxia and the supplementary motor area. Arch Neurol 43:787–792, 1986.
44. Sánchez-Pernaute R, Künig G, del Barrio A, de Yébenes JG, Vontobel P, Leenders KL. Bradykinesia in early Huntington's disease. Neurology 54:119–125, 2000.

12

Animal Models of Parkinson's Disease and Related Disorders

Giselle M. Petzinger and Michael W. Jakowec
University of Southern California Keck School of Medicine, Los Angeles, California, U.S.A.

INTRODUCTION

Animal models of neurological disorders are critical for determining underlying disease mechanisms and developing new therapeutic modalities. In general, the utility of an animal model for a particular disease is often dependent on how closely the model replicates all or part of the human condition. In Parkinson's disease (PD) and related parkinsonian disorders there now exists a variety of animal models, each of which makes a unique contribution to our understanding of the human condition.

These models have been derived in a variety of species (pig, nonhuman primate, rodent, and cat) using multiple techniques, including (1) surgical lesioning, (2) pharmacological manipulation, (3) administration of neuro-toxicants, and (4) genetic alterations. While these models are not identical to the human condition with respect to behavioral characteristics, brain anatomy, or disease progression, they have provided significant advancements in our understanding of the underlying mechanisms and treatment of movement disorders such as PD.

PD is characterized by bradykinesia, rigidity, postural instability, and resting tremor. The primary pathological and biochemical features of PD are the loss of nigrostriatal dopaminergic neurons in the substantia nigra, the appearance of intracellular inclusions called Lewy bodies, and the depletion of striatal dopamine. Clinical features are apparent when striatal dopamine depletion reaches 80% despite the fact that 45–60% of nigrostriatal dopaminergic neurons still remain (1). Since the destruction of the nigrostriatal system and consequent depletion of striatal dopamine are key features in the human condition, attempts have been made in animal models to disrupt an analogous anatomical area through surgical, pharmacological, or neurotoxicant manipulation.

The purpose of this chapter is to introduce the many different animal models utilized in PD research. Each model, when applicable, will be discussed with respect to its development, behavioral profile, biochemical and neuropathological alterations, and contribution to the field.

PHARMACOLOGICALLY INDUCED MODELS OF PARKINSON'S DISEASE

Reserpine

The first animal model for PD was demonstrated by Carlsson in the 1950s using rabbits treated with reserpine. Reserpine is a catecholamine-depleting agent that blocks vesicular storage of monoamines. The akinetic state, resulting from reserpine-induced dopamine depletion in the caudate and putamen, led Carlsson to speculate that PD was due to striatal dopamine depletion. This speculation was supported by the discovery of striatal dopamine depletion in postmortem brain tissue of PD patients and led to the subsequent use of levodopa (in conjunction with a peripheral dopa-decarboxylase inhibitor) for symptomatic treatment of PD (2,3). Thus, the initial observations derived from an animal model led to an important clinical therapy that remains a gold standard.

Alpha-Methyl-para-Tyrosine

Although less commonly used, alpha-methyl-para-tyrosine (AMPT), like reserpine, serves as an effective catecholamine-depleting agent (4). By directly inhibiting tyrosine hydroxylase (the rate-limiting enzyme in dopamine biosynthesis), the nascent synthesis of dopamine in neurons of the substantia nigra pars compacta and ventral tegmental area is prevented.

Both reserpine and AMPT have been used to discover new dopaminomimetics for the treatment of PD, but since their effects are transient (hours to days), these models are primarily useful for acute studies. In addition, neither agent can duplicate the extensive biochemical and pathological changes seen in PD. Consequently, other models with long-lasting behavioral alterations have been sought using site-specific neurotoxicant injury.

NEUROTOXICANT-INDUCED MODELS OF PARKINSON'S DISEASE

6-Hydroxydopamine

6-Hydroxydopamine (6-OHDA or 2,4,5-trihydroxyphenylethylamine) is a specific catecholaminergic neurotoxin structurally analogous to both dopamine and noradrenaline. Acting as a "false-substrate," 6-OHDA is rapidly accumulated in catecholaminergic neurons. The mechanism of 6-OHDA toxicity is complex and involves (1) alkylation, (2) rapid auto-oxidization (leading to the generation of hydrogen peroxide, superoxide, and hydroxyl radicals), and (3) impairment of mitochondrial energy production (5,6). The 6-OHDA–induced rat model of PD was initially carried out by Ungerstedt in 1968, using stereotactic bilateral intracerebral injections into the substantia nigra or lateral hypothalamus (medial forebrain bundle) (7). The bilateral administration of 6-OHDA resulted in catalepsy, generalized inactivity, aphagia, and adipsia, and a high degree of animal morbidity and mortality. Consequently, the administration of 6-OHDA was modified to a unilateral intracerebral lesion (targeting the substantia nigra and/or medial forebrain bundle). With unilateral lesioning there was (1) minimal postoperative morbidity, (2) behavioral asymmetry, and (3) a nonlesioned side to serve as a control (8,9). An additional modification of 6-OHDA administration was chronic low-dose striatal injections. This led to progressive dopaminergic cell death that more closely resembled the human condition (10).

A distinctive behavioral feature of the unilateral lesioned model is rotation (11,12). This motor feature is due to asymmetry in dopaminergic neurotransmission between the lesioned and intact sides. Specifically, animals rotate away from the side of greater dopaminergic activity. Nomenclature describes the direction of rotation as either ipsilateral or contralateral to the lesioned side. Initial reports of rotation examined both spontaneous and pharmacologically manipulated rotation. Spontaneous rotation consists of ipsilateral rotation (towards the lesioned side), while pharmacologically induced rotation may be either contra- or ipsilateral rotation. For example, apomorphine and other dopamine agonists induce contralateral rotation (away from the lesioned side). This is due to their direct action on supersensitized dopaminergic receptors on the lesioned side. Conversely, d-amphetamine phenylisopropylamine (AMPH) induces ipsilateral rotation by blocking dopamine reuptake and increasing dopamine receptor activity on the nonlesioned side. In general, a greater than 80% depletion of dopamine is necessary to manifest rotation in this model (4,13) Circling behavior can be measured either by observation or by special devices called rotometers. The rate of rotation correlates with the severity of the lesion, and animals with more extensive striatal dopamine depletions are less likely to show behavioral recovery. This simple model of rotation away from the side with the most dopamine receptor occupancy has recently proven much more complex and less predictable than previously thought, especially in the context of various pharmacological treatments and neuronal transplantation. In addition to rotation, other behavioral assessments in the 6-OHDA model may include tests of forelimb use, bilateral tactile stimulation, single limb akinesia, and bracing (for review see Ref. 14).

The 6-OHDA–lesioned rat model has proven to be a valuable tool in evaluating (1) the pharmacological action of new drugs on the dopaminergic system, (2) the mechanisms of motor complications, (3) the neuroplasticity of the basal ganglia in response to nigrostriatal injury, and (4) the safety and efficacy of neuronal transplantation in PD. Extensive pharmacological studies have utilized the 6-OHDA–lesioned rat to investigate the role of various dopamine receptor (D1–D5) agonists and antagonists and other neurotransmitter systems (including glutamate, adenosine, nicotine, or opiods) in modulating dopamine neurotransmission. These studies elucidate the role of these compounds in electrophysiological, behavioral, and molecular (signal transduction) properties of the basal ganglia. A review of the vast amount of pharmacological literature regarding this model is beyond the scope of this chapter (see Ref. 12).

The 6-OHDA–lesioned rat model has also been an important tool in elucidating the mechanism(s) underlying motor complications. The chronic administration of levodopa (over a period of weeks) to the 6-OHDA rat has been demonstrated to lead to a shortening response similar to the wearing-off complication in idiopathic PD (15). This altered motor response occurs when greater than 95% of nigrostriatal cells are lost. Studies using glutamate antagonists have demonstrated improvement in the wearing-off response and have implicated the role of glutamate receptor subtypes in the development of motor complications (16–18). These findings have been supported by molecular studies that demonstrate alterations in the phosphorylation state of glutamate receptor subunits of the NMDA subtype (19). Unlike the wearing-off phenomenon, 6-OHDA lesioned rats do not develop typical dyskinesias (20).

In the context of neuroplasticity, the 6-OHDA–lesioned rat model demonstrates behavioral recovery and has been instrumental in characterizing the neurochemical, molecular, and morphological alterations within the basal ganglia in response to nigrostriatal dopamine depletion (21). These mechanisms of neuroplasticity in surviving dopaminergic neurons and their striatal terminals include (1) increased turnover of dopamine and its metabolites, (2) alterations in the expression of tyrosine hydroxylase, the rate-limiting step in dopamine biosynthesis, (3) decreased dopamine uptake through altered dopamine transporter expression, (4) alterations in the electrophysiological phenotype (both pattern and rate of neuronal firing) of substantia nigra neurons, and (5) sprouting of new striatal dopaminergic terminals. These molecular mechanisms may provide new targets for novel therapeutic interventions such as growth factors to enhance the function of surviving dopaminergic neurons.

The 6-OHDA–lesioned rat model has also been useful for determining important parameters for successful transplantation. These parameters include (1) target site (striatum versus substantia nigra), (2) volume of innervation at the target site, (3) number of cells transplanted, (4) type and species of cells transplanted including fetal mesencephalon, engineered cell lines, and stem cells, (5) age of host and donor tissues, (6) pretreatment of transplant tissue or host with neurotrophic factors, antioxidants, immuno-suppressive therapy, or neuroprotective pharmacological agents, and (7) surgical techniques including needle design, cell suspension media, and transplant cell delivery methods (22,23). The near absence of dopaminergic neurons and terminals within the striatum due to 6-OHDA lesioning provide a template for the assessment of sprouting axons and terminals from the transplant. Measures of transplant success in this model include reduction in the rotational behavior and the survival, sprouting and innervation (synapse formation) of dopaminergic fibers within the denervated striatum. The reduction of rotational behavior suggests increased striatal dopamine production originating from the transplanted tissue. Interestingly, not all behavioral measures appear to respond to transplant. The advancements made in the 6-OHDA–lesioned rat provide a framework for the further testing of transplantation in nonhuman primates and future human clinical trials.

While the 6-OHDA–lesioned rat model has many advantages, it serves primarily as a model of dopamine dysfunction. Lesioning with 6-OHDA is highly specific for catecholaminergic neurons and does not replicate many of the behavioral, neurochemical, and pathological features of human PD. For example, the 6-OHDA lesioned rat does not manifest alterations in the cholinergic and serotonergic neurotransmitter systems, which are commonly affected in PD. Stereotactic injections of 6-OHDA to precise targets does not replicate the extensive pathology of PD where other anatomical regions of the brain (including the locus coeruleus, nucleus basalis of Meynert, and raphe nuclei) are affected. In addition, Lewy body formation, a pathological hallmark of PD, has not been reported in this model. Interestingly, a recent report using a regimen of chronic administration of 6-OHDA into the third ventricle did show a more extensive lesioning pattern reminiscent of human PD (24). In addition to the rat, other species including the nonhuman primate have served as models for 6-OHDA lesioning (25). Lesioning in nonhuman primates provides for the analysis of behaviors not observed in the rat, such as targeting and retrieval tasks of the arm and hand.

Overall, lesioning with 6-OHDA has provided a rich source of information regarding the consequences of precise dopamine depletion and its effects on rotational behavior, dopamine biosynthesis, biochemical and morphological aspects of recovery, and serves as an excellent template to study both pharmacological and transplantation treatment modalities for PD.

The Neurotoxin 1-Methyl-4-phenyl-1,2,3,6-tetrahydropyridine

The inadvertent self-administration of 1-methyl-4-phenyl-1,2,3,6-tetrahydropyridine (MPTP) by heroin addicts in the 1980s induced an acute form of parkinsonism, whose clinical and biochemical features were indistinguishable from idiopathic PD (26,27). Like PD, this MPTP cohort demonstrated an excellent response to levodopa and dopamine agonist treatment but developed motor complications within a short period of time (over weeks). The rapidity with which these motor complications appeared presumably reflected the severity of substantia nigra neuronal degeneration induced by MPTP. Given the above similarities between the human model of MPTP-induced parkinsonism and PD, it became evident that MPTP could be used to develop animal models of PD.

The subsequent administration of MPTP to a number of different animals has demonstrated a wide variety of sensitivity to the toxic effects of MPTP. These differences were shown to be species, strain, and age dependent. For example, the nonhuman primate is the most sensitive to the toxic effects of MPTP. The mouse, cat, dog, and guinea pig are less sensitive, and the rat is the least sensitive. Even within species there are strain differences. For example, the C57BL/6 mouse is the most sensitive of all mouse strains tested, while strains such as CD-1 appear almost resistant (28,29). Some differences amongst strains may also depend on the supplier; this may account for differences seen with the Swiss Webster mouse (30). In addition to strain, animal sensitivity to the neurotoxicant effects of MPTP may be influenced by the animal's age, with older mice, for example, being more sensitive (31,32). Studies suggest that age-dependent differences may be due to differences in MPTP metabolism (33).

The mechanism of MPTP toxicity has been thoroughly investigated. The meperidine analog 1-methyl-4-phenyl-1,2,3,6-tetrahydropyridine (MPTP) is converted to 1-methyl-4-pyridinium (MPP$^+$) by monoamine oxidase B. MPP$^+$ acts as a substrate of the dopamine transporter (DAT), leading to the inhibition of mitochondrial complex I, the depletion of adenosine triphosphate (ATP), and cell death of dopaminergic neurons. MPTP administration to mice and nonhuman primates selectively destroys dopaminergic neurons of the substantia nigra pars compacta (SNpc), the same neurons affected in PD (34). Similar to PD, other catecholaminergic neurons, such as those in the ventral tegmental area (VTA) and locus coeruleus, may be affected to a lesser degree. In addition, dopamine depletion occurs in both the putamen and caudate nucleus. The preferential lesioning of either the putamen or caudate nucleus may depend on animal species and regimen of MPTP administration (35–37). Unlike PD, Lewy bodies have not been reported, but eosinophilic inclusions (reminiscent of Lewy bodies) have been described in aged nonhuman primates (38). The time course of MPTP-induced neurodegeneration is rapid and therefore represents a major difference from idiopathic PD, which is a chronic progressive disease. Interestingly, data from humans exposed to MPTP indicate that the toxic effects of MPTP may be more protracted than initially believed (39). Details of MPTP toxicity and utility are described in Refs. 40 and 41.

The MPTP-Lesioned Mouse Model

The administration of MPTP to mice results in behavioral alterations that may resemble human parkinsonism. For example hypokinesia, bradykinesia, and akinesia can be observed through various behavioral analyses including open field activity monitoring, swim test, pole test, grip coordination, and rotorod. Whole body tremor and postural abnormalities have also been reported, but primarily in the acute phase (42). In general, these behavioral alterations tend to be highly variable, with some mice showing severe deficits while others show little or no behavioral change (for review see Ref. 42). This behavioral variability may be due to a number of factors, including the degree of lesioning, mouse strain, time course after lesioning, and the reliability and validity of the behavioral analysis.

The MPTP-lesioned mouse model has proven valuable to investigate potential mechanisms of neurotoxic induced dopaminergic cell death. For example, mechanisms under investigation have included mitochondrial dysfunction, energy (ATP) depletion, free-radical production, apoptosis, and glutamate excitotoxicity (41). In addition to its utility in studying acute cell death, the MPTP-lesioned model also provides an opportunity to study injury-induced neuroplasticity. The MPTP-lesioned mouse displays the return of striatal dopamine several weeks to months after lesioning (35,37,43). The molecular mechanism of this neuroplasticity of the injured basal ganglia is an area of investigation in our laboratory and in others and appears to encompass both neurochemical and morphological components. In addition, work in our laboratory has shown that this plasticity may be facilitated through activity-dependent processes using treadmill training.

MPTP-Lesioned Nonhuman Primate

Administration of MPTP to nonhuman primates results in parkinsonian symptoms including bradykinesia, postural instability, and rigidity. In some species resting or action/postural tremor has been observed (44). Similar to PD, the MPTP-lesioned nonhuman primate responds to traditional antiparkinsonian therapies such as levodopa and dopamine receptor agonists. Following the administration of MPTP, the nonhuman primate progresses through acute (hours), subacute (days), and chronic (weeks) behavioral phases of toxicity that are due to the peripheral and central effects of MPTP. The acute phase is characterized by sedation, and a hyperadrenergic state, the subacute phase by the development of varying degrees of parkinsonian features, and the chronic phase by initial recovery (by some, but not all animals) followed by the stabilization of motor deficits (45). In general, the behavioral response to MPTP lesioning may vary at both the inter- and intraspecies levels. Variability may be due to age and species phylogeny. For example, older animals and Old World monkeys (such as rhesus *Macaca mulatta*, or African Green *Cercopithecus aethiops*) tend to be more sensitive than young and New World monkeys (such as the squirrel monkey, *Saimiri sciureus*, or marmoset, *Callithrix jacchus*) (46–48).

Behavioral recovery after MPTP-induced parkinsonism has been reported in most species of nonhuman primates. The degree and time course of behavioral recovery is dependent on age, species, and mode of MPTP administration (45). In general the more severely affected animal is less likely to recover (44). The molecular mechanisms underlying behavioral recovery of the nonhuman primate is a major focus of our laboratory. Results of our work and others have identified that the mechanisms underlying recovery may include (1) alterations in dopamine biosynthesis (increased tyrosine hydroxylase protein and mRNA expression) and turnover, (2) downregulation of dopamine transporter, (3) increased dopamine metabolism, (4) sprouting and branching of tyrosine hydroxylase fibers, (5) alterations of other neurotransmitter systems, including glutamate and serotonin, and (6) alterations of signal transduction pathways in both the direct (D1) and indirect (D2) pathways (49).

The administration of MPTP through a number of different dosing regimens has led to the development of several distinct models of parkinsonism in the nonhuman primate. Each model is characterized by unique behavioral and neurochemical parameters. As a result, numerous studies addressing a variety of hypotheses have been conducted. These studies consist of new pharmacological treatments, transplantation, mechanisms of motor complications, deep brain stimulation, behavioral recovery, cognitive impairment, and the development of novel neuroprotective and restorative therapies. For example, in some models there is profound striatal dopamine depletion and denervation with little or no dopaminergic axons or terminals remaining. This model provides an optimal setting to test fetal tissue grafting since the presence of any tyrosine hydroxylase positive axons or sprouting cells would be due to transplanted tissue survival. Other models have less extensive dopamine depletion and only partial denervation with a modest to moderate degree of dopaminergic axons and terminals remaining. This partially denervated model best resembles mild to moderately affected PD patients. Therefore, sufficient dopaminergic neurons and axons as well as compensatory mechanisms are likely to be present. The effects of growth factors (inducing sprouting) or neuroprotective factors (promoting cell survival) are best evaluated in this situation. The following section reviews the most commonly used MPTP-lesioned nonhuman primate models.

In the *systemic lesioned* model, MPTP may be administered via intramuscular, intravenous, intraperitoneal, or subcutaneous injection (50–53). This leads to bilateral depletion of striatal dopamine and nigrostriatal cell death. A feature of this model is that the degree of lesioning can be titrated, resulting in a range (mild to severe) of parkinsonian symptoms. The presence of clinical asymmetry is common, with one side more severely affected. Levodopa administration leads to the reversal of all behavioral signs of parkinsonism in a dose-dependent fashion. After several days to weeks of levodopa administration, animals develop reproducible motor complications, both wearing-off and dyskinesia. Animal behavior in this model and others may be assessed using (1) cage-side or video-based observation, (2) automated activity measurements in the cage through infrared based motion detectors or accelerometers, and (3) examination of hand-reaching movement tasks. The principal advantage of this model is that the behavioral syndrome closely resembles the clinical features of idiopathic PD. The systemic model has partial dopaminergic denervation bilaterally and probably best represents the degree of loss seen in all stages of PD, including end-stage disease where some dopaminergic neurons are still present. This model is well suited for therapeutics that interact with remaining dopaminergic neurons, including growth factors, neuroprotective agents, and dopamine modulation. The easily reproducible dyskinesia in this model allows for extensive investigation of its underlying mechanism and treatment. Disadvantages of this model include spontaneous recovery in mildly affected animals. Alternatively, bilaterally severely affected animals may require extensive veterinary care and dopamine supplementation.

Administration of MPTP via unilateral intracarotid infusion has been used to induce a hemiparkinsonian state in the primate, called the *hemi-lesioned* model (54). The rapid metabolism of MPTP to MPP^+ in the brain may account for the localized toxicity to the hemisphere ipsilateral to the infusion. Motor impairments appear primarily on the contralateral side. Hemi-neglect, manifested by a delayed motor reaction time, also develops on the contralateral side. In addition, spontaneous ipsilateral rotation may develop. Levodopa administration reverses the parkinsonian symptoms and induces contralateral rotation. Substantia nigra neurodegeneration and striatal dopamine depletion (>99%) on the ipsilateral side to the injection is more extensive than seen in the systemic model. The degree of unilateral lesioning in this model is dose dependent.

Major advantages of the *hemi-lesioned* model include (1) the ability for animals to feed and maintain themselves without supportive care, (2) the availability of the unaffected limb on the ipsilateral side to serve as a control, and (3) the utility of the dopamine-induced rotation for pharmacological testing. In addition, due to the absence of dopaminergic innervation in the striatum, *the hemi-lesioned* model is well suited for examining neuronal sprouting of transplanted tissue. A disadvantage of this model is that only a subset of parkinsonian features is evident, which are restricted to one side of the body, a situation never seen in advanced PD.

The *bilateral intracarotid* model employs an intracarotid injection of MPTP followed several months later by another intracarotid injection on the opposite side (55). This model combines the less debilitating features of the carotid model as well as creating bilateral clinical features, a situation more closely resembling idiopathic PD. The advantage of this model is its prolonged stability and limited inter-animal variability. Similar to the hemi-lesioned model, where there is extensive striatal dopamine depletion and denervation, the bilateral intracarotid model is well suited for evaluation of transplanted tissue. However, levodopa administration may result in only partial improvement of parkinsonian motor features and food retrieval tasks. This can be a disadvantage since high doses of test drug may be needed to demonstrate efficacy, increasing the risk for medication related adverse effects.

A novel approach to MPTP lesioning is the administration of MPTP via intracarotid infusion followed by a systemic injection. This *overlesioned* model is characterized by severe dopamine depletion ipsilateral to the

MPTP-carotid infusion and a partial depletion on the contralateral side due to the systemic MPTP injection. Consequently, animals are still able to maintain themselves due to a relatively intact side. The behavioral deficits consist of asymmetrical parkinsonian features. The more severely affected side is contralateral to the intracarotid injection (56). Levodopa produces a dose-dependent improvement in behavioral features, but the complications of levodopa therapy such as dyskinesia have not been as consistently observed. This model combines some of the advantages of both the systemic and intracarotid MPTP models, including stability. This model is suitable for both transplant studies, utilizing the more depleted side, and neuroregeneration with growth factors, utilizing the partially depleted side where dopaminergic neurons still remain.

Finally, the *chronic low-dose* model consists of intravenous injections of a low dose of MPTP administration over a 5- to 13-month period (57). This model is characterized by cognitive deficits consistent with frontal lobe dysfunction reminiscent of PD or normal aged monkeys. These animals have impaired attention and short-term memory processes and perform poorly in tasks of delayed response or delayed alternation. Since gross parkinsonian motor symptoms are essentially absent, at least in early stages, this model is well adapted for studying cognitive deficits analogous to those that accompany idiopathic PD.

The MPTP-lesioned nonhuman primate has provided a valuable tool for investigating potential mechanisms underlying motor complications related to long-term levodopa use in human idiopathic PD. The MPTP-lesioned nonhuman primate has been shown to demonstrate both wearing-off and dyskinesia. Although the etiology of dyskinesia is unknown, electrophysiological, neurochemical, molecular, and neuroimaging studies in the nonhuman primate models suggest that the pulsatile delivery of levodopa may lead to (1) changes in the neuronal firing rate and pattern of the globus pallidus and subthalamic nucleus, (2) enhancement of D1- and/or D2-receptor–mediated signal transduction pathways, (3) super-sensitivity of the D2 receptor; (4) alterations in the phosphorylation state and subcellular localization of glutamate (NMDA subtype) receptors, (5) modifications in the functional links between dopamine receptor subtypes (D1 and D2, and D1 and D3), (6) changes in glutamate receptors (AMPA and NMDA receptor subtypes), and (7) enhancement of opiod-peptide–mediated neurotransmission (58–62).

While the presence of a nigral lesion has long been considered an important prerequisite for the development of dyskinesia in the MPTP model, recent studies demonstrate that even normal nonhuman primates when given sufficiently large doses of levodopa (with a peripheral decarboxylase inhibitor) over 2–8 weeks may develop peak-dose dyskinesia

(63). The high levels of plasma levodopa in this dosing regimen may serve to exhaust the buffering capacity within the striatum of the normal animal and therefore lead to pulsatile delivery of levodopa and priming of postsynaptic dopaminergic sites for dyskinesia.

In addition to its central effects, the administration of MPTP may lead to systemic effects, which may prove detrimental to any animal during the induction of a parkinsonian state. For example, the peripheral conversion of MPTP to MPP^+ in the liver could lead to toxic injury of the liver and heart. To address these potential peripheral effects of MPTP, squirrel monkeys were administered MPTP (a series of 6 subcutaneous injections of 2 mg/kg, free-base, 2 weeks apart) and were given a comprehensive exam 1, 4, and 10 days after each injection. This exam included measurements of body weight, core body temperature, heart rate, blood pressure, liver and kidney function, and white blood cell count. Biochemical markers of hepatocellular toxicity were evident within days of MPTP lesioning and persisted for several weeks after the last injection. In addition, animals had significant hypothermia within 48 hours after lesioning that persisted for up to 10 days after the last MPTP injection. The pathophysiology of these effects may be directly related to MPTP itself and/or its metabolites. The systemic effects of MPTP on animal models should be taken into consideration during the design of any pharmacological study.

Methamphetamine

Amphetamine and its derivatives (including methamphetamine) lead to long-lasting depletion of both dopamine and serotonin when administered to rodents and nonhuman primates (64,65). Methamphetamine (METH), one of the most potent of these derivatives, leads to terminal degeneration of dopaminergic neurons in the caudate-putamen, nucleus accumbens, and neocortex. In contrast to MPTP, the axonal trunks and soma of SNpc and VTA neurons are spared (66). However, there have been occasional reports of METH-induced cell death in the substantia nigra (67). In general, the effects of severe METH lesioning are long-lasting. There is evidence of recovery of dopaminergic innervation depending on the METH regimen and species used (68). Despite the severe depletion of striatal dopamine, the motor behavioral alterations seen in rodents and nonhuman primates are subtle (69).

The neurotoxic effects of METH are dependent on the efflux of dopamine since agents that deplete dopamine or block its uptake are neuroprotective (70,71). The metabolic mechanisms underlying METH-induced neurotoxicity involve the perturbation of antioxidant enzymes such as glutathione peroxidase or catalase, leading to the formation of reactive oxygen/nitrogen species including H_2O_2, superoxide, and hydroxyl radicals (72–76). The administration of antioxidant therapies or overexpression of superoxide dismutase (SOD) in transgenic mice models is neuroprotective against METH toxicity (77,78). In addition, both glutamate receptors and nitric oxide synthase (NOS) are important to METH-induced neurotoxicity since the administration of either NMDA receptor antagonists or NOS inhibitors are also neuroprotective (79). Other factors important to METH-induced neurotoxicity include the inhibition of both tyrosine hydroxylase and dopamine transporter activity and METH-induced hyperthermia (75).

The administration of METH to adult animals has played an important role in testing the molecular and biochemical mechanisms underlying dopaminergic and serotonergic neuronal axonal degeneration, especially the role of free radicals and glutamate neurotransmission. Understanding these mechanisms has led to testing different neuroprotective therapeutic modalities. An advantage of the METH model over MPTP is that the serotonergic and dopaminergic systems can be lesioned in utero during the early stages of the development of these neurotransmitter systems. Such studies have indicated that there is a tremendous degree of architectural rearrangement that occurs within the dopaminergic and serotonergic systems of injured animals as they develop. These changes may lead to altered behavior in the adult animal (80).

In light of the toxic nature of these compounds in animals, studies in humans have suggested that abusers of METH and substituted amphetamines (including MDMA, "ecstasy") may suffer from the long-lasting effects of these drugs (81,82). Specifically, these individuals may be prone to develop parkinsonism (83).

Rotenone

Epidemiological studies have suggested that environmental factors such as pesticides may increase the risk for PD (84). The demonstration of specific neurochemical and pathological damage to dopaminergic neurons by the application of various pesticides such as rotenone (an inhibitor of mitochondrial complex I) have supported these epidemiological findings. For example, using a chronic rotenone infusion paradigm, Greenamyre and colleagues reported degeneration of a subset of nigrostriatal dopaminergic neurons, the formation of cytoplasmic inclusions, and the development of parkinsonian behavioral features (including hunched posture, rigidity, unsteady movement, and paw tremor) in the rat (85). Studies examining the effects of various pesticide applications in animal models may lead to insights into the mechanisms of neuronal death in PD (86).

GENETIC MODELS OF PARKINSON'S DISEASE

In addition to pharmacological and neurotoxicant models of PD, there are spontaneous rodent (such as the *weaver* mouse and *AS/AGU* rat) and transgenic mouse (including parkin, α-synuclein) models that provide important avenues to investigate the basal ganglia.

Spontaneous Rodent Models for Parkinson's Disease

There are several naturally occurring spontaneous mutations in rodents that are of particular interest in PD. Spontaneous rodent models include the *weaver, lurcher, reeler, Tshr*[hyt], *tottering, coloboma* mice and the *AS/AGU* and *circling* (*ci*) rat. These models possess unique characteristics that may provide insight into neurodegenerative processes of PD and related disorders. Several of these spontaneous rodent models display altered dopaminergic function or neurodegeneration and have deficits in motor behavior (87). For example, the *weaver* mouse displays cell death of dopaminergic neurons while the *tottering* mouse displays tyrosine hydroxylase hyperinnervation. The *AS/AGU* rat is a spontaneous model characterized by progressive rigidity, staggering gait, tremor, and difficulty in initiating movements (88). Microdialysis in the *AS/AGU* rat model has revealed that even prior to dopaminergic neuronal cell death, there is dysfunction in dopaminergic neurotransmission that correlates with behavioral deficits. Another potentially interesting rodent model is the *circling* (*ci*) rat (89). This animal model displays spontaneous rotational behavior as a result of an imbalance in dopaminergic neurotransmission despite the absence of asymmetrical nigral cell death.

Transgenic Mouse Models

The development of transgenic animal models is dependent on identifying genes of interest. A transgenic mouse is an animal in which a specific gene of interest has been altered through one of several techniques including: (1) the excision of the host gene (knock-out), (2) the introduction of a mutant gene (knock-in), and (3) the alteration of gene expression (knock-down). In PD, one source of transgenic targeting is derived from genes identified through epidemiological and linkage analysis studies. α-Synuclein and parkin are examples of genes that have been identified through linkage analysis. Other transgenic animals have been developed based on the identification of genes important for normal basal ganglia and dopaminergic function. These transgenic mouse lines target several genes, including superoxide dismutase (SOD), glutathione reductase, monoamine oxidase (MAO), dopamine receptors (D1, D2), dopamine transporter (DAT), caspases, neurotrophic factors (BDNF and GDNF), and neurotransmitter receptors (NMDA and AMPA). Once the transgene has been constructed, the degree of its expression and its impact on the phenotype of the animal depends on many factors, including the selection of sequence (mutant versus wild-type), site of integration, number of copies recombined, selection of transcription promoter, and upstream controlling elements (enhancers). Other important factors may include the background strain and age of the animal. These different features may account for some of the biochemical and pathological variations observed among transgenic mouse lines. Two examples of recent transgenic mouse lines are discussed.

Parkin

An autosomal recessive form of juvenile parkinsonism (AR-JP) led to the identification of a gene on chromosome 6q27 called parkin (90,91). Mutations in parkin may account for the majority of autosomal recessive familial cases of PD. Parkin protein has a large N-terminal ubiquitin-like domain and C-terminal cysteine ring structure and is expressed in the brain (92–94). Recent biochemical studies indicate that Parkin protein may play a critical role in mediating interactions with a number of different proteins involved in the proteasome-mediated degradation pathway, including α-synuclein (95,96). Mutations of the parkin gene have been introduced into transgenic mice. At present there is very little known about pathological or behavioral alterations due to mutations in Parkin protein. However, parkin transgenic models enable investigation of the ubiquitin-mediated protein degradation pathways and their relationship to neurodegenerative disease.

α-Synuclein

Rare cases of autosomal dominant familial forms of PD (the Contursi and German kindreds) have been linked to point mutations in the gene encoding α-synuclein (97). The normal function of α-synuclein is unknown, but its localization and developmental expression suggests a role in neuroplasticity (98,99). The disruption of normal neuronal function may lead to the loss of synaptic maintenance and subsequent degeneration. It is interesting that mice with knockout of α-synuclein are viable, suggesting that a "gain-in-function" phenotype or other protein-protein interactions may contribute to neurodegeneration. Although no mutant forms of α-synuclein have been identified in idiopathic PD, its localization to Lewy bodies (including PD and related disorders) has suggested a patho-physiological link between α-synuclein aggregation and neurodegenerative disease. To investigate these potential mechanisms, several groups have developed transgenic mouse models. An interesting caveat is that the mutant allele of α-synuclein in the Contursi kindred is identical to the wild-type mouse, suggesting that protein expression and/or protein-protein interactions may be more important than loss of function due to missense mutation. Therefore, transgenic mouse models developed for α-synuclein focus on altered protein expression through the use of different promoters and gene cassette constructs. Some transgenic mouse lines show pathological changes in dopaminergic neurons (including inclusions, decreased striatal dopamine, and loss of striatal tyrosine hydroxylase immunoreactivity), behavioral deficits (rotorod and attenuation of dopamine-dependent locomotor response to amphetamine), while other lines show no deficits (100–102). No group has reported the loss of substantia nigra dopaminergic neurons. This range of results with different α-synuclein constructs from different laboratories underscores the important link between protein expression (mutant vs. wild-type alleles) and pathological and behavioral outcome. Important applications of α-synuclein transgenic mice are occurring at the level of understanding the role of this protein in basal ganglia function. For example, the response of α-synuclein expression to neurotoxic injury as well as interactions with other proteins, including parkin, will provide valuable insights into mechanisms important to neurodegeneration (95).

Invertebrate Models

Recent developments of invertebrate transgenic models (such as in *Drosophila melanogaster*) for α-synuclein, parkin, and other genes of interest provide another avenue to investigate the function of proteins of interest in PD. In addition, the application of dopaminergic-specific toxins, such as 6-OHDA to *Caenorhabditis elegans*, may provide another tool for understanding mechanisms of cell death (103). Unlike mammalian animal models, invertebrate models tend to be less expensive and greater numbers can be generated in shorter periods of time. These advantages offer a means for high-volume screening of pharmacological agents for the treatment of PD (104,105).

MODELS OF PD VARIANTS

While the models discussed in the above sections provide insights into PD as well as related disorders such as multisystem atrophy (MSA) and progressive supranuclear palsy (PSP), other models have been developed that share a greater similarity with these variants.

Multisystem Atrophy and Striatonigral Degeneration

Multisystem atrophy (MSA) is a variant of PD characterized by a combination of clinical symptoms involving cerebellar, extrapyramidal, and autonomic systems. The predominant subtype of MSA is striatonigral degeneration (SND), a form of levodopa-unresponsive parkinsonism. Neuropathological changes of SND include degeneration of the nigrostriatal pathway, medium spiny striatal GABAergic projection pathways (putamen greater than caudate), as well as other regions of the brain stem, cerebellum, and spinal cord. Inclusion-like aggregates that immuno-stain for ubiquitin and α-synuclein are seen in oligodendrocytes and neurons.

The basis for developing an animal model for SND emerged from established animal models for both parkinsonian (having SNpc pathology) and Huntington's disease (HD) (having striatal pathology). For example, rodent models for SND have been generated through sequential stereotactic injections of 6-OHDA and quinolinic acid (QA) into the medial forebrain bundle and striatum, respectively, or striatal injections of MPP^+ and 3-nitropropionic acid (3-NP)(106–108). These double-lesioning models are characterized morphologically by neuronal degeneration in the SNpc and ipsilateral striatum. The order of neurotoxic lesioning may influence the degree of nigral or striatal pathology. For example, animals receiving 6-OHDA prior to QA exhibit predominantly nigral pathology, while animals receiving QA prior to 6-OHDA show predominantly striatal pathology. This may be due to QA-induced terminal damage or other complex interactions after lesioning that reduce terminal uptake of 6-OHDA. Glial inclusions have not been reported in any of these models indicating a significant difference compared with the human condition.

Motor deficits in models for MSA and SND are assessed by ipsilateral and contralateral motor tasks (including stepping response, impaired paw reaching, and balance) and drug-induced circling behavior. As described earlier, characteristic drug-induced circling behavior occurs after 6-OHDA lesioning resulting in ipsilateral rotation in response to amphetamine and contralateral rotation in response to apomorphine. The subsequent striatal lesioning with QA diminishes (or has no effect on) amphetamine-induced ipsilateral rotation and reduces (or abolishes) apomorphine-induced contralateral rotation. This observation may be mediated by dopamine release on the intact side (in response to amphetamine) and/or the loss of dopamine receptor activation on the lesioned side (in response to apomorphine). The lack of response to apomorphine has been shown to correlate with the volume of the striatal lesion and is analogous to the diminished efficacy of levodopa therapy observed in the majority of SND patients.

A nonhuman primate (*Macaca fasicularis*) model of SND has been generated through the sequential systemic administration of MPTP and 3-NP (106,109). The parkinsonian features after MPTP lesioning are levodopa responsive, but subsequent administration of 3-NP worsens motor symptoms and nearly eliminates the levodopa response. Levodopa occasionally induces facial dyskinesia as sometimes seen in human MSA. Similar to SND morphological changes include cell loss in the SNpc (typical of MPTP-lesioning) and severe circumscribed degeneration of striatal GABAergic projection neurons (typical of 3-NP lesioning). Despite the similarities with the human condition, the MSA model is characterized by an equal degree of lesioning in the putamen and caudate nucleus, while in human SND the putamen is more affected. In addition, inclusion bodies that may underlie the pathogenesis of SND have not been reported in the nonhuman primate model.

The Tauopathies Including Progressive Supranuclear Palsy and Other Tau-Related Disorders

The low molecular weight microtubule-associated protein tau has been implicated in a number of neurodegenerative diseases, including Alzheimer's disease, progressive supranuclear palsy (PSP), Pick's disease, frontotemporal dementia with parkinsonism (FTDP), and amyotrophic lateral sclerosis/parkinsonism-dementia complex (ALS/PDC) of Guam. Together these neurodegenerative diseases comprise what is referred to as tauopathies, since they share common neuropathological features including abnormal hyperphosphorylation and filamentous accumulation of aggregated tau proteins. Reports in the literature have implicated either alternative RNA splicing (generating different isoforms) or missense mutations as mechanisms underlying many of the tauopathies. Therefore, transgenic mice have been generated that overexpress specific splice variants or missense mutations of tau (110). One such transgenic line has been developed to overexpress the shortest human tau isoform (111). These mice showed progressive motor weakness, intraneuronal and intra-axonal inclusions (detectable by 1-month postnatal), and reduced axonal transport. Fibrillary tau inclusions developed in the neocortical neurons after 18 months of age implicating age-specific processes in the pathogenesis of fibrous tau inclusions. An interesting tau transgenic line has been developed in *Drosophila melanogaster*, where expression of a tau missense mutation showed no evidence of large filamentous aggregates (neurofibrillary tangles). However, aged flies showed evidence of vacuolization and degeneration of cortical neurons (112). These observations suggest that tau-mediated neurodegeneration is age-dependent and may take place independent of protein aggregation.

CONCLUSIONS

Our understanding of Parkinson's disease and related disorders has been advanced through animal models using surgical, pharmacological, and neurotoxicant manipulation. The nonhuman primate, rodent, cat, and pig models have contributed to the development of symptomatic (dopamine modulation), neuroprotective (antioxidants, free-radical scavengers), and restorative (growth factors, transplantation) therapies. In addition, these animal models have furthered our understanding of motor complications (wearing off and dyskinesia), neuronal cell death, and neuroplasticity of the basal ganglia. Future direction in PD research is through the continued development of animal models with altered genes and proteins of interest. In conjunction with existing models, these genetic-based models may lead to the eventual cure of PD and related disorders.

ACKNOWLEDGMENTS

We would like to thank our colleagues at the University of Southern California for their support. Thank you to Beth Fisher, Mickie Welsh, Tom McNeill, and Mark Lew for their suggestions. Studies in our laboratory were made possible through the generous support of the Parkinson's Disease Foundation, The Baxter Foundation, The Zumberge Foundation, The Lisette and Norman Ackerberg Foundation, friends of the USC Parkinson's Disease Research Group, and NINDS Grant RO1 NS44327-01 (to MWJ). Thank you to Nicolaus, Pascal, and Dominique for their patience and encouragement.

REFERENCES

1. Jellinger K. Pathology of Parkinson's syndrome. In: D Calne, ed. Handbook of Experimental Pharmacology. Berlin: Springer 1988:47–112.
2. Birkmayer W, Hornykiewicz O. Der 1-3, 4-Dioxy-phenylanin (1-DOPA)-effekt bei der Parkinson-Akinesia Klin Wochenschr 1961; 73:787.
3. Ehringer H, Hornykiewicz O. Verteilung von Noradrenalin und Dopamin (3-Hydroxytyramin) in gehrindes Menschen und ihr Verhalten bei Erkrankungen des extrapyramidalen Systems. Klin Wochenschr 1960; 38:1238–1239.
4. Schultz W. Depletion of dopamine in the striatum as an experimental model of Parkinsonism: direct effects and adaptive mechanisms. Prog Neurobiol 1982; 18:121–166.
5. Glinka Y, Youdim MBH. Mechanisms of 6-hydroxydopamine neurotoxicity. J Neural Transm 1997; 50:55–66.
6. Blum D, Torch S, Lambeng N, Nissou M, Benabid A, Sadoul R, Verna J. Molecular pathways involved in the neurotoxicity of 6-OHDA, dopamine and

MPTP: contribution to the apoptotic theory in Parkinson's disease. Prog Neurobiol 2001; 6+5:135–172.

7. Ungerstedt U. 6-Hydroxy-dopamine induced degeneration of central mono-amine neurons. Eur J Pharmacol 1968; 5:107–110.

8. Ungerstedt U, Arbuthnott G. Quantitative recording of rotational behavior in rats after 6-hydroxydopamine lesions of the nigrostriatal dopamine system. Brain Res 1970; 24:485–493.

9. Ungerstedt U. Postsynaptic supersensitivity after 6-hydroxydopamine induced degeneration of the nigro-striatal dopamine system. Acta Physiol Scand 1971; 367 suppl:69–93.

10. Sauer H, Oertel WH. Progressive degeneration of nigrostriatal dopamine neurons following intrastriatal terminal lesions with 6-hydroxydopamine: a combined retrograde tracing and immunocytochemical study in the rat. Neuroscience 1994; 59:401–415.

11. Schwarting RKW, Huston JP. The unilateral 6-hydroxydopamine lesion model in behavioral brain research. Analysis of functional deficits, recovery and treatments. Prog Neurobiol 1996; 50:275–331.

12. Schwarting RK, Huston JP. Unilateral 6-hydroxydopamine lesions of meso-striatal dopamine neurons and their physiological sequelae. Prog Neurobiol 1996; 49:215–266.

13. Schwarting RK, Huston JP. The unilateral 6-hydroxydopamine lesion model in behavioral brain research. Analysis of functional deficits, recovery and treatments. Prog Neurobiol 1996; 20:275–331.

14. Shallert T, Tillerson JL. Interventive strategies for degeneration of dopamine neurons in parkinsonism: optimizing behavioral assessment of outcome. In: Emerich DF, Dean RL, Sanberg PR, eds. Central Nervous System Diseases. Totowa, NJ: Human Press 2000:131–151.

15. Papa SM, Engber TM, Kask AM, Chase TN. Motor fluctuations in levodopa treated parkinsonian rats: relation to lesion extent and treatment duration. Brain Res 1994; 662:69–74.

16. Papa SM, Boldry RC, Engber TM, Kask AM, Chase TN. Reversal of levodopa-induced motor fluctuations in experimental parkinsonism by NMDA receptor blockade. Brain Res 1995; 701:13–18.

17. Chase TN, Engber TM, Mouradian MM. Contribution of dopaminergic and glutamatergic mechanisms to the pathogenesis of motor response complications in Parkinson's disease. Adv Neurol 1996; 69:497–501.

18. Chase TN, Konitsiotis S, Oh JD. Striatal molecular mechanisms and motor dysfunction in Parkinson's disease. Adv Neurol 2001; 86:355–360.

19. Oh JD, Russell D, Vaughan CL, Chase TN. Enhanced tyrosine phosphoryla-tion of striatal NMDA eceptor subunits: effect of dopaminergic denervation and L-DOPA administration. Brain Res 1998; 813:150–159.

20. Henry B, Crossman AR, Brotchie JM. Characterization of enhanced behavioral responses to L-DOPA following repeated administration in the 6-hydroxydopamine-lesioned rat model of Parkinson's disease. Exp Neurol 1998; 151:334–342.

21. Zigmond MJ, Abercrombie ED, Berger TW, Grace AA, Sticker EM. Compensations after lesions of central dopaminergic neurons: some clinical and basic implications. Trends Neurosci 1990; 13:290–295.

22. Winkler C, Kirik D, Bjorklund A, Dunnett SB. Transplantation in the rat model of Parkinson's disease: ectopic versus homotopic graft placement. Prog Brain Res 2000; 127:233–265.

23. Nikkhah G, Olsson M, Eberhard J, Bentlage C, Cunningham MG, Bjorklund A. A microtransplantation approach for cell suspension grafting in the rat Parkinson model: a detailed account of the methodology. Neuroscience 1994; 63:57–72.

24. Rodriguez M, Barroso-Chinea P, Abdala P, Obeso J, Gonzalez-Hernandez T. Dopamine cell degeneration induced by intraventricular administration of 6-hydroxydopamine in the rat: similarities with cell loss in Parkinson's disease. Exp Neurol 2001; 169:163–181.

25. Annett LE, Rogers DC, Hernandez TD, Dunnett SB. Behavioral analysis of unilateral monoamine depletion in the marmoset. Brain 1992; 115:825–856.

26. Davis GC, Williams AC, Markey SP, Ebert MH, Caine ED, Reichert CM, Kopin IJ. Chronic parkinsonism secondary to intravenous injection of meperidine analogues. Psychiatry Res 1979; 1:249–254.

27. Langston JW, Ballard P, Tetrud JW, Irwin I. Chronic parkinsonism in humans due to a product of meperidine-analog synthesis. Science 1983; 219:979–980.

28. Muthane U, Ramsay KA, Jiang H, Jackson-Lewis V, Donaldson D, Fernando S, Ferreira M, Srzedborski S. Differences in nigral neuron number and sensitivity to 1-methyl-4-phenyl-1,2,3,6-tetrahydropyris in C57/bl and CD-1 mice. Exp Neurol 1994; 126:195–204.

29. Hamre K, Tharp R, Poon K, Xiong X, Smeyne RJ. Differential strain susceptibility following 1-methyl-4-phenyl-1,2,3,6-tetrahydropyridine (MPTP) administration acts in an autosomal dominant fashion: quantitative analysis in seven strains of Mus musculus. Brain Res 1999; 828:91–103.

30. Heikkila RE. Differential neurotoxicity of 1-methyl-4-phenyl-1,2,3,6-tetrahydropyridine (MPTP) in Swiss-Webster mice from different sources. Eur J Pharmacol 1985; 117:131–133.

31. Jarvis MF, Wagner GC. Age-dependent effects of 1-methyl-4-phenyl-1,2,3,6-tetrahydropyridine (MPTP). Neuropharmacology 1985; 24:581–583.

32. Ali SF, David SN, Newport GD, Cadet JL, Slikker W. MPTP-induced oxidative stress and neurotoxicity are age-dependent: evidence from measures of reactive oxygen species and striatal dopamine levels. Synapse 1994; 18:27–34.

33. Saura J, Richards J, Mahy N. Age-related changes on MAO in Bl/C57 mouse tissues: a quantitative radioautographic study. J Neural Transm 1994; 41:89–94.

34. Jackson-Lewis V, Jakowec M, Burke RE, Przedborski S. Time course and morphology of dopaminergic neuronal death caused by the neurotoxin 1-methyl-4-phenyl-1,2,3,6-tetrahydropyridine. Neurodegen 1995; 4:257–269.

35. Ricaurte GA, Langston JW, DeLanney LE, Irwin I, Peroutka SJ, Forno LS. Fate of nigrostriatal neurons in young mature mice given 1-methyl-4-phenyl-1,2,3,6-tetrahydropyridine: a neurochemical and morphological reassessment. Brain Res 1986; 376:117–124.
36. Kalivas PW, Duffy P, Barrow J. Regulation of the mesocorticolimbic dopamine system by glutamic acid receptor subtypes. J Pharm Exp Therap 1989; 251:378–387.
37. Bezard E, Dovero S, Imbert C, Boraud T, Gross CE. Spontaneous long-term compensatory dopaminergic sprouting in MPTP-treated mice. Synapse 2000; 38:363–368.
38. Forno LS, Langston JW, DeLanney LE, Irwin I, Ricaurte GA. Locus ceruleus lesions and eosinophilic inclusions in MPTP-treated monkeys. Ann Neurol 1986; 20:449–455.
39. Langston JW, Forno LS, Tetrud J, Reeves AG, Kaplan JA, Karluk D. Evidence of active nerve cell degeneration in the substantia nigra of humans years after 1-methyl-4-phenyl-1,2,3,6-tetrahydropyridine exposure. Ann Neurol 1999; 46:598–605.
40. Przedborski S, Jackson-Lewis V, Naini AB, Jakowec M, Petzinger G, Miller R, Akram M. The parkinsonian toxin 1-methyl-4-phenyl-1,2,3,6-tetrahydropyridine (MPTP): a technical review of its utility and safety. J Neurochem 2001; 76:1265–1274.
41. Royland JE, Langston JW. MPTP: A dopamine neurotoxin. In: RM Kostrzewa, ed. Highly Selective Neurotoxins. Totowa, NJ: Human Press 1998:141–194.
42. Sedelis M, Schwarting RK, Huston JP. Behavioral phenotyping of the MPTP mouse model of Parkinson's disease. Behav Brain Res 2001; 125:109–125.
43. Ho A, Blum M. Induction of interleukin-1 associated with compensatory dopaminergic sprouting in the denervated striatum of young mice: model of aging and neurodegenerative disease. J Neurosci 1998; 18:5614–5629.
44. Taylor JR, Elsworth JD, Roth RH, Sladek JR, Redmond DE. Severe long-term 1-methyl-4-phenyl-1,2,3,6-tetrahydropyridine-induced parkinsonism in the vervet monkey (Cercopithecus aethiops sabaeus). Neuroscience 1997; 81:745–755.
45. Petzinger GM, Langston JW. The MPTP-lesioned non-human primate: A model for Parkinson's disease. In: J Marwah, H Teitelbbaum, eds. Advances in Neurodegenerative Disease. Vol. I: Parkinson's Disease. Scottsdale, AZ: Prominent Press 1998:113–148.
46. Rose S, Nomoto M, Jackson EA, Gibb WRG, Jaehnig P, Jenner P, Marsden CD. Age-related effects of 1-methyl-4-phenyl-1,2,3,6-tetrahydropyridine treatment of common marmosets. Eur J Pharm 1993; 230:177–185.
47. Gerlach M, Reiderer P Animal models of Parkinson's disease: an empirical comparison with the phenomenology of the disease in man. J Neural Transm 1996; 103:987–1041.
48. Ovadia A, Zhang, Gash DM. Increased susceptibility to MPTP toxicity in middle-aged rhesus monkeys. Neurobiol Aging 1995; 16:931–937.

49. Bezard E, Gross C. Compensatory mechanisms in experimental and human parkinsonism: towards a dynamic approach. Prog Neurobiol 1998; 55:96–116.

50. Tetrud JW, Langston JW. MPTP-induced parkinsonism as a model for parkinson's disease. Acta Neurol Scand 1989; 126:35–40.

51. Elsworth JD, Deutch AY, Redmond DE, Sladek JR, Roth RH. MPTP-induced parkinsonism: relative changes in dopamine concentration in subregions of substantia nigra, ventral tegmental area and retrorubal field of symptomatic and asymptomatic vervet monkeys. Brain Res 1990; 513:320–324.

52. Waters CM, Hunt SP, Jenner P, Marsden CD. An immunohistochemical study of the acute and long-term effects of 1-methyl-4-phenyl-1,2,3,6-tetrahydropyridine in the marmoset. Neuroscience 1987; 23:1025–1039.

53. Eidelberg E, Brooks BA, Morgan WW, Walden JG, Kokemoor RH. Variability and functional recovery in the N-methyl-4-phenyl-1,2,3,6-tetrahydropyridine model of parkinsonism in monkeys. Neuroscience 1986; 18:817–822.

54. Bankiewicz KS, Oldfield EH, Chiueh CC, Markey SP, Burns RS, Johannessen JN, Pert A, Kopin IJ, Doppman JL, Jacobowitz DM, Kopin IJ. Hemiparkinsonism in monkeys after unilateral internal carotid infusion of 1-methyl-4-phenyl-1,2,3,6-tetrahydropyridine. Life Sci 1986; 39:7–16.

55. Smith R, Zhang Z, Kurlan R, McDermott M, Gash D. Developing a stable bilateral model of parkinsonism in rhesus monkeys. Neuroscience 1993; 52.7–16.

56. Eberling JL, Jagust WJ, Taylor S, Bringas J, Pivirotto P, VanBrocklin HF, Bankiewicz KS. A novel MPTP primate model of Parkinson's disease: neurochemical and clinical changes. Brain Res 1998; 805:259–262.

57. Bezard E, Imbert C, Deloire X, Bioulac B, Gross CE. A chronic MPTP model reproducing the slow evolution of Parkinson's disease: evolution of motor symptoms in the monkey. Brain Res 1997; 766:107–112.

58. Bezard E, Brotchie JM, Gross CE. Pathophysiology of levodopa-induced dyskinesia: potential for new therapies. Nat Rev Neurosci 2001; 2:577–588.

59. Hurley MJ, Mash DC, Jenner P. Dopamine D(1) receptor expression in human basal ganglia and changes in Parkinson's disease. Brain Res Mol Brain Res 2001; 87:271–279.

60. Papa SM, Chase TN. Levodopa-induced dyskinesias improved by a glutamate antagonist in parkinsonian monkeys. Ann Neurol 1996; 39:574–578.

61. Bedard PJ, Mancilla BG, Blanchette P, Gagnon C, Di Paolo T. Levodopa-induced dyskinesia: facts and fancy. What does the MPTP monkey model tell us? Can J Neurol Sci 1992; 19:134–137.

62. Calon F, Morissette M, Ghribi O, Goulet M, Grondin R, Blanchet PJ, Bedard PJ, Di Paola T. Alteration of glutamate receptors in the striatum of dyskinetic 1-methyl-4-phenyl-1,2,3,6-tetrahydropyridine-treated monkeys following dopamine agonist treatment. Prog Neuropsychopharm Biol Psych 2002; 26:127–138.

63. Pearce RK, Heikkila M, Linden IB, Jenner P. L-Dopa induces dyskinesia in normal monkeys: behavioral and pharmacokinetic observations. Psychopharmacology (Berl) 2001; 156:402–409.

64. Ricaurte GA, Schuster CR, Seiden LS. Long-term effects of repeated methylamphetamine administration on dopamine and serotonin neurons in the rat brain: a regional study. Brain Res 1980; 193:153–63.

65. Ricaurte GA, Guillery RW, Seiden LS, Schuster CR, Moore RY. Dopamine nerve terminal degeneration produced by high doses of methylamphetamine in the rat brain. Brain Res 1982; 235:93–103.

66. Kim BG, Shin DH, Jeon GS, Seo JH, Kim YW, Jeon BS, Cho SS. Relative sparing of calretinin containing neurons in the substantia nigra of 6-OHDA treated rat parkinsonian model. Brain Res 2000; 855:162–165.

67. Sonsalla PK, Jochnowitz ND, Zeevalk GD, Oostveen JA, HE D. Treatment of mice with methamphetamine produces cell loss in the substantia nigra. Brain Res 1996; 738:172–175.

68. Harvey DC, Lacan G, Melega WP. Regional heterogeneity of dopaminergic deficits in vervet monkey striatum and substantia nigra after methamphetamine exposure. Exp Brain Res 2000; 133:349–358.

69. Walsh SL, Wagner GC. Motor impairments after methamphetamine-induced neurotoxicity in the rat. J Pharmacol Exp Ther 1992; 263:617–626.

70. Westphale RI, Stadlin A. Dopamine uptake blockers nullify methamphetamine-induced decrease in dopamine uptake and plasma membrane potential in rat striatal synaptosomes. Ann NY Acad Sci 2000; 914:187–193.

71. Fumagalli F, Gainetdinov RR, Valenzano, Caron MG. Role of dopamine transporter in methamphetamine-induced neurotoxicity: evidence from mice lacking the transporter. J Neurosci 1998; 18:4861–4869.

72. Cubells JF, Rayport S, Rajendran G, Sulzer D. Methamphetamine neurotoxicity involves vacuolation of endocytic organelles and dopamine-dependent intracellular oxidative stress. J Neurosci 1994; 14:2260–2271.

73. Gluck MR, Moy LY, Jayatilleke E, Hogan KA, Manzino L, Sonsalla PK. Parallel increases in lipid and protein oxidative markers in several mouse brain regions after methamphetamine treatment. J Neurochem 2001; 79:152–160.

74. Yamamoto BK, Zhu W. The effects of methamphetamine on the production of free radicals and oxidative stress. J Pharmacol Exp Ther 1998; 287:107–114.

75. Imam SZ, el-Yazal J, Newport GD, Itzhak Y, Cadet JL, Slikker WJ, Ali SF. Methamphetamine-induced dopaminergic neurotoxicity: role of peroxynitrite and neuroprotective role of antioxidants and peroxynitrite decomposition catalysts. Annals NY Acad Sci 2001; 939:366–380.

76. Davidson C, Gow AJ, Lee TH, Ellinwood EH. Methamphetamine neurotoxicity: necrotic and apoptotic mechanisms and relevance to human abuse and treatment. Brain Res Brain Res Rev 2001; 36:1–22.

77. Cadet JL, Ladenheim B, Baum I, Carlson E, Epstein C. CuZn-superoxide dismutase (CuZnSOD) transgenic mice show resistance to the lethal effects of methylenedioxyamphetamine (MDA) and of methylenedioxymethamphetamine (MDMA). Brain Res 1994; 655:259–262.

78. Hirata H, Ladenheim B, Carlson E, Epstein C, Cadet JL. Autoradiographic evidence for methamphetamine-induced striatal dopaminergic loss in mouse brain: attenuation in CuZn- superoxide dismutase transgenic mice. Brain Res 1996; 714:95–103.

79. Sonsalla PK, Riordan DE, Heikkila RE. Competitive and noncompetitive antagonists at N-methyl-D-asparate receptors protect against methamphetamine-induced dopaminergic damage in mice. J Pharm Exp Therap 1991; 256:506–512.

80. Frost DO, Cadet JL. Effects of methamphetamine-induced neurotoxicity on the development of neural circuitry: a hypothesis. Brain Res Brain Res Rev 2000; 34:103–118.

81. McCann UD, Wong DF, Yokoi F, Villemagne V, Dannals RF, Ricaurte GA. Reduced striatal dopamine transporter density in abstinent methamphetamine and methcathinone users: evidence from positron emission tomography studies with [11C]WIN-35,428. J Neurosci 1998; 18:8417–8422.

82. Paulus MP, Hozack NE, Zauscher BE, Frank L, Brown GG, Braff DL, Schuckit MA. Behavioral and functional neuroimaging evidence for prefrontal dysfunction in methamphetamine-dependent subjects. Neuropsychopharmacology 2002; 26:53–65.

83. Guilarte TR. Is methamphetamine abuse a risk factor in parkinsonism? Neurotoxicology 2001; 22:725–731.

84. Tanner CM, Ottman R, Goldman SM, Ellenberg J, Chan P, Mayeux R, Langston JW. Parkinson disease in twins: an etiologic study. JAMA 1999; 281:341–346.

85. Betarbet R, Sherer TB, MacKenzie G, Garcia-Osuna M, Panov AV, Greenamyre JT. Chronic systemic pesticide exposure reproduces features of Parkinson's disease. Nat Neurosci 2000; 3:1301–1306.

86. Thiruchelvam M, Richfield EK, Baggs RB, Tank AW, Cory-Slechta DA. The nigrostriatal dopaminergic system as a preferential target of repeated exposures to combined paraquat and maneb: implications for Parkinson's disease. J Neurosci 2000; 20:9207–9214.

87. Heintz N, Zoghbi HY. Insights from mouse models into the molecular basis of neurodegeneration. Ann Rev Physiol 2000; 62:779–802.

88. Payne AP, Campbell JM, Russell D, Favor G, Sutcliffe RG, Bennett NK, Davies RW, Stone TW. The AS/AGU rat: a spontaneous model of disruption and degeneration in the nigrostriatal dopaminergic system. J Anat 2000; 196:629–633.

89. Richter A, Ebert U, Nobrega JN, Vallbacka JJ, Fedrowitz M, Loscher W. Immunohistochemical and neurochemical studies on nigral and striatal functions in the circling (ci) rat, a genetic animal model with spontaneous rotational behavior. Neuroscience 1999; 89:461–471.

90. Kitada T, Asakawa S, Hattori N, Matsumine H, Yamamura Y, Minoshima S, Yokochi M, Mizuno Y, Shimizu N. Mutations in the parkin gene cause autosomal recessive juvenile parkinsonism. Nature 1998; 392:605–608.

91. Hattori N, Kitada T, Matsumine H, Asakawa S, Yamamura Y, Yoshino H, Kobayashi T, Yokochi M, Wang M, Yoritaka A, Kondo T, Kuzuhara S, Nakamura S, Shimizu N, Mizuno Y. Molecular genetic analysis of a novel Parkin gene in Japanese families with autosomal recessive juvenile parkinsonism: evidence for variable homozygous deletions in the Parkin gene in affected individuals. Ann Neurol 1998; 44:935–941.

92. Fallon L, Moreau F, Croft BG, Labib N, Gu WJ, Fon EA. Parkin and CASK/LIN-2 associate via a PDZ-mediated interaction and are co-localized in lipid rafts and postsynaptic densities in brain. J Biol Chem 2002; 277:486–491.

93. Huynh DP, Dy M, Nguyen D, Kiehl TR, Pulst SM. Differential expression and tissue distribution of parkin isoforms during mouse development. Brain Res Dev Brain Res 2001; 130:173–181.

94. Solano SM, Miller DW, Augood SJ, Young AB, Penney JBJ. Expression of alpha-synuclein, parkin, and ubiquitin carboxy-terminal hydrolase L1 mRNA in human brain: genes associated with familial Parkinson's disease. Ann Neurol 2000; 47:201–210.

95. Shimura H, Schlossmacher MG, Hattori N, Frosch MP, Trockenbacher A, Schneider R, Mizuno Y, Kosik KS, Selkoe DJ. Ubiquitination of a new form of {alpha}-synuclein by parkin from human brain: Implications for Parkinson's disease. Science 2001; 293:263–269.

96. Tanaka K, Suzuki T, Chiba T, Shimura H, Hattori N, Mizuno Y. Parkin is linked to the ubiquitin pathway. J Mol Med 2001; 79:482–494.

97. Polymeropoulos M, Lavendan C, Leroy E, Ide S, Dehejia A, Dutra A, Pike B, Root H, Rubenstein J, Boyer R, Stenroos E, Chandrasekharappa S, Athanassiasdou A, Papapetropoulos T, Johnson W, Lazzarini A, Duvoisin R, Di Iorio G, Golbe L, Nussbaum R. Mutation in the α-synuclein gene identified in families with Parkinson's disease. Science 1997; 276:2045–2047.

98. George JM, Jin H, Woods WS, Clayton DF. Characterization of a novel protein regulated during the critical period for song learning in the zebra finch. Neuron 1995; 15:361–372.

99. Jakowec MW, Donaldson DM, Barba J, Petzinger GM. The postnatal expression of α-synuclein in the substantia nigra and striatum of the rodent. Dev Neurosci 2001; 23:91–99.

100. Abeliovich A, Schmitz Y, Farinas I, Choi- Lundberg D, Ho WH, Castillo PE, Shinsky N, Verdugo JM, Armanini M, Ryan A, Hynes M, Phillips H, Sulzer D, Rosenthal A. Mice lacking alpha-synuclein display functional deficits in the nigrostriatal dopamine system. Neuron 2000; 25:239–252.

101. Masliah E, Rockenstein E, Veinbergs I, Mallory M, Hashimoto M, Takeda A, Sagara Y, Sisk A, Mucke L. Dopaminergic loss and inclusion body formation in alpha-synuclein mice: implications for neurodegenerative disorders. Science 2000; 289:1265–1269.

102. Kahle PJ, Neumann M, Ozmen L, Muller V, Jacobsen H, Schindzielorz A, Okochi M, Leimer U, van Der Putten H, Probst A, Kremmer E, Kretzschmar HA, Haass C. Subcellular localization of wild-type and Parkinson's disease-

associated mutant alpha -synuclein in human and transgenic mouse brain. J Neurosci 2000; 20:6365–6373.

103. Nass R, Hall DH, Miller DMr, Blakely RD. Neurotoxin-induced degeneration of dopamine neurons in Caenorhabditis elegans. Proc Natl Acad Sci USA 2002; 99:3264–3269.

104. Feany MB, Bender WW. A Drosophila model of Parkinson's disease. Nature 2000; 404:394–398.

105. Pendleton G, Parvez F, Sayed M, Hillman R. Effects of pharmacological agents upon a transgenic model of Parkinson's disease in Drosophila melanogaster. J Pharmacol Exp Ther 2002; 300:91–96.

106. Ghorayeb I, Puschban Z, Fernagut PO, Scherfler C, Rouland R, Wenning GK, Tison F. Simultaneous intrastriatal 6-hydroxydopamine and quinolinic acid injection: a model of early-stage striatonigral degeneration. Exp Neurol 2001; 167:133–147.

107. Wenning GK, Granata R, Puschban Z, Scherfler C, Poewe W. Neural transplantation in animal models of multiple system atrophy: a review. J Neural Transm 1999; (suppl 55):103–113.

108. Scherfler C, Puschban Z, Ghorayeb I, Goebel GP, Tison F, Jellinger K, Poewe W, Wenning GK. Complex motor disturbances in a sequential double lesion rat model of striatonigral degeneration (multiple system atrophy). Neuroscience 2000; 99:42–54.

109. Ghorayeb I, Fernagut PO, Aubert I, Bezard E, Poewe W, Wenning GK, Tison F. Toward a primate model of L-dopa-unresponsive parkinsonism mimicking striatonigral degeneration. Mov Disord 2000; 15:531–536.

110. Barbieri S, Hofele K, Wiederhold KH, Probst A, Mistl C, Danner S, Kauffmann S, Sommer B, Spooren W, Tolnay M, Bilbe G, van der Putten H. Mouse models of alpha-synucleinopathy and Lewy pathology. Alpha-synuclein expression in transgenic mice. Adv Exp Med Biol 2001; 487:147–167.

111. Ishihara T, Hong M, Zhang B, Nakagawa Y, Lee MK, Trojanowski JQ, Lee VM. Age-dependent emergence and progression of a tauopathy in transgenic mice overexpressing the shortest human tau isoform. Neuron 1999; 24:751–762.

112. Wittmann CW, Wszolek MF, Shulman JM, Salvaterra PM, Lewis J, Hutton M, Feany MB. Tauopathy in Drosophila: neurodegeneration without neurofibrillary tangles. Science 2001; 293:711–714.

13

Dopamine Receptor Diversity: Anatomy, Function, and Relevance to Parkinson's Disease

Deborah C. Mash
University of Miami School of Medicine, Miami, Florida, U.S.A.

INTRODUCTION

The importance of dopamine in the motor functions of the striatum is evident in Parkinson's disease (PD). The striatum controls motor activity by processing the flow of information arising from the cerebral cortex and projecting via direct and indirect pathways to the output nuclei of the basal ganglia. The degenerative loss of dopamine is a hallmark of this disease and leads to severe motor impairments that are relieved by dopamine agonists. However, dopamine plays a role not only in the execution of complex movement, but also in higher-order cognitive processes, including motor planning and sequencing, motor learning, and motivational drive and affect. Of the biogenic amine neurotransmitters, dopamine has been the best studied in the central nervous system (CNS). The actions of dopamine are segregated in different neural circuits. For example, dopamine in the nigrostriatal pathway is involved in the generation and execution of voluntary movement. In this function, dopamine is a prime modulator of various other basal ganglia neurotransmitters, including gamma-aminobu-tyric acid (GABA), acetylcholine, glutamate, enkephalin, and substance P. Dopamine in the mesolimbic pathway plays a role in the control of various cognitive functions, including drive, reinforcement, attention, and in the addiction to psychostimulants.

Five different receptor subtypes that are members of the large G-protein–coupled receptor superfamily mediate the central effects of dopamine. Dopamine receptors are divided into two major subclasses, D1-like and D2-like receptors, which differ in their second messenger transduction systems and anatomical locations. The cloning of these receptors and their genes in the last decade has led to the identification of multiple dopamine receptor subtypes termed D1, D2, D3, D4, and D5. The D1 and D5 subtypes of dopamine receptors exhibit overlapping functional and pharmacological properties that are related to the D1 receptor (D1-like), whereas the remaining members of this receptor family share pharmacological characteristics that are similar to the D2 receptor subtype (D2-like). The two receptor families have overlapping but distinct neuroanatomical distributions as determined by radioligand binding autoradiography and immunocytochemical localization. Thus, the various functions of dopaminergic neurotransmission appear to be mediated by the regional expression of these different receptor subtypes.

The molecular cloning of dopamine receptor subtype genes and the identification of their different locations in the brain and distinct pharmacology has advanced medication development for the treatment of PD and serious mental illnesses. The focus on dopaminergic neurotransmission as a target for medication development is due largely to the recognition that alterations in dopamine function are involved in neurodegenerative and psychiatric brain disorders. Degeneration of the nigral dopamine-containing neurons contributes to the pathogenesis of PD (1). The antiparkinson effects of the indirect dopamine agonist levodopa and other direct-acting agonists are mediated by dopamine receptors localized to striatal neurons (for review, see Ref. 2). The chorea of Huntington's disease is due to a deterioration of the dopaminoceptive cells localized to the striatum. Schizophrenia and other psychotic disorders are thought to be due to an imbalance in corticolimbic dopamine signaling. Dopamine receptor antagonists are used for the clinical management of these disorders (3–5). Chronic dopamine receptor blockade leads to a dysregulation of central dopaminergic tone and the development of extrapyramidal syndromes, while involuntary movements and psychosis are observed with chronic administration of the indirect-acting agonist levodopa in PD (2). Antipsychotic medications act through the D2-like family of receptors. Although none of the dopamine receptor subtypes have been linked to the etiology of schizophrenia, the distinct regional locations of D3 and D4 receptors in cerebral cortical and associated subcortical limbic brain areas suggest that subtype-selective neuroleptics that lack extrapyramidal side effects may be developed. The advent of new subtype-selective dopamine receptor agonists may provide neuroprotective effects in PD and modify symptom progression (for review, see Ref. 6).

MOLECULAR SUBTYPES OF DOPAMINE RECEPTORS

The molecular cloning and characterization of dopamine receptor heterogeneity was advanced by the early recognition that G-protein–coupled receptors are evolutionarily related (for review, see Ref. 7). The existence of a G-protein–coupled receptor supergene was proposed based on the reported sequences for rhodopsin and beta$_2$-adrenergic receptors (7). Both of these receptors have a membrane typology of seven highly conserved transmembrane domains of amino acid residues. Several structural features are common to all biogenic amine receptors. These include the specific aspartate and serine residues that interact with the neurotransmitter, sites for N-linked glycosylation located on putative extracellular regions, and consensus sites for phosphorylation by protein kinase A or C found on putative intracellular domains. These similarities suggested that all G-protein–coupled receptors had similar structural characteristics, a hypothesis that was immediately strengthened by the cloning and sequencing of the m2 muscarinic receptor (8). The identification of primary shared sequence homologies among G-protein–coupled receptors advanced the development of technical approaches for, first, the cloning of the D2 receptor (9) and, then, the D1 receptor (10,11) subtypes.

The complementary deoxyribonucleic acid (cDNA) for the D2 receptor was first isolated in 1988 (9), and subsequently alternative splice variants were identified (12,13). The cDNA encodes a protein of 415 amino acids, with three glycosylation sites in the N-terminus, a large third intracellular loop between transmembrane regions 5 and 6, and a short C-terminus. The D3 receptor was isolated by screening rat libraries with the known D2 sequence followed by polymerase chain reaction (PCR) extension (14). The topography of the D3 receptor includes a glycoprotein of 400 amino acids with a glycosylation site in the N-terminus and a short C-terminus. The D4 receptor was cloned by screening a library from the human neuroblastoma cell line SK-N-MC (15). The D4 glycoprotein is 387 amino acid residues in length with the characteristic seven transmembrane spanning domains, a large third intracellular loop, and a short C-terminus. The dopamine D1 (or D1$_a$) receptor was independently cloned by four separate groups of investigators (10,11,16,17). The isolation of cDNAs or genes from rat or human DNA libraries was done by homology screening with a D2 receptor probe and by polymerase chain reaction with degenerate primers. Both the rat and human D1 receptor genes encode a protein that is 91% homologous for amino acid sequence. The second member of the D1-like receptor family, D5 was isolated using the sequence of the D1 receptor (18). The coding region for the carboxy terminal of the protein is about seven times longer for D1-like than for the D2-like receptors (19,20). The cloned D1 and D5 receptors are 446 residues in length and exhibit 91% amino acid sequence homology within the highly conserved seven transmembrane spanning regions.

The gene structure of D2 receptors demonstrated that the coding region contains six introns, the D3 receptor contains five introns, and the D4 has three introns (19,20). The presence of introns within the coding region of the D2 receptor family allows generation of splice variants of the receptor. For example, alternative splicing of the D2 receptor at the exon between introns 4 and 5 results in functional D2S (short) and D2L (long) isoforms (13). Putative nonfunctional proteins encoded by alternative splice variants of the D3 receptor also have been demonstrated (22–24). The human D4 receptor gene, located on the short arm of chromosome 11, has eight different polymorphic variants. The existence of polymorphic variations within the coding sequence of the D4 receptor demonstrated a 48-base-pair sequence in the third cytoplasmic loop that exists with multiple repeated sequences (25). The number of repeated sequences is related to ethnicity, with most humans (70%) having four repeats. Nonfunctional, truncated isoforms of the D5 receptor have been reported on human chromosomes 1 and 2 (20,25,26).

NEUROANATOMICAL LOCALIZATION OF DOPAMINE
RECEPTOR PROTEIN AND MESSAGE

The dopaminergic systems in the brain comprise three distinct pathways, including the nigrostriatal, mesocortical, and mesolimbic projections (27). The nigrostriatal pathway originates in the ventral tier of neurons of the substantia nigra pars compacta and terminates in the striatum. The mesolimbic pathway originates in the ventral tegmental area (VTA) and paranigral area and projects to the limbic sectors of the striatum, amygdala, and olfactory tubercle. The mesocortical pathway originates in the VTA and terminates within particular sectors of the cerebral cortical mantle, including the prefrontal, orbitofrontal cingulate, and entorhinal cortices.

D1-like and D2-like receptors and message are abundant in the CNS, having a widespread distribution across the three dopaminergic projection systems. The anatomical localization of D1 receptors correlates with dopamine-stimulated adenylyl cyclase and radioligand-binding activities.

High densities of radioligand-binding sites are found within the caudate, putamen, and nucleus accumbens with lower levels in the thalamus and cerebral cortex (Fig. 1). D1 receptor messenger ribonucleic acid (mRNA) is localized to medium-sized neurons of the striatonigral projection that also express substance P (28). D5 mRNA is distributed in a more restricted pattern than D1 mRNA with the highest expression seen in limbic and cerebral cortical brain areas (29). Very low levels of D5 mRNA are found within the rat and human striatum.

Radioligand binding and mRNA studies have demonstrated a good correlation for the D2-like receptors. D2 receptors and message are found in the striatum and substantia nigra of the rat and human brain (Fig. 1). D2 receptors are expressed by medium spiny neurons containing enkephalin that project to the external segment of the globus pallidus (28). The globus pallidus is a major efferent projection system of the striatum that has high densities of D2 receptors (29). However, neurons expressing D2 receptor mRNA are lower in the globus pallidus than in the caudate and putamen, suggesting that most of the D2 protein is located on projections extrinsic to this structure. D2 receptor mRNA is co-localized with enkephalin expression cells in many brain areas, including the periaquaductal grey, suggesting a role for these sites in the modulation of analgesia.

The D3 dopamine receptor is highly expressed in limbic brain and has low expression in motor divisions of the striatum (6,30). In vitro receptor autoradiography demonstrates that D3 receptors in the human brain have a distinct localization pattern that is less dense than either D1 or D2 binding sites (Fig. 1). The highest densities of D3 receptors are seen over subcortical limbic brain regions. Low levels of D3 binding sites are seen over the ventromedial (limbic) sectors of the striatum. The highest levels of D3 message expression are found within the telencephalic areas receiving mesocortical dopaminergic inputs, including the islands of Calleja, bed nucleus of the stria terminalis, hippocampus, and hypothalamus. In the cerebellum, Purkinje cells lobules IX and X express abundant D3 mRNA, whereas binding sites are only found in the molecular layer (30,31). Since no known dopaminergic projections are known to exist in this area, it has been suggested that the D3 receptor may mediate the nonsynaptic (paracrine) actions of dopamine (31). D4 receptor message is localized to dopamine cell body fields of the substantia nigra and VTA. This pattern suggests that the D4 receptor protein may function as a presynaptic autoreceptor in dendrites and/or presynaptic terminals (32). The highest areas of D4 expression are found in the frontal cortex, amygdala, and brainstem areas. The very low levels of D4 receptor message in the terminal fields of the striatum are in keeping with the lack of extrapyramidal side effects observed following treatment with putative D4 selective atypical neuroleptics.

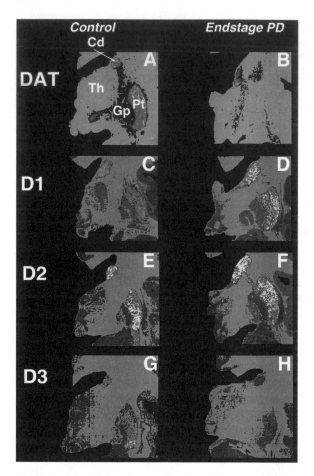

FIGURE 1   Autoradiographic localization of the distribution of D1, D2, and D3 receptors in representative coronal half-hemisphere sections of the human brain. Brain autoradiograms are shown in pseudocolor codes corresponding to a rainbow scale (red = high densities; green = intermediate densities; purple = low densities) for a control subject (male, age 72 yrs) and a patient with Parkinson's disease (male, age 67 yrs). The dopamine transporter was labeled with [3H]WIN 35, 428 (panels A and E) and shows the severity of the loss of dopamine terminals in end-stage Parkinson's disease. Panels B and F illustrate the distribution of D1 receptors with 1 nM [^{3}H]SCH 23390 in the presence of 10 nM mianserin to occlude labeling of the 5-HT$_2$ receptor. Panels C and G show the distribution of D2 receptors labeled with 2 nM [^{3}H] raclopride. Panels D and H illustrate the distribution of D3 receptors labeled with [^{3}H]7OH DPAT. Panels C and F show the distribution of D3 receptors labeled with [3H]7OH-DPAT (for method see Ref. 68). Cd, caudate; Gp, globus pallidus; Pt, putamen; Th, thalamus. (See color insert.)

Previous studies have suggested that D1-like and D2-like receptors may be colocalized in a subpopulation of the same neostriatal cells (33). This hypothesis has been questioned by recent data from Gerfen and coworkers (34), which demonstrated that the interactions may occur at an intercellular level as opposed to an intracellular second messenger integration. This latter hypothesis suggests that the D1-like and D2-like receptor proteins are on distinct populations of neurons with extensive axon collateral systems subserving the integration across neural subfields. However, there is considerable evidence from anatomical and electrophysiological studies that direct cointegration may occur at the single cell level (32,33). This anatomical arrangement would afford D1-mediated cooperative/synergistic control of D2-mediated motor activity and other psychomotor behaviors. Most studies have demonstrated opposing roles of D1 and D2 receptor–mediated actions in the striatum resulting from the stimulation and inhibition of adenylyl cyclase, respectively (35). While more studies are needed to clarify the precise nature and extent of these functional interactions on cyclic adenosine monophosphate (cAMP) second messenger systems, species-specific differences may limit the extrapolation of rodent studies to monkeys and humans (36).

Isolated activation of D1 and D2 dopamine receptors produces short-term effects on striatal neurons, whereas the combined stimulation of dopamine and glutamate receptors produces long-lasting modification in synaptic excitability (37). Dopamine terminals arising from the substantia nigra constitute, along with corticostriatal afferents containing glutamate, the majority of axon terminals in the striatum. Morphological studies have demonstrated close proximity of glutamatergic and dopaminergic synaptic boutons contacting dendritic spines of striatal spiny neurons (for review, see Ref. 38). Repetitive stimulation of both glutamate and dopamine receptors produces either long-term depression (LTD) or long-term potentiation (LTP) of excitatory synaptic transmission (37). Corticostriatal synaptic plasticity is severely impaired following dopaminergic denervation. The physiological and pharmacological features of corticostriatal transmission as an excitatory drive to striatal cells is important for understanding development of dyskinesias and treatment-related fluctuations in PD. D1 receptor occupation by dopamine stimulates adenylyl cyclase activity and augments the direct striatal output pathway, while D2 receptors inhibit adenylyl cyclase and inhibit neurons projecting from the external segment of the globus pallidus forming the first neuron in the indirect pathway. Pathological inhibition of striatal output neurons may be due to repetitive D1 receptor stimulation and functional uncoupling of D1 and D2 receptor subtypes from their respective second messenger pathways (39).

SECOND MESSENGER PATHWAYS

Dopamine receptors transduce the effects of agonists by coupling to specific heterotrimeric guanosine triphosphate (GTP) binding proteins (i.e., G-proteins) consisting of alpha, beta, and gamma subunits (for review, see Ref. 40). Within the dopamine receptor family, the adenylyl cyclase stimulatory receptors include the D1 and D5 subtypes. Although the D1 and D5 share sequence homology that is greater than 80%, the receptors display 50% overall homology at the amino acid level (41). D5 receptors have been suggested to have higher affinity toward dopamine and lower affinity for the antagonist (+) butaclamol. However, when the D1 and D5 subtypes are expressed in transfected cell lines derived from the rat pituitary, both D1 and D5 receptors stimulate adenylyl cyclase and have identical affinities for agonists and antagonists (for review, see Ref. 42). Studies done in transfected cell lines are complicated by the fact that transection systems may not express the relevant complement of G-proteins as in the native tissue environment. In the primate brain, there is an overlap in the regional brain expression of D1 and D5 receptors. Thus, because of the identical affinities of D1 and D5 receptors for agonists and antagonists and the lack of subtype selective drugs that fully discriminate between these receptor subtypes, it is not yet possible to assign with certainty specific functions to D1 vs. D5 receptor activation.

Although G-protein–coupled receptors were initially believed to selectively activate a single effector, they are now known to have an intrinsic ability to generate multiple signals through an interaction with different α subunits (43). D1 and D5 receptors have been shown by a variety of methodologies to couple to the Gsα subunit of G-proteins. The Gsα subunit has been linked to the regulation of Na^+, Ca^+, and K^+ channels, suggesting that D1 receptor activation affects the functional activity of these ion channels. To complicate this picture, D1 receptors inactivate a slow K^+ current in the resting state of medium spiny neurons in the striatum (44) through an activation of Goα in the absence of D1 receptor Gsα coupling (42,45). These studies provide evidence for the involvement of this G-protein subunit in the D1-mediated regulation of diverse ion channels.

The ability of the D5 receptor to stimulate adenylyl cyclase predicts that this subtype couples to Gsα. D5 receptors inhibit catecholamine secretion in bovine chromaffin cells (46). The negligible dopamine stimulation of adenylyl cyclase demonstrated in these cells suggests the possibility that this activity of the D5 receptor is mediated by a different G-protein. Recent studies have demonstrated that the D5 receptor can couple to a novel G-protein termed Gzα (47), which is abundantly expressed in neurons. Thus, despite similar pharmacological properties, differential coupling of D1 and D5 receptors to distinct G-proteins can transduce varied signaling responses by dopamine stimulation. However, since the precise function of $Gz\alpha$ has not been established, the molecular implications of D5/$Gz\alpha$ coupling is not yet known. For example, $Gz\alpha$ has been shown to inhibit adenylyl cyclase activity in certain cell types (48). Even though it is unclear which signaling pathways are linked to D_5/$Gz\alpha$ coupling, the co-localization of D5, $Gz\alpha$, and specific cyclase subtypes may provide a clue to the physiological relevance. For example, $Gz\alpha$ inhibits adenylyl cyclase type I and V (48). Both type V cyclase and D1 receptors are expressed in very high amounts in striatum, which has rich dopaminergic input (49). D1 receptor activation in the striatum is known to stimulate the activity of adenylyl cyclase type V (50). In contrast, the hippocampus is rich in D5 but not in D1 receptors, and type I cyclase is abundantly expressed in this brain region (51). Taken together, these studies suggest the functional relevance of co-localization of specific cyclases with a particular member of the D1-like receptor family.

D2, D3, and D4 receptors have introns in their coding region and exist in various forms by alternate splicing in the region of the third cytoplasmic loop. These receptors produce rapid physiological actions by two major mechanisms, involving either the activation of inward K^+ channels or the inhibition of voltage-dependent Ca^+ channels, or involving activation of Gi/Go proteins to inhibit adenylyl cyclase activity (20). D2 and D4 receptors inhibit adenylyl cyclase by coupling to inhibitory G-proteins of the Gi/Go family (20,21), whereas D3 receptors demonstrate weak inhibition of adenylyl cyclase activity (52). This weak effect on inhibiting cAMP production led to the conclusion that the D3 receptor does not couple to G-proteins (21,52). Both isoforms of the D2 receptor inhibit adenylyl cyclase activity, although the short isoform requires lower concentrations of agonist to cause half maximal inhibition than the long isoform expressed in transfected cell lines (53,54). The short D2 receptor isoform couples to K^+ currents via a pertussis-toxin–insensitive mechanism (55), whereas the long isoform couples to the same current via a pertussis-toxin–sensitive mechanism (56). Thus, D2 receptors, if expressed by the same cells, can influence transmembrane currents in similar ways, but through independent transduction pathways. D2-like receptors that couple to G-proteins modulate a variety of other second messenger pathways, including ion channels, Ca^+ levels, K^+ currents, arachidonic acid release, phosphoinositide hydrolysis, and cell growth and differentiation (for review, see Ref. 57).

PHARMACOLOGICAL SELECTIVITY

Central dopamine systems have properties that make them unique in comparison to other neurotransmitter systems. For example, dopaminergic projections are mainly associated with diffuse neural pathways. This anatomical arrangement argues for dopamine to act as a neuromodulatory molecule in addition to its role as a neurotransmitter in brain. Dopamine neurons are highly branched with elongated axons capable of releasing neurotransmitters from many points along their terminal networks en route to the striatum (58,59). This mode of volumetric transmission of action potentials suggests that dopamine release mediates paracrine (i.e., neuro-humoral) signals across the network. This view is supported by the observation that dopamine is released by axon terminals and dendrites, providing a double polarity for regulating basal ganglia function, simultaneously gating signaling at nigral, striatal, and pallidal levels. These properties have important implications in the clinical expression of human disorders involving dopamine neuron dysfunction.

The members of the D1 receptor subfamily have several characteristics that distinguish them from the D2 subfamily. All members of the D1 subfamily bind benzazepines with high affinity and bind butyrophenones and benzamides with low affinity (12). Subtypes in the D1 family have approximately 50% homology overall and 80% homology in the highly conserved transmembrane region. All of the receptors in this family have short third intracellular loops and a long carboxy terminus. These regions are important for the generation of second messenger signals as explained above. D5 and the rat D1b are species homologs because they map to the same chromosomal locus (26). D5 and D1b have a 10-fold higher affinity for dopamine, suggesting that D5 receptors are activated at neurotransmitter concentrations that are subthreshold for the D1 receptor (21). The D2-like receptors bind butyrophenones and benzamides with high affinity and bind benzazepines with low affinity (10,15,16).

The pharmacological distinction of dopamine receptor subtypes holds tremendous potential for treatment of nervous system dysfunction. Dopamine receptors are the primary targets for the pharmacological treatment of PD, schizophrenia, and several other nervous system disorders. Presently used drugs have significant limitations that are in part due to their nonselective binding to many receptor subtypes. For example, drug-related side effects, including dyskinesias and delirium, are frequent and important problems in parkinsonian patients receiving levodopa or dopamine agonist therapy. These adverse effects result from stimulation of dopamine receptors in motor and cognitive circuits, respectively (21). Conversely, treatment of schizophrenia with dopaminergic antagonists, although intended to selectively block receptors in cortical and limbic circuits, may induce parkinsonian symptoms or even tardive dyskinesias by interaction with dopamine receptor subtypes in motor pathways. Clearly, drugs aimed at molecular subtypes of dopamine receptors offer the potential for specific therapeutic interventions for motor and psychiatric disorders of the nervous system.

Although there are agonists and antagonists that are highly selective and that can discriminate between D1-like and D2-like receptor subfamilies, there are few agents that are highly selective for the individual receptor subtypes (Table 1). Some progress has been made in the development of antagonists for the D2 receptor family. For the D1/D5 receptor subtypes, there are currently no compounds that exhibit high selectivity. Thus, the high overall sequence homology between dopamine receptors of the same subfamily have made it difficult to develop specific ligands that do not interact with related receptors. The high affinity of the "atypical" neuroleptic, clozapine, for D4 receptors and the low level of D4 receptor expression in the striatum and high levels in the cerebral cortex and certain limbic brain areas led to the suggestion that the antipsychotic properties of the neuroleptics may be mediated through blockade of D4 receptors, whereas the side effects may be mediated through blockade of D2 receptors (15,60). This hypothesis was strengthened by the low incidence of extrapyramidal side effects for clozapine. However, clozapine at therapeutic doses also blocks many other types of receptors in addition to D4 receptors making it difficult to draw definitive conclusions. For example, clozapine binds to muscarinic acetylcholine receptors and is 20- to 50-fold more potent at these sites than at D2 receptors (for review, see Ref. 61)

Recently, it has been suggested that clozapine and other related antipsychotic drugs that elicit little or no parkinsonism bind more loosely than dopamine to brain D2 receptors, yet have high occupancy of these receptors (61). By determining fractional occupancies of receptors bound by therapeutic drug levels, it has been demonstrated that the dominant factor for deciding if a particular antipsychotic drug will elicit parkinsonism is whether it binds more tightly or more loosely than dopamine at the D2 receptor subtype. Thus, for those antipsychotic drugs that elicit little or no parkinsonism, it appears that the high endogenous dopamine in the human striatum must outcompete the more loosely bound neuroleptic at the striatal D2 receptor subtype. Dopamine less readily displaces the more hydrophobic radioligands of the haloperidol type, providing an additional correlate between the magnitude of in vivo competition with endogenous agonists and parkinsonism. The separation of antipsychotic drugs into "loose" and "tight" binding to D2 receptors is consistent with the observation that catalepsy induced by olanzapine and loxapine (more loosely bound than

TABLE 1 Properties of Dopamine Receptor Subtypes

Receptor subtype	D1-like		D2-like		
	D1	D5	D2	D3	D4
Amino acids	446	477	443	400	387
Chromosome	5q35.1	4p15.1-16.1	11q22-23	3p13.3	11p15.5
Second messenger	cAMP	cAMP	cAMP K$^+$ channel Ca$^+$	K$^+$ channel Ca$^+$ channel	cAMP K$^+$ channel
mRNA	Striatum	Hippocampus Kidney	Striatum	Nucleus Accumbens	Cerebral cortex
Selective agonists	SKF38393	SKF38393	Bromocriptine Butaclamol Pergolide Ropinirole	7-OH-DPAT Pramipexole Pergolide Ropinirole PD128,907	—
Selective antagonists	SCH23390	SCH23390	Spiperone Raclopride Sulpiride	Spiperone Raclopride Sulpiride Nafodotride	Spiperone Clozapine

Source: Data from Refs. 15,16,19,68.

dopamine) but not haloperidol (more tightly bound than dopamine to D2 receptors) was fully reversible (61). Taken together, these observations suggest that D2 blockade may be necessary for achieving antipsychotic action. This suggestion is in keeping with the observation that many patients will suddenly relapse when stopping clozapine, perhaps due to a sudden pulse of endogenous dopamine arising from emotional or physical activity which displaces the loosely bound neuroleptic from the receptor. Clinical dosing schedules can be adjusted to obtain sufficient but low occupancies of D2 receptors in order to minimize the development of parkinsonism. The psychosis caused by levodopa or bromocriptine can be readily treated by low doses of either clozapine or remoxipride (62), since there is very little endogenous dopamine to compete with the antagonist. Further studies are needed to determine whether newer antipsychotic drugs with low affinity for D2 receptors and with low risk for parkinsonism will cause less tardive dyskinesia.

The success of treating parkinsonian symptoms with dopamine precursor amino acid levodopa is due to its ability to reverse the dopamine deficiency. Unfortunately, treatment complications emerge shortly after beginning levodopa therapy. In the DATATOP study (63), almost half of the patients developed wearing off (loss of efficacy towards the end of a dosing interval), about one third showed dyskinesias, and about one fourth were showing early signs of freezing (sudden loss of capacity to move) with a mean duration of treatment of only 18 months. Modern pharmacological treatment of PD has been advanced by the increased understanding of the complexity of dopamine receptor pharmacology and the ability to screen drug candidates in vitro against cloned and expressed human dopamine receptor subtypes (2,21).

Symptoms of parkinsonism in primate models are treated with agonists that activate the D2-like receptor subfamily. D2 agonists with long half-lives can relieve parkinsonism in these animals with little risk of motor side effects, while repetitive levodopa doses will induce motor fluctuations and dyskinesias (64). In dyskinetic animals that had received levodopa doses, D2 agonists that had few side effects on their own, now elicit dyskinesias. These observations suggest that repetitive co-activation of denervated striatal dopamine receptor subtypes initiates the development of these disabling side effects by nonselective activation of postsynaptic D1 and D2/D3 receptors. Pramipexole is a novel dopamine agonist with preferential affinity for D3 receptors (Table 1). It has little affinity for the D1-like receptors, and within the D2 receptor subfamily it exhibits its highest affinity at the D3 receptor subtype, distinguishing it from all other dopamine agonists currently used for the treatment of PD (2,65). As PD progresses, there is marked reduction of D3 receptors in the caudal sectors of the putamen (Fig. 1H).

Dopamine normally inhibits striatal GABAergic cells of the indirect pathway by stimulating D2 receptors and stimulates GABAergic cells of the direct pathway by activating D1 and D3 receptors. These effects result in the inhibition of the globus pallidus (GPi). In PD, when dopamine innervation has been lost, the GPi fires at very high rates to inhibit thalamic relay neurons resulting in bradykinesia (for review, see Ref. 66). Pramipexole stimulates D3 receptors that directly inhibit GPi neurons, removing its inhibitory gate on thalamocortical motor pathways, and stimulates D2 receptors to indirectly inhibit GPi neurons (66). Thus, pramipexole has two synergistic mechanisms to mimic dopamine and restore function in PD. While D3 receptors have a lower density in the striatum as compared to D2 receptors (Fig. 1E and G), chronic administration of indirect-acting agonists may cause an upregulation in the number of D3 binding sites (67). In keeping with this suggestion, chronic cocaine abusers have elevated densities of D3 receptor sites in limbic sectors of the striatum and nucleus accumbens (68). It is not known if this regulatory change occurs in the denervated striatum, early in the course of agonist replacement for PD. However, pramipexole has shown efficacy for the treatment of depression in PD, in keeping with its postsynaptic effects on limbic targets (69). Thus, pramipexole has clinically meaningful antidepressant activity in moderate depression, a property that is possibly tied to its preferential binding to the D3 receptor subtype.

Joyce (6) has suggested that the D3 receptor may provide neuroprotective effects in PD and modify clinical symptoms that D2 receptor–preferring drugs cannot provide. Although D3 receptors are confined to the limbic sectors of the striatum, they may play a role in PD because the limbic striatum is involved in aspects of movement, including the execution of goal-directed behaviors requiring locomotor activity. Experimental models of PD suggest that D3-preferring agonists do act through D3 receptors to provide relief of akinesia (6). The nucleus accumbens, a region rich in D3 receptors that remains relatively spared in advanced PD (Fig. 1), is involved in behavioral sensitization to psycho-stimulants and changes in affective state. Thus, D3 agonists could modulate the effects of dopamine afferents originating from the medial substantia nigra.

The primary dopamine receptors mediating the antiparkinson effects of levodopa and other direct-acting dopamine agonists are D1 and D2 receptors. D3 receptors afford a novel target for medication development in PD. Whether or not other novel subtypes of dopamine receptors exist in the brain is unknown. However, rapid advances in molecular cloning may reveal additional heterogeneity in the expression of synaptic proteins involved in dopaminergic neurotransmission. At this time, five cloned and expressed dopaminergic receptor proteins provide a complex molecular basis for a variety of neural signals mediated by a single neurotransmitter. At least three of these receptor subtypes are relevant for understanding the pathophysiology and treatment of PD.

ACKNOWLEDGMENTS

This work was funded by the National Parkinson Foundation, Inc., Miami, FL.

REFERENCES

1. Hornykiewicz O. Dopamine (3-hydroxytyramine) and brain function. Pharmacol Rev 1966; 18:925–964.
2. Factor SA. Dopamine agonists. Med Clin North Am 1999; 83:415–443.
3. Carlsson A. The current status of the dopamine hypothesis of schizophrenia. Neuropsychopharmacology 1988; 1:179 186.
4. Creese I, Burt DR, Snyder SH. Dopamine receptor binding predicts clinical and pharmacological potencies of antischizophrenic drugs. Science 1976; 192:481–483.
5. Seeman P, Lee T, Chau-Wong M, Wong K. Antipsychotic drug doses and neuroleptic/dopamine receptors. Nature 1976; 261:717–719.
6. Joyce JN. Dopamine D3 receptor as a therapeutic target for antipsychotic and antiparkinsonian drugs. Pharmacol Ther 2001; 90:231–259.
7. Dohlman HG, Caron MG, Lefkowitz RJ. A family of receptors coupled to guanine nucleotide regulatory proteins. Biochemistry 1987; 26:2657–2664.
8. Dixon, RA, Kobilka BK, Strader DJ, et al., Cloning of the gene and cDNA for mammalian beta-adrenergic receptor and homology with rhodopsin. Nature 1986; 321:75–79.
9. Kubo T, Maeda A, Sugimoto K, Akiba I, Mikami A, Takahashi H, Haga T, Haga K, Ichiyama A, et al. Primary structure of porcine cardiac muscarinic receptor deduced from the cDNA sequence. FEBS Lett 1986; 209:367–372.
10. Bunzow JR, Van Tol HH, Grandy DK, Albert P, Salon J, Christie M, Machida CA, Neve KA, Civelli O. Cloning and expression of a rat D_2 dopamine receptor cDNA. Nature 1988; 336:783–787.
11. Dearry A, Gingrich JA, Falardeau P, Fremeau RT, Bates MD, Caron MG. Molecular cloning and expression of the gene for a human D_1 dopamine receptor. Nature 1990; 347:72–76.
12. Monsma FJ Jr, Mahan LC, McVittie LD, Gerfen CR, Sibley DR. Molecular cloning and expression of a D_1 dopamine receptor linked to adenylyl cyclase activation. Proc Natl Acad Sci USA 1990; 87:6723–6727.

13. Dal Toso R, Sommer B, Ewart M, Herb A, Pritchett DB, Bach A, Shivers BD, Seeburg PH. The dopamine D2 receptor: two molecular forms generated by alternative splicing. EMBO J 1989; 8:4025–4034.

14. Monsma FJ Jr, McVittie LD, Gerfen CR, Mahan LC, Sibley DR. Multiple D_2 dopamine receptors produced by alternative RNA splicing. Nature 1989; 342:926–929.

15. Sokoloff P, Giros B, Martres MP, Bouthenet ML, Schwartz JC. Molecular cloning and characterization of a novel dopamine receptor (D-3) as a target for neuroleptics. Nature 1990; 347:146–151.

16. Van Tol HH, Bunzow JR, Guan HC, Sunahara RK, Seeman P, Niznik HB, Civelli O. Cloning of the gene for a human dopamine D_4 receptor with high affinity for the antipsychotic clozapine. Nature 1991; 350:610–614.

17. Sunahara RK, Niznik HB, Weiner DM, Stormann TM, Brann MR, Kennedy JL, Gelernter JE, Rozmahel R, Yang YL, Israel Y, Seeman P, O'Down BF. Human dopamine D_1 receptor encoded by an intronless gene on chromosome 5. Nature 1990; 347:80–83.

18. Zhou QY, Grandy DK, Thambi L, Kushner JA, Van Tol HH, Cone R, Pribnow D, Salon J, Bunzow JR, Civelli O. Cloning and expression of human and rat D_1 dopamine receptors. Nature 1990; 347:76–80.

19. Sunahara RK, Guan HC, O'Dowd BF, Seeman P, Laurier LG, Ng G, George SR, Torchia J, Van Tol HH, Niznik HB. Cloning of the gene for a human dopamine D_5 receptor with higher affinity for dopamine than D_1. Nature 1991; 350:614–619.

20. O'Dowd BF. Structures of dopamine receptors. J Neurochem 1993; 60:804–816.

21. Lachowicz JE, Sibley DR. Molecular characteristics of mammalian dopamine receptors. Pharmacol Toxicol 1997; 81:105–113.

22. Snyder LA, Roberts JL, Sealfon SC. Alternative transcripts of the rat and human dopamine D3 receptor. Biochem Biophys Res Commun 1991; 180:1031–1035.

23. Fishburn CS, Belleli D, David C, Carmon S, Fuchs S. A novel short isoform of the D3 dopamine receptor generated by alternative splicing in the third cytoplasmic loop. J Biol Chem 1993; 268:5872–5878.

24. Giros B, Martres MP, Pilon C, Sokoloff P, Schwartz JC. Shorter variants of the D3 dopamine receptor produced through various patterns of alternative splicing. Biochem Biophys Res Commun 1991; 176:1584–1592.

25. Van Tol HH, Wu CM, Guan HC, Ohara K, Bunzow JR, Civelli O, Kennedy J, Seeman P, Niznik HB, Jovanovic V. Multiple dopamine D4 receptor variants in the human population. Nature 1992; 358:149–152.

26. Weinshank RL, Adham N, Macchi M, Olsen MA, Branchek TA, Hartig PR. Molecular cloning and characterization of a high affinity dopamine receptor (D1 beta) and its pseudogene. J Biol Chem 1991; 266:22427–22435.

27. Bjorklund A, Lindvall O. Dopamine-containing systems in the CNS. In: Bjorklund A, Hokfelt T, eds. Handbook of Chemical Neuroanatomy, Vol. 2.

Classical Transmitters in the CNS Part I. Amsterdam, NY: Elsevier 1994:55–122.

28. Le Moine C, Normand E, Guitteny AF, Fouque B, Teoule R, Bloch B. Dopamine receptor gene expression by enkephalin neurons in rat forebrain. Proc Natl Acad Sci USA 1990; 87(1):230–234.

29. Diaz J, Levesque D, Griffon N, Lammers CH, Martres MP, Sokoloff P, Schwartz JC. Opposing roles for dopamine D2 and D3 receptors on neurotensin mRNA expression in nucleus accumbens. Eur J Neurosci 1994; 6:1384–1387.

30. Diaz J, Levesque D, Lammers CH, Griffon N, Martres MP, Schwartz JC, Sokoloff P. Phenotypical characterization of neurons expressing the dopamine D3 receptor in the rat brain. Neuroscience 1995; 65:731–745.

31. Bouthenet ML, Souil E, MP, Martres M, Sokoloff P, Giros B, Schwartz JC. Localization of dopamine D3 receptor mRNA in the rat brain using in situ hybridization histochemistry: comparison with dopamine D2 receptor mRNA. Brain Res 1991; 64:203 19.

32. Le Moine C, Bloch B. Anatomical and cellular analysis of dopmaine receptor gene expression. In: Ariano MA, Sermeir DJ, eds. Molecular and Cellular Mechanisms of Neostriatal Function. New York: Springer-Verlag, 1995:45–58.

33. Surmeier DJ, Eberwine J, Wilson CJ, Cao Y, Stefani A, Kitai ST. Dopamine receptor subtypes colocalize in rat striatonigral neurons. Proc Natl Acad Sci USA 1992; 89:10178–10182.

34. Gerfen CR, Keefe KA, Steiner H. Dopamine-mediated gene regulation in the striatum. Adv Pharmacol 1998; 42:670–673.

35. Waddington JL, O'Boyle KM. Drugs acting on brain dopamine receptors a conceptual reevaluation five years after the first selective D1 antagonist. Pharmacol Ther 1989; 43:1–52.

36. Loschmann PA, Smith LA, Lange KW, Jaehnig P, Jenner P, Marsden CD. Motor activity following the administration of selective D-1 and D-2 dopaminergic drugs to normal common marmosets. Psychopharmacology 1991; 105:303–309.

37. Centonze D, Picconi B, Gubellini P, Benardi G, Calabresi P. Dopaminergic control of synaptic plasticity in the dorsal striatum. Eur J Neurosci 2001; 13:1071–1077.

38. Smith AD, Bolan JP. The neural network of the basal ganglia as revealed by the study of synaptic connentions of the identified neurones. Trends Neurosci 1990; 13:259–265.

39. Wooten GF. Anatomy and function of dopamine receptors: understanding the pathophysiology of fluctations in Parkinson's disease. Parkinsonism Reatl Disord 2001; 8:79–83.

40. Hepler JR, Gilman AG. G proteins. Trends Biochem Sci 1992; 17:383–387.

41. Grandy DK, Zhang Y, Bouvier C, Zhou QY, Johnson RA, Allen L, Buck K, Bunzow JR, Salon J, Civelli O. Multiple human D5 dopamine receptor genes:

a functional receptor and two pseudogenes. Proc Natl Acad Sci USA 1991; 88:9175–9179.

42. Sidhu A. Coupling of D1 and D5 dopamine receptors to multiple G proteins: implications for understanding the diversity in receptor-G protein coupling. Mol Neurobiol 1998; 16:125–134.

43. Birnbaumer L, Abramowitz J, Brown AM. Receptor-effector coupling by G proteins. Biochim Biophys Acta 1990; 1031:163–224.

44. Kitai ST, Surmeier DJ. Cholinergic and dopaminergic modulation of potassium conductances in neostriatal neurons. Adv Neurol 1993; 60:40–52.

45. Kimura K, White BH, Sidhu A. Coupling of human D1 dopamine receptors to different guanine nucleotide binding proteins. Evidence that D1 dopamine receptors can couple to both Gs and G(o). J Biol Chem 1995; 270:14672–14678.

46. Dahmer MK, Senogles SE. Dopaminergic inhibition of catecholamine secretion from chromaffin cells: evidence that inhibition is mediated by D4 and D5 dopamine receptors. J Neurochem 1996; 66:222–232.

47. Sidhu A. Regulation and expression of D-1, but not D-5, dopamine receptors in human SK-N-MC neuroblastoma cells. J Recep Signal Transduct Res 1997; 17:777–784.

48. Kozasa T, Gilman AG. Purification of recombinant G proteins from Sf9 cells by hexahistidine tagging of associated subunits: characterization of alpha 12 and inhibition of adenylyl cyclase by Gzα. J Biol Chem 1995; 270:1734–1741.

49. Glatt CE, Snyder SH. Cloning and expression of an adenylyl cyclase localized to the corpus striatum. Nature 1993; 361:536–538.

50. Yoshimura M, Ikeda H, Tabakoff B. mu-Opioid receptors inhibit dopamine-stimulated activity of type V anenylyl cyclase and enhance dopamine-stimulated activity of type VII adenylyl cyclase. Mol Pharmacol 1996; 50:43–51.

51. Cooper DM, Mons N, Karpen JW. Adenylyl cyclases and the interaction between calcium and cAMP signaling. Nature 1995; 374:421–424

52. McAllister G, Knowles MR, Ward-Booth SM, Sinclair HA, Patel S, Marwood R, Emms F, Patel S, Smith A, Seabrook GR, Freedman SB. Functional coupling of human D2, D3, and D4 dopamine receptors in HEK293 cells. J Recept Signal Tranducts Res 1995; 15:267–281.

53. Hayes G, Biden TJ, Selbie LA, Shine J. Structural subtypes of the dopamine D2 receptor are functionally distinct: expression of the cloned D2A and D2B subtypes in a heterologous cell line. Mol Endocrinol 1992; 6:920–926.

54. Montmayeur JP, Borelli E. Trascription mediated by a cAMP-responsive promoter element is reduced upon activation of dopamine D2 receptors. Proc Natl Acad Sci USA 1991; 88:3135–3139.

55. Castellano MA, Liu LX, Monsma FJ Jr, Sibley DR, Kapatos G, Chiodo LA. Transfected D2 short dopamine receptors inhibit voltage-dependent potassium current in neuroblastoma x glioma hybrid (NG108-15) cells. Mol Pharmacol 1993; 44:649–656.

56. Liu LX, Monsma FJ Jr, Sibley DR, Chiodo LA. Coupling of D2-long receptor isoform to K^+ currents in neuroblastoma x glioma (NG108-15) cells. Soc Neurosci 1993; 19:79.

57. Jaber M, Robinson SW, Missale C, Caron MG. Dopamine receptors and brain function. Neuropharmacology 1996; 35:1503–1519.

58. Levey AI, Hersch SM, Rye DB, et al., Localization of D1 and D2 receptors in brain with subtype-specific antibodies. Proc Natl Acad Sci USA 1993; 90:8861–8865.

59. Tiberi M, Jarvie KR, Silvia C, Falardeau P, Gingrich JA, Godinot N, Bertrand L, Yang-Feng TL, Fermeau RT Jr, Caron MG. Cloning, molecular characterization and chromosomal assignment of a gene encoding a second D1 dopamine receptor subtype: differential expression pattern in rat brain compared with the D1 receptor. Proc Natl Acad Sci USA 1991; 88:7491–7495.

60. Gerlach J, Behnke K, Heltberg J, Munk-Anderson E, Nielsen H. Sulpiride and haloperidol in schizophrenia: a double-blind cross-over study of therapeutic effect, side effects and plasma concentrations. Br J Psychiatry 1985; 147:283–288.

61. Seeman P, Tallerico T. Antipsycholtic drugs which elicit little or no parkinsonism bind more loosely to brain D2 receptors, yet occupy high levels of these receptors. Mol Psychiatry 1998; 3:123–134.

62. Sandor P, Lang AE, Singal S, Angus C. Remoxipride in the treatment of levodopa-induced psychosis. J Clin Psychopharmacol 1996; 16:395–399.

63. Parkinson Study Group. Impact of deprenyl and tocopherol treatment in progression of disability in early Parkinson's disease. N Engl J Med 1993; 328:176–183.

64. Blanchet PJ, Calon F, Martel JC, Bedard PJ, DiPaolo T, Walters RR, Piercey MF. Continuous administration decreases and pulsatile administration increases behavioral sensitivity to a novel dopamine D2 agonist (U-91356A) in MPTP-exposed monkeys. J Pharmacol Exp Ther 1995; 272:854–859.

65. Bennett JP Jr., Piercy MF. Pramipexole—a new dopamine agonist for the treatment of Parkinson's disease. J Neurol Sci 1999; 163:25–31.

66. Piercey MF, Hyslop DK, Hoffmann WE. Excitation of type II anterior caudate neurons by stimulation of dopamine D3 receptors. Brain Res 1997; 762:19–28.

67. Goetz CG, Shannon KM, Tanner CM, Carroll VS, Klawans HL. Agonist substitution in advanced Parkinson's disease. Neurology 1989; 39:1121–1122.

68. Staley JK, Mash DC. Adaptive increase in D3 dopamine receptors in the brain reward circuits of human cocaine fatalities. J Neurosci 1996; 16:6100–6106.

69. Szegedi A, Wetzel H, Hillert A, Kleiser E, Gaebel W, Benkert O. Pramipexole, a novel seletive dopamine agonist in major depression. Mov Disord 1996; 11(suppl 1):266.

14

Genetics

Zbigniew K. Wszolek and Matthew Farrer
Mayo Clinic, Jacksonville, Florida, U.S.A., and Mayo Medical School, Rochester, Minnesota, U.S.A

INTRODUCTION

Despite considerable progress in the understanding of clinical and pathological features of Parkinson's disease (PD), the etiology of this condition remains unknown (1,2). There are two major plausible explanations on which current working hypotheses are based. The "environmental hypothesis," widely propagated in the 1980s, appears to have had only limited influence (3). The scope of environmental factors on causation of PD is discussed in Chapter 15. The "genetic hypothesis," which was popular in the 1990s, stemmed from significant progress in the development of new molecular genetic techniques and from the description of several large families with a phenotype closely resembling that of sporadic PD (4,5). However, genetic factors still do not explain the etiology of all cases of PD (6). It is reasonable to assume that a combination of environmental and inherited risk factors plays the crucial role in developing disease in most cases of parkinsonism. The era of exploration of these intermingling influences and factors is just beginning.

Understanding the etiology of PD is further complicated by a lack of in vivo biological markers for a diagnosis of PD, requiring reliance on clinical or pathological criteria (7). In addition, PD is probably not a uniform clinical entity but rather represents a heterogeneous syndrome (8). In this chapter we will discuss the contributions of epidemiological, twin, kindred, and association studies to the support of the genetic hypothesis of PD and related parkinsonism-plus syndromes (PPS).

EPIDEMIOLOGICAL STUDIES

Epidemiological studies indicate a genetic contribution to the etiology of PD. According to a study conducted by Lazzarini and colleagues (9) in New Jersey, the chance of having PD at age 80 years is about 2% for the general population and about 5–6% if a parent or sibling is affected. However, if both a parent and a sibling are affected, the probability of having PD increases further, reaching 20–40%. Marder and colleagues (10) assessed the risk of PD among first-degree relatives from the same geographic region (northern Manhattan, New York). The cumulative incidence of PD to age 75 years among first-degree relatives of patients with PD was 2% compared with 1% among first-degree relatives of controls. The risk of PD was higher in male than in female first-degree relatives [relative risk, 2.0; 95% confidence interval (CI), 1.1–3.4]. The risk of PD in any first-degree relative was also higher for whites than for African-Americans and Hispanics (relative risk, 2.4; 95% CI, 1.4–4.1).

In an Italian case-control study (11), history of familial PD was the most relevant risk factor (odds ratio, 14.6; 95% CI, 7.2–29.6). In a Canadian study of PD patients (12), the prevalence rate of PD in first- and second-degree relatives was more than five times higher than that of the general population. Even patients who reported a negative family history of PD actually had a prevalence rate of PD in relatives more than three times higher than that in the general population. A study of the Icelandic population (13) revealed the presence of genetic as well as environmental components in the etiology of late-onset PD (onset at >50 years of age). The risk ratio for PD was 6.7 (95% CI, 1.2–9.6) for siblings, 3.2 (95% CI, 1.2–7.8) for offspring, and 2.7 (95% CI, 1.6–3.9) for nephews and nieces of patients with late-onset PD. The most recent epidemiological study, conducted by Maher and colleagues (14) on 203 sibling pairs with PD, also supported a genetic contribution to the etiology of PD. This study showed that sibling pairs with PD were more similar in age at symptomatic disease onset than in year of symptomatic disease onset. The frequency of PD in parents (7.0%) and siblings (5.1%) was greater than that in spouses (2%).

TWIN STUDIES

Studies of twins can provide a powerful confirmation of the genetic contribution to the etiology of a neurodegenerative condition. If a genetic component is present, concordance will be greater in monozygotic (MZ) than in dizygotic (DZ) twins. If a disorder is exclusively genetic in origin and the diagnosis is not compounded by age-associated penetrance or stochastic or environmental factors, MZ concordance may be close to 100%.

Although earlier twin studies in PD were inconclusive (15 17), the most recent twin study, conducted by Tanner and colleagues (18) on a large cohort of twins, demonstrated the presence of genetic factors in the etiology of PD if disease begins at or before age 50 years. This was a study of twins enrolled in the National Academy of Science/National Research Council World War II Veteran Twin Registry. No genetic component was evident when the onset of symptoms occurred after age 50 years. However, twin studies such as this one, which was based exclusively on clinical observations, may require extended longitudinal follow-up to confirm the presence of PD in a co-twin (19).

Positron emission tomography (PET) studies with [18F]6-fluorodopa (6FD) may in part circumvent the need for extended follow-up. Indeed, reduced striatal uptake of 6FD has been demonstrated in some clinically asymptomatic co-twins (20). Using longitudinal evaluation with measurement of 6FD, Piccini and colleagues (21) demonstrated 75% concordance of PD in MZ twins versus 22% in DZ twins.

EVALUATION OF KINDREDS

Kindreds with a parkinsonian phenotype have been reported in the world literature since the nineteenth century (22,23). In a review of literature in 1926, Bell and Clark (24) described 10 families with "shaking palsy" believed to exist on a hereditary basis. They also provided 20 references of earlier accounts of familial paralysis agitans. In 1937, Allen (25) detailed an additional 25 families with inherited parkinsonism and speculated that in approximately two thirds of these kindreds the inheritance was autosomal dominant and probably the result of a "single autosomal gene." In 1949, a monograph by Mjönes (26) detailed eight pedigrees with inherited parkinsonism, some with atypical features such as myoclonic epilepsy. In the levodopa era, a number of reports described families with PD and PPS (22), including two very large multigenerational kindreds known as Contursi and Family C (German-American) (27,28). With progress in molecular genetic techniques, the importance of collecting data from parkinsonian families with PD and PPS phenotypes has grown exponentially.

Table 1 summarizes the status of current knowledge of the genetics of PD and related conditions. It shows the types of inheritance and the location of known chromosomal loci and mutations. The key literature references are also provided.

ASSOCIATION STUDIES

Despite substantial progress in identification, the number of known large pedigrees with PD or PPS is still small. Furthermore, genetic linkage studies, which use "identity-by-descent" mapping, have been hampered because the amount of DNA available from affected pedigree members is limited, generally as a result of death, lack of consent, or geographic dispersion. Association or "identity-by-state" mapping is an alternate approach employing groups of unrelated individuals. Association studies measure differences in genetic variability between a group with the disease in question and a group of matched, normal individuals. This method is most powerful in implicating genes for multigenic traits in homogeneous population isolates. However, many past studies have been confounded by misconceived, a priori notions of disease etiology and by clinical, locus, and allelic heterogeneity. Studies must be reproducible, preferably in different ethnic populations, and the genetic variability should have some functional consequence (either directly or in disequilibrium) that alters gene expression or the resultant protein.

The genes for α-synuclein, ubiquitin C-terminal hydrolase, parkin, and tau harbor mutations that segregate with parkinsonism in large multiply affected kindreds (31,33,34,37,43) (Fig. 1). Although the relevance of these findings for sporadic PD is unclear, there is no doubt that these genes mark a pathway that is perturbed in both familial and sporadic PD. Understanding the components of this pathway and its regulation is the first step in elucidating the molecular etiology of parkinsonism (48). In some studies, common genetic variability in genes for α-synuclein (49,50), ubiquitin C-terminal hydrolase (51–53), and tau (54–56) has now been implicated in sporadic PD by association methods. It is clear that these genes contribute to risk in at least a subset of patients with idiopathic PD.

Other contributing genes are likely to be identified through family studies, ultimately facilitating molecular rather than clinicopathological diagnosis. Mutations in genes implicated in parkinsonism have already been used to create in vivo models that are providing powerful insights into neuronal degeneration (57–61). Much as in Alzheimer's disease, these new tools bring the hope of novel therapies designed to address the causes rather than merely the symptoms of disease (62).

TABLE 1 Familial Parkinsonism with Reported Mutations/Loci

Chromosome	Gene	Locus	Age at onset, range, y(mean)	Phenotype	Response to levodopa	Ref.
Autosomal dominant						
1p32	Unknown	PARK9	NA (65)	PD, pathology unknown	Good	29
2p13	Unknown	PARK3	36–89 (58)	PD, with LBs	Good	28,30
4p14–15	UCH-L1 (3 mutations)	PARK5	49–51 (50)	PD, pathology unknown	Good	31
4p15	Unknown	PARK4	24–48 ($\approx$30)	PD and D, with LBs	Good	23,32
4q21	α-Synuclein (2 mutations)	PARK1	20–85 (46)	PD and D, with LBs	Good	33,34
12p11.2-q13.1	Unknown	PARK8	38–68 (53)	PD, pathology unknown	Good	M. Hasegawa, personal communication, 2001
12q23-24.1	SCA2 (ataxin-2)	SCA2	19–61 (39)	PD, PD and A, without LBs	Fair	35
14q32.1	SCA3 (ataxin-3)	SCA3	31–57 (42)	PD and A, without LBs	Good	36
17q21-22	Tau (>20 mutations)	FTDP-17	25–76 (49)	FTD, PD, PSP, CBGD, ALS with tau pathology	Poor	37,38
19q13	Unknown	DYT12	12–45 (23)	Rapid-onset dystonia—parkinsonism, pathology unknown	Poor	39

TABLE 1 (continued)

Chromosome	Gene	Locus	Age at onset, range, y(mean)	Phenotype	Response to levodopa	Ref.
Autosomal recessive						
1p35-36	Unknown	PARK6	32–68 (45)	PD, probably with LBs	Good	40,41
1p36	Unknown	PARK7	27–40 (33)	PD, probably with LBs	Good	42
6q25.2–27	*Parkin* (>32 mutations)	PARK2	6–58 (26)	PD, sometimes with LBs	Good	43 (reviewed in Ref. 44)
X-linked recessive						
Xq13.1	Unknown	DYT3	12–48 (35)	Dystonia-parkinsonism, without LBs	Poor	45
Mitochondrial						
Complex 1	*ND4*	Unknown	(31)	PD, D, dystonia, and ophthalmoplegia without LBs	Fair	46
Complex 1	Unknown	Unknown	35–79 (42)	PD, pathology unknown	Good	47

A, ataxia; AD, autosomal dominant; ALS, amyotrophic lateral sclerosis; AR, autosomal recessive; CBGD, corticobasal ganglionic degeneration; D, dementia; FTD, frontotemporal dementia; FTDP-17, frontotemporal dementia and parkinsonism linked on chromosome 17; LBs, Lewy bodies; NA, not available; PD, Parkinson's disease; PSP, progressive supranuclear palsy; UCH-L1, ubiquitin carboxy-terminal hydrolase L1.

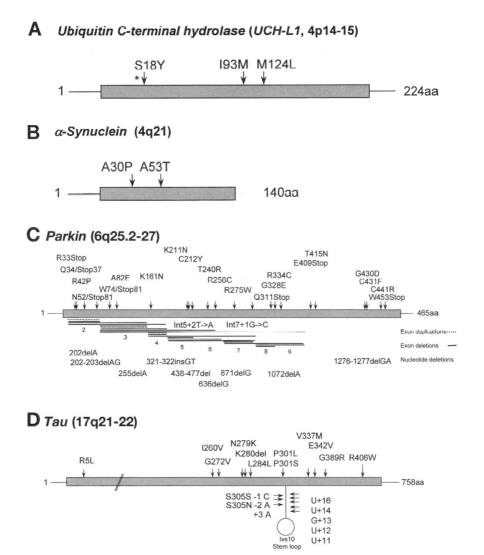

FIGURE 1 Genes and mutations associated with parkinsonism. Gene names are indicated in italics with their chromosomal assignment. (A) *Ubiquitin C-terminal hydrolase*; (B) α-*Synuclein*; (C) *Parkin*; (D) *Tau*. Boxes represent the coding sequence. Amino acids (aa) are shown N′ to C′ terminal. Coding mutations are indicated above; splice-site mutations and exonic and nucleotide deletions are represented below (not to scale). *Coding polymorphism associated with disease.

CLINICAL MOLECULAR GENETIC TESTING

At present, diagnostic molecular genetic testing is not commercially available and not clinically recommended for patients with sporadic PD or for those with a positive family history of PD. However, if patients express interest in research, they may be directed to centers where molecular genetic screening for PD is conducted. There are many such centers in the United States, Europe, Asia, and Australia.

SUMMARY

It is apparent that the genetics of PD and related conditions is complex, even in monogenic parkinsonism. The discovery of mutations in the genes for α-synuclein, ubiquitin C-terminal hydrolase, parkin, and tau has created a unique glimpse into the basic mechanisms responsible for neurodegenerative processes (43). Further genetic studies of already known PD/PPS loci will undoubtedly uncover more mutations. Subsequent clinical correlation aids in understanding the pathogenetic mechanisms and events that underlie cell dysfunction and death.

A large number of families have been described for which the genetic etiology is still to be explored. The study of these families—and those waiting to be discovered—will further enhance our knowledge of the biology of this neurodegenerative disease. Based on this background, an understanding of gene-gene and gene-environment interactions is also emerging. After almost 180 years, only short-term palliative remedies are presently available, but hope exists that this work will lead to curative treatments for PD and related conditions.

ACKNOWLEDGMENTS

The authors wish to thank patients with Parkinson's disease and their families for their cooperation, patience, and continued support for genetic research on parkinsonian conditions.

REFERENCES

1. Gelb DJ, Oliver E, Gilman S. Diagnostic criteria for Parkinson disease. Arch Neurol 56:33–39, 1999.
2. Mizuno Y, Mori H, Kondo T. Parkinson's disease: from etiology to treatment. Intern Med 34:1045–1054, 1995.
3. Kopin IJ. Tips from toxins: the MPTP model of Parkinson's disease. In: G Jolles, JM Stutzman, eds. Neurodegenerative Diseases. San Diego: Academic Press Limited, 1994, pp 143–154.

4. Golbe LI. Alpha-synuclein and Parkinson's disease. Mov Disord 14:6–9, 1999.
5. Wszolek ZK, Uitti RJ, Markopoulou K. Familial Parkinson's disease and related conditions. Clinical genetics. Adv Neurol 86:33–43, 2001.
6. Payami H, Zareparsi S. Genetic epidemiology of Parkinson's disease. J Geriatr Psychiatry Neurol 11:98–106, 1998.
7. Brooks DJ. Parkinson's disease—a single clinical entity? QJM 88:81–91, 1995.
8. Calne DB. Parkinson's disease is not one disease. Parkinsonism Relat Disord 7:3–7, 2000.
9. Lazzarini AM, Myers RH, Zimmerman TR Jr, Mark MH, Golbe LI, Sage JI, Johnson WG, Duvoisin RC. A clinical genetic study of Parkinson's disease: evidence for dominant transmission. Neurology 44:499–506, 1994
10. Marder K, Tang MX, Mejia H, Alfaro B, Cote L, Louis E, Groves J, Mayeux R. Risk of Parkinson's disease among first-degree relatives: a community-based study. Neurology 47:155–160, 1996.
11. De Michele G, Filla A, Volpe G, De Marco V, Gogliettino A, Ambrosio G, Marconi R, Castellano AE, Campanella G. Environmental and genetic risk factors in Parkinson's disease: a case-control study in southern Italy. Mov Disord 11:17–23, 1996.
12. Uitti RJ, Shinotoh H, Hayward M, Schulzer M, Mak E, Calne DB. "Familial Parkinson's disease"—a case-control study of families. Can J Neurol Sci 24:127–132, 1997.
13. Sveinbjornsdottir S, Hicks AA, Jonsson T, Petursson H, Gugmundsson G, Frigge ML, Kong A, Gulcher JR, Stefansson K. Familial aggregation of Parkinson's disease in Iceland. N Engl J Med 343:1765–1770, 2000.
14. Maher NE, Golbe LI, Lazzarini AM, Mark MH, Currie LJ, Wooten GF, Saint-Hilaire M, Wilk JB, Volcjak J, Maher JE, Feldman RG, Guttman M, Lew M, Schuman S, Suchowersky O, Lafontaine AL, Labelle N, Vieregge P, Pramstaller PP, Klein C, Hubble J, Reider C, Growdon J, Watts R, Montgomery E, Baker K, Singer C, Stacy M, Myers RH. Epidemiologic study of 203 sibling pairs with Parkinson's disease: the GenePD study. Neurology 58:79–84, 2002.
15. Duvoisin RC, Eldridge R, Williams A, Nutt J, Calne D. Twin study of Parkinson disease. Neurology 31:77–80, 1981.
16. Ward CD, Duvoisin RC, Ince SE, Nutt JD, Eldridge R, Calne DB. Parkinson's disease in 65 pairs of twins and in a set of quadruplets. Neurology 33:815–824, 1983.
17. Johnson WG, Hodge SE, Duvoisin R. Twin studies and the genetics of Parkinson's disease—a reappraisal. Mov Disord 5:187–194, 1990.
18. Tanner CM, Ottman R, Goldman SM, Ellenberg J, Chan P, Mayeux R, Langston JW. Parkinson disease in twins: an etiologic study. JAMA 281:341–346, 1999.
19. Dickson D, Farrer M, Lincoln S, Mason RP, Zimmerman TR Jr, Golbe LI, Hardy J. Pathology of PD in monozygotic twins with a 20-year discordance interval. Neurology 56:981–982, 2001.

20. Laihinen A, Ruottinen H, Rinne JO, Haaparanta M, Bergman J, Solin O, Koskenvuo M, Marttila R, Rinne UK. Risk for Parkinson's disease: twin studies for the detection of asymptomatic subjects using [^{18}F]6-fluorodopa PET. J Neurol 247(suppl 2):II110–II113, 2000.

21. Piccini P, Burn DJ, Ceravolo R, Maraganore D, Brooks DJ. The role of inheritance in sporadic Parkinson's disease: evidence from a longitudinal study of dopaminergic function in twins. Ann Neurol 45:577–582, 1999.

22. Wszolek ZK, Pfeiffer RF. Heredofamilial parkinsonian syndromes. In: RL Watts, WC Koller, eds. Movement Disorders: Neurologic Principles and Practice. New York: McGraw-Hill, 1997, pp 351–363.

23. Muenter MD, Forno LS, Hornykiewicz O, Kish SJ, Maraganore DM, Caselli RJ, Okazaki H, Howard FM Jr, Snow BJ, Calne DB. Hereditary form of parkinsonism—dementia. Ann Neurol 43:768–781, 1998.

24. Bell J, Clark AJ. A pedigree of paralysis agitans. Ann Eugenics 1:455–462, 1926.

25. Allen W. Inheritance of the shaking palsy. Arch Intern Med 60:424–436, 1937.

26. Mjönes H. Paralysis agitans. A clinical and genetic study. Acta Psychiatr Neurol Scand Suppl 54:1–195, 1949.

27. Golbe LI, Di Iorio G, Bonavita V, Miller DC, Duvoisin RC. A large kindred with autosomal dominant Parkinson's disease. Ann Neurol 27:276–282, 1990.

28. Wszolek ZK, Cordes M, Calne DB, Munter MD, Cordes I, Pfeifer RF. Hereditary Parkinson disease: report of 3 families with dominant autosomal inheritance [German]. Nervenarzt 64:331–335, 1993.

29. Hicks A, Pétursson H, Jónsson T, Stefánsson H, Jóhannsdóttir H, Sainz J, Frigge ML, Kong A, Gulcher JR, Stefánsson K, Sveinbjörndóttir S. A susceptibility gene for late-onset idiopathic Parkinson disease successfully mapped (abstr). Am J Hum Genet 69(suppl):200, 2001.

30. Gasser T, Muller-Myhsok B, Wszolek ZK, Oehlmann R, Calne DB, Bonifati V, Bereznai B, Fabrizio E, Vieregge P, Horstmann RD. A susceptibility locus for Parkinson's disease maps to chromosome 2p13. Nat Genet 18:262–265, 1998.

31. Leroy E, Boyer R, Auburger G, Leube B, Ulm G, Mezey E, Harta G, Brownstein MJ, Jonnalagada S, Chernova T, Dehejia A, Lavedan C, Gasser T, Steinbach PJ, Wilkinson KD, Polymeropoulos MH. The ubiquitin pathway in Parkinson's disease (letter). Nature 395:451–452, 1998.

32. Farrer M, Gwinn-Hardy K, Muenter M, DeVrieze FW, Crook R, Perez-Tur J, Lincoln S, Maraganore D, Adler C, Newman S, MacElwee K, McCarthy P, Miller C, Waters C, Hardy J. A chromosome 4p haplotype segregating with Parkinson's disease and postural tremor. Hum Mol Genet 8:81–85, 1999.

33. Polymeropoulos MH, Lavedan C, Leroy E, Ide SE, Dehejia A, Dutra A, Pike B, Root H, Rubenstein J, Boyer R, Stenroos ES, Chandrasekharappa S, Athanassiadou A, Papapetropoulos T, Johnson WG, Lazzarini AM, Duvoisin RC, Di Iorio G, Golbe LI, Nussbaum RL. Mutation in the alpha-synuclein gene identified in families with Parkinson's disease. Science 276:2045–2047, 1997.

34. Kruger R, Kuhn W, Muller T, Woitalla D, Graeber M, Kosel S, Przuntek H, Epplen JT, Schols L, Riess O. Ala30Pro mutation in the gene encoding alpha-synuclein in Parkinson's disease (letter). Nat Genet 18:106–108, 1998.

35. Gwinn-Hardy K, Chen JY, Liu HC, Liu TY, Boss M, Seltzer W, Adam A, Singleton A, Koroshetz W, Waters C, Hardy J, Farrer M. Spinocerebellar ataxia type 2 with parkinsonism in ethnic Chinese. Neurology 55:800–805, 2000.

36. Gwinn-Hardy K, Singleton A, O'Suilleabhain P, Boss M, Nicholl D, Adam A, Hussey J, Critchley P, Hardy J, Farrer M. Spinocerebellar ataxia type 3 phenotypically resembling Parkinson disease in a black family. Arch Neurol 58:296–299, 2001.

37. Hutton M, Lendon CL, Rizzu P, Baker M, Froelich S, Houlden H, Pickering-Brown S, Chakraverty S, Isaacs A, Grover A, Hackett J, Adamson J, Lincoln S, Dickson D, Davies P, Petersen RC, Stevens M, de Graaff E, Wauters E, van Baren J, Hillebrand M, Joosse M, Kwon JM, Nowotny P, Che LK, Norton J, Morris JC, Reed LA, Trojanowski J, Basun H, Lannfelt L, Neystat M, Fahn S, Dark F, Tannenberg T, Dodd PR, Hayward N, Kwok JBJ, Schofield PR, Andreadis A, Snowden J, Craufurd D, Neary D, Owen F, Oostra BA, Hardy J, Goate A, van Swieten J, Mann D, Lynch T, Heutink P. Association of missense and 5'-splice-site mutations in tau with the inherited dementia FTDP-17. Nature 393:702–705, 1998.

38. Wszolek ZK, Tsuboi Y, Farrer MJ, Uitti RJ, Hutton ML. Hereditary tauopathies and parkinsonism. Adv Neurol 91:153–163, 2002.

39. Kramer PL, Mineta M, Klein C, Schilling K, de Leon D, Farlow MR, Breakefield XO, Bressman SB, Dobyns WB, Ozelius LJ, Brashear A. Rapid-onset dystonia-parkinsonism: linkage to chromosome 19q13. Ann Neurol 46:176–182, 1999.

40. Valente EM, Bentivoglio AR, Dixon PH, Ferraris A, Ialongo T, Frontali M, Albanese A, Wood NW. Localization of a novel locus for autosomal recessive early-onset parkinsonism, PARK6, on human chromosome 1p35-p36. Am J Hum Genet 68:895–900, 2001.

41. Valente EM, Brancati F, Ferraris A, Graham EA, Davis MB, Breteler MM, Gasser T, Bonifati V, Bentivoglio AR, De Michele G, Durr A, Cortelli P, Wassilowsky D, Harhangi BS, Rawal N, Caputo V, Filla A, Meco G, Oostra BA, Brice A, Albanese A, Dallapiccola B, Wood NW; The European Consortium on Genetic Susceptibility in Parkinson's Disease. PARK6-linked parkinsonism occurs in several European families. Ann Neurol 51:14–18, 2002.

42. van Duijn CM, Dekker MC, Bonifati V, Galjaard RJ, Houwing-Duistermaat JJ, Snijders PJ, Testers L, Breedveld GJ, Horstink M, Sandkuijl LA, van Swieten JC, Oostra BA, Heutink P. Park7, a novel locus for autosomal recessive early-onset parkinsonism, on chromosome 1p36. Am J Hum Genet 69:629–634, 2001.

43. Kitada T, Asakawa S, Hattori N, Matsumine H, Yamamura Y, Minoshima S, Yokochi M, Mizuno Y, Shimizu N. Mutations in the parkin gene cause autosomal recessive juvenile parkinsonism. Nature 392:605–608, 1998.

44. West A, Periquet M, Lincoln S, Lücking CB, Nicholl D, Bonifati V, Rawal N, Gasser T, Lohmann E, Deleuze J-F, Maraganore D, Levey A, Wood N, Dürr A, Hardy J, Brice A, Farrer M, and the French Parkinson's Disease Genetics Study Group and the European Consortium on Genetic Suscept- ibility on Parkinson's Disease. Complex relationship between Parkin mutations and Parkinson's disease. Am J Med Genet 114: 584–591, 2002.

45. Haberhausen G, Schmitt I, Kohler A, Peters U, Rider S, Chelly J, Terwilliger JD, Monaco AP, Muller U. Assignment of the dystonia-parkinsonism syndrome locus, DYT3, to a small region within a 1.8-Mb YAC contig of Xq13.1. Am J Hum Genet 57:644–650, 1995.

46. Simon DK, Pulst SM, Sutton JP, Browne SE, Beal MF, Johns DR. Familial multisystem degeneration with parkinsonism associated with the 11778 mitochondrial DNA mutation. Neurology 53:1787–1793, 1999.

47. Swerdlow RH, Parks JK, Davis JN 2nd, Cassarino DS, Trimmer PA, Currie LJ, Dougherty J, Bridges WS, Bennett JP Jr, Wooten GF, Parker WD. Matrilineal inheritance of complex I dysfunction in a multigenerational Parkinson's disease family. Ann Neurol 44:873–881, 1998.

48. Hardy J. Pathways to primary neurodegenerative disease. Mayo Clin Proc 74:835–837, 1999.

49. Farrer M, Maraganore DM, Lockhart P, Singleton A, Lesnick TG, de Andrade M, West A, de Silva R, Hardy J, Hernandez D. Alpha-synuclein gene haplotypes are associated with Parkinson's disease. Hum Mol Genet 10:1847– 1851, 2001.

50. Krüger R, Vieira-Saecker AM, Kuhn W, Berg D, Müller T, Kühn N, Fuchs GA, Storch A, Hungs M, Woitalla D, Przuntek H, Epplen JT, Schöls L, Riess O. Increased susceptibility to sporadic Parkinson's disease by a certain combined alpha-synuclein/apolipoprotein E genotype. Ann Neurol 45:611– 617, 1999.

51. Maraganore DM, Farrer MJ, Hardy JA, Lincoln SJ, McDonnell SK, Rocca WA. Case-control study of the ubiquitin carboxy-terminal hydrolase L1 gene in Parkinson's disease. Neurology 53:1858–1860, 1999.

52. Zhang J, Hattori N, Leroy E, Morris HR, Kubo S, Kobayashi T, Wood NW, Polymeropoulos MH, Mizuno Y. Association between a polymorphism of ubiquitin carboxy-terminal hydrolase L1 (UCH-L1) gene and sporadic Parkinson's disease. Parkinsonism Relat Disord 6:195–197, 2000.

53. Satoh J, Kuroda Y. A polymorphic variation of serine to tyrosine at codon 18 in the ubiquitin C-terminal hydrolase-L1 gene is associated with a reduced risk of sporadic Parkinson's disease in a Japanese population. J Neurol Sci 189:113–117, 2001.

54. Golbe LI, Lazzarini AM, Spychala JR, Johnson WG, Stenroos ES, Mark MH, Sage JI. The tau A0 allele in Parkinson's disease. Mov Disord 16:442– 447, 2001.

55. Maraganore DM, Hernandez DG, Singleton AB, Farrer MJ, McDonnell SK, Hutton ML, Hardy JA, Rocca WA. Case-control study of the extended tau gene haplotype in Parkinson's disease. Ann Neurol 50:658–661, 2001.

56. Martin ER, Scott WK, Nance MA, Watts RL, Hubble JP, Koller WC, Lyons K, Pahwa R, Stern MB, Colcher A, Hiner BC, Jankovic J, Ondo WG, Allen FH Jr, Goetz CG, Small GW, Masterman D, Mastaglia F, Laing NG, Stajich JM, Ribble RC, Booze MW, Rogala A, Hauser MA, Zhang F, Gibson RA, Middleton LT, Roses AD, Haines JL, Scott BL, Pericak-Vance MA, Vance JM. Association of single-nucleotide polymorphisms of the tau gene with late-onset Parkinson disease. JAMA 286:2245–2250, 2001.

57. Yamazaki K, Wakasugi N, Tomita T, Kikuchi T, Mukoyama M, Ando K. Gracile axonal dystrophy (GAD), a new neurological mutant in the mouse. Proc Soc Exp Biol Med 187:209–215, 1988.

58. Saigoh K, Wang YL, Suh JG, Yamanishi T, Sakai Y, Kiyosawa H, Harada T, Ichihara N, Wakana S, Kikuchi T, Wada K. Intragenic deletion in the gene encoding ubiquitin carboxy-terminal hydrolase in GAD mice. Nat Genet 23:47–51, 1999.

59. Masliah E, Rockenstein E, Veinbergs I, Mallory M, Hashimoto M, Takeda A, Sagara Y, Sisk A, Mucke L. Dopaminergic loss and inclusion body formation in alpha-synuclein mice: implications for neurodegenerative disorders. Science 287:1265–1269, 2000.

60. Kahle PJ, Neumann M, Ozmen L, Muller V, Odoy S, Okamoto N, Jacobsen H, Iwatsubo T, Trojanowski JQ, Takahashi H, Wakabayashi K, Bogdanovic N, Riederer P, Kretzschmar HA, Haass C. Selective insolubility of alpha-synuclein in human Lewy body diseases is recapitulated in a transgenic mouse model. Am J Pathol 159:2215–2225, 2001.

61. Hutton M, Lewis J, Dickson D, Yen SH, McGowan E. Analysis of tauopathies with transgenic mice. Trends Mol Med 7:467–470, 2001.

62. Schenk D, Barbour R, Dunn W, Gordon G, Grajeda H, Guido T, Hu K, Huang J, Johnson-Wood K, Khan K, Kholodenko D, Lee M, Liao Z, Lieberburg I, Motter R, Mutter L, Soriano F, Shopp G, Vasquez N, Vandevert C, Walker S, Wogulis M, Yednock T, Games D, Seubert P. Immunization with amyloid-beta attenuates Alzheimer-disease-like pathology in the PDAPP mouse. Nature 400:173–177, 1999.

15

Environmental Risk Factors for Parkinson's Disease

Jay M. Gorell

Henry Ford Health Sciences Center, Henry Ford Health System, and Wayne State University, Detroit, Michigan, U.S.A.

Benjamin A. Rybicki

Henry Ford Health Sciences Center, Henry Ford Health System, Detroit, Michigan, U.S.A.

INTRODUCTION

The vast majority of Parkinson's disease (PD) is etiologically multifactorial, with important contributions from both genetic and environmental determinants. Very few cases of PD can be attributed to single gene disorders (1–5). For PD without single gene Mendelian inheritance, relative risks as high as 14 for first-degree relatives of PD cases have been reported (6), but most studies have found more modest risks, on the order of two- to fourfold (7–10). Tanner et al. (11), in a study of a World War II cohort of monozygotic (MZ) and dizygotic (DZ) twins, with at least one of each pair with PD, found no difference in concordance between MZ and DZ twins diagnosed after the age of 50, when most PD occurs (12–15). While these studies suggest that, on a population level, a major genetic contribution to

PD is unlikely, there is a potentially important role for genetic susceptibility to environmental exposures in both sporadic and familial cases (16–18). Therefore, to increase our understanding of the etiology of PD, future analytical PD epidemiological studies must focus on better defining environmental factors that confer risk or protection, identifying genetic factors that modify risk, and determining the roles played by these factors, alone and interactively. In this chapter, we will review research on environmental factors implicated in PD, initially with a focus on methodology, and thereafter with a concentration on selected analytical epidemiological studies.

ENVIRONMENTAL FACTORS ASSOCIATED WITH PD

Retrospective Assessment of Occupational Risks: The Paradigm of Metal Exposures

Determining the most suitable methods to assess past occupational exposures, which is essential in all retrospective case-control studies, is an important subject of ongoing research. It is inherently more difficult to evaluate exposures under these circumstances than in a prospective cohort, for which current occupational environments can be assessed and exposures determined directly. The use of expert review of job histories for retrospectively assessing occupationally related exposures has long been used in the field of cancer epidemiology (19,20). Taking a cue from that experience, our group was the first to apply such methodology to the field of neuroepidemiology (21–24).

In our study of occupational metal exposures and PD (21), a case-blind industrial hygienist assessed metal exposure in all jobs held for 6 months or longer for all subjects throughout adult life. The hygienist considered subjects' tasks involving specific metals, the tools used, the ambient environment, and measures taken for protection from exposure. In a parallel methodological study (22), we compared assessment by self-report, job titles linked to a job exposure matrix (JEM) (25), and assignment by an industrial hygienist. Data derived from self-report and a JEM separately, as well as information from both methods, were not comparable with industrial hygienist assessment. Taking industrial hygienist exposure assessment as the gold standard, we showed that the method of exposure assessment can have a large influence on the association between a disease outcome and exposure. This was further highlighted in a recent reanalysis (J. M. Gorell et al., in preparation) of our original published data (21). We found that, if we had relied on self-report alone instead of an industrial hygienist's case-blind rating of factors associated with exposure, no significant results would have emerged. Moreover, had we only assessed ever-exposure to metals instead of also evaluating chronic exposure, no significant findings would have been seen. As opposed to self-report, our expert assessment methodology was very amenable to evaluating exposure duration, which, in hindsight, was critical in teasing apart the PD-occupational metal exposure association.

Despite what appears to be an advantage of expert assessment of metal exposures, similarly trained industrial hygienists can reach different conclusions in reviews of the same data set (19,23,26,27). This issue of subjectivity suggests that it is difficult to reliably transform an occupational history into an estimate of exposure, and implies that it may be desirable to combine such assessments with a more objective measure of chronic exposure to metals, if this is available. Wherever possible, it would seem desirable to compare such data with exposure measurements (e.g., blood and/or bone lead or other metal determinations, or assessments of ambient air, water or soil concentration of toxicants, as appropriate) taken at the time of presumed risk.

As an extension of our experience with retrospective metal exposure assessment, we suggest that employing industrial hygienists or occupational toxicologists with expertise in other fields (e.g., agricultural chemical, soil, water and farming lifestyle exposures; mixing, loading, applying or otherwise using pesticides, metals or organic solvents, etc.) will improve upon self-report or the use of a JEM. Resulting exposure assignments should be compared with specific records of relevant exposures at the time at risk, if available. Finally, it may be helpful to construct a cumulative lifetime exposure history to a toxicant of interest in order to best assess its dose effect on disease outcome.

Occupational Metal Exposure

Metals may be involved in the etiology and/or pathogenesis of PD. For example, manganese (28), copper (29), lead (28), and iron (30) have been shown to promote oxidative stress by free radical generation, an ongoing process in the PD substantia nigra (SN) (30). Iron (as Fe^{3+} and total levels) has been reported to be elevated in the PD SN (31), but copper has either been reported to be increased (32) or decreased (33,34). Manganese may have a role in catecholamine autoxidation (35), in the formation of neuromelanin (36), and, perhaps, in the production of Lewy bodies (37). Copper(II) can react with ascorbate (38) or levodopa (39) to produce genotoxic free radicals. Lead(II) may be directly genotoxic, as it inhibits DNA polymerase (40), possibly hampering DNA repair. This potential action of lead (41) may be particularly important in a neurodegenerative disease associated with aging.

The relationship between occupational exposure to specific metals and PD has been examined infrequently in case-control studies with sizable populations (21,42–46). Results in these studies have varied, likely because of differences involving the means of exposure assessment, the duration of exposure, as well as the populations studied.

Occupational Exposure to Selected Metals and PD

Manganese.   Semchuk et al. (42), in a population-based case-control study in Calgary, Alberta, reported no increase of PD risk for ever-exposure to manganese, assessed by self-report. Seidler et al. (43), in a case-control study of nine German clinics, reported no significant association of PD with any occupational exposure to manganese, assessed by a JEM. Gorell et al. (21) found a significant association of more than 20 years of occupational exposure to manganese [odds ratio (OR) = 10.61], though caution is needed in the interpretation of the relationship, as it was driven by just three cases and one control subject with chronic manganese exposure. Finally, when considering manganese exposure as a risk factor for PD, it is important not to reject a potential association because of confusion with the severe poisoning seen in manganism, in which there is preferential affection of the globus pallidus rather than the SN, with clinical dystonic parkinsonism produced most often (44,45).

Mercury.   Ohlson and Hogstedt (46), in a hospital-based case-control study in Sweden, found no group difference in occupational exposure to mercury, assessed by self-report. Seidler et al. (43) found elevated, but nonsignificant, ORs with respect to neighborhood controls when assessing any occupational contact with mercury. Gorell et al. (21) found no significant association of PD with any occupational exposure to mercury. However, Ngim and Devathasan (47), in a hospital-based case-control study in Singapore, found a significant association between mercury exposure and PD, assessed by self-report. They also found a dose-response relationship when comparing blood mercury levels from the highest tertile (OR = 9.4; 95% CI 2.5–35.9) and middle tertile (OR = 8.5; 95% CI 2.2–33.2) with the lowest tertile of subjects. The lack of consistency in reports regarding an association between mercury exposure and PD weakens the likelihood of its biological significance. However, it is possible that differences in genetic susceptibility among ethnic or racial groups, or different routes of mercury exposure (e.g., ingestion of contaminated foods or medications), may account for the variability in the conclusions of studies thus far.

Iron, Copper, Lead, and Zinc. A potential relationship between occupational exposure to iron, copper, lead, or zinc with PD has been infrequently studied. Seidler et al. (43) did not assess a possible role of iron exposure, but found a slightly elevated, nonsignificant association with any occupational zinc exposure and no relation with copper exposure. However, these authors did find that ever-exposure to lead was associated with PD, though significantly only with reference to one of their two control groups. Gorell et al. (21) reported no association of more than 20 years of occupational zinc exposure with PD, a borderline association with lead alone ($p = 0.059$), and a significant association with more than 20 years of occupational exposure to copper (OR $- 2.49$; 95% CI 1.06–5.89).

Combinations of Metals. Zayed et al. (48), in a study in southern Quebec, reported that, among 42 cases and 84 controls, assessed by self-report, there was a significant association between PD and occupational exposure to a combination of manganese, iron, and aluminum, particularly for more than 30 years (OR $= 13.64$; 95% CI 1.52–76.28). However, the magnitude of contribution of individual metals to the risk of PD could not be determined. Semchuk et al. (42) did not find a significant association of aluminum exposure with PD, evaluated by self-report. In the only study thus far to assess occupational exposure to cadmium, nickel or arsenic, Seidler et al. (43) found no association with PD. Finally, Gorell et al. (21) found that greater than 20 years of occupational exposure to combinations of lead-copper (OR $= 5.24$; 95% CI 1.59–17.21), lead-iron (OR $= 2.83$; 95% CI 1.07–7.50), and iron-copper (OR $= 3.69$; 95% CI 1.40–9.71) were associated with PD. These combined metal exposure results showed a greater association with PD than did any metal alone.

To our knowledge, no investigators have assessed potential genetic risk factors as modifiers of occupational metal exposures, and further research is needed. However, we did evaluate risk modification by a history of PD in first- and second-degree relatives of subjects (10). Among participants in the study of Gorell et al. (21) with a PD family history, occupational exposure to copper, lead, or iron increased the risk, albeit nonsignificantly (OR $= 3.0$; 95% CI 0.7–13.3), but no such trend was found in those without a family history (OR $= 1.1$; 95% CI 0.7–1.6).

Pesticide Exposure

Certain human and animal models of PD have been produced only by exogenous toxicants, highlighting the potential importance of environmental factors in the etiology of the human disease. For example, parkinsonism has been produced by the intravenous injection of the meperidine analog, 1-methyl-4-phenyl-1,2,3,6-tetrahydropyridine (MPTP)

(49), which is chemically similar to the herbicide paraquat (50). MPTP exposure is associated with nigral neuronal death and mimicry of the clinical symptoms and signs and the neurochemical pathology of PD (49–55). MPTP is converted in the brain into 1-methyl-4-phenylpyridinium [MPP$^+$] by astrocytic monoamine oxidase B [MAO-B] (54). MPP$^+$ then enters nigral neurons through the dopamine transporter and is concentrated in mitochondria, where it inhibits Complex I, reduces adenosine triphosphate (ATP) levels, and produces cyto-destructive free radicals (55). Another animal model of PD has recently been produced by rotenone, an insecticide that binds to the same Complex I site as does MPP$^+$, causing nigral neuronal loss thereby (56) and, perhaps, by other biochemical mechanisms (57). Fleming et al. (58) found a significant association between PD, diagnosed postmortem, and the presence of the organochlorine insecticide dieldrin in these brains, and Corrigan et al. (59) confirmed these findings. Finally, exposure of animals to combinations of agents such as the herbicide paraquat and the fungicide maneb (60) also causes nigral neuronal loss. The latter observation suggests that multiple agents may be required to achieve, or to accelerate, the biochemical processes that produce PD.

We surveyed case-control investigations in which queries about pesticide use extended at least to the class level (i.e., insecticides, herbicides, fungicides, etc.), and were not listed simply as "pesticides" or "pesticides/ herbicides." All such studies were limited by one or more of the following factors: (1) poor recall of subjects of particular pesticides to which they might have been exposed; for example, both Semchuck et al. (61,42) and Gorell et al. (62) found no better than 40% recall of specific agents, despite the fact that subjects were given extensive lists of potential pesticides from which to choose; (2) assessment by self-report, rather than by case-blind determinations by agricultural industrial hygienists or agronomists; and (3) lack of validation of self-reported exposure histories.

Several investigations have shown an association between PD and pesticide classes such as insecticides or herbicides (42,61–63), though this has not always been found, and only rarely has the association held for specific agents (e.g., paraquat) (64). For example, Semchuk et al. (61), in Alberta, found in univariate analyses of self-reported exposures an association with insecticides (OR = 2.05; 95% CI 1.03–4.07) and a further increase after more than 46 years of contact (OR = 3.50; 95% CI 1.03– 11.96). In the case of herbicide exposure, the overall crude OR was 3.06 (95% CI 1.34–7.00), and the association also increased with many years of contact (26–35 years: OR = 4.82; 95% CI 1.51–15.35). Moreover, Semchuk et al. (61) found that occupational herbicide exposure remained significant (OR = 3.06; 95% CI 1.34–7.00) after multiple logistical regression analyses that adjusted for other associated factors. Interestingly, this association held against other, more general risk factors (i.e., head injury and a family history of PD) in a test of a multifactorial etiological hypothesis (42). In contrast, Hertzman et al. (65), in a population-based study in British Columbia in 1994, found no significant self-reported associations with insecticides, herbicides, or fungicides, as classes, nor did they find associations with more specific subclasses (i.e., chlorphenoxy herbicides, organochlorines, organophosphates, carbamates, borates, or copper salts). Seidler et al. (43), in a nine clinic–based study in Germany, with results assessed by self report, found no consistent relationship of PD with exposure to insecticides or herbicides, as classes, and associations varied between PD and different control groups for specific agents (i.e., organochlorines, alkylated phosphates, and carbamates). Gorell et al. (62) found significant associations with occupational (not residential) exposure to insecticides (OR = 3.55; 95% CI 1.75–7.18) and herbicides (OR = 4.10; 95% CI 1.37–12.24), but no relationship with fungicide exposure. Finally, a recent investigation of signs of parkinsonism among career orchardists, professional pesticide applicators, and pesticide plant workers in Washington State (66) found an association with long-term pesticide and insecticide use, but no specific pesticides were identified as risk factors. Clearly, further studies that assess exposure to specific agents will be important, as will expert evaluations of such exposures over time.

One study (67) has assessed a potential association of pesticide exposure with polymorphisms of genes that metabolize such agents. These authors, in a study of just 95 PD patients and 95 controls from a variety of university clinic, hospital, and community settings in Australia, found no association between *GST P1* variants and PD. However, when they restricted their analysis to subjects with pesticide exposure (39 cases and 26 controls), a statistically significant ($p = 0.009$) relationship between *GST P1* variants and PD emerged. This work needs confirmation in a larger study.

Farming

The wide variation in the reported association of farming with PD has largely hinged on the definition of farming, whether the duration of farming was studied, and whether farming was examined independently of pesticide exposure. We surveyed case-control studies in which farming was defined by specific areas of work.

Tanner et al. (68), in a study of subjects in neurology clinics in Beijing or Guangzhou, China, found protective, self-reported associations with pig raising (OR = 0.17; $p < 0.001$), wheat growing (OR = 0.4; $p < 0.02$), and chicken raising (OR = 0.53; $p < 0.05$), but no association with corn growing (OR = 0.54; NS), soybean raising (OR = 0.67; NS), fruit growing

(OR = 1.00), rice growing (OR = 1.29; NS), or livestock raising (OR = 0.63; NS). In 1990, Hertzman et al. (69), in a population-based study of self-reported activities among subjects in a mountainous region of British Columbia, Canada, found an age- and sex-adjusted association of orchard work with PD (OR = 4.45; $p = 0.003$), as well as with planer mill work (OR = 3.89; $p < 0.05$). Semchuk et al. (61), in a population-based study in Alberta, Canada, found self-reported ever-farming in the areas of field crop farming, grain farming, market gardening, wood processing, or commercial greenhouse work to be unassociated with PD in overall univariate analyses. However, these authors also found a dose-response relationship with PD for the ages of exposure and duration of farming. That is, with exposure at ages 16–25 (10 years' exposure), ages 16–35 (20 years' exposure), and at ages 16–45 (30 years' exposure), for any form of agricultural work, the OR increased from 1.65 to 2.45 to 3.48. For field crop farming, the OR increased from 1.49 to 2.50 to 3.84; and for grain farming, the OR increased from 1.39 to 2.39 to 4.44. However, after multiple logistical regression, none of these areas of farming was statistically significant ($p < 0.05$), whereas only occupational exposure to herbicides survived these multiple adjustments (OR = 3.06; 95% CI 1.34–7.00). In contrast, Hertzman et al., in 1994 (65), did not find a significant association with PD in their study in a defined horticultural region of British Columbia, whether farming was evaluated overall, or whether animal farming, crop farming, mixed farming, or soft or hard fruit orchard farming were analyzed; this study, then, did not replicate their 1990 results (69) with orchardist activities. Gorell et al. (62) evaluated, as a single category, activities reported as either grain or vegetable farming, fruit or nut farming, field crop farming, diversified crop farming, domestic animal farming, domestic fowl farming and general farming, using codes in the *Dictionary of Occupational Titles* (70). Farming as an occupation after age 18, following adjustment for sex, race, age, and smoking status, was associated with PD (OR = 2.79; 95% CI 1.03–7.55). Moreover, in joint models with occupational exposure to herbicides and fungicides, farming remained significant after adjustment for occupational herbicide exposure, though it was of borderline significance ($p = 0.052$) after adjustment for occupational insecticide exposure. Our results suggest that pesticide exposure could not account for all the risk conferred by farming and that other lifestyle and environmental exposures related to farming need to be considered in future work.

Rural Living

This category of exposure is vague and has been variably defined. It has been difficult to find consistency in results. We reviewed studies in which some attempt at definition was made.

Rajput et al. (71) found a significant ($p = 0.015$) association between PD among 15 cases with onset under age 40 and living in communities in Saskatchewan of less than 140 persons. Tanner et al. (68), in a study in China, defined "rural" as a history of living in a village; so designated, the association with PD was protective ($OR = 0.57$; $p < 0.05$). In contrast, Koller et al. (72), in a study in Kansas, considered subjects who lived in a town with a population less than 2500 (U.S. Census Bureau criterion) and found a positive association with PD ($OR = 1.9$; $p = 0.01$). Butterfield et al. (63), working with several clinic and support group populations in Oregon and Washington, defined "rural" as living in a locale with less than 10,000 people at the time of diagnosis, and reported an OR of 2.72 ($p = 0.27$). Gorell et al. (62) defined "rural" as living in a "small town or less populated area" and found no association, nor was there a relationship with living or working on a farm (namely, independent of farming as an occupation).

Well Water Consumption

The study of Tanner et al. (68), in China, found no significant association of well water consumption and PD, and neither did Zayed et al. (48), in Quebec, Semchuck et al. (73) in Alberta, Butterfield et al. (63) in Oregon and Washington, Hertzman et al. (65) in British Columbia, Seidler et al. (43) in Germany, and Gorell et al. (62) in Michigan. In contrast, Koller et al. (72) in Kansas (OR 1.7; $p = 0.03$) and Jimenez-Jimenez et al. (74) in Madrid, Spain ($p < 0.02$), did find a relationship.

Smoking

Morens et al. (75) reviewed 35 separate case-control studies published by others through 1993, and found 34 reporting an inverse relationship with PD and smoking. Typically, the effect was robust, with odds ratios of about 0.5. Since then, Hellenbrand et al. (76), in a case-control study in Germany, found an inverse dose-response relationship relating never-smokers to ex-smokers and current smokers, stratified according to the pack-years smoked prior to diagnosis in cases versus neighborhood or regional controls. Gorell et al. (77) also found an inverse dose-response effect with PD, with those who were heavy, current smokers (>30 pack-years) being most protected ($OR = 0.08$ vs. never-smokers), and former smokers having an intermediate degree of protection. Nelson et al. (78) also showed an inverse dose-response effect, with a greater decrease with increased duration of smoking or pack-years. In contrast, Benedetti et al. (79), in Olmsted county, Minnesota, found no association of PD with smoking.

To our knowledge, the potential modification of smoking risk by specific genetic factors has not been studied. However, several investigations have used family history as a potential surrogate for genetic risk. For example, Rybicki et al. (10) found that ever smoking cigarettes was inversely associated with PD in those without a PD family history (OR = 0.6; 95% CI 0.4–0.9), but was positively associated with PD in those with a PD family history (OR = 1.7; 95% CI 0.5–5.9). Elbaz et al. (80), in the Europarkinson Study Group's case-control investigation of the relationship between a family history of PD in first-degree relatives and smoking, found interesting results. That is, among individuals over the age of 75, exposure to both factors gave an OR of 17.6 (95% CI 1.9–160.5), whereas among younger subjects the OR for joint exposure was not significant. Results of these studies (10,80) suggest that one or more genetic or (unmeasured) environmental factors reverse the usual inverse relationship between smoking and PD, though the determination of the time during adult life when such factors act as modifiers will require further research.

Finally, findings concerning smoking among monozygotic (MZ) and dizygotic (DZ) twins in the World War II cohort have been published (81). There was a high within-pair correlation of smoking among MZ twins but not among DZ twins. Analysis of smoking among 33 MZ and 39 DZ twin pairs discordant for PD, in which at least one twin of each pair smoked, revealed that twins without PD had smoked more pack-years than those who had the disease. This effect was more marked among MZ pairs, implying that sharing a greater number of genes, of unspecified identity, magnifies the PD-smoking relationship.

The usual controversy in retrospective case-control studies involving smoking is whether the inverse association with PD that has been found most often is biologically meaningful or an artifact of study design. Potential artifactual explanations might include: (1) selective mortality of smokers who were destined to acquire PD, resulting in fewer smoking PD subjects available to recruit, (2) suppression of PD signs and symptoms by smoking, allowing PD cases to masquerade as controls, (3) a cause-effect bias, in which previous smokers who acquired PD would quit smoking after becoming symptomatic or being diagnosed with the condition, or (4) unmeasured confounding factors (e.g., premorbid personality factors; depletion of nonstriatal brain dopamine; an undiscovered genetic risk factor; consumption of alcohol or coffee; etc.) that may reduce the likelihood of smoking.

Despite such concerns, prospective cohort studies have supported conclusions reached in most case-control investigations regarding smoking and PD. For example, the Honolulu Asia-Aging Study, a prospective cohort investigation since 1965 of 8006 males of Japanese ancestry (82), reported an inverse dose-response relation with PD, depending on the history of pack-years smoked. Morens et al. (83), from the same group, found that age-specific mortality trends for smokers with and without PD was mostly associated with the illness itself and not with smoking. Recently, Hernan et al. (84) reported analyses of data from the Nurses Health Study (1976–1996) and the Health Professionals Follow-Up Study (1986–1996). These authors found, in women, age-adjusted rate ratios for PD for past smokers versus never-smokers of 0.7 (95% CI 0.5–1.0) and 0.4 (0.2–0.7) for current smokers. In men, age adjusted rate ratios for PD in past smokers versus never-smokers were 0.5 (0.4–0.7) and 0.3 (0.1–0.8) for current smokers. Data from both cohorts revealed an inverse association with time since quitting among former smokers, which was strengthened considering the number of cigarettes smoked by current smokers and considering the number of pack-years smoked.

Possible biological explanations for a protective effect of smoking include: (1) the reduction of MAO B activity in smokers (85), which might slow dopamine catabolism (86) or diminish activation of MPTP-like neurotoxicants (87); (2) catecholamine stimulation by nicotine (88); (3) nicotine-induced production of neurotrophic factors that stimulate dopaminergic neuron survival (89); and (4) nicotine-induced attenuation of the expected dopaminergic cell loss from MPP^+ in mesencephalic neuron cultures (90) and nigral neuronal damage in animal models of parkinsonsim (91 94). Behavioral explanations, such as risk avoidance among persons who may be prone to PD (95), also deserve consideration, though definitive data are lacking. Finally, Ross et al. (96), in a postmortem study of Lewy body counts in SN from PD in the Honolulu Asia-Aging Study, were unable to find a relationship with lifetime smoking histories. However, there appears to be a PD-protective effect in the (indirect) action of a MAO-B G allele (97), which deserves further study.

Caffeine

There is evidence that caffeine is a significant protective factor in PD (79,98–100), inasmuch as its effects appear to be independent after adjustments for smoking are made. In the Honolulu Asia-Aging Study (99), among 102 incident PD cases in a cohort of 8006 Japanese-American men, the age-adjusted incidence of PD declined consistently with increased amounts of coffee intake, from 10.4 per 10,000 person-years in men who drank no coffee to 1.9 per 10,000 person-years in men who drank at least 28 oz./day. Similar trends were seen with total caffeine intake. Ascherio et al. (100) reported data from two prospective cohorts, the Health Professionals Follow-Up Study and the Nurses Health Study, with a total of 47,351 men and 88,565 women. Among men, after adjustment for age and smoking, there was a relative risk of PD of 0.42 for those in the top one fifth of caffeine intake compared with those in the bottom fifth. Similar trends were seen for coffee and tea, considered separately. Among women, the relationship between caffeine or coffee intake and the risk of PD was U-shaped, with the lowest risk seen with moderate intake, equivalent to 1–3 cups of coffee/day, or the third quintile of caffeine consumption.

The mechanism underlying the action of caffeine in PD is not established, though recent work in animals (101) suggests that caffeine protects against MPTP-parkinsonism by antagonism of brain adenosine A2A receptors.

Alcohol

There is less consistency among reports of the relationship between alcohol intake and PD. Hellenbrand et al. (98) found an inverse association with beer and spirits, but not with wine. Nelson et al. (78) found a significant inverse association of alcohol intake just preceding the diagnosis of PD, as well as a significant inverse dose-response trend relating weekly alcohol consumption to PD risk. However, Gorell et al. (77) reported that both light to moderate and heavy drinkers had an inverse relationship with PD, though neither value was statistically significant, nor was there a dose-response trend between alcohol use and PD risk. In the latter study, alcohol attenuated, but did not abolish, the inverse association of PD with smoking. Clearly, further work will be needed to clarify these differing results.

Diet

Retrospective dietary assessments are notoriously difficult, but may give acceptable levels of misclassification for periods of food consumption up to 10 years before the time when questioning occurs (102). This may often be adequate since dietary habits rarely change significantly over the course of adult life, except during episodes of severe general medical illnesses or depression. However, we should remember that study participants are typically asked to mentally project themselves back in time to a period before the diagnosis was made. Such a procedure may be inaccurate. Moreover, there remains some concern that having the preclinical illness may change dietary habits. If that were to occur, there could be a bias because of systematic misclassification of cases relative to control subjects, whether the nutrient(s) in question was/were or was/were not related to the disease etiology. A final methodological point is that the more recent use of food frequency questionnaires that reduce food or nutritional supplement consumption to nutrients from all sources (103,104) appears to be an advance. However, unless all nutrients are included in assessment software programs, there is a possibility that data derived from food or supplement intake may not disclose relationships involving potentially important, unmeasured factors.

In the field of nutritional epidemiology in PD, there has been a continuing interest in a potential relationship between intake of antioxidant foods and/or supplements and the disease. However, there are inconsistent reports of a relationship between dietary intake of vitamin E–rich foods or vitamin E itself and PD, with most studies finding no association (105–111). Others have found an association of PD with the intake of carotenoids (106,109), as well as with lutein, individually (110). Two studies have had divergent results regarding whether iron intake differs between cases and controls, with Logroscino et al. (106) finding no such relationship and Johnson et al. (110) finding that iron intake was greater among PD patients in the highest quartile of consumption.

There is some suggestion of an elevated PD risk related to diets with high fat content (106,110,111), and with cholesterol, specifically (110). More studies will be needed to clarify this important area of PD epidemiology.

Head Trauma

There have been inconsistent associations of head trauma with PD (112,113). One important methodological issue is the frequent lack of specification of the neurological consequences of the injury. For example, there are reports of parkinsonism with other deficits (e.g., corticospinal, cognitive, and other functional disorders) in some case series. Moreover, much work involves the study of prevalent cases and the use of convenience controls (e.g., spouses, not sex-matched subjects), raising questions about the interpretation of results that have been found. Most authors recognize the potential of recall bias among cases, particularly if the injuries were dramatic, and especially in retrospective case-control series.

Semchuk et al. (42), in a population-based case-control study in Alberta, found head injury, without specification as to its neurological severity, to confer significant risk of PD (OR 3.67; 95% CI 1.86–7.26). Moreover, head injury was retained in a logistical regression model containing a number of unrelated risk factors found in univariate analyses. We also assessed head injury as a potential risk factor for PD (Gorell et al., in preparation), and required that it be associated with loss of consciousness, but found no significant relationship with the disease (OR = 1.07; 95% CI 0.64–1.76). We cannot account for the difference between our research and that of Semchuk et al. (42), but suggest that future work try to grade the severity of injury, particularly whether consciousness was lost and whether there were significant cognitive or motor complications.

Infectious Disease

This category of prior illness has been discussed as a potential risk factor since the occurrence of encephalitis lethargica in the early years of the twentieth century (114). Because of the circumstantial association of postencephalitic parkinsonism with the influenza pandemic in 1918–1919 (115), attempts to isolate influenza A virus from PD brain (116), or to show a positive case-control difference in serum levels of antibody (117,118), were made, without success. Epidemiological studies by Kessler (119,120), in both hospital- and community-based settings, suggested that PD cases were less likely than matched controls to have had self-reported infections with measles, mumps, German measles and chickenpox, though no associations reached statistical significance. Sasco and Paffenbarger (121), in a case-control study that followed two cohorts of college undergraduates through adult life, found a significant inverse association of PD with measles prior to college entrance (OR = 0.53; 95% CI 0.31–0.93). However, this finding has remained unexplained.

More recently, a temporarily levodopa-responsive movement disorder in mice induced by *Nocardia asteroides* has been described in a group of infected animals with a head tremor (122). These mice had a loss of tyrosine hydroxylase-bearing neurons in the SN and ventral tegmental brain regions, with inclusions that resembled Lewy bodies in some respects. However, there were no specific remnants of nocardial infection, pathologically, at the time of the movement disorder. These intriguing results have not been matched with epidemiological support in the only study done so far (123).

Solvent Exposure

This potentially important area has not been explored very thoroughly. A few studies (43,46) found no overall association with solvent exposure. However, Smargiassi et al. (124) found a relationship with a broad category of "industrial chemicals" (OR = 2.13; 95% CI 1.16–3.91), and a more recent study (125), focusing on hydrocarbon exposure, reported a suggestive correlation with PD severity ($r = 0.311$) and an inverse relationship with disease latency ($r = -0.252$). More research involving specific exposures is warranted.

SUMMARY

Several risk and protective environmental factors for PD have been discovered. However, many areas of uncertainty remain, partly because of methodological issues:

1. Many studies have had small samples, often using tertiary medical referral or other convenience subjects and inappropriately chosen controls.
2. The diagnostic accuracy of PD cases has been variable.

3. Most studies have enrolled prevalent rather than incident or near-incident cases, raising the issue of not having identified etiologically relevant risk factors but, rather, factors related to survival with the disease.
4. Exposures have often been defined in broad categories, not at the level of specific agents, and objective, validated measures of exposures have rarely been found or tested.
5. Only a few cohort studies of PD that provide prospective risk factor data have been performed.

More sophistication can be expected in analytical PD epidemiology in the future. Thus far, it has been easier to measure genetic than environmental risk factors in PD. A sense of certainty seems to attach to identification of a potential genetic risk factor because a specific assay has been performed on some tissue sample (e.g., blood, postmortem brain tissue), whereas environmental risk factors have been assessed with variable methodology and sophistication. However, more complexity in both genetic and environmental research can be expected in the future. For example, it is likely that multiple genes helping to determine a phenotypic outcome, and the interactive, quantitative effects of gene activation or suppression, rather than only the presence or absence of polymorphisms of portions of genes, will be studied. In addition, increasingly sophisticated environmental measures of ever more specific risk and protective factors by experts such as industrial hygienists, agronomists, and occupational toxicologists will be done. Advances in molecular biology and further insights into toxicant exposure assessment may provide better biomarkers of chronic exposure. More analytical studies will become population-based (126) and will employ suitable samples of cases and controls. Reviewers of evidence for and against potential risk factors for PD will consider the adequacy of methods used by investigators in studies surveyed for such updates. More studies will investigate both environmental and genetic factors together, rather than simply evaluating one or the other influence on disease etiology. Finally, it will be appreciated that, to study gene-environment interactions properly, populations will need to be large enough to have sufficient statistical power to study environmental and genetic factors present at low frequency (127,128).

ACKNOWLEDGMENTS

This work was supported by the National Institute of Environmental Health Sciences (ES 06418) award to JMG, as well as by the William T. Gossett Parkinson's Disease Center and Louis Hayman Parkinson's Disease

Research Fund, both of the Department of Neurology, Henry Ford Health System.

REFERENCES

1. Polymeropoulos MH, Lavedan C, Leroy E, Ide SE, Dehejia A, Dutra A, Pike B, Root H, Rubenstein J, Boyer R, Stenroos ES, Chandrasekharappa S, Athanassiadou A Papapetropoulos T, Johnson WG, Lazzarini AM, Duvoisin RC, Di Iorio G, Golbe LI, Nussbaum RL, et al. Mutation in the α-synuclein gene identified in families with Parkinson's disease. Science 1997; 276:2045–2047.
2. Kruger R, Kuhn W, Muller T, Woitalla D, Graeber M, Kosel S, Przuntek H, Epplen JT, Schols L, Riess O. Ala30Pro mutation in the gene encoding α-synuclein in Parkinson's disease. Nat Genet 1998; 18:106–108.
3. Gasser T, Muller-Myhsok B, Wszolek ZK, Oehlmann R, Calne DB, Bonifati V, Bereznai B, Fabrizio E, Vieregge P, Horstmann RD. A susceptibility locus for Parkinson's disease maps to chromosome 2p13. Nat Genet 1998; 18:262–265.
4. Vaughan JR, Davis MB, Wood NW. Genetics of parkinsonism: a review. Ann Hum Genet 2001; 65: 111–120.
5. Mouradian MM. Recent advances in the genetics and pathogenesis of Parkinson disease. Neurology 2002; 58:179–185.
6. De Michele G, Filla A, Volpe G, De Marco V, Gogliettino A, Ambrosio G, Marconi R, Castellano AE, Campanella G. Environmental and genetic risk factors in Parkinson's disease: a case-control study in southern Italy. Mov Disord 1996; 11:17–23.
7. Payami H, Larsen K, Bernard S, Nutt J. Increased risk of Parkinson's disease in parents and siblings of patients. Ann Neurol 1994; 36:659–661.
8. Plante-Bordeneuve V, Taussig D, Thomas F, Ziegler M, Said G. A clinical and genetic study of familial cases of Parkinson's disease. J Neurol Sci 1995; 133:164–172.
9. Marder K, Tang MX, Mejia H, Alfaro B, Cote L, Louis E, Groves J, Mayeux R. Risk of Parkinson's disease among first-degree relatives: a community-based study. Neurology 1996; 47:155–160.
10. Rybicki BA, Johnson CC, Peterson EL, Kortsha GX, Gorell JM. A family history of Parkinson's disease (PD) and its effect on other PD risk factors. Neuroepidemiology 1999; 18:270–278.
11. Tanner CM, Ottman R, Goldman SM, Ellenberg J, Chan P, Mayeux R, Langston JW. Parkinson disease in twins: an etiologic study. JAMA 1999; 281:341–346.
12. De Rijk MC, Breteler MMB, Graveland GA, Ott A, Grobbee DE, van der Meche FGA, Hofman A. Prevalence of Parkinson's disease in the elderly: The Rotterdam Study. Neurology 1995; 45:2143–2146.
13. Mayeux R, Marder K, Cote LJ, Denaro J, Hemenegildo N, Mejia H, Tang M-X, Lantingua R, Wilder D, Gurland B, Hauser A. The frequency of idiopathic

Parkinson's disease by age, ethnic group, and sex in northern Manhattan, 1988–1993. Am J Epdemiol 1995; 142:820–827.

14. Fall P-A, Axelson O, Fredriksson M, Hanson G, Lindvall B, Olsson J-E, Granerus A-K. Age standardized incidence and prevalence of Parkinson's disease in a Swedish community. J Clin Epidemiol 1996; 49:637–641.

15. Morens DM, Davis JW, Grandinetti A, Ross GW, Popper JS, White LR. Epidemiologic observations on Parkinson's disease: incidence and mortality in a prospective study of middle-aged men. Neurology 1996; 46:1044–1050.

16. Barbeau A, Roy M, Bernier G, Campanella G, Paris S. Ecogenetics of Parkinson's disease: prevalence and environmental aspects in rural areas. Can J Neurol Sci 1987; 14:36–41.

17. Costa LG. The emerging field of ecogenetics. NeuroToxicology 2000; 21:85–90.

18. Gorell JM, Checkoway H. Parkinson's disease, environment and genes. Epidemiological studies: risk factors. Session IV Summary and Research Needs. NeuroToxicology 2001; 22:837–844.

19. Gerin M, Siemiatycki J, Kemper H, Begin D. Obtaining occupational exposure histories in epidemiologic case-control studies. J Occup Med 1985; 27:420–426.

20. Siemiatycki J, Day NE, Fabry J, Cooper JA. Discovering carcinogens in the occupational environment: a novel epidemiologic approach. J Natl Cancer Inst 1981; 66:217 225.

21. Gorell JM, Johnson CC, Rybicki BA, Peterson EL, Kortsha GX, Brown GG, Richardson RJ. Occupational exposures to metals as risk factors for Parkinson's disease. Neurology 1997; 48:650–658.

22. Rybicki BA, Johnson CC, Peterson EL, Kortsha GX, Gorell JM. Comparability of different methods of retrospective exposure assessment of metals in manufacturing industries. Am J Ind Med 1997; 31:36–43.

23. Rybicki BA, Peterson EL, Johnson CC, Kortsha GX, Cleary WM, Gorell, JM. Intra- and inter-rater agreement in the assessment of occupational exposure to metals. Int J Epidemiol 1998; 27:269–273.

24. Gorell JM, Rybicki BA, Johnson CC, Peterson EL. Occupational metal exposures and the risk of Parkinson's disease. Neuroepidemiology 1999; 18:303–308.

25. Sieber WKJ, Sundin DS, Frazier TM, Robinson CF. Development, use, and availability of a job exposure matrix based on national occupational hazard survey data. Am J Ind Med 1991; 20:163–174.

26. Goldberg MS, Siemiatycki J, Gerin M. Inter-rater agreement in assessing occupational exposure in a case-control study. Br J Ind Med 1986; 43:667–676.

27. Siemiatycki J, Fritschi L, Nadon L, Gerin, M. Reliability of an expert rating procedure for retrospective assessment of occupational exposures in community-based case-control studies. Am J Ind Med 1997; 31:280–286.

28. Kawanishi S. Role of active oxygen species in metal-induced DNA damage. In: RA Goyer, MG Cherian, eds. Handbook of Experimental Pharmacology,

Vol. 115. Toxicology of Metals—Biochemical Aspects. New York: Springer-Verlag, 1995:349–371.

29. Goldstein S, Czapski G. The role and mechanism of metal ions and their complexes in enhancing damage in biological systems or in protecting these systems from the toxicity of O_2. J Free Radic Biol Med 1986; 2:3–11.

30. Gerlach M, Ben-Shachar D, Riederer P, Youdim MBH. Altered brain metabolism of iron as a cause of neurodegenerative diseases? J Neurochem 1994; 63:793–807.

31. Sofic E, Paulus W, Jellinger K, Riederer P, Youdim MB. Selective increase of iron in substantia nigra zona compacta of parkinsonian brains. J Neurochem 1991; 56:978–982.

32. Riederer P, Sofic E, Rausch WD, Schmidt B, Reynolds GP, Jellinger K, Youdim MB. Transition metals, ferritin, glutathione, and ascorbic acid in parkinsonian brains. J Neurochem 1989; 52:515–520.

33. Dexter DT, Wells FR, Lees AJ, Agid F, Jenner P, Marsden CD. Increased nigral iron content and alterations in other metal ions occurring in brain in Parkinson's disease. J Neurochem 1989; 52:1830–1836.

34. Uitti RJ, Rajput AH, Rozdilsky B, Bickis M, Wollin T, Yuen WK. Regional metal concentrations in Parkinson's disease, other chronic neurological diseases, and control brains. Can J Neurol Sci 1989; 16:310–314.

35. Archibald FS, Tyree C. Manganese poisoning and the attack of trivalent manganese upon catecholamines. Arch Biochem Biophys 1987; 256:638–650.

36. Graham DG. Oxidative pathways for catecholamines in the genesis of neuromelanin and cytotoxic quinones. Mol Pharmacol 1978; 14:633–643.

37. Montine TJ, Farris DB, Graham DG. Covalent crosslinking of neurofilament proteins by oxidized catechols as a potential mechanism of Lewy body formation. J Neuropathol Exp Neurol 1995; 54:311–319.

38. Stich HF, Wei L, Whiting RF. Enhancement of the chromosome-damaging action of some reducing agents. Cancer Res 1979; 39:4115–4151.

39. Spencer JP, Jenner A, Aruoma OI, Evans PJ, Kaur H, Dexter DT, Jenner P, Lees AJ, Marsden CD, Halliwell B. Intense oxidative DNA damage promoted by L-dopa and its metabolites. Implications for neurodegenerative disease. FEBS Lett 1994; 353:246–250.

40. Popenoe EA, Schmaeler MA. Interaction of human DNA polymerase beta with ions of copper, lead and cadmium. Arch Biochem Biophys 1979; 106:190–201.

41. Rao KS. Genomic damage and its repair in young and aging brain. Mol Neurobiol 1993; 7:23–48.

42. Semchuk KM, Love EJ, Lee RG. Parkinson's disease: a test of the multifactorial etiologic hypothesis. Neurology 1993; 43:1173–1180.

43. Seidler A, Hellenbrand W, Robra BP, Vieregge P, Nischan P, Joerg J, Oertel WH, Ulm G, Schneider E. Possible environmental, occupational and other etiologic factors for Parkinson's disease: a case-control study in Germany. Neurology 1996; 46:1275–1284.

44. Cook DG, Fahn S, Brait KA. Chronic manganese intoxication. Arch Neurol 1974; 30:59–64.
45. Calne DB, Chu NS, Huang CC, Lu CS, Olanow CW. Manganism and idiopathic Parkinsonism: similarities and differences. Neurology 1994; 44:1583–1586.
46. Ohlson CG, Hogstedt C. Parkinson's disease and occupational exposure to organic solvents, agricultural chemicals and mercury: A case-referent study. Scand J Work Environ Health 1981; 7:252–256.
47. Ngim CII, Devathasan G. Epidemiologic study on the association between body burden mercury level and idiopathic Parkinson's disease. Neuroepidemiology 1989; 8:128–141.
48. Zayed J, Ducic S, Campanella G, Panisset JC, Andre P, Masson H, Roy M. Facteurs environnementaux dans l'étiologie de la maladie de Parkinson. Can J Neurol Sci 1990; 17:286–291.
49. Langston JW, Ballard PA, Tetrud JW, Irwin I. Chronic parkinsonism in humans due to a product of meperidine analog synthesis. Science 1983; 219:979–980.
50. Burns RS, Chiueh CC, Markey SP, Ebert MII, Jacobowitz DM, Kopin IJ. A primate model of parkinsonism: selective destruction of dopaminergic neurons in the pars compacta or the substantia nigra by N-methyl-4-phenyl-1,2,3,6-tetrahydropyridine. Proc Natl Acad Sci USA 1983; 80:4546–4550.
51. Singer TP, Castagnoli N Jr, Ramsay RR, Trevor AJ. Biochemical events in the development of parkinsonism induced by 1-methyl-4-phenyl-1,2,3,6-tetrahydropyridine. J Neurochem 1987; 49:1–8.
52. Nicklas WJ, Vyas I, Heikkila RE. Inhibition of NADH-linked oxidation in brain mitochondria by 1-methyl-4-phenyl-pyridine, a metabolite of the neurotoxin 1-methyl-4-phenyl-1,2,3,6-tetrahydropyridine. Life Sci 1985; 36:2503–2508.
53. Temlett JA, Landsberg JP, Watt F, Grime GW. Increased iron in the substantia nigra compacta of the MPTP-lesioned hemiparkinsonian African green monkey: evidence from proton microprobe elemental microanalysis. J Neurochem 1994; 62:134–146.
54. Swerdlow RH, Parks JK, Miller SW, Tuttle JB, Trimmer PA, Sheehan JP, Bennett JP Jr, Davis RE, Parker WD Jr. Origin and functional consequences of Complex I defect in Parkinson's disease. Ann Neurol 1996; 40:663–671.
55. Schapira AHV, Cooper JM, Dexter D, Clark JB, Jenner P, Marsden CD. Mitochondrial complex I deficiency in Parkinson's disease. J Neurochem 1990; 54:823–827.
56. Betarbet R, Sherer TB, MacKenzie G, Garcia-Osuna M, Panov AV, Greenamyre JT. Chronic systemic pesticide exposure reproduces features of Parkinson's disease. Nat Neurosci. 2000; 3:1301–1306.
57. Gao H-M, Hong J-S, Zhang W, Liu B. Distinct role for microglia in rotenone-induced degeneration of dopaminergic neurons. J Neurosci 2002; 22:782–790.

58. Fleming L, Mann JB, Bean J, Briggle T, Sanchez-Ramos JR. Parkinson's disease and brain levels of organochlorine pesticides. Ann Neurol 1994; 36:100–103.

59. Corrigan FM, Wienburg CL, Shore RF, Daniel SE, Mann D. Organochlorine insecticides in substantia nigra in Parkinson's disease. J Toxicol Environ Health, Part A 2000; 59:229–234.

60. Thiruchelvam M, Brockel BJ, Richfield EK, Baggs RB, Cory-Slechta DA. Potentiated and preferential effects of combined paraquat and maneb on nigrostriatal dopamine systems: environmental risk factors for Parkinson's disease. Brain Res 2000; 873:225–234.

61. Semchuk KM, Love EJ, Lee RG. Parkinson's disease and exposure to agricultural work and pesticide chemicals. Neurology 1992; 42:1328–1335.

62. Gorell JM, Johnson CC, Rybicki BA, Peterson EL, Richardson RJ. The risk of Parkinson's disease with exposure to pesticides, farming, well water, and rural living. Neurology 1998; 50:1346–1350.

63. Butterfield PG, Valanis BG, Spencer PS, Lindeman CA, Nutt JG. Environmental antecedents of young-onset Parkinson's disease. Neurology 1993; 43:1150–1158.

64. Liou HH, Tsai MC, Chen CJ, Jeng JS, Chang YC, Chen SY, Chen RC. Environmental risk factors and Parkinson's disease: a case-control study in Taiwan. Neurology 1997; 48:1583–1588.

65. Hertzman D, Wiens M, Snow B, Kelly, Calne DB. A case-control study of Parkinson's disease in a horticultural region of British Columbia. Mov Disord 1994; 9:69–75.

66. Engel LS, Checkoway H, Keifer MC, Seixas NS, Longstreth WT Jr., Scott KC, Hudnell K, Anger WK, Camicioli R. Parkinsonism and occupational exposure to pesticides. Occup Environ Med 2001; 58:582–589.

67. Menegon A, Board PG, Blackburn AC, Mellick GD, Le Couteur DG. Parkinson's disease, pesticides, and glutathione transferase polymorphisms. Lancet 1998; 352:1344–1346.

68. Tanner CM, Chen B, Wang W, Peng M, Liu Z, Liang X, Kao LC, Gilley DW, Goetz CG, Schoenberg BS. Environmental factors and Parkinson's disease: a case-control study in China. Neurology 1989; 39:660–664.

69. Hertzman C, Wiens M, Bowering D, Snow B, Calne D. Parkinson's disease: a case-control study of occupational environmental risk factors. Am J Ind Med 1990; 17:349–355.

70. Dictionary of Occupational Titles, 4th ed. U.S. Department of Labor, Employment, and Training Administration. Lanham, MD: Bernan Press, 1991.

71. Rajput AH, Uitti RJ, Stern W, Laverty W, O'Donnell K, O'Donnell D, Yuen WH, Dua A. Geography, drinking water chemistry, pesticides and herbicides and the etiology of Parkinson's disease. Can J Neurol Sci 1987; 14:414–418.

72. Koller W, Vetere-Overfield B, Gray C, Alexander C, Chin T, Dolezal J, Hassanein R, Tanner C. Environmental risk factors in Parkinson's disease. Neurology 1990; 40:1218–1221.

73. Semchuk KM, Love EJ, Lee RG. Parkinson's disease and exposure to rural environmental factors: a population based case-control study. Can J Neurol Sci 1991; 18:279–286.

74. Jimenez-Jimenez FJ, Mateo D, Gimenez-Roldan S. Exposure to well water and pesticides in Parkinson's disease: a case-control study in the Madrid area. Mov Disord 1992; 7:149–152.

75. Morens DM, Grandinetti A, Reed D, White LR, Ross GW. Cigarette smoking and protection from Parkinson's disease: false association or etiologic clue? Neurology 1995; 45:1041–1051.

76. Hellenbrand W, Seidler A, Robra BP, Vieregge P, Oertel WH, Joerg J, Nischan P, Schneider E, Ulm G. Smoking and Parkinson's disease: a case-control study in Germany. Int J Epidemiol 1997; 26:328–339.

77. Gorell JM, Rybicki BA, Johnson CC, Peterson EL. Smoking and Parkinson's disease: a dose-response relationship. Neurology 1999; 52:115–119.

78. Nelson LM, Van den Eeden SK, Tanner CM, Bernstein AL, Harrington DP. Association of alcohol and tobacco consumption with Parkinson's disease: a population-based study. Neurology 1999; 52(suppl 2):A538–539.

79. Benedetti MD, Bower JH, Maraganore DM, McDonnell SK, Peterson BJ, Ahlskog JE, Schaid DJ, Rocca WA. Smoking, alcohol, and coffee consumption preceding Parkinson's disease: a case-control study. Neurology 2000; 55:1350–1358.

80. Elbaz A, Manubens-Bertran JM, Baldereschi M, Breteler MMB, Grigoletto F, Lopez-Pousa S, Dartigues J-F, Alperovitch A, Rocca WA, Tzourio C. Parkinson's disease, smoking, and family history. J Neurol 2000; 247:793–798.

81. Tanner CM, Goldman SM, Aston DA, Ottman R, Ellenberg J, Mayeux R, Langston JW. Smoking and Parkinson's disease in twins. Neurology 2002; 58:581–588.

82. Grandinetti A, Morens DM, Reed D, MacEachern D. Prospective study of cigarette smoking and the risk of developing idiopathic Parkinson's disease. Am J Epidemiol 1994; 139:1129–1138.

83. Morens DM, Grandinetti A, Davis JW, Ross GW, White LR, Reed D. Evidence against the operation of selective mortality in explaining the association between cigarette smoking and reduced occurrence of idiopathic Parkinson disease. Am J Epidemiol 1996; 144:400–404.

84. Hernan MA, Zhang SM, Rueda-de Castro AM, Colditz GA, Speizer FE, Ascherio A. Cigarette smoking and the incidence of Parkinson's disease in two prospective studies. Ann Neurol 2001; 50:780–786.

85. Fowler JS, Volkow ND, Wang GJ, Pappas N, Logan J, MacGregor R, Alexoff D, Shea C, Schyler DJ, Wolf AP, Warner D, Zezulkova I, Cilento R. Inhibition of monoamine oxidase B in the brains of smokers. Nature 1996; 379:733–736.

86. Riederer P, Konradi C, Hebestreit C, Youdim MBH. Neurochemical perspectives to the function of monoamine oxidase. Acta Neurol Scand 1989; 126:41–45.

87. Chiba K, Trevor A, Castagnoli N. Metabolism of the neurotoxic tertiary amine, MPTP, by brain monoamine oxidase. Biochem Biophys Res Commun 1984; 120:574–578.

88. Seppa T, Ahtee L. Comparison of the effects of epibatidine and nicotine on the output of dopamine in the dorsal and ventral striatum of freely-moving rats. Naunyn Schmiedebergs Arch Pharmacol 2000; 362:444–447.

89. Maggio R, Riva M, Vaglini F, Fornai F, Molteni R, Armogida M, Racagni G, Corsini GU. Nicotine prevents experimental parkinsonism in rodents and induces striatal increase of neurotrophic factors. J Neurochem 1998; 71:2439–2446.

90. Quik M, Jeyarasasingam G. Nicotinic receptors and Parkinson's disease. Eur J Pharmacol 2000; 393:223–2230.

91. Janson AM, Moller A. Chronic nicotine treatment counteracts nigral cell loss induced by a partial mesodiencephalic hemitransection: an analysis of the total number and mean volume of neurons and glia in substantia nigra of the male rat. Neuroscience 1993; 57:931–941.

92. James JR, Nordberg A. Genetic and environmental aspects of the role of nicotinic receptors in neurodegenerative disorders: emphasis on Alzheimer's disease and Parkinson's disease. Behav Genet 1995; 25:149–159.

93. Lange KW, Kornhuber J, Riederer P. Dopamine/glutamate interactions in Parkinson's disease. Neurosci Behav Rev 1997; 21:393–400.

94. Costa G, Abin-Carriquiry JA, Dajas F. Nicotine prevents striatal dopamine loss produced by 6-hydroxydopamine lesion in the substantia nigra. Brain Res 2001; 888:336–342.

95. Paulson GW, Dedmehr N. Is there a premorbid personality typical for Parkinson's disease? Neurology 1991; 41(suppl 2):73–76.

96. Ross GW, White LR, Petrovitch H, Davis DG, Hardman J, Nelson J, Markesbery W, Morens DM, Grandinetti A. Association of midlife smoking and coffee consumption with presence of Lewy bodies in the locus ceruleus or substantia nigra at autopsy. Neurology 1999; 52(suppl 2):A539.

97. Checkoway H, Franklin GM, Costa-Mallen P, Smith-Weller T, Dilley J, Swanson PD, Costa LG. A genetic polymorphism of MAO-B modifies the association of cigarette smoking and Parkinson's disease. Neurology 1998; 50:1458–1461.

98. Hellenbrand W, Seidler A, Boeing H, Robra BP, Vieregge P, Nischan P, Joerg J, Oertel WH, Schneider E, Ulm G. Diet and Parkinson's disease. I: A possible role for the past intake of specific foods and food groups. Results from a self-administered food-frequency questionnaire in a case-control study. Neurology 1996; 47:636–643.

99. Ross GW, Abbott RD, Petrovitch H, Morens DM, Grandinetti A, Tung KG, Tanner CM, Masaki KH, Blanchette PL, Curb JD, Popper JS, White LR. Association of coffee and caffeine intake with the risk of Parkinson's disease. JAMA 2000; 283:2674–2679.

100. Ascherio A, Zhang SM, Hernan MA, Kawachi I, Colditz GA, Speizer FE, Willett WC. Prospective study of caffeine consumption and risk of Parkinson's disease in men and women. Ann Neurol 2001; 50:56–63.
101. Chen J-F, Xu K, Petzer JP, Staal R, Xu YH, Beilstein M, Sonsalla PK, Castagnoli K, Castagnoli N Jr, Schwarzschild MA. Neuroprotection by caffeine and A2A receptor inactivation in a model of Parkinson's disease. J Neurosci 2001; 21:RC143:1 6.
102. Willett W. Recall of remote diet. In: Willett W, ed. Nutritional Epidemiology. 2nd ed. New York. Oxford University Press, 1998:148 156.
103. Willett WC, Sampson ML, Browne MJ, Stampfer Rosner B, Hennekens CH, Speizer FE. The use of a self-administered questionnaire to assess diet four years in the past. Am J Epidemiol 1988; 127:188–199.
104. Block G, Coyle LM, Hartman AM, Scoppa SM. Revision of dietary analysis software for the Health Habits and History Questionnaire. Am J Epidemiol 1994; 139:1190–1196.
105. Golbe LI, Farrell TM, Davis PH. Follow-up study of early-life protective and risk factors in Parkinson's disease. Mov Disord 1990; 5:66–70.
106. Logroscino G, Marder K, Cote L, Tang MX, Shea S, Mayeux R. Dietary lipids and antioxidants in Parkinson's disease: a population-based case-control study. Ann Neurol 1996; 39:89–94.
107. Hellenbrand W, Boeing H, Robra BP, Seidler A, Vieregge P, Nischan P, Joerg J, Oertel WH, Schneider E, Ulm G. Diet and Parkinson's disease. II: A possible role for the past intake of specific nutrients. Results from a self-administered food-frequency questionnaire in a case-control study. Neurology 1996; 47:644–650.
108. Morens DM, Grandinetti A, Waslien CI, Park CB, Ross GW, White LR. Case-control study of idopathic Parkinson's disease and dietary vitamin E intake. Neurology 1996; 46:1270–1274.
109. Scheider WL, Hershey LA, Vena JE, Holmlund T, Marshall JR, Freudenheim JL. Dietary antioxidants and other dietary factors in the etiology of Parkinson's disease. Mov Disord 1997; 12:190–196.
110. Johnson CC, Gorell JM, Rybicki BA, Sanders K, Peterson EL. Adult nutrient intake as a risk factor for Parkinson's disease. Int J Epidemiol 1999; 28:1102–1109.
111. Anderson C, Checkoway H, Franklin G, Beresford S, Smith-Weller T, Swanson PD. Dietary factors in Parkinson's disease: the role of food groups and specific foods. Mov Disord 1999; 14:21–27.
112. Factor SA, Weiner WJ. Prior history of head trauma in Parkinson's disease. Mov Dis 1991; 6:225–229.
113. Lees AJ. Trauma and Parkinson's disease. Rev Neurol (Paris) 1997; 153:541–546.
114. Poskanzer DC, Schwab RS. Cohort analysis of Parkinson's syndrome. Evidence for a single etiology related to subclinical infection about 1920. J Chron Dis 1963; 16:961–973.

115. Ravenholt RT, Foege WH. 1918 influenza, encephalitis lethargica, parkinsonism. Lancet 1982; 2:860–864.
116. Schwartz J, Elizan TS. Search for viral particles and virus-specific products in idiopathic Parkinson's disease brain material. Ann Neurol 1979; 6:261–263.
117. Marttila RJ, Halonen P, Rinne UK. Influenza virus antibodies in parkinsonism. Arch Neurol 1977; 34:99–100.
118. Elizan TS, Madden DL, Noble GR, et al. Viral antibodies in serum and CSF of parkinsonian patients and controls. Arch Neurol 1979; 36:529–534.
119. Kessler II. Epidemiologic studies of Parkinson's disease II. A hospital-based survey. Am J Epidemiol 1972; 95:308–318.
120. Kessler II. Epidemiologic studies of Parkinson's disease III. A community-based survey. Am J Epidemiol 1972; 96:242–254.
121. Sasco AJ, Paffenbarger RS. Measles infection and Parkinson's disease. Am J Epidemiol 1986; 122:1017–1031.
122. Kohbata S, Beaman BL. L-Dopa-responsive movement disorder caused by *Nocardia asteroides* localized in the brains of mice. Infect and Immun 1991; 59:181–191.
123. Hubble JP, Cao T, Kjelstrom JA, Koller WC, Beaman BL. *Nacardia* species as an etiologic agent in Parkinson's disease: serological testing in a case–control study. J Clin Microbiol 1995; 33:2768–2769.
124. Smargiassi A, Mutti A, De Rosa A, De Palma G, Negrotti A, Calzetti S. A case-control study of occupational and environmental risk factors for Parkinson's disease in the Emilia-Romagna region of Italy. Neurotoxicology 1998; 4–5:709–712.
125. Pezzoli G. Canesi M, Antonini A, Righini A, Perbellini L, Barichella M, Mariani CB, Tenconi F, Tesei S, Zecchinelli A, Leenders KL. Hydrocarbon exposure and Parkinson's disease. Neurology 2000; 55:667–673.
126. K Rothman, S Greenland. Case-Control Studies. In: K Rothman, S Greenland. Modern Epidemiology. 2nd ed. Philadelphia: Lippincott-Raven, 1998:93–114.
127. Hwang SJ, Beaty TH, Liang KY, Coresh J, Khoury MJ. Minimum sample size estimation to detect gene-environment interaction in case-control design. Am J Epidemiol 1994; 140:1029–1037.
128. Garcia-Closas M, Lubin JH. Power and sample size calculations in case control studies of gene-environment interactions: comments on different approaches. Am J Epidemiol 1999; 149:689–692.

16

Amantadine and Anticholinergics

Joseph S. Chung, Allan D. Wu, and Mark F. Lew
University of Southern California–Keck School of Medicine,
Los Angeles, California, U.S.A.

INTRODUCTION

Amantadine and anticholinergics have been used for several decades as therapy for Parkinson's disease (PD). In spite of reduced interest in these compounds with the advent of more specific dopaminergic therapies, there remain clinical situations where amantadine and anticholinergics retain clinical usefulness and a role in the contemporary treatment of PD.

AMANTADINE

History

Amantadine (Symmetrel®) was initially marketed in the 1960s as an antiviral agent. Its use as an antiparkinsonian agent was first described in 1969 when a woman with advanced PD serendipitously noted transient relief of tremor, rigidity, and bradykinesia during a 6-week course of flu prophylaxis with amantadine (1). Since that time, further studies confirmed a mild antiparkinsonian effect for amantadine (2). For years, amantadine was generally used either in early PD or as a mild adjunctive agent in later stage PD. The use of amantadine has remained limited in PD. This has been likely due to (1) the development of dopamine agonists, (2) better tolerance of levodopa with the advent of carbidopa, and (3) the misconception of transient benefit, known as tachyphylaxis. Investigators have sought to confirm or document the potential clinical uses of amantadine. Modulating effects of amantadine on motor complications in later stage PD have been documented in several studies (3–5).

Many different mechanisms of action have been proposed for the antiparkinsonian effects of amantadine, but clear attribution has remained obscure. Traditional mechanisms for amantadine were usually ascribed to dopaminergic or anticholinergic mechanisms such as the proposed mechanism of promoting endogenous dopamine release (6). However, further studies have demonstrated a variety of biological effects beyond these systems. For instance, recent studies have suggested that amantadine possesses glutamate blocking activity (7), a mechanism of substantial current interest in neurology for its role in a variety of different conditions.

Pharmacokinetics and Dosing

Amantadine is an aliphatic primary amine formulated as a hydrochloride salt for clinical use as an oral preparation. It is a relatively inexpensive drug available as a 100 mg tablet or 50 mg/mL liquid. Other than some anticholinergics and apomorphine, it is also one of the few PD medications available in a parenteral formulation (amantadine-sulfate). This intravenous preparation, however, is not available for use in the United States (8).

The bioavailability of amantadine is nearly 100% in oral form. It is excreted virtually unmetabolized via the kidneys and has a large volume of distribution. In fasting, healthy patients, peak plasma concentration was found 1–4 hours after a single oral dose of 2.5–5 mg/kg. Plasma half-life in healthy elderly men has been reported between 18 to 45 hours, suggesting that steady state may take up to 9 days (9). Serum amantadine levels are not routinely drawn and are probably of limited clinical utility. Pharmacological studies have reported serum levels between 0.2 and 0.9 µg/mL at dosages of 200 mg/day (10). Fahn et al. reported a case of one patient with psychosis following acute intoxication with amantadine who was found to have a level of 2.37 µg/mL (11).

Few drug interactions have been reported with amantadine. Other than a case report suggesting amantadine toxicity from an interaction with hydrochlorothiazide-triamterene (12), little else has been reported in the literature.

Routine dosing starts at 100 mg twice daily. Because of the relatively long half-life, increases are generally not recommended any sooner than once per week. Doses up to 500 mg have been reported for the use of diminishing motor complications in PD patients (13). The maximum tolerable doses are suggested at 400–500 mg each day in patients with normal renal function (14). Doses over 400 mg produce no added benefit and an increased incidence of side effects.

Clinical Uses

Early Parkinson's Disease

Amantadine is generally considered a mild antiparkinsonian agent with effects on rigidity and bradykinesia and a very well tolerated side effect profile. In this context, major uses have been in early treatment of PD or as a mild adjunctive agent in moderate PD. Its use in early PD may be helpful when considering levodopa-sparing strategies or when symptoms are mild and do not warrant more aggressive therapy. Amantadine has been studied in early PD as monotherapy and in combination with anticholinergics in limited series and small controlled studies with relatively short follow-up (15–17).

Part of the rationale for considering amantadine monotherapy are suggestions that amantadine itself may have neuroprotective properties to slow the progression of PD. Uitti and colleagues (18) found that amantadine use was an independent predictor of improved survival in a retrospective analysis of all parkinsonism patients (92% PD) treated with amantadine compared to those not using this medication. The results are suggestive of either an ongoing symptomatic improvement or the presence of an inherent neuroprotective property. There has been no confirmatory evidence to suggest neuroprotection from studies in PD patients, although basic science work on potential neuroprotective mechanisms with amantadine remains intriguing (see below).

In the 2002 American Academy of Neurology (AAN) guidelines on initiation of PD treatment, amantadine is not mentioned. The bulk of discussion has now focused on current literature involving selegiline, levodopa, and dopamine agonists (19).

Moderate Parkinson's Disease

In moderate PD, where symptoms necessitate treatment with levodopa or dopamine agonists, amantadine may be of benefit as an adjunctive medication.

Many patients report that they may be initial non-responders to amantadine, but that they may respond at a later point in time as their PD progresses (20). Patients with moderate PD who require additional mild benefit to their existing dopaminergic therapy are good candidates for amantadine.

Late Parkinson's Disease

Use of amantadine in managing late-stage PD motor complications was first described in 1987 by Shannon et al. (3) in a small open-label study. They reported improved motor fluctuations using a qualitative scale weighing changes in relative "on" and "off" function in 20 PD patients. This notion has gained further support from Metman et al. (21), who reported the results of double-blind, placebo-controlled, crossover studies of amantadine in 14 PD patients. They described a 60% reduction in both peak dose "on" choreiform dyskinesias and severity of "off" periods along with a decreased duration of "off" time (21). One year later, these patients had maintained significant benefit (5).

The above studies by Metman et al. did not distinguish between types of dyskinesia. The recognition of different motor dyskinesia phenomenology may be potentially important in the response to amantadine. For instance, dystonic dyskinesias have shown varied interindividual effects (some improving, some worsening) with amantadine in a few studies (3,4). Specific efficacy for sudden "on-offs" or biphasic dyskinesias has not been formally investigated.

Evidence suggests that amantadine produces antidyskinetic effects via a glutamate N-methyl-D-aspartate (NMDA) antagonism (22). This independence from dopaminergic mechanisms was proposed as an explanation for the ability of amantadine to ameliorate levodopa-induced dyskinesias without worsening parkinsonism (21).

Miscellaneous Considerations

One frequent assumption about amantadine is that it offers only transient efficacy, typically lasting less than a year. However, this apparent loss of efficacy for ameliorating parkinsonian symptoms has been reviewed and was attributed largely to the progression of the disease itself. It has also been reported that early-stage PD patients may be treated effectively for years with amantadine and still find that their symptoms noticeably worsen following drug withdrawal (13).

Side Effects

Amantadine is generally well tolerated with a favorable side effect profile. The most common idiosyncratic side effects include livedo reticularis and pedal edema. Livedo reticularis is a mottled bluish-red reticular skin discoloration, which blanches to pressure. It is more common in women (23) and is usually predominant in the lower extremies. The appearance is nonspecific and skin biopsies of the area are normal (24). Livedo reticularis usually appears after weeks of treatment and is of unclear etiology. The cosmetic appearance is usually far more apparent than any physical adverse effects.

Pedal edema can also appear idiosyncratically and is independent of either renal or cardiac failure. Its presence has generally been attributed to a redistribution of fluid and does not appear to represent a fluid excess. Quinn reported a few cases of congestive heart failure occurring in association with the use of amantadine, but this appears to be an exception to routine clinical use (25).

The presence of either livedo reticularis or pedal edema does not always necessitate discontinuation of amantadine. There is no specific treatment for the cosmetic discoloration associated with livedo reticularis. Diuretics may be used if the pedal edema is uncomfortable, though specific benefit tends to be uncertain. Symptoms are generally expected to resolve with discontinuation of the drug, but may take up to several weeks. Rarely, these conditions may be severe and associated with leg ulceration and peripheral neuropathy (26). A prudent combination of discontinuing the drug and of providing appropriate referrals to exclude important secondary causes (such as a superimposed renal failure, cardiac failure, autoimmune or vasculitic livedo, and ruling out deep vein thrombosis) must be an important part of continued clinical follow-up for patients on amantadine.

Nonspecific symptoms such as lightheadedness, insomnia, jitteriness, depression, and concentration difficulties are potential side effects of amantadine (9). Amantadine itself also possesses mild anticholinergic properties, which contribute to further reported side effects such as dry mouth, orthostatic hypotension, constipation, dyspepsia, and urinary retention. Therefore, reasonable care should be taken when administering amantadine in conjunction with anticholinergics (27). Cardiac arrhythmias have been reported with amantadine in one report (8). Amantadine is not recommended during pregnancy as it has more teratogenic potential than other PD medications (28).

Acute toxicity presenting as delirium (15) and psychosis (11) has been reported. Abrupt withdrawal has also been reported to produce delirium (29) as well as neuroleptic malignant syndrome (30). In many of these cases patients had either baseline cognitive deficits, psychiatric background, or excessive amantadine use. In general, the cognitive side effects such as confusion and concentration difficulties are more common in those with underlying, preexisting cognitive dysfunction. In advanced PD, amantadine may even carry comparable propensity for cognitive side effects to levodopa

(31). As such, conservative use in the elderly and avoidance of use even in the mildly cognitively impaired patient is necessary.

Because of the renal predominant excretion of amantadine, patients with impaired kidney function carry a higher risk of toxicity. Dosing schedules have been developed for patients with poor renal function according to creatinine clearance (32). However, as a practical matter, with the availability of many other antiparkinsonian agents, it is best to avoid the use of amantadine in patients with poor renal clearance. In the event of suspected toxicity, dialysis is not helpful in decreasing toxic levels, probably due to extensive tissue binding (33).

Mechanisms of Action

Many studies have suggested putative mechanisms of action for amantadine that may explain antiparkinsonian effects, but the clinical significance of any given individual mechanism remains uncertain. It seems likely that amantadine has a combination of multiple effects on both dopaminergic and nondopaminergic systems.

Dopaminergic mechanisms described for amantadine include findings of increased dopamine release (34), increased dopamine synthesis (35), inhibition of dopamine reuptake (36) and modulation of dopamine D2 receptors producing a high affinity state (37). This latter effect may speculatively play a role in modulating levodopa-induced dyskinesias. The relevance of these dopaminergic mechanisms is uncertain given that studies have demonstrated that the antiparkinsonian effects can occur without changes in brain concentrations of dopamine or its metabolites (38) and without evidence for dopamine synthesis or release (39).

Other neurotransmitter effects reported with amantadine include serotonergic, noradrenergic, anticholinergic, and antiglutaminergic properties (40). The anticholinergic properties suggest a well-described antiparkinsonian interaction (41,42). Renewed interest has arisen in the antiglutamate properties of amantadine. These can be attributed to two important clinical implications. First, it may provide a putative neuroprotective mechanism and be added to the list of drugs that may be examined for such clinical effects. Second, converging lines of evidence provide support to the idea that the antiglutamate properties of amantadine may be important for modulating motor complications in late-stage PD.

Amantadine possesses mild anti-NMDA properties that have led to the suggestion that the drug may contribute to a possible neuroprotective effect in PD (43,44). Glutamate excitotoxicity, mediated via persistent or sustained activation of NMDA receptors, produces an excess calcium influx activating a cascade of molecular events leading to the common final pathway of neuronal death. Blockade of NMDA glutamate receptors has been shown to experimentally diminish the excitotoxic effects of this cascade of reactions (45,46). In cell cultures, preexposure of substantia nigra dopaminergic neurons to glutamate antagonists provided protection when subsequently exposed to MPP^+ (1-methyl-4-phenyl-pyridium ion, the active metabolite of MPTP), a common specific nigral toxin used to produce animal models of PD (47). Extension of these preclinical findings to clinical applicability in PD patients remains speculative, but probably best serves a role to stimulate future studies.

The anti-NMDA properties of amantadine have also been implicated in its role modulating motor complications. Evidence has accumulated that glutamate NMDA receptors may play a significant role in the pathogenesis of motor complications. Loss of striatal dopamine and nonphysiological stimulation by extrinsic levodopa both cause sensitization of NMDA receptors on striatal medium spiny neurons in animal models (22). This sensitization may play a key role in altering normal basal ganglia responses to cortical glutaminergic input and produce the disordered motor output that leads to motor complications. Recent studies have reported that striatal injection or systemic administration of glutamate antagonists in primate and rodent models of PD can decrease levodopa motor complications without decreasing benefits of dopaminergic treatment (7,48–51).

Summary

With improved management options for PD, patients are living longer, and, as a result, more are suffering from long-term complications of disease and therapy. Although the influx of new medications has changed the landscape of pharmacological options for PD patients, a reexamination of older medications such as amantadine can offer evident benefit.

Amantadine retains its primary utility as a mild antiparkinsonian agent to be used mostly as adjunctive therapy and occasionally in early monotherapy as a means to avoid early use of levodopa. It is frequently being utilized as the only available antiparkinsonian agent to diminish dyskinesia and offer improvement of PD symptoms simultaneously (52).

ANTICHOLINERGICS

History

Anticholinergics are among the earliest class of pharmaceuticals used for the management of PD. Naturally occurring anticholinergics, such as the belladonna alkaloids, have been used for centuries to treat a variety of ailments. Since the mid-1900s and until the development of dopaminergic agents, anticholinergics were a major component of therapy for PD (53). In the 1940s, synthetic anticholinergics were introduced with trihexyphenidyl (Artane®) and similar agents replacing impure herbal preparations of belladonna alkaloids in the treatment of PD. Eventually, a wide variety of different anticholinergics, each with varying receptor specificities, blood-brain barrier penetration, and side effect profiles became available. Historically and by physician preference, certain medications have gained popularity or notoriety for treating PD. This has varied throughout the decades (54).

With recent developments in PD therapy, anticholinergics have been relegated to a less prominent role. In particular, levodopa and dopamine agonists have largely replaced anticholinergics as major antiparkinsonian agents. Contemporary reviews and investigations continue to support anticholinergic use in certain clinical situations such as PD-associated tremor or dystonia. Side effects have always been a prominent concern with anticholinergics, particularly in susceptible individuals such as the elderly. As such, careful risk-benefit assessment in anticholinergic use remains a prudent routine practice in PD patients.

Pharmacokinetics and Dosing

Anticholinergics are a diverse group of medications. The majority of the anticholinergic medications have good oral absorption. In general, most have half-lives requiring at least twice and usually three times a day dosing.

The antiparkinsonian effect of anticholinergics is largely attributed to centrally acting acetylcholine receptors that can cross the blood-brain barrier (55). Most synthetic (tertiary) anticholinergics used in PD are predominantly in this class: biperiden (Akineton®), trihexyphenidyl (Artane®), benztropine (Cogentin®), procyclidine (Kemadrin®). Benztropine has useful central effects that can be used for PD management, is more potent than trihexyphenidyl, but has less sedating effects than antihistamines (56).

Anticholinergic effects are often seen as side effects for many other groups of medications. Exploiting these secondary side effects when choosing medications for other indications is a common practice, especially when their anticholinergic effects assist in managing PD symptoms. These include tricyclic antidepressants like amitriptyline, antihistamines like diphenhydramine, and atypical antipsychotics like olanzapine or quetiapine.

Recommended doses vary by practitioner, but one rule is to start with a low dose and increase slowly and conservatively (Table 1). Maximum dosing is limited by the side effect profile of these medications. Individual

TABLE 1 Common Anticholinergics Used in Parkinson's Disease

Name	Mechanisms	Preparations	Initial dose	Escalation schedule	Maximum dose per day	Comments
Primary anticholinergics						
Trihexyphenidyl (Artane)	Central antimuscarinic	2, 5 mg tabs; 2 mg/5 ml elixir	1 mg qd-bid	Increase to tid; every 3–4 days increase by 1/2–1 mg each dose	2–3 mg tid	First synthetic anticholinergics
Benztropine (Cogentin)	Central antimuscarinic	0.5,1,2 mg tablets; injection 1 mg/mL	0.5 mg bid	Increase to tid; every 3–4 days increase by 1/2–1 mg each dose	2 mg tid	Also available parenterally
Biperiden (Akineton)	Central antimuscarinic	2 mg tablets & 5 mg/mL ampules	1 mg bid	Increase to tid; every 3–4 days increase by 1/2–1 mg each dose	3 mg tid	Also available parenterally
Ethopropazine (Parsidol, Parsitan)	Central antimuscarinic	50 mg tablets	12.5 mg tid/qid	Increase to tid; every 3–4 days increase by 12.5 mg each dose	50 mg tid-qid	Approved by FDA; not available in U.S.
Secondary anticholinergic effects						
Diphenhydramine (Benadryl)	Antihistamine	12.5, 25 mg tablets; 12.5 mg liquid	25 mg qhs	Increase by 25 mg every 3–4 days	25 mg tid or 25–100 mg qhs	H1 blocker, also available parenterally
Amitriptyline (Elavil)	Tricyclic antidepressant	10, 25, 50, 75, 100, 150 tablets; injection 10 mg/mL	12.5 mg qhs	Increase by 12.5 mg every 2–3 nights	150 mg	
Clozapine (Clozaril)	Atypical antipsychotic	25 mg tablets	6.25–12.5 mg	Increase by 6.25–12.5 mg every 2–3 nights	100 mg	May cause paradoxical increased salivation

practitioners usually have particular anticholinergics they prefer to use due to their clinical impression or experience.

Clinical Uses

Since the advent of specific dopaminergic therapy for PD in the 1960s, the usefulness and popularity of anticholinergics waned dramatically. However, they are still used among many clinicians in certain situations.

Tremor Predominant Parkinson's Disease

The most recognized use of this class of medication is to treat tremor in early- or young-onset PD representing a levodopa-sparing strategy. In general, it appears that anticholinergics help tremor but do not significantly affect other akinetic or rigid features of PD. Original AAN practice parameters in 1993 stated that there was a common use for anticholinergic agents for initial therapy of tremor predominant PD, but concluded on the basis of class II evidence* that anticholinergics are probably no better than levodopa for tremor. Schrag et al. found equivalent reductions in tremor with a single dose of either apomorphine or biperiden, but only the dopamine agonist reduced rigidity and akinesia (58). Although anti-cholinergics do not appear to have significant effects on akinesia and rigidity as therapy, deterioration of all parkinsonian symptoms has been described following abrupt withdrawal (59).

Anticholinergics are useful in the early treatment of tremor predominant PD in young or mild patients if the primary indication for symptomatic therapy is tremor, and there are relatively minimal associated signs of rigidity or bradykinesia. Anticholinergics can also offer a useful adjunctive option if additional tremor relief beyond the patient's existing antiparkinsonian regimen is needed. Anticholinergics should be avoided in patients with baseline cognitive deficits, significant orthostatic hypotension, or urinary retention as these patients are at higher risk for exacerbation of these symptoms. For similar reasons, anticholinergics are reserved for rare use in elderly PD patients.

Parkinson's Disease–Associated Dystonia

Dystonia can occur in association with PD. Anticholinergics can play an adjunctive role in managing such dystonia. Most PD-associated dystonia occurs in the context of motor complications, but it can occur even in

---

Evidence provided by one or more well-designed clinical studies such as case control, cohort studies, and so forth (57). The AAN 1993 practice parameters summary statement has since been revised (19).

levodopa-naïve patients. Most commonly, an "off" dystonia characteristically causes painful foot and toe posturing when dopaminergic medication wears off in the morning. Levodopa-induced "on" dystonias can follow either biphasic or peak-dose patterns. Poewe et al. (60) suggest that anticholinergics can play a role in helping relieve the severity of episodic dystonia in PD. However, limb dystonia as an early symptom in levodopa-naive patients tended not to respond as well compared to dystonia associated with motor fluctuations.

Miscellaneous Considerations

Often anticholinergic agents can be used to treat miscellaneous indications. In this setting, agents are often chosen on the basis of secondary anticholinergic side effects. For example, if antidepressants are needed, a tricyclic antidepressant such as amitriptyline might be chosen for its anticholinergic properties to assist with insomnia or PD-related tremor. Diphenhydramine (Benadryl) is an antihistamine commonly prescribed for allergies or insomnia and possesses mild anticholinergic side effects that can be used for PD-associated sialorrhea and may help reduce tremor. Regarding sialorrhea, atropine drops in 1.0% solution administered sublingually twice daily have been reported as beneficial with no significant mental state changes (61).

Another class of medications commonly used in PD is the atypical antipsychotics. Clozapine, in particular, has significant anticholinergic-attributed sedation, but also can reduce tremor (62) and produce paradoxical increased salivation and drooling. Amantadine, discussed earlier in this chapter, shows modest anticholinergic properties, although its antiparkinsonian use is commonly chosen on its own merits (63).

A partial list of commonly used medications with either primary or secondary anticholinergic properties and their use is shown in Table 1.

Side Effects

Side effects of anticholinergic agents are a significant clinical concern, which can limit their usefulness in the treatment of PD symptoms. Most antiparkinsonian effects are assumed to be mediated via central muscarinic acetylcholine receptors. Side effects may occur as either additional unintended central muscarinic effects or as incidental autonomic effects attributed to peripheral binding to muscarinic and nicotinic acetylcholine receptors. In general, most side effects are dose-dependent and respond to dose reductions.

Central Side Effects

Sedation, confusion, memory difficulties, and psychosis are well-described adverse events attributed to central nervous system anticholinergic toxicity. An anticholinergic, scopolamine (Transderm-Scop®), in normal controls was found to have effects on cognitive activities requiring rapid information processing (64). Bedard et al. found a transient induction of executive dysfunction in nondemented PD subjects with an acute subclinical dose of scopolamine (65). These findings underscore the necessity to be aware that even in early PD patients with no clinical intellectual dysfunction, anticholinergics may have adverse effects on cognition. These drug-induced cognitive deficits are reversible. In patients taking anticholinergics who develop psychosis, increased memory difficulties, and confusion, anticholinergic agents should be withdrawn promptly.

Peripheral Side Effects

Peripheral anticholinergic effects can produce a variety of autonomic dysfunction including, but not limited to, dry mouth, orthostatic hypotension, and urinary retention. Rare but potentially serious side effects such as narrow-angle glaucoma have been described.

Similar to central effects, peripheral effects are often exacerbated in PD patients due to an underlying baseline autonomic dysfunction or an increased susceptibility due to advanced age. Concomitant dopaminergic medications may further exacerbate anticholinergic symptoms such as orthostatic hypotension, constipation, or sedation. Orthostatic hypotension is a common problem in PD and can be exacerbated by addition of anticholinergic agents.

Dry mouth due to parasympathetic depression of salivary glands is an extremely common and potentially uncomfortable side effect (66). In some patients with drooling, this effect may be advantageous. The severity of dry mouth also improves with a decrease in anticholinergic dose and may improve with prolonged exposure. Anticholinergics can also result in urinary retention due to excess parasympathetic inhibition, so caution must be exercised. Risks are particularly great in elderly men due to bladder outlet obstruction from benign prostate hypertrophy. If there is any history of urinary hesitancy or urgency, a urology evaluation is reasonable prior to initiation of anticholinergic therapy.

Blurred vision is another common side effect with anticholinergics. This symptom is often attributed to relatively reduced accommodation due to parasympathetic blockade and excessive dryness of the cornea. For persistent symptoms, consultation with an ophthalmologist may be appropriate. Rarely, anticholinergic therapy can precipitate narrow angle glaucoma (closed angle glaucoma), an ophthalmic emergency. The acute increase in intraocular pressure presents with pain and redness in the affected eye. In practice, this condition is extremely rare. Risk of narrow angle glaucoma is minimal if there are normal pupillary responses and intact vision. Ophthalmology consultation should be sought during anticholinergic treatment should vision diminish or pupillary responses become abnormal. In contrast, the more common open angle glaucoma presents minimal risk for treatment with anticholinergics (54).

Careful consideration of risk-benefit analysis is needed when prescribing anticholinergic medications. Patients should be counseled about the potential for side effects and instructed to call with any problems. In younger patients without comorbidity besides mild PD, anticholinergics are generally very well tolerated and represent a viable option for tremor-predominant symptoms. In more susceptible patients with clinically relevant autonomic dysfunction, cognitive dysfunction or advanced age, anticholinergics should be used very sparingly.

Mechanisms of Action

Antiparkinsonian benefit is generally attributed to inhibition of central muscarinic acetylcholine receptors. For instance, Duvoisin and Katz (55) reported an antiparkinsonian benefit to benztropine and scopolamine, both centrally acting anticholinergics, with an exacerbation of parkinsonism after a trial of physostigmine, a centrally acting anticholinesterase. In contrast, peripheral anticholinergics (methyl scopolamine and propantheline) and a peripheral anticholinesterase (edrophonium) did not affect parkinsonian symptoms (55). Details of how centrally acting anticholinergics can modify PD symptoms, usually attributed to dopaminergic deficiency, remain unclear.

Abnormalities in the central acetylcholine neurotransmitter system have been described in PD patients (67,68). An oversimplified but clinically useful conceptualization is that the anticholinergic use corrects an imbalance between dopamine and acetylcholine (69). The depleted nigro-striatal dopaminergic system in PD causes a relative increase in striatal acetylcholine-dopamine ratio, which can be normalized by use of anticholinergics. Other miscellaneous proposed mechanisms include inhibition of dopamine reuptake (70) and mild NMDA glutamate antagonism (71). The clinical significance of these findings remains to be determined.

Summary

Anticholinergics have relatively few clinical uses in PD other than the treatment of tremor in young-onset patients. Anticholinergics can be used in younger patients with problematic PD-associated dystonia unresponsive to or intolerant of dopaminergic manipulation. Secondary anticholinergic effects may occasionally be helpful for insomnia, sialorrhea, or urinary frequency. Appropriate caution remains in judging risks of side effects versus benefits in anticholinergic use, particularly in patients who may be more susceptible to either the central or peripheral anticholinergic effects.

SUMMARY

With the advent of specific dopaminergic agents, the roles of amantadine and anticholinergics have taken a back seat. Traditional uses still dominate with amantadine used as a mild antiparkinsonian agent with a well-tolerated side effect profile and anticholinergics used to treat tremor predominant PD. In addition, evidence that amantadine has efficacy in the modulation of later stage PD motor complications is clinically helpful information. Careful judgment of use of both of these agents related to their respective side effect profiles remains a concern, particularly with anticholinergics in susceptible elderly patients. In summary, amantadine and anticholinergics are helpful agents in the practicing clinician's arsenal when dealing with particular clinical PD scenarios.

REFERENCES

1. Schwab RS, England AC, Jr., Poskanzer DC, Young RR. Amantadine in the treatment of Parkinson's disease. Jama 208(7):1168–1170, 1969.
2. Danielczyk W. Twenty-five years of amantadine therapy in Parkinson's disease. J Neural Transm Suppl 46:399–405, 1995.
3. Shannon KM, Goetz CG, Carroll VS, Tanner CM, Klawans HL. Amantadine and motor fluctuations in chronic Parkinson's disease. Clin Neuropharmacol 10(6):522–526, 1987.
4. Adler CH, Stern MB, Vernon G, Hurtig HI. Amantadine in advanced Parkinson's disease: good use of an old drug. J Neurol 244(5):336–337, 1997.
5. Metman LV, Del Dotto P, LePoole K, Konitsiotis S, Fang J, Chase TN. Amantadine for levodopa-induced dyskinesias: a 1-year follow-up study. Arch Neurol 56(11):1383–1386, 1999.
6. Farnebo LO, Fuxe K, Goldstein M, Hamberger B, Ungerstedt U. Dopamine and noradrenaline releasing action of amantadine in the central and peripheral nervous system: a possible mode of action in Parkinson's disease. Eur J Pharmacol 16(1):27–38, 1971.

7. Greenamyre JT, O'Brien CF. N-Methyl-D-aspartate antagonists in the treatment of Parkinson's disease. Arch Neurol 48(9):977–981, 1991.

8. Ruzicka E, Streitova H, Jech R, Kanovsky P, Roth J, Rektorova I, Mecir P, Hortova H, Barcs M, Hejdukova B, Rektor I. Amantadine infusion in treatment of motor fluctuations and dyskinesias in Parkinson's disease. J Neural Transm 107(11):1297–1306, 2000.

9. Aoki FY, Sitar DS. Clinical pharmacokinetics of amantadine hydrochloride. Clin Pharmacokinet 14(1):35–51, 1988.

10. Pacifici GM, Nardini M, Ferrari P, Latini R, Fieschi C, Morselli PL. Effect of amantadine on drug-induced parkinsonism: relationship between plasma levels and effect. Br J Clin Pharmacol 3(5):883–889, 1976.

11. Fahn S, Craddock G, Kumin G. Acute toxic psychosis from suicidal overdosage of amantadine. Arch Neurol 25(1):45–48, 1971.

12. Wilson TW, Rajput AH. Amantadine-dyazide interaction. Can Med Assoc J 129(9):974–975, 1983.

13. Factor SA, Molho ES. Transient benefit of amantadine in Parkinson's disease: the facts about the myth. Mov Disord 14(3):515–517, 1999.

14. Greulich W, Fenger E. Amantadine in Parkinson's disease: pro and contra. J Neural Transm Suppl 46:415–421, 1995.

15. Butzer JF, Silver DE, Sahs AL. Amantadine in Parkinson's disease. A double-blind, placebo-controlled, crossover study with long-term follow-up. Neurology 25(7):603–606, 1975.

16. Dallos V, Heathfield K, Stone P, Allen FA. Use of amantadine in Parkinson's disease. Results of a double-blind trial. Br Med J 4(726):24–26, 1970.

17. Mann DC, Pearce LA, Waterbury LD. Amantadine for Parkinson's disease. Neurology 21(9):958–962, 1971.

18. Uitti RJ, Rajput AH, Ahlskog JE, Offord KP, Schroeder DR, Ho MM, Prasad M, Rajput A, Basran P. Amantadine treatment is an independent predictor of improved survival in Parkinson's disease. Neurology 46(6):1551–1556, 1996.

19. Miyasaki JM, Martin W, Suchowersky O, Weiner WJ, Lang AE. Practice parameter: initiation of treatment for Parkinson's disease: an evidence-based review: report of the Quality Standards Subcommittee of the American Academy of Neurology. Neurology 58(1):11–17, 2002.

20. Fahn S, Isgreen WP. Long-term evaluation of amantadine and levodopa combination in parkinsonism by double-blind crossover analyses. Neurology 25(8):695–700, 1975.

21. Verhagen Metman L, Del Dotto P, van den Munckhof P, Fang J, Mouradian MM, Chase TN. Amantadine as treatment for dyskinesias and motor fluctuations in Parkinson's disease. Neurology 50(5):1323–1326, 1998.

22. Chase TN, Oh JD. Striatal mechanisms and pathogenesis of parkinsonian signs and motor complications. Ann Neurol 47(4 suppl 1):S122–129; discussion S129–130, 2000.

23. Timberlake WH, Vance MA. Four-year treatment of patients with parkinsonism using amantadine alone or with levodopa. Ann Neurol 3(2):119–128, 1978.

24. Vollum DI, Parkes JD, Doyle D. Livedo reticularis during amantadine treatment. Br Med J 2(762):627–628, 1971.

25. Quinn NP. Anti-parkinsonian drugs today. Drugs 28(3):236–262, 1984.

26. Shulman LM, Minagar A, Sharma K, Weiner WJ. Amantadine-induced peripheral neuropathy. Neurology 53(8):1862–1865, 1999.

27. Schwab RS, Poskanzer DC, England AC, Jr., Young RR. Amantadine in Parkinson's disease. Review of more than two years' experience. Jama 222(7):792–795, 1972.

28. Hagell P, Odin P, Vinge E. Pregnancy in Parkinson's disease: a review of the literature and a case report. Mov Disord 13(1):34–38, 1998.

29. Factor SA, Molho ES, Brown DL. Acute delirium after withdrawal of amantadine in Parkinson's disease. Neurology 50(5):1456–1458, 1998.

30. Simpson DM, Davis GC. Case report of neuroleptic malignant syndrome associated with withdrawal from amantadine. Am J Psychiatry 141(6):796–797, 1984.

31. Cummings JL. Behavioral complications of drug treatment of Parkinson's disease. J Am Geriatr Soc 39(7):708–716, 1991.

32. Wu MJ, Ing TS, Soung LS, Daugirdas JT, Hano JE, Gandhi VC. Amantadine hydrochloride pharmacokinetics in patients with impaired renal function. Clin Nephrol 17(1):19–23, 1982.

33. Blye E, Lorch J, Cortell S. Extracorporeal therapy in the treatment of intoxication. Am J Kidney Dis 3(5):321–338, 1984.

34. Stromberg U, Svensson TH. Further studies on the mode of action of amantadine. Acta Pharmacol Toxicol 30(3):161–171, 1971.

35. Scatton B, Cheramy A, Besson MJ, Glowinski J. Increased synthesis and release of dopamine in the striatum of the rat after amantadine treatment. Eur J Pharmacol 13(1):131–133, 1970.

36. Von Voigtlander PF, Moore KE. Dopamine: release from the brain in vivo by amantadine. Science 174(7):408–410, 1971.

37. Allen RM. Role of amantadine in the management of neuroleptic-induced extrapyramidal syndromes: overview and pharmacology. Clin Neuropharmacol 6(suppl 1):S64–S73, 1983.

38. Quack G, Hesselink M, Danysz W, Spanagel R. Microdialysis studies with amantadine and memantine on pharmacokinetics and effects on dopamine turnover. J Neural Transm Suppl 46:97–105, 1995.

39. Maj J, Sowinska H, Baran L. The effect of amantadine on motor activity and catalepsy in rats. Psychopharmacologia 24(2):296–307, 1972.

40. Huber TJ, Dietrich DE, Emrich HM. Possible use of amantadine in depression. Pharmacopsychiatry 32(2):47–55, 1999.

41. Stoof JC, Booij J, Drukarch B, Wolters EC. The anti-parkinsonian drug amantadine inhibits the N-methyl-D-aspartic acid-evoked release of acet-

ylcholine from rat neostriatum in a non-competitive way. Eur J Pharmacol 213(3):439–443, 1992.

42. Lupp A, Lucking CH, Koch R, Jackisch R, Feuerstein TJ. Inhibitory effects of the antiparkinsonian drugs memantine and amantadine on N-methyl-D-aspartate-evoked acetylcholine release in the rabbit caudate nucleus in vitro. J Pharmacol Exp Ther 263(2):717–724, 1992.

43. Danysz W, Parsons CG, Kornhuber J, Schmidt WJ, Quack G. Aminoadamantanes as NMDA receptor antagonists and antiparkinsonian agents — preclinical studies. Neurosci Biobehav Rev 21(4):455–468, 1997.

44. Kornhuber J, Bormann J, Hubers M, Rusche K, Riederer P. Effects of the 1-amino-adamantanes at the MK-801-binding site of the NMDA-receptor-gated ion channel: a human postmortem brain study. Eur J Pharmacol 206(4):297–300, 1991.

45. Albin RL, Greenamyre JT. Alternative excitotoxic hypotheses. Neurology 42(4):733–738, 1992.

46. Blandini F, Porter RH, Greenamyre JT. Glutamate and Parkinson's disease. Mol Neurobiol 12(1):73–94, 1996.

47. Turski L, Bressler K, Rettig KJ, Loschmann PA, Wachtel H. Protection of substantia nigra from MPP + neurotoxicity by N-methyl-D-aspartate antagonists. Nature 349(6308):414–418, 1991.

48. Shoulson I et al. A randomized, controlled trial of remacemide for motor fluctuations in Parkinson's disease. Neurology 56(4):455–462, 2001.

49. Marin C, Papa S, Engber TM, Bonastre M, Tolosa E, Chase TN. MK-801 prevents levodopa-induced motor response alterations in parkinsonian rats. Brain Res 736(1–2):202–205, 1996.

50. Papa SM, Boldry RC, Engber TM, Kask AM, Chase TN. Reversal of levodopa-induced motor fluctuations in experimental parkinsonism by NMDA receptor blockade. Brain Res 701(1–2):13–18, 1995.

51. Blanchet PJ, Konitsiotis S, Chase TN. Amantadine reduces levodopa-induced dyskinesias in parkinsonian monkeys. Mov Disord 13(5):798–802, 1998.

52. Ferreira JJ, Rascol O. Prevention and therapeutic strategies for levodopa-induced dyskinesias in Parkinson's disease. Curr Opin Neurol 13(4):431–436, 2000.

53. Olanow CW, Watts RL, Koller WC. An algorithm (decision tree) for the management of Parkinson's disease (2001): treatment guidelines. Neurology 56(11 suppl 5):S1–S88, 2001.

54. Friedman Z, Neumann E. Benzhexol-induced blindness in Parkinson's disease. Br Med J 1(800):605, 1972.

55. Duvoisin RC, Katz R. Reversal of central anticholinergic syndrome in man by physostigmine. JAMA 206(9):1963–1965, 1968.

56. de Leon J, Canuso C, White AO, Simpson GM. A pilot effort to determine benztropine equivalents of anticholinergic medications. Hosp Community Psychiatry 45(6):606–607, 1994.

57. Practice parameters: initial therapy of Parkinson's disease (summary statement). Report of the Quality Standards Subcommittee of the American Academy of Neurology. Neurology 43(7):1296–1297, 1993.

58. Schrag A, Schelosky L, Scholz U, Poewe W. Reduction of Parkinsonian signs in patients with Parkinson's disease by dopaminergic versus anticholinergic single-dose challenges. Mov Disord 14(2):252–255, 1999.

59. Weiner WJ, Lang AE. *Parkinson's disease*. In Movement Disorders, A Complete Survey. New York: Futura Publishing Co., 1989, p. 95.

60. Poewe WH, Lees AJ, Stern GM. Dystonia in Parkinson's disease: clinical and pharmacological features. Ann Neurol 23(1):73–78, 1988.

61. Hyson HC, Jog MS, Johnson A. Sublingual atropine for sialorrhea secondary to parkinsonism (abstr). Parkinsonism Related Disord 7(suppl.):P-TU-194, 2001.

62. Marjama-Lyons J, Koller W. Tremor-predominant Parkinson's disease. Approaches to treatment. Drugs Aging 16(4):273–278, 2000.

63. Nastuk WL, Su P, Doubilet P. Anticholinergic and membrane activities of amantadine in neuromuscular transmission. Nature 264(5581):76–79, 1976.

64. Wesnes K, Warburton DM. Effects of scopolamine and nicotine on human rapid information processing performance. Psychopharmacology 82(3):147–150, 1984.

65. Bedard MA, Lemay S, Gagnon JF, Masson H, Paquet F. Induction of a transient dysexecutive syndrome in Parkinson's disease using a subclinical dose of scopolamine. Behav Neurol 11(4):187–195, 1998.

66. Burke RE, Fahn S. Pharmacokinetics of trihexyphenidyl after short-term and long-term administration to dystonic patients. Ann Neurol 18(1):35–40, 1985.

67. Whitehouse PJ, Hedreen JC, White CL, 3rd, Price DL. Basal forebrain neurons in the dementia of Parkinson disease. Ann Neurol 13(3):243–248, 1983.

68. Ruberg M, Ploska A, Javoy-Agid F, Agid Y. Muscarinic binding and choline acetyltransferase activity in Parkinsonian subjects with reference to dementia. Brain Res 232(1):129–139, 1982.

69. Barbeau A. The pathogenesis of Parkinson's disease: a new hypothesis. Canad Med Ass J 87:802–807, 1962.

70. Coyle JT, Snyder SH. Antiparkinsonian drugs: inhibition of dopamine uptake in the corpus striatum as a possible mechanism of action. Science 166(907):899–901, 1969.

71. Olney JW, Price MT, Labruyere J, Salles KS, Frierdich G, Mueller M, Silverman E. Anti-parkinsonian agents are phencyclidine agonists and N-methyl-aspartate antagonists. Eur J Pharmacol 142(2):319–320, 1987.

17

Levodopa

Anthony J. Santiago and Stewart A. Factor
Albany Medical Center, Albany, New York, U.S.A.

INTRODUCTION AND HISTORY

Parkinson's disease (PD), like other neurodegenerative disorders, is clinically heterogeneous (1). Age of onset, the relative prominence of certain signs and symptoms, course and rate of progression, and the responsiveness to therapy are variable but still assist in differentiating it from atypical forms of parkinsonism (2). Mainly described by its cardinal motor manifestations (bradykinesia/akinesia, rigidity, resting tremor, and postural instability), progression is inevitable, as there is a continuous loss of nigrostriatal dopaminergic neurons in the substantia nigra pars compacta (SNpc) (3).

Before 1918, treatment was primarily supportive (4). However, the encephalitis epidemic of 1917–1926 and the emergence of the postencephalitic form of parkinsonism led to a more aggressive pursuit of effective therapies. The pursuit initially focused on the development of an effective vaccine, and then necessarily toward symptomatic therapy (5,6). As we cannot, at this time, halt the progression of PD, symptomatic relief remains the only available proven approach to care. While this is at times inadequate, the available symptomatic therapies for PD are far more effective than those available for any other neurodegenerative disease (3).

A number of natural remedies have been tried to treat the symptoms of PD over the last century and a half. Charcot, in the latter half of the nineteenth century, described the use of potato plant extracts, such as Bulgarian belladonna and atropine, to treat PD. These were initially received with great promise, but fell short of expectations. In the decade following the emergence of postencephalitic parkinsonism, many studies were published comparing the various plant extracts, evaluating the effectiveness of certain agents for specific symptoms; for example, stramonium was felt to be effective for rigidity and hyoscine for tremor (4).

By the early 1950s, synthetic drugs became available to treat the symptoms of PD. Trihexyphenidyl hydrochloride, a synthetic anticholinergic, was highly touted for its effectiveness for relieving rigidity, tremor, akinesia, and oculogyric crisis. It was heralded as more effective than the plant extracts and better tolerated than other early synthetic preparations (4,7,8). While still used today, its limitations in treating all the symptoms of PD were recognized even then.

Levodopa (LD) has become the cornerstone of symptomatic therapy. It is a metabolic precursor of the neurotransmitter dopamine (see below). D/L Dopa was first synthesized in 1911 (9). Guggenhiem, in 1913, isolated LD from the broad bean plant (10). Its use in PD only emerged after the important works of various researchers in the late 1950s and early 1960s that demonstrated that dopamine depletion was characteristic of PD. Carrlson in 1957 and 1958 (11,12) demonstrated in animal models that the akinetic effects of reserpine (an agent known to deplete dopamine) could be reversed by LD. In addition, Carrlson reported that the striatum was a site of dopamine concentration (11,12). Hornykiewicz in 1960 showed that the striatum of parkinsonian brains were depleted of dopamine and 2 years later that intravenous doses of LD (50 mg) had anti-parkinsonian effects (13). However, studies in the early and mid-1960s showed variable results, and, in fact, treatment with LD was almost abandoned. It was the seminal work of Cotzias, who examined the role of high-dose oral LD in modifying parkinsonism, that dramatically changed the landscape of PD treatment (14,15). LD was ultimately approved by the U.S. Food and Drug Administration (FDA) for use in PD in 1970, 60 years after its discovery and more than 10 years after the realization that dopamine depletion was the key abnormality in PD (16). In 1973, the combined use of a peripheral aromatic amino acid decarboxylase inhibitor (AADI) with LD was reported. Its use resulted in a decrease in peripheral metabolism of LD to dopamine and fewer peripheral side effects such as hypotension and nausea

(17). Controlled-release formulations were tested in the 1980s to treat fluctuations (see below), and one was approved in the United States in 1991 (3).

Still regarded as the most potent symptomatic therapy for PD, LD has its drawbacks. Late complications such as motor fluctuations and dyskinesias are associated with chronic administration. Neuropsychiatric disturbances can be frequent and serious adverse effects. Questions have arisen regarding its potential toxicity to nigrostriatal neurons as well as a possible association with melanoma. The question of when to initiate therapy with LD is still ongoing. This chapter will review the pharmacology of LD, its role in the emergence and progression of motor complications, its possible toxicity, whether tolerance develops, if it can be of assistance in diagnosing PD, and its effect on mortality of PD.

PHARMACOLOGY

Dopamine depletion, particularly in the striatum, is the neurochemical hallmark responsible for the motor features of PD. However, dopamine cannot be utilized as a treatment because it does not cross the blood-brain barrier (BBB), and its use is associated with several side effects. On the other hand, LD, an aromatic amino acid and precursor to dopamine, readily crosses the BBB. When it is administered orally, it is converted to dopamine in the extracerebral tissues via decarboxylation. To lessen the peripheral effects of dopamine and increase the brain bioavailability of LD, it is often co-administered with AADIs like carbidopa or benserazide. AADIs do not cross the BBB and therefore will not affect conversion to dopamine in the brain. Their use reduces the amount of LD required to attain an adequate response by approximately 75% and increases its plasma half-life from 50 to 90 minutes.

Two major enzymatic pathways for LD exist leading to the formation of 3-O-methyldopa (3-OMD), both peripherally and centrally (Fig. 1). Dopamine is subsequently converted to 3,4-dioxyphenylacetic acid (DOPAC) and homovanillic acid (HVA) in the central nervous system (CNS).

Transport of LD across the gut mucosa and BBB involves an energy-dependent carrier-mediated system. Large neutral amino acids (LNAA) compete for transport at the same sites. When oral LD was administered with a high-protein meal, there was an overall reduction in its plasma level. When IV LD was administered with a high-protein meal, the anticipated clinical response was diminished, indicating an effect at the BBB as well (18). Upon entering the CNS, LD is converted to dopamine in dopaminergic neurons and probably other cells containing dopa decarboxylase.

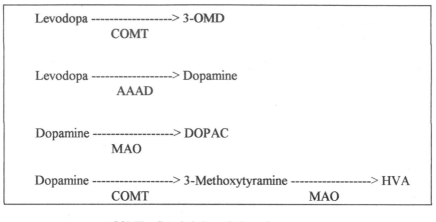

COMT = Catechol-O-methyltransferase
MAO = Monoamine oxidase

FIGURE 1 Levodopa metabolism. 3-OMD = 3-O-methyldopa, AAAD = arometic amino acid decarboxylase, DOPAC = 3,4-dioxyphenylacetic acid, HVA = homovanillic acid.

MOTOR FLUCTUATIONS AND DYSKINESIAS: DEFINITIONS

It is established that a loss of 50–60% of nigrostriatal neurons or a reduction in striatal dopamine concentrations of approximately 80% is required to cause clinical symptoms (19). The surviving neurons can initially compensate but subsequently, with continued disease progression, fail. The loss of the ability to store and release dopamine appropriately results in less reliable responses to LD (20). Glial cells can also convert LD to dopamine, but they lack the machinery for appropriate regulation (21). In PD, the loss of nigrostriatal innervation is associated with putaminal D2 receptor upregulation with a subsequent decline, possibly below baseline, which may be related to both disease and treatment (22).

These presynaptic and postsynaptic changes are important not only for responsiveness to LD but also the occurrence of motor fluctuations (wearing-off, dyskinesias, unpredictable responses). Historical literature suggests that the rate is approximately 50% for motor fluctuations and dyskinesias after 5 years of disease duration and as high as 90% for patients with onset of PD under age 40 (23). Ahlskog and Muenter compared more recent literature to older studies and found that the rate is probably 35–40% after 4–6 years of disease duration (24). These figures vary depending on the study, and these variances may relate to definitions and measuring tools.

The response to LD treatment is complex, and understanding it requires many considerations. Muenter and Tyce defined the long-duration response (LDR) as the gradual motor improvement seen after repeated dosing and subsequent decline over days upon LD withdrawal. This effect remains present even after long-term chronic therapy (20). The short-duration response (SDR) is defined as that which parallels the plasma concentrations of LD. It seems to be present to some extent from the beginning of therapy (22). Nutt and colleagues showed that after a 3-day withdrawal of LD, a patient receiving a single dose would have a full SDR only, without a LDR. It may be that the LDR leads to the remarkable early responsiveness to LD and its loss results in the subsequent dependency on the SDR for symptomatic relief (25,26). A negative or inhibitory response has also been described; it is a worsening of motor function occurring prior to the SDR. It can last minutes to hours and has been termed a "super-off" (27). These three responses are imposed on a diurnal pattern of motor function (better performance in the morning with subsequent decline throughout the day) and on top of the continued endogenous dopamine activity (28,29). Nutt and colleagues propose that the residual endogenous dopamine activity as well as the LDR essentially determine the off-time (25).

Several patterns of motor fluctuations have been described. They progress from simple predictable patterns early on to more complicated unpredictable ones and, as expected, become more difficult to treat. The earliest type is the end of dose wearing-off effect. With this pattern, the antiparkinsonian effect of LD wears off toward the end of dose in a predictable fashion. This has also been referred to as end-of-dose failure. This is followed by complicated wearing-off where the duration of response of LD becomes more variable so that the timing of wearing off becomes less predictable. At this point, patients begin to experience delayed-on (a delay in onset of effect of LD) and dose failures (otherwise know as no-on). The random on-off effect is when LD response varies in an unpredictable manner unrelated to timing of the dose. This often happens suddenly like a light switch being turned on and off. Dyskinesias can also occur in various patterns. Most common are peak dose dyskinesias. With this, choreic movements occur when plasma LD levels are at their peak. Usually the patient has an on time with no dyskinesias, but as they reach peak effect they develop the involuntary movements. Diphasic dyskinesias are when choreic or dystonic movements occur at the beginning and end of dose. The legs seem to be more involved. Some patients have dyskinesias for the entire time they are on (square wave dyskinesias). Dyskinesias may occur in the off state as well, and this is usually in the guise of dystonia. The patterns include early morning dystonia and off period dystonia. Finally, patients may fluctuate abruptly from severe immobility to severe dyskinesia known as yo-yoing.

CLINICAL TRIALS OF LEVODOPA

Early Trials

The initial studies of LD as first line therapy for PD were carried out in the late 1960s to early 1970s. These studies were quite different from modern ones in that the patients had varying durations of disease, some quite advanced, and standard measures such as the Unified Parkinson's Disease Rating Scale (UPDRS) were not yet devised. The results, however, were dramatic. The breakthrough report was that by Cotzias et al. (14). After conflicting findings and consideration of abandoning dopa therapy, Cotzias was able to demonstrate the definitive effectiveness of LD (as opposed to the D/L-Dopa). These investigators examined 28 patients in an open-label manner with intermittent replacement with placebo and utilized LD without a dopa decarboxylase inhibitor. The duration of disease ranged from 1 to 30 years (mean 10 years), and they used a 0–4 scale. All patients responded with 20 of them having a marked to dramatic improvement, and some returned to work. All motor features improved. Some patients developed fluctuations and dyskinesias quickly, and it was suggested that these problems related to duration of disease. Many studies followed that supported these findings (30,31). Sweet and McDowell (32) studied 100 patients treated for up to 5 years in an open-label fashion. Forty-seven of them completed the whole 5 years. The patients improved remarkably by 6 months (60% of patients were more than 50% improved), and despite worsening over the next 4.5 years the Cornell weighted scale scores remained significantly better than that seen at baseline. All the signs of PD improved, and some patients were able to resume working. The severity of the parkinsonian features at initiation of therapy had little bearing on the ultimate response. This remarkable result was observed despite the fact that more than half the patients being treated suffered from concomitant dementia. It became clear that LD was not a cure for PD (as previously hoped) as it did not stop progression of disease and was associated with several late complications. In particular, motor fluctuations and dyskinesias were observed from the beginning with LD therapy. Five-year estimates based on these early studies were approximately 50% for both (31,32). Three issues regarding early LD therapy may have impacted on these figures. First, patients with advanced disease were included, and they certainly were more susceptible to the onset of late complications. Second, dopa decarboxylase inhibitors were not used in a majority of patients since they were not widely available. It was later shown that these inhibitors decreased the frequency of fluctuations. Finally, patients were treated with the maximum tolerated dose. This use of high doses may have increased the likelihood of dyskinesias and fluctuations. Some studies have indicated that lower doses of LD bring about a similar response but fewer complications (33), while others were not in agreement (34). Nevertheless, clinicians tend to use the lowest possible effective dose.

Recent Trials

Several studies have been completed in the last decade that provide more information about the effectiveness of LD therapy. They include comparisons of immediate-release and controlled-release formulations and comparisons of LD and dopamine agonists. The populations of patients are more homogeneous than in the early trials as the patients are primarily those with early disease (<5 years). Recent studies have shown more varied frequencies of late complications. The variances probably relate to the manner in which they are defined and detected. The CR First study (35) was a 5-year, randomized, double-blind study comparing controlled release and standard formulation carbidopa/levodopa in 618 LD-naive patients (mean duration of disease of 2.3 years). The primary endpoint was the time until onset of motor fluctuations. The definitions of motor fluctuations included that reported in patient completed diaries or observations of investigators in the clinic recorded on a standard questionnaire. The time until the onset of fluctuations was the earlier of two consecutive diary periods demonstrating their presence with either $\geqslant 10\%$ of the waking day with dyskinesias or $\geqslant 20\%$ in the off state. It could also be the time until onset of fluctuations based on the investigator questionnaire. This definition would indicate that they were not just testing for first onset of fluctuations but instead onset of functionally meaningful symptoms. Sixty percent of patients completed 5 years. Mean dose of LD in both groups was low (400–500 mg/day). There were no differences between the two formulations with regard to efficacy or frequency of motor fluctuations. Despite low doses there was a significant improvement of the UPDRS motor score that gradually diminished over time but was still better than the baseline score as seen in the earlier studies. However, only about 20% of patients in each group developed wearing off and dyskinesias, far lower than prior numbers. The CALM-PD study (36,37), a parallel-group, double-blind, randomized trial consisting of both clinical and imaging substudies, compared the rates of dopaminergic motor complications and dopamine neuron degeneration (primary endpoints), respectively, after initial treatment of early PD with pramipexole versus LD. The clinical 2-year data reported that 28% of patients assigned to pramipexole developed motor complications compared with 51% of patients assigned to LD ($p < 0.001$). However, the mean improvement in UPDRS score was significantly greater in the LD group compared with pramipexole (9.2 vs. 4.5; $p < 0.001$). When extended to 4 years, slightly more than half (52%) of the patients initially assigned to the pramipexole group developed motor complications compared with 74% of the LD-treated patients ($p < 0.0001$). The mean improvement in UPDRS scores from baseline through 48 months was significantly greater in the LD group (3.6) than the pramipexole group (-0.98; $p < 0.01$). The imaging portion of the study (38,39) included 82 patients who underwent four sequential [123]I B-CIT single photon emission computed tomography (SPECT) scans over a 46-month period to compare the rate of nigrostriatal dopaminergic degeneration between the treatment groups. It is assumed that a reduction in striatal [123]I B-CIT uptake is a marker of dopamine neuron degeneration. The authors report a 40% relative reduction in the rate of loss of uptake when comparing pramipexole to LD. Whether this suggests a protective effect of the dopamine agonist with respect to LD or that LD may accelerate the rate of loss of uptake or that this is a pharmacological effect is not clear given the limits of the study design. A similar 5-year comparison of ropinirole and LD in 268 patients was reported in 2001 (40). Approximately half of the patients withdrew by the end of 5 years. At a mean dose of 16.5 mg/day, ropinirole monotherapy was well tolerated and could be maintained in 16% of patients. The primary endpoint was the appearance of dyskinesias as measured by item 32 on the UPDRS. They were shown to occur earlier and more frequently in patients treated with LD than ropinirole. Regardless of LD supplementation, 20% of ropinirole subjects experienced dyskinesias by the end of 5 years versus 45% of LD subjects. Prior to the addition of LD, 5% of the ropinirole group and 36% of the LD group developed dyskinesias. The differences were statistically significant. The change from baseline of the UPDRS activities of daily living (ADL) score was similar between the two groups, but there was a significant difference in favor of the LD group for the change from baseline of the UPDRS motor score, which improved by approximately four times compared to the ropinirole group. This difference in efficacy was reported in the 6-month interim report published earlier (41). LD treatment is associated with greater therapeutic benefit (both early in the course of disease as well as later), and at least half of the patients developed motor complications after several years regardless of initial treatment.

Thirty years of experience and literature have led to several conclusions regarding LD therapy in PD. It is currently the most potent symptomatic therapy for PD. We have learned quite a bit about the nuances of treatment such that our goals have changed. We now treat with the lowest effective dose, not the highest tolerated one, we avoid frequent small doses, which only add to the unpredictable responses seen, and we have developed adjunctive therapies that complement LD. In short, we have become better at utilizing LD to treat our patients. The outcome is fewer late complications, though we do not state that these are no longer a problem.

DOES LEVODOPA CAUSE MOTOR FLUCTUATIONS?

It has been well known since the early days of LD that motor fluctuations and dyskinesias relate to therapy (2). Barbeau referred to it as the long-term levodopa syndrome (42). At that time, with no alternative treatments available, he indicated that its existence did not counterbalance the great usefulness of the drug. But what causes its onset and progression? The debate addresses whether it is disease progression or primarily LD itself or both. The answer is not totally clear but this question has been examined extensively in two ways: (1) evaluating patient populations and examining which of the two factors correlates with the onset of fluctuations and dyskinesias; (2) examining the actual response fluctuations in a controlled setting to determine possible etiological explanations. The conclusion to this debate is now more important than ever since alternative therapies are becoming available and the choice of which drug to use first is in question.

In a retrospective study, Lesser et al. (43) collected data from 131 PD patients relating to severity of disease and late complications and assessed whether these problems were attributed to duration of disease or LD therapy. A relationship was seen between the presence of fluctuations and duration of therapy whereby those with fluctuations tended to be treated for 4 years or more. This was not true for dyskinesias. They, therefore, associated fluctuations with LD therapy but did not rule out the possibility that those receiving LD longer had a more progressive disease. It was recommended that initiation of therapy be delayed until the patient "begins to function unsatisfactorily in occupational or social situations." This is perhaps the most frequently quoted paper on the subject, but the authors themselves pointed out the flaws in a retrospective study and indicated the need for a prospective evaluation of the problem. In another retrospective study, de Jong et al. (44) examined 129 patients to determine the role of age of onset, predominant symptom (tremor vs. akinetic rigid PD vs. all three together), duration of therapy, and disease severity in the occurrence of motor fluctuations. There was no significant effect of age of onset, predominant symptom, and duration of disease prior to LD therapy (but there was a trend). However, those patients with later therapy showed a lower frequency of fluctuations. Those patients treated in the earlier stages of disease (Hoehn and Yahr stages 1 and 2) did significantly worse with regard to the onset of fluctuations than patients initiating therapy in later stages (Hoehn and Yahr stages 3 and 4), suggesting that LD should not be started until stage 3 disease.

Several studies have since been published which contradict these findings. Cedarbaum et al. (45) questioned the papers described above, indicating that the patients treated earlier had to be because of more severe disease prior to initiating therapy, continued to progress faster, and thus were more prone to the onset of motor fluctuations. They suggested that LD was not the cause of the late complications, nor did the drug itself lead to loss of efficacy. In their own retrospective study, 307 patients were surveyed or interviewed with regard to motor fluctuations and various demographic features and records were reviewed. Patients were evaluated as a whole and were divided into several subgroups based on duration of disease and duration of therapy. Analyses failed to show an association between initiation of LD therapy and fluctuations or dyskinesias. Both the duration of disease and duration of therapy were longer in the patients with motor fluctuations and dyskinesias than in the group as a whole. Despite these findings, detailed statistical analyses of subgroups failed to demonstrate that age of onset and duration of therapy influenced the occurrence of fluctuations and dyskinesias. Mean delay in LD therapy was the same for fluctuators and nonfluctuators. However, patients with dyskinesias were more than three times as likely to have had initiation of LD delayed more than 2 years from diagnosis. These authors did not advocate delaying LD therapy because it, in fact, increased the chances of dyskinesias. Blin et al. (46) agreed that the apparent acceleration of progression of disease after initiation of LD therapy related to the rapidity of progression prior to LD therapy and not the therapy itself. They also found that delayed initiation of LD led to quicker onset of dyskinesia. Caraceni et al. (47) performed a prospective study on 125 patients. The study followed patients for a mean of 6 years from initiation of LD therapy to evaluate any risk factors for motor fluctuations and dyskinesias. All patients were started on LD at first diagnosis. Using a multivariable analysis, they found the risk of late complications was greater in those with akinetic-rigid PD, younger-onset age, greater disability and duration of disease, and longer interval between initiation of disease onset and LD therapy. Duration and dose of LD therapy were not associated with onset of late complications. They concluded that LD did not accelerate the appearance of motor fluctuations and that these complications relate to the severity and progression of PD. Thus, they also concluded that there is no need to delay LD treatment. Hoehn (48) indicated, based on her comparison of patients in pre- and post-levodopa eras, that a delay in the introduction of LD but not duration of treatment was associated with a poorer outcome. Horstink et al. (49) examined the relationship of duration of disease and duration of LD therapy and onset of peak dose dyskinesias in 54 PD patients and found that both duration of disease and LD therapy were greater in the dyskinetic group. The two variables are closely linked, so they then studied patients with significantly asymmetrical dyskinesias and found dyskinesia. to be most prominent on the worst side, suggesting that disease severity is an important risk factor for dyskinesias, not duration of LD therapy. Roos et al. (50) retrospectively studied 89 PD patients and several clinical correlates with onset of response fluctuations (age of onset of PD, the presenting symptom, the duration of illness, stage of illness at initiation of LD, mean and last dose of LD). They used survival and covariate analyses. No correlation was found between the dose of LD and the onset of fluctuations. However, a rapid increase in LD dose rather than the total dose seemed to determine the onset of fluctuations. They suggested that this meant that fluctuations occurred in patients with a more rapidly progressive disease requiring a more rapid escalation in LD dose. They also concluded that there are no good reasons to delay LD therapy if disability dictates its need. Finally, Kostic et al. (51) recently examined the effect of stage of disease at initiation of LD on the development of motor complications. Of 40 consecutive PD patients, 17 were treated in stage 1, 13 at stage 2, and 10 at stage 3. They found that severity of disease was an important factor in the onset of fluctuations and dyskinesias. Those patients initially treated at stage 3 developed dyskinesias and fluctuations significantly earlier than patients did in stages 1 and 2. However, latencies from disease onset to development of fluctuations and dyskinesias were no different between groups. This suggested that onset of late complications relate to disease duration and severity and not LD therapy.

While questions remain, these data suggest that disease duration, progression, and severity are important risk factors in the development of motor fluctuations and dyskinesias. In accepting this conclusion one would agree that, based on the occurrence of motor complications, there is no reason to delay LD therapy. In fact, two of the studies indicate that a delay would increase the likelihood of dyskinesias. These findings are consistent with reports of patients with late-stage PD (1) or severe parkinsonism secondary to 1-methyl-4-phenyl-1,2,3,6-tetrahydropyridine (MPTP) developing fluctuations soon after the initiation of therapy. This has also been seen in MPTP-treated nonhuman primates (52) and postencephalitic parkinsonism (53).

Several groups have studied the mechanism of motor fluctuations. The findings suggest that both duration of disease and LD therapy play a role. Work by Fabbrini and colleagues (54) has demonstrated that perhaps the initial feature that leads to onset of fluctuations is the degeneration of nigral dopaminergic neurons to a threshold level. Once this level is reached, motor fluctuations begin with wearing off. In their studies, they examined four groups of patients: levodopa-naive, levodopa-treated stable responders (nonfluctuators), patients with wearing-off, and patients with unpredictable on/off. They treated each patient with a continuous intravenous infusion of LD for 16 hours and then abruptly stopped it. They found that there was no change in pharmacokinetics of LD in the more advanced patients. However, it was noted that there was a decay of antiparkinsonian effect, which worsened as the patients advanced from being LD-naive to having on/off phenomenon. The authors concluded from the study that the wearing-off effect is probably initiated as a consequence of the marked loss of presynaptic dopaminergic neurons. With loss to a threshold number of neurons, the dopamine system loses its ability to store and release dopamine and, thus, buffer fluctuations in serum and cerebral LD and dopamine levels. It is believed that LD is converted to dopamine in nondopaminergic cells that lack the ability to store and release it in the normally tonic fashion (21). Stimulation at postsynaptic dopamine receptors then becomes intermittent as a reflection of the peak and trough profile of oral LD therapy. It appears that as soon as this intermittent stimulation of dopamine receptors begins, postsynaptic changes are initiated. Studies have demonstrated a narrowing of the therapeutic window, alteration of threshold for onset of dyskinesias, and steepening of the anti-PD response slope, all which underlie progression toward a more unstable response to LD (55,56). These findings support the involvement of postsynaptic mechanisms, reflecting an increased sensitivity of clinical response to small fluctuations in dopamine levels and differing pharmacological mechanisms for antiparkinsonian response and dyskinesias.

In trials comparing LD to dopamine agonists, LD therapy leads to earlier onset and more frequent occurrence of dyskinesias and wearing-off. This would suggest that either the agonist prevents the onset of these problems or that LD therapy does have some role in causing them. Disease progression with loss of nigrostriatal dopaminergic neurons to a threshold level appears to be at the root of onset of motor fluctuations. LD plays a role, via intermittent stimulation of postsynaptic receptors, in the progression of fluctuations to a more unpredictable pattern. One needs to consider that onset and progression are probably caused by different scenarios. Delaying LD may delay this progression, but the symptoms would come on sooner after LD initiation, as previously demonstrated. The delay of therapy would deprive the patient of a period of known good response. Mouradian et al. (57) demonstrated that continuous infusion of LD can reverse motor fluctuations and dyskinesias. The same can be said about subthalamic nucleus (STN) stimulation. Some indicate that the reversibility of fluctuations implicates LD in the cause of the fluctuations (58,59) but that is not the only interpretation. It can also mean that the role LD plays in motor fluctuations is potentially reversible.

IS LEVODOPA TOXIC?

It has been suggested that LD may be toxic to dopaminergic neurons, leading to more rapid degeneration. This notion is based on the oxyradical hypothesis. There is evidence that oxyradicals play a role in the pathogenesis of cell death in PD (60). Dopamine, when metabolized by MAO or autooxidized, forms H_2O_2, a precursor to the toxic hydroxyl radical. In PD, after loss of a substantial number of nigral cells, those surviving cells increase their dopamine metabolism, possibly increasing the risk of further degeneration, especially in an environment where protective mechanisms, such as glutathione, are diminished and iron has accumulated. The use of LD may lead to an increase in dopamine formation and, in turn, an increase in dopamine metabolism with greater free radical formation (61). While this theory has widespread appeal, and while laboratory evidence supports this possibility, the theory remains controversial (62). However, detailed reviews on the subject (63–65) have indicated that there is no convincing evidence to suggest that levodopa is toxic to our patients and that this concern should not govern how we treat our patients.

The evaluations for LD toxicity have included both in vitro (cell culture) and in vivo animal studies. In the cell culture studies, various cell types were used including fetal mesencephalic cells, neuroblastoma, fetal fibroblasts, pheochromocytoma PC12 cells, chick sympathetic neurons, and others (66). Results of these studies were variable because of the LD concentrations used and culture conditions. High doses of LD are toxic to dopaminergic neurons in pure neuronal cultures. Mechanisms of toxicity include oxyradicals, mitochondrial toxicity, or apoptosis (67–69). However, as the conditions are set to more accurately reflect in vivo systems, the toxicity disappears and the neurons are more able to resist injury. In fact, with exposure to medium doses (20–100 µm) and with glial cells present, LD actually has a trophic influence. The glial cells contain the protective enzymes catalase and glutathione peroxidase and provide a nutritive and protective environment. LD exposure to these cultures actually increases cellular concentrations of reduced glutathione peroxidase and may have other neurotrophic properties. At levels that are likely present in the extracellular fluid in the striatum of patients, as measured in animals by microdialysis (picomolar levels), it is unlikely that LD has any effect (65).

In vivo studies have included both unlesioned and lesioned animals. Several studies involved giving healthy animals LD for up to 18 months, and they demonstrated no loss of dopaminergic neurons (70,71). In one study, Cotzias et al. actually reported that mice given LD lived longer than controls not given LD (72). However, a controversy surrounds previously lesioned animals. Fahn (66) reviewed more than 15 studies of in vivo effects of LD and dopamine. Four studies are of particular relevance to the issue of early LD therapy for PD. Blunt et al. (73) lesioned rats with 6-hydroxydopamine (6-OHDA) and gave LD to some. They then counted tyrosine hydroxylase (TH)–stained cells in the substantia nigra (SN) and ventral tegmental area (VTA). The unlesioned (healthy) side was unaffected by the LD, supporting the prior studies. The SN on the lesioned side lost 96% of its cells from the 6-OHDA. The VTA was less affected, with 23–65% of cells remaining. LD further reduced surviving cell numbers to 10–35%. They concluded that either LD suppressed TH activity or caused increased cell death, a conclusion that has been questioned (74). Fukuda et al. (75) used MPTP-lesioned mice and examined the effect of LD and bromocriptine on total and TH+ cell counts. LD further reduced cell counts in MPTP-treated mice but it was in TH– cells. TH+ cells were unaffected. Bromocriptine had no effect, but combined LD and bromocriptine resulted in a significant increase in surviving cells. Murer et al. (74) examined the effects of LD on nigrostriatal and VTA cells in rats with moderate and severe 6-OHDA lesions and sham-lesioned animals. They measured three dopaminergic markers—TH, dopamine transporter (DAT), and vesicular monoamine transporter (VMAT2)—via radio-immunohistochemistry in the SN, VTA, and striatum. They also examined rotational behavior to assess pharmacologically relevant doses and postsynaptic receptor binding. The study failed to demonstrate any significant difference on cell counts in SNpc and VTA in LD-treated animals compared to those treated with vehicle using all three markers. There was a trend toward increased TH staining in the SNpc of the moderately lesioned animals. At the level of striatum there was no effect of LD treatment in the sham-lesioned and severely lesioned animals, but in the moderate lesioned animals there was partial recovery of nerve terminals in the damaged area, suggesting a neuroprotective potential. The increased immunostaining in this region reached statistical significance compared to those rats treated with vehicle. It was suggested that this increased striatal activity with LD related to partial recovery via axonal sprouting by the remaining neurons. LD also tended to reverse increased binding (upregulation) of dopamine receptors and diminished the development of behavioral supersensitivity, indicating that the doses of LD were pharmacologically effective. These results indicate that LD did not damage the neurons or their terminals in normal and moderately or severely lesioned animals. It may promote compensatory mechanisms at the terminals and thus recovery of innervation of the striatum. Datla et al. (76) demonstrated similar findings. In the rats with 6-OHDA and ferric chloride ($FeCl_3$) lesions, LD had no short-term or long-term effects on the number of TH+ cells. In contrast, in the 6-OHDA model there may have been a protective effect since there was an increase in TH+ cells after 24 weeks. While results of these animal studies appear to be conflicting, the latter studies seem to provide evidence that LD is not toxic. One could conclude that LD has no detrimental effect on dopaminergic neurons in healthy and compromised animals.

Human studies have also been nonsupportive for the possibility of LD toxicity. Quinn et al. (77) reported on the treatment of a non-PD patient who received high-dose LD for 4 years. Autopsy results demonstrated a normal SN. Rajput et al. (78) reported on five patients with similar results. Three patients had essential tremor, one had dopa-responsive dystonia, and the other was nonprogressive. Autopsies in two were normal. None of the essential tremor patients developed parkinsonism; the two other patients showed no progression of disease clinically. This would indicate that LD is not detrimental to patients with normal or dysfunctional SN. Yahr et al. (79) compared postmortem results in patients treated and never treated with LD and reported no difference in the pathology of the SNpc. Gwinn-Hardy et al. (80) examined the effect of LD on a family with autosomal dominant LD responsive parkinsonism (mutation on chromosome 4p). There were 12 affected individuals, and survival duration and disease progression were compared in those treated and not treated. Survival was significantly different between the two groups, as was progression of disease, both in favor of LD therapy. Finally, a recent neuroimaging study compared progression of PD with a dopamine agonist versus LD (38,39). It utilized B-CIT SPECT imaging comparing LD and pramipexole. The decrease in binding was less over several years for the agonist than for LD. This may be an indicator that LD is toxic, that the agonist is neuroprotective, or it may reflect a differential pharmacological effect. At this point the answer is unknown.

When one looks at the data from cell culture, animals, and humans, there is so far no support for the notion that LD is toxic. There should be no concern about this when considering therapy in PD patients.

DOES TOLERANCE DEVELOP FROM LEVODOPA?

The lay literature is replete with information suggesting that LD loses its effect after about 5 years. This leads to some trepidation on the part of the patient and physician in initiating therapy. If that were the case, it would indicate that tolerance is a possible concern and such an occurrence would argue for delaying treatment. It is conceivable that, when all nigrostriatal cells are depleted, LD would lose all effectiveness since these are the cells that convert LD and release dopamine. Lesser et al. (43) found that longer duration of disease did not appear to adversely affect response to LD at the time of initiation of therapy, yet they demonstrated a deterioration in response that did not correlate with duration of disease. Those receiving LD longer had more severe disease. The assumption made by the authors was that PD patients developed tolerance. Despite these findings, the authors did not rule out the possibility that those receiving LD longer had a more progressive disease. However, Blin et al. (46) noted that chronic treatment does not lead to decreased effectiveness. Evidence indicates that conversion of dopa to dopamine can occur at sites other than dopaminergic terminals in the striatum (43,54,58). Thus, LD continues to be effective throughout the course of disease. The potency of LD does not change with chronic use. Markham and Diamond (81,82) demonstrated this when they studied three groups of patients; those starting LD after 1–3 years of disease, 4–6 years, and 7–9 years. In this manner they could assess whether the apparent loss of efficacy could relate to the disease duration or the duration of drug therapy. After 6 years of follow-up they noted the following:

1. The disability scores were different for the three groups at initiation of LD and remained different thereafter.
2. Disability scores were the same for the three groups when they were matched for disease duration despite varied durations of therapy.
3. There was no significant difference with respect to the incidence of dyskinesias.

In projecting the course of disease it was found that all three groups ultimately followed the same predictable course of progression independent of the duration of LD therapy. This was confirmed after 12 years of follow-up of the first group (81,82). The authors concluded that LD works at all stages of PD, does not result in tolerance over time, but does not stop progression of disease. In other words, changes in disability of PD are related to duration of disease and not duration of therapy or tolerance to LD. Aside from progression of disease, another cause of the apparent loss of efficacy relates to narrowing of the therapeutic window—increased sensitivity to adverse effects such as dyskinesias and hallucinations (45,46). The worsening of disease also comes from the onset and progression of symptoms not attributable to dopamine systems, such as postural instability, freezing, and dementia (46).

MORTALITY OF PD WITH LEVODOPA

Several studies performed in the 1970s demonstrated that LD therapy improves mortality in PD. These studies compared the survival of LD-treated patients to the mortality rate demonstrated in the pre-levodopa Hoehn and Yahr study (2), which demonstrated that mortality was three times greater than in the normal population. Nearly all studies indicated that LD improved survival with rates of 1.4–2.4 (83,84). Some investigators suggested that survival approached normal, while others indicated that the effect was only seen early in therapy and then disappeared. However, many of the studies have been criticized due to methodological flaws, problems with patient selection, and possible biases. One study of particular interest (83) utilized a population-based study design (retrospective) to avoid many of these flaws and examine the change in survival related to LD therapy. The study included patients treated from 1964 to 1978 to include patients treated early and late as well as untreated cases. Results indicated that survival for all patients was significantly poorer than that of the general population but was better in treated than in untreated PD. The improved survival over time was not linear. Throughout the entire 17 years of follow-up there was reduced risk of death with LD therapy.

One other area of interest relates to the timing of LD therapy. Does early or later intervention affect the survival rates? Diamond et al. (81,82) examined this question looking at 359 patients treated between 1968 and 1977. They divided patients into three groups: group one, 1–3 years of PD; group two, 4–6 years of PD; group three, 7–9 years of PD. They used observed-to-expected death rate (from a group of similar make-up in the general population) ratios as measures of survival. When duration of therapy is held constant at 15 years, the ratio was higher for patients with longer duration of disease. When duration of disease was held constant at 17 years, the patients in group one had a better mortality ratio than the other two groups. Thus, early initiation of LD therapy was beneficial to life expectancy. They suggested that the improved survival related to the symptomatic effect of the drug, keeping patients more active in the earlier years. In another study, Scigliano et al. (84) studied 145 patients seen from 1970 to 1983. Of those, 98 were treated for 2 or more years while 47 were treated for <2 years. Mortality was found to be 2.5 times greater among the patients treated later, but a multivariate analysis taking into account age and disease severity made the difference nonsignificant. However, there were biases that led to an underestimation of mortality in the delayed treatment group, including 47 patients who were lost to follow-up. They concluded that survival from early LD initiation is the same or better than late. Uitti et al. (85) examined the duration of the interval from onset of disease to treatment and found that it had no influence on subsequent mortality.

IS THERE AN ASSOCIATION BETWEEN LD THERAPY AND MELANOMA?

Previous reports as well as the *Physician's Desk Reference* caution against the use of LD in PD patients with a history of melanoma. As recently as 1998, Pfutzner and Przybilla reported that while no causal relationship has been proven, patients with a history of malignant melanoma receiving LD therapy should be carefully followed for the development of new pigmented lesions (86). Anecdotal reports exist in the literature of the potential carcinogenic effects of LD therapy and its potential to activate malignant melanoma (87). Because dopamine acts on and is produced by pigmented neurons, it has been proposed that levodopa may affect the activity of melanocytes, possibly promoting malignant transformation.

Weiner et al. in 1993 (88) reviewed the literature and concluded that there is anecdotal evidence at best to support a link between LD and melanoma. They reported on nine patients with PD and a history of melanoma who were treated with LD, none of whom had a recurrence. They concluded that LD therapy could be used safely in PD patients with melanoma. Woofter and Manyam (87) reported on a 74-year-old man with PD who was treated with LD and whose malignant melanoma was later discovered. Prior to the diagnosis of melanoma, it was estimated that the patient received 5.7 kg of LD over a 6-year period. The patient continued with LD treatment for more than 10 years, with an additional 4.3 kg LD prescribed, and no recurrence of his melanoma was observed. They concluded that withholding LD therapy for fear of accelerating melanoma was unwarranted (87). Siple et al. reviewed 34 case reports found by literature review (January 1966–September 1999) and indicated that the association between LD and induction or exacerbation of malignant melanoma was unlikely (89).

Thus, despite the continued warning appearing in the prescribing literature for LD, there appears to be no causal relationship between LD therapy in PD and the occurrence of malignant melanoma. A history of melanoma in a PD patient should not prohibit the use of LD.

LEVODOPA CHALLENGE TEST

It can be difficult to accurately differentiate PD from other forms of parkinsonism, especially during early presentation. LD administration can be used for diagnostic purposes as PD patients respond more frequently and robustly to LD compared with other forms of parkinsonism.

Clarke and Davies recently published a review of 13 studies that examined whether an acute LD or apomorphine challenge test could aid in the diagnosis of PD (90). Four studies examined de novo patients and nine examined patients with clinically established idiopathic PD. Although there was significant variability in the methodologies employed, abstracted sensitivity and specificity data were summarized from the studies and the two challenge tests compared as to their ability to accurately predict patients' diagnosis. The sensitivity for the diagnosis of established PD for apomorphine was 0.86 (95% CI), acute levodopa 0.75 (95% CI), and chronic levodopa therapy 0.91 (95% CI). The specificity for the diagnosis of established PD was apomorphine 0.85 (95% CI), acute levodopa 0.87 (95% CI), and chronic levodopa therapy 0.77 (95% CI). The number of patients positive for each test divided by the number with clinically diagnosed de novo disease was apomorphine 0.63 (95% CI), acute levodopa therapy 0.69 (95% CI), and chronic levodopa therapy 0.76 (95% CI). Twenty-one chronic LD patients described as having positive response were initially negative via acute LD.

The authors concluded that the accuracy of the acute levodopa and apomorphine tests was similar but not superior than that of chronic levodopa therapy and that these were not more accurate than the established accuracy of clinical diagnosis of PD (75–80% accuracy). In addition, given the additional costs and adverse effects associated with their use, they could not recommend using the challenge tests.

Rossi et al. (91) reported on the use of acute challenge with apomorphine and LD in patients with clinically defined forms of parkinsonism to assess the potential accuracy of the tests with regards to diagnosis. Motor responses to the acute administration of LD and apomorphine were analyzed in a series of 134 parkinsonian patients (83 with a clinical diagnosis of idiopathic PD, 28 patients with multiple system atrophy, 6 with progressive supranuclear palsy and 17 unclassified patients). The duration of disease or the clinical stage of the patients was not described. Patients received LD/AADI (250/25 mg) or subcutaneous apomorphine (1.5, 3, 4.5 mg). UPDRS motor scores were evaluated 1 hour following LD administration and 20 minutes after apomorphine injection. The motor evaluation was matched with the clinical diagnosis and the response to chronic LD therapy. Those patients who had improvement of at least 16% on their UPDRS were more likely to have PD when compared to non-PD patients. When comparing PD with MSA patients, those who improved at least 18% on their UPDRS were more likely to have PD rather than MSA. If a patient responded to the challenge test with at least 14.5% improvement in UPDRS, they were more likely to respond favorably to chronic LD therapy. The authors conclude that use of the challenge test was helpful in making treatment decisions regarding long-term LD therapy (91). It appears that an acute LD test is not very useful in improving our ability to diagnose PD. Questions remain about its use in making treatment decisions.

ACKNOWLEDGMENTS

This work was supported by the Riley Family Chair of Parkinson's Disease (SAF), The Phyllis Dake Neurosciences Fellowship (AJS), and the Albany Medical College Parkinson's Research Fund.

REFERENCES

1. Parkinson J. An Essay on the Shaking Palsy. London: Sherwood, Neely and Jones, 1817.
2. Hoehn MM, Yahr MD. Parkinsonism: onset, progression, and mortality. Neurology 1967; 17:427–442.
3. Factor SA. Parkinson's disease: initial treatment with levodopa or dopamine agonists. Curr Treat Options 2001; 3:479–493.
4. Doshay L, Constable K. Newer drugs in the treatment of Parkinsonism. Neurology 1951; 1:68–74.
5. Epidemic Encephalitis. Report of a Survey by the Matheson Commission, New York, Columbia University Press, 1939.
6. Von Witzleben H. Methods of Treatment in Postencephalitic Parkinsonism. New York: Grune & Stratton, Inc., 1942.
7. Doshay L. Recent trends in the treatment of epidemic encephalitis. NYS J Med 1934; 34:707.
8. Foley P. The L-dopa story revisited. Further surprises to be expected? J Neur Transm Suppl 2000; 60:1–20.
9. Funk C. Synthase des d,1–3–4,Dioxyphenylalanins. Chem Zentralbl I, 1911.
10. Guggenhiem M. Dioxyphenylalanin, eine neue Aminosäure aus Vicia faba. Z Phys Chem, 1913.
11. Carrlson A, Lindqvist M, Magmusson T. 3,4-Dihydroxyphenylalanine and 5-hydroxytriptophan as reserpine antagonists. Nature (London) 1957; 180:1200.
12. Carrlson A, Linqvist M, Magmussen T, Waldbeck B. On the presence of 3-hydroxytyramine in the brain. Science 1958; 127:471.
13. Ehringer H, Hornykiewicz O. Verteilung von Noradrenalin und Dopamin im Gehirn des Menschwen und ihr Verhalten bei Erkränkungen des extrapyramidalen Systems. Klin Wochenscher 1960; 38:1236–1239.
14. Cotzias G, Van Woert M, Schiffer L. Aromatic amino acids and modification of parkinsonism. N Engl J Med 1967; 276:374–379.
15. Cotzias G, Papavasiliou P, Gellene R. Modification of parkinsonism—chronic treatment with L-DOPA. N Engl J Med 1969; 280:337–345.
16. Kapp W. The history of drugs for the treatment of Parkinson's disease. J Neural Transm 1992; 38:1–6.

17. Rinne U, Sonninen V, Siirtola T. Treatment of parkinsonian patients with levodopa and estracerebral decarboylase inhibitor, Ro 4-4062. Adv Neurol 1973; 3:59–71.

18. Nutt JG, Woodward WR, Hammerstad JP, Carter JH, Anderson JL. The "on-off" phenomenon in Parkinson's disease. Relation to levodopa absorption and transport. N Engl J Med 1984; 310(8):483–488.

19. Bernheimer H, Birkmayer W, Hornykiewicz O, Jellinger K, Seitelberger F. Brain dopamine and syndromes of Parkinson and Huntington. J Neurol Sci 1975; 30:415–455.

20. Muenter M, Tyce G. L-dopa therapy of Parkinson's disease: plasma L-dopa concentration, therapeutic response and side effects. Mayo Clin Proc 1971; 46:231–239.

21. Melamed E, Hefti F, Wurtman RJ. Nondopaminergic striatal neurons convert exogenous L-dopa to dopamine in parkinsonism. Ann Neurol 1980; 8:558–563.

22. Poewe W, Wenning G. Levodopa. Parkinson's disease: mechanisms of action, pathophysiology of late failure. In: Parkinson's Disease and Movement Disorders. Jankovic J, Tolosa E, eds. Baltimore: Williams and Wilkins, 1998, pp 177–190.

23. Fahn S. Parkinson's disease, the effect of levodopa and the ELLDOPA trial. Arch Neurol 1999; 56:529–535.

24. Ahlskog JE, Muenter MD. Frequency of levodopa-related dyskinesias and motor fluctuations as estimated from the cummulative literature. Mov Disord 2001; 16(3):448–458.

25. Nutt J, Carter J, Woodward W. Long-duration response to levodopa. Neurology 1995; 45:1613–1616.

26. Nutt J. Motor Fluctuations and dyskinesia in Parkinson's disease. Parkinsonism Relat Disord 2001; 8:101–108.

27. Nutt J. Pharmacodynamics of levodopa in Parkinson's disease. Clin Exp Pharmacol Physiol 1995; 22:837–840.

28. Nutt J, Gancher S, Woodward W. Does an inhibitory action of levodopa contribute to motor fluctuations? Neurology 1988; 38:1553–1557.

29. Merello M, Hughes A, Colosimo C, Hoffman M, Starkstein S, Leiguarda R. Sleep benefit in Parkinson's disease. Mov Disord 1997; 12:506–508.

30. Simuni T, Hurtig H. Levodopa: 30 years of progress. In: Parkinson's Disease: Diagnosis and Clinical Management. Factor SA, Weiner WJ, eds. New York: Demos, 2002:339–356.

31. Yahr MD. Levodopa. Ann Int Med 1975; 83:677–682.

32. Sweet RD, McDowell FH. Five years' treatment of Parkinson's disease with levodopa: therapeutic results and survival of 100 patients. Ann Int Med 1975; 83:456–463.

33. Rajput AH, Stern W, Laverly WH. Chronic low-dose levodopa therapy in Parkinson's disease: an argument for delaying levodopa therapy. Neurology 1984; 34:991–996.

34. Poewe WH, Lees AJ, Stern GM. Low dose L-dopa therapy in Parkinson's disease: a 6-year follow-up study. Neurology 1986; 36:1528–1530.

35. Koller WC, Hutton JT, Tolosa E, Capilldeo R, and the Carbidopa/Levodopa Study Group. Immediate-release and controlled-release carbidopa/levodopa in PD: a 5-year randomized multicenter study. Neurology 1999; 53:1012–1019.
36. Parkinson Study Group. Pramipexole versus levodopa as initial treatment for Parkinson's disease: a randomized controlled trial. JAMA 2000; 284:1931–1938.
37. Holloway RG. Pramipexole versus levodopa as initial treatment for Parkinson's disease: a four-year randomized controlled trial. Neurology 2002; 58(suppl 3):A81–82.
38. Parkinson Study Group. Dopamine transporter brain imaging to assess the effects of pramipexole versus levodopa on Parkinson disease progression. JAMA 2002; 287:1653–1661.
39. Marek K. Pramipexole versus levodopa: effects on Parkinson disease progression assessed by dopamine transporter imaging. Neurology 2002; 58(suppl 3):A82.
40. Rascol O, Brooks DJ, Korczyn AD, et al. A five-year study of the incidence of dyskinesia in patients with early Parkinson's disease who were treated with ropinirole or levodopa. N Engl J Med 2000; 42:1484–1491.
41. Rascol O, Brooks DJ, Brunt ER, et al. Ropinirole in the treatment of early Parkinson's disease: a 6-month interim report of a 5-year levodopa controlled study. Mov Disord 1998; 13:39–45.
42. Barbeau A. Long-term appraisal of levodopa therapy. Neurology 1972; 22(suppl):22–24.
43. Lesser RP, Fahn S, Snider SR, et al. Analysis of the clinical problems in parkinsonism and the complications of long term therapy. Neurology 1979; 29:1253–1260.
44. de Jong GJ, Meerwaldt JD, Schmitz PIM. Factors that influence the occurence of response variations in Parkinson's disease. Ann Neurol 1987; 22:4–7.
45. Cedarbaum JM, Gandy SE, McDowell FH. "Early" initiation of levodopa treatment does not promote the development of motor response fluctuations, dyskinesia or dementia in Parkinson's disease. Neurology 1991; 41:622–629.
46. Blin J, Bonnet A-M, Agid Y. Does levodopa aggravate Parkinson's disease? Neurology 1988; 38:1410–1416.
47. Caraceni T, Scigliano G, Musicco M. The occurrence of motor fluctuations in parkinsonian patients treated long term with levodopa: role of early treatment and disease progression. Neurology 1991; 41:380–384.
48. Hoehn MM. Parkinsonism treated with levodopa: progression and mortality. J Neural Transm 1983; 19:253–264.
49. Horstink MWIM, Zijlmans JCM, Pasman JW, Berger HJC, van't Hof MA. Severity of Parkinson's disease is a risk factor for peak dose dyskinesia. J Neurol Neurosurg Psychiatry 1990; 59:224–226.
50. Roos RAC, Vredevoogd CB, van der Velde EA. Response fluctuations in Parkinson's disease. Neurology 1990; 40:1344–1346.

51. Kostic VS, Marinkovic J, Svetel M, Stfanova E, Przedborski S. The effect of stage of Parkinson's disease at the onset of levodopa therapy on development of motor complications. Eur J Neurol 2000; 9:9–14.

52. Langston JW. The impact of MPTP on Parkinson's disease research: past, present and future. In: Parkinson's Disease: Diagnosis and Clinical Management. Factor SA, Weiner WJ, eds. New York: Demos, 2002:299–329.

53. Fahn S. Welcome news about levodopa, but uncertainty remains. Ann Neurol 1998; 43:551–554.

54. Fabbrini G, Mouradian MM, Juncos JL, et al. Motor fluctuations in Parkinson's disease. central pathophysiological mechanisms, part 1. Ann Neurol 1988; 24:366–371.

55. Bravi D, Mouradian MM, Roberts JW, Davis TL, Sohn YH, Chase TN. Wearing-off fluctuations in Parkinson's disease: contributions of postsynaptic mechanisms. Ann Neurol 1994; 36:27–31.

56. Mouradian MM, Juncos JL, Fabbrini G, et al: Motor fluctuations in Parkinson's disease: central pathophysiological mechanisms, part II. Ann Neurol 1988; 24:372–378.

57. Mouradian MM, Heuser JE, Baronti F, Chase TN. Modification of central dopaminergic mechanisms by continuous levodopa therapy for advanced Parkinson's disease. Ann Neurol 1990; 27:18–23.

58. Melamed E. Initiation of levodopa therapy in parkinsonian patients should be delayed until advanced stages of the disease. Arch Neurol 1986; 43:402–405.

59. Shulman LM. Levodopa toxicity in Parkinson's disease: reality or myth? Reality—practice patterns should change. Arch Neurol 2000; 57:406–407.

60. Fahn S, Cohen G. The oxidant stress hypothesis in Parkinson's disease: evidence supporting it. Ann Neurol 1992; 32:804.

61. Olanow CW. Oxidation reactions in Parkinson's disease. Neurology 1990; 40(suppl 3):32–37.

62. Calne DB. The free radical hypothesis in Parkinson's disease: evidence against it. Ann Neurol 1992; 32:799.

63. Agid Y. Levodopa: is toxicity a myth? Neurology 1998; 50:858–863.

64. Agid Y, Chase T, Marsden D. Adverse reactions to levodopa: drug toxicity or progression of disease? Lancet 1998; 351:851–852.

65. Agid Y, Ahlskog E, Albanese A, et al. Levodopa in the treatment of Parkinson's disease: a consensus meeting. Mov Disord 1999; 14:911–913.

66. Fahn S. Is levodopa toxic? Neurology 1996; 47(suppl 3):S184–S195.

67. Olney JW, Zorumski CF, Stewart GR, et al. Excitotoxicity of L-DOPA and 6-OH-DOPA: implications for Parkinson's and Huntington's diseases. Exp Neurol 1990; 108:269–272.

68. Przedborski S, Jackson-Lewis V, Muthane U, et al. Chronic levodopa administration alters cerebral mitochondrial respiratory chain activity. Ann Neurol 1993; 34:715–723.

69. Ziv I, Zilkha-Falb R, Shirvan A, Barzilai A, Melamed E. Levodopa induces apoptosis in cultured neuronal cells-a possible accelerator of nigrostriatal degeneration in Parkinson's disease? Mov Disord 1997; 12:17–23.

70. Hefti F, Melamed E, Bhawan J, Wurtman RJ. Long-term administration of levodopa does not damage dopaminergic neurons in the mouse. Neurology 1981; 31:1194–1195.
71. Perry TL, Yong VW, Ito M, et al. Nigrostriatal dopaminergic neurons remain undamaged in rats given high doses of L-dopa and carbidopa chronically. J Neurochem 1984; 43:990–993.
72. Cotzias GC, Miller ST, Tang LC, Papavasiliou PS. Levodopa, fertility and longevity. Science 1977; 196:549–551.
73. Blunt SB, Jenner P, Marsden CD. Suppressive effect of L-dopa on dopamine cells remaining in the ventral tegmental area of rats previously exposed to the neurotoxin 6-hydroxydopamine. Mov Disord 1993; 8:129–133.
74. Murer MG, Dziewczapolski G, Menalled, et al. Chronic levodopa is not toxic for remaining dopamine neurons, but instead promotes their recovery, in rats with moderate nigrostriatal lesions. Ann Neurol 1998; 43:561–575.
75. Fukuda T, Watabe K, Tanaka J. Effects of bromocriptine and/or L-DOPA on neurons in substantia nigra of MPTP-treated C57BL/6 mice. Brain Res 1996; 728:274–276.
76. Datla KP, Blunt SB, Dexter DT. Chronic L-DOPA administration is not toxic to the remaining dopaminergic neurons, but instead may promote their functional recovery, in rats with partial 6-OHDA or FeCl3 nigrostriatal lesions. Mov Disord 2001; 16:424–434.
77. Quinn NP, Parkes D, Janota I, Marsden CD. Case report: preservation of the substantia nigra and locus ceruleus in a patient receiving levodopa (2 g) plus a decarboxylase inhibitor over a four-year period. Mov Disord 1986; 1:65–68.
78. Rajput AH, Fenton ME, Birdi S, Macaulay R. Is levodopa toxic to human substantia nigra? Mov Disord 1997; 12:634–638.
79. Yahr MD, Wolf A, Antunes J-L, et al. Autopsy findings in parkinsonism following treatment with levodopa. Neurology 1972; 22(suppl):56–71.
80. Gwinn-Hardy K, Evidente VGH, Waters C, Muenter MD, Hardy J. L-dopa slows the progression of familial parkinsonism. Lancet 1999; 353:1850–1851.
81. Markham CH, Diamond SG. Evidence to support early levodopa therapy in Parkinson's disease. Neurology 1981; 31:125–131.
82. Markham CH, Diamond SG. Long-term follow-up of early dopa treatment in Parkinson's disease. Ann Neurol 1986; 19:365–372.
83. Diamond SG, Markham CH, Hoehn MM, McDowell FH, Muenter MD. Multi-center study of Parkinson mortality with early versus later dopa treatment. Ann Neurol 1987; 22:8–12.
84. Scigliano G, Musicco M, Soliveri P, et al. Mortality associated with early and late levodopa therapy initiation in Parkinson's disease. Neurology 1990; 40:265–269.
85. Uitti RJ, Ahlskog JE, Maraganore DM, et al. Levodopa therapy and survival in idiopathic Parkinson's disease: Olmsted County project. Neurology 1993; 43:1918–1926.

86. Pfutzner W, Przybilla B. Malignant melanoma and levodopa: is there a relationship? Two new cases and a review of the literature. J Am Acad Dermatol 1998; 38:782–784.

87. Woofter M, Manyam B. Safety of long-term levodopa therapy in malignant melanoma. Clin Neuropharmacol 1994; 17:315–319.

88. Weiner W, Singer C, Sanchez-Ramos J, Goldenberg J. Levodopa, melanoma and Parkinson's Disease. Neurology 1993; 43:674–677.

89. Siple J, Schneider D, Wanlass W, Rosenblatt B. Levodopa therapy and the risk of malignant melanoma. Ann Pharmacother 2000; 34:382–385.

90. Clarke C, Davies P. Systematic review of acute levodopa and apomorphine challenge tests in the diagnosis of idiopathic Parkinson's disease. J Neurol Neurosurg Psychiatry 2000; 69:590 594.

91. Rossi P, Colosimo C, Moro E, Tonali P, Albanese A. Acute challenge with apomorphine and levodopa in parkinsonism. Eur Neurol 2000; 43:95–101.

18

Dopamine Agonists

Mark A. Stacy
Barrow Neurological Institute,
Phoenix, Arizona, U.S.A.

INTRODUCTION

Dopamine agonists (DA) have been used to treat symptoms of Parkinson's disease (PD) since the late 1970s (1). These agents were initially introduced to supplement the beneficial effect and possibly reduce the incidence of long-term complications of levodopa. In the last 30 years, methodical investigations of DA have demonstrated therapeutic benefit in all stages of PD both in combination with levodopa and as monotherapy. More recently, positron emission tomography (PET) and single photon emission computed tomography (SPECT) imaging have demonstrated possible benefit in patients randomized to a DA when compared to subjects receiving levodopa (2–4). Increasingly, clinical, animal model, and cellular data suggest not only a levodopa-sparing effect and a delay in the incidence of motor fluctuations, but also a potential neuroprotective effect (5). A number of hypotheses regarding this phenomenon have been proposed. These include reduction of free radical formation by limiting levodopa exposure or increase in the activity of radical-scavenging systems, perhaps by changing mitochondrial membrane potential. In addition, some investigators suggest that DA may enhance neurotrophic activity. However, there is currently no evidence of neurological improvement clinically, using trial designs with sufficient duration and washout periods to assess neurological status beyond therapeutic response.

This chapter will review the history of DA usage in the treatment of PD and provide a summary of data concerning efficacy, treatment approaches, and comparison between commonly prescribed DA. In addition, data suggesting long-term favorability when compared to levodopa will be reviewed. Lastly, similarly designed clinical trials will be discussed with direct comparative trials in an effort to better define the relative efficacy of these agents.

DOPAMINE AGONISTS AND DOPAMINE RECEPTORS

The DA most often used in treating symptoms of PD include apomorphine, bromocriptine, cabergoline, lisuride, pergolide, pramipexole, and ropinirole. All of these agents activate D_2 receptors, while pergolide has been shown to be a mild D_1 agonist, and pramipexole may have higher affinity for D_3 (Table 1). Five subtypes of DA receptors have been identified and may be classified into striatal (D_1 and D_2) receptors or cortical (D_3, D_4, and D_5) receptors. The D_{3-5} receptors are present in the limbic system and other dopaminergic pathways. Although the different roles of D_1 and D_2 receptors in regulation of striatal function are more fully outlined elsewhere in this volume, the D_1 receptor ($D_{1,5}$) family is associated with activation of adenylate cyclase, and dopamine and DA activate the D_2 receptor family (D_{2-4}) (6). Postmortem examination of brains of subjects with PD reveal upregulation of striatal D_2 and downregulation of the D_1 receptors. It is postulated that these changes lead to alteration of the indirect D_2-mediated pathway and disinhibition of the subthalamic nucleus. Intracortical inhibition studies comparing apomorphine, a rapid-acting DA, to deep brain stimulation found comparable changes in Unified Parkinson's Disease Rating Scale (UPDRS) and intracortical inhibition with bilateral sub-thalamic nuclei or globus pallidus stimulation or with apomorphine infusion, suggesting a connection between the nigral dopaminergic pathway and the thalamo-cortical motor pathway (7).

Apomorphine

Because of the powerful emetic action of apomorphine, clinical usage of this compound in treating PD has been avoided (8). More recently, this short-acting DA has been developed as injectable and sublingual forms to be used in "rescuing" PD patients from unpredictable off-periods. This therapy may

TABLE 1 Dopamine Agonists in Parkinson's Disease

Dopamine agonist	D$_1$	D$_2$	D$_3$	D$_4$	D$_5$	5-HT	NE	ACh
Dopamine	+	++	+++	++	+++	0	0	0
Bromocriptine	−	++	+	+	+	−	+	0
Pergolide	+	+++	+++	+++	+	0	+	0
Pramipexole	0	+++	+++	++	0	+	+	+
Ropinirole	0	+++	+++	0	0	0	0	0

D = dopamine; 5-HT = 5 hydroxytryptamine; NE − norepinephrine; ACh − acetylcholine.
Source: Adapted from Ref. 6.

require initial treatment with domperidone, a peripheral DA receptor blocking antiemetic agent. Dewey et al. (9) demonstrated a 62% improvement in off-state UPDRS scores in subjects with advanced PD 20 minutes after subcutaneously injecting apomorphine in a 2:1 randomized placebo-controlled trial. This agent has been demonstrated to be effective as a subcutaneously administered agent in 30 patients for up to 5 years of therapy (10), and some follow-up studies of up to 8 years have demonstrated long-term persistence of apomorphine efficacy. In a subset of patients who could no longer tolerate subcutaneous injections, an intravenous (IV) preparation is being evaluated. In one study of five subjects with severe subcutaneous nodule formation who were followed for a mean of 7 months (range 0.5–18 months) IV administered apomorphine appeared to produce more consistent motor abilities, allowed for a reduction in oral medications by an average of 59%, and decreased off time from 5.4 to 0.5 hours per day. However, unanticipated intravascular thrombotic complications, secondary to apomorphine crystal accumulation, were seen in two subjects (11).

Bromocriptine

Bromocriptine was first approved in the United States in 1978. This ergot alkaloid is a partial D$_2$ agonist and a mild adrenergic agonist. It also has mild D$_1$ and 5-hydroxytryptamine (5-HT) antagonist properties (Table 1). When taken orally, bromocriptine is rapidly absorbed and 90% degraded through first-pass hepatic metabolism. Peak drug levels are achieved in 70–100 minutes, and it has a half-life of 3–8 hours. Less than 5% of the drug is excreted into the urine, and bromocriptine is highly protein bound. The drug is formulated into 2.5 mg scored tablets and 5 mg capsules (1). Dosing titration usually begins at 1.25 mg/day and increases to a recommended

20 mg/day over the course of 7 weeks; however, successful treatment with dosages higher than 60 mg/day has been reported (12) (Table 2).

While the side effects of the various DA are similar, only the ergot-derived compounds have been associated with retroperitoneal fibrosis, a rare but serious condition associated with severe pulmonary and renal complications (13). Erythromelalgia, a painful discoloration of the shins, may also be more prevalent in patients taking ergoline DA. The side effects of nausea, vomiting, sleepiness, orthostatic hypotension, and hallucinations are common to all DA, but in pivotal trials using bromocriptine they were 8–12% more common than in subjects receiving placebo (14) (Table 3).

Bromocriptine has been investigated extensively in de novo and levodopa-treated populations. A recent systematic review of all randomized controlled trials of bromocriptine monotherapy compared with levodopa (LD) monotherapy in PD found that although numerous small trials have been reported, methodological factors or lack of a control population has led to a lack of evidence basis for clinical decisions (15–17). From 1974 to

TABLE 2 Agonist Titration Schedule

Time	Bromocriptine	Pergolide	Pramipexole	Ropinirole
Week 1	1.25 mg qd	0.05 mg qd	0.125 mg tid	0.25 mg tid
Week 2	1.25 mg bid	0.05 mg tid	0.25 mg tid	0.50 mg tid
Week 3	1.25 mg tid	0.10 mg tid	0.50 mg tid	0.75 mg tid
Week 4	2.50 mg tid	0.15 mg tid	0.75 mg tid	1.00 mg tid
Week 5	3.75 mg tid	0.25 mg tid	1.00 mg tid	2.00 mg tid
Week 6	5.00 mg tid	0.50 mg tid		3.00 mg tid
Week 7	5.00 mg qid	0.75 mg tid		4.00 mg tid
Week 8		1.00 mg tid		
Maximum dosage	15.0 mg qid	2.00 mg qid	1.5 mg tid	8.00 mg tid

Source: Adapted Ref. 12.

TABLE 3 Dopamine Agonists in Parkinson's Disease

Dopamine agonist	$t_{1/2}$ (h)	Metabolism	Percentage				
			N	S	H	OH	RPF
Bromocriptine	3–8	Hepatic	37	8	12	44	2–5
Pergolide	27	Hepatic	24	6	14	2	2–5
Pramipexole	8–12	Renal	18	13	19	16	0
Ropinirole	4–6	Hepatic	20	12	15	17	0

N = nausea; S = somnolence; H = hallucinations; OH = orthostatic hypotension; RPF = retroperitoneal or pulmonary fibrosis.
Source: Adapted from Ref. 1. Additional data from published package inserts.

January 1999, six studies randomizing more than 850 patients to a bromocriptine or a levodopa regimen are in the literature, but only two trials were performed according to a double-blind design (16). These studies indicate a reduced frequency of dyskinesias, and there was a trend toward less wearing-off and fewer on-off problems in the bromocriptine group. However, the statistically larger number of dropouts in the bromocriptine group leaves these data subject to varied interpretations. In the treatment of early PD bromocriptine may be beneficial in delaying motor complications and dyskinesias with comparable effects on impairment and disability in those patients who tolerate the drug.

Bromocriptine is well accepted as a treatment in advancing PD. Although numerous studies have demonstrated this benefit in the past, a more recent, well-designed, multicenter trial comparing bromocriptine to placebo in patients with motor fluctuations has been reported. In this 9-month study there was a 14% improvement in UPDRS activities of daily living, and a 23.8% improvement in motor score. The bromocriptine arm also demonstrated a 29.7% reduction in off-time while taking a mean dosage of 22.8 mg/day (18).

Pergolide

Pergolide, an ergoline-derived DA, was approved for usage in the United States in 1989. It is 10 times more potent than bromocriptine. Like bromocriptine, pergolide has high affinity for the D_2 receptor and mild α_2-adrenergic activity, but it does not have 5-HT activity. In addition, pergolide has significant D_3 activity and is the only DA with D_1 agonist activity, although this is mild (1) (Table 1). Pergolide is available in three tablet sizes—0.05, 0.25, and 1.0 mg—and is usually titrated to an effective dosage or an initial maximum dosage of 3 mg daily over the course of 6–8 weeks (12) (Table 2). If clinical benefit is seen at 3 mg daily, this dosage may be increased with disease progression to a typical maximum dosage of 6–8 mg/day. Pergolide is rapidly absorbed from the gut and reaches a peak plasma concentration in 1–3 hours. While the duration of action is typically 4–8 hours, the half-life ranges from 15 to 42 hours, with a mean of 27 hours. Pergolide is highly protein bound, and >50% is excreted through the kidney (1). Side effects associated with pergolide are similar to bromocriptine and include retroperitoneal fibrosis, erythromelalgia, somnolence, orthostatic hypotension, and hallucinations (14,19) (Table 3).

Pergolide has been demonstrated effective in both early- and late-stage PD (20). In an open-label trial, Mizuno et al. demonstrated mild to moderate to marked benefit in 47.5% of patients after 8 weeks of pergolide at dosages up to 5 mg/day (21). Another open-label trial of 20 PD subjects reported benefit in 7 subjects with a mean dosage of 0.85 mg/day. These subjects were followed for 3 years. By 30 months, 7 subjects required supplementation with levodopa, and by the end of the study the mean dosage of pergolide had increased to 2.15 mg/day (19). A more recent de novo PD study (PELMOPET-trial), with randomization to levodopa or pergolide and concurrently evaluated using PET scanning, suggests a more robust therapeutic effect. In this double-blind study, 294 subjects were randomized to pergolide ($n = 148$) or levodopa ($n = 146$) and treated without levodopa rescue for 36 months (4). An early report indicated that 77 subject (52%) receiving pergolide compared to 90 subjects (61.6%) treated with levodopa completed the study. Mean dosages for pergolide were 3.23 mg/day and for levodopa were 504 mg/day. Although no statistical significance was seen in study completers, differences were noted in change from baseline UPDRS motor score (13.4 ± 8.8 pergolide vs. 18.1 ± 10.1 levodopa). As expected, dyskinesias were three times more frequent and motor complications more severe in the levodopa group as captured by the UPDRS, part IV. In addition, 88 subjects were followed by 18F-Dopa PET scans. Early reports of these results show a decrease in uptake in the putamen of 7.9% in the pergolide group and 14.5% in the levodopa group, but these differences were nonsignificant ($p = 0.288$) (Table 4). Evidence-based treatment data for pergolide therapy in patients with motor fluctuations on levodopa are available. In general, numerous small trials found data similar to those reported by Olanow et al. (22). In this report of a 24-week, double-blind trial of 377 subjects randomized to pergolide (189) or placebo (187), significant improvements were seen in motor scores and off-time, and levodopa dosages were reduced by approximately 25% in the pergolide group (Table 5).

   A review comparing efficacy data in adjunct therapy trials of pergolide and bromocriptine found that pergolide was superior to bromocriptine in

TABLE 4 Relative Potencies of Dopamine Agonists in Early Parkinson's Disease

	Effective dose (mg/d)	Relative potency	Relative dose range	UPDRS III Benefit vs. levodopa	UPDRS III monoRx
Bromocriptine	15–60	1:1	15–60	n/a	+0.2
Pergolide	1.5–8	10:1	15–80	+3.0 vs – 2.5[a]	n/a
Pramipexole	1.5–4.5	10:1	15–45	– 3.4 vs – 7.3[b]	– 6.0
Ropinirole	9–24	2:1	18–48	– 0.8 vs – 4.8[c]	– 4.5

[a] 36-month study.
[b] 23-month study.
[c] 40-month study.

TABLE 5 Relative Potencies of Dopamine Agonists in Advanced Parkinson's Disease

	Effective dose (mg/d)	LD↓ (mg/d)	Off-time decrease (%)	UPDRS III Benefit
Bromocriptine	22.6	ns-30%	0–30	−3.0 (24%)
Pergolide	2.9	235 (20%)	32	n/a (35%)
Pramipexole	3.4	(22%)	15	−4.0 (35%)
Ropinirole	7.5–24	191 (25%)	7	n/a

regard to improvements in motor function and activities of daily living (23). In addition, more patients reported a "marked" or "moderate improvement" with pergolide than with bromocriptine. However, no significant difference in motor fluctuations, dyskinesias, levodopa dose reduction, dropouts, or adverse events was found.

Pramipexole

Pramipexole was approved for use in the United States in July 1997. It is a synthetic, nonergot DA. Like the ergot-derived DA, this agent is active at the D_2, D_3, and D_4 receptors. Pramipexole also has affinity for α- and β-adrenoreceptors, acetylcholine receptors, and 5-HT receptors (Table 1). The drug is available in 0.125, 0.25, 0.5, 1.0, and 1.5 mg tablets, and the usual dosage is 3.0 mg/day over 5 weeks (12) (Table 2). When ingested, this drug reaches peak plasma levels within 1–3 hours and has an elimination half-life of 8–12 hours. The agent is excreted mostly unchanged in the urine, and <20% of pramipexole is protein bound. Pivotal trials with pramipexole report nausea, vomiting, somnolence, and orthostatic hypotension 0–13%, higher than in subjects randomized to placebo (14) (Table 3). A condition described as an "unexpected sleep episode" has been described and has also been seen with other dopamine agents (24,25). In addition, pathological gambling has been reported (26,27).

Pramipexole has been thoroughly studied in de novo and adjunctive populations. Three major trials have evaluated the effectiveness of pramipexole as monotherapy in early PD (28–31). A large dose ranging trial ($n = 264$) conducted by the Parkinson Study Group found that most patients tolerated dosages of 6 mg or less of pramipexole. In this 10-week study, 98% (placebo), 81% (1.5 mg/day), 92% (3.0 mg/day), 78% (4.5 mg/day) and 67% (6.0 mg/day) of subjects tolerated drug to study conclusion (28). A 20% benefit in motor score was seen in all active treatment groups, and it was determined that the optimum dosage range was 1.5 4.5 mg/day. In a 6-month study, 335 subjects were randomized to pramipexole ($n = 164$)

or placebo ($n = 171$). Investigators reported a greater than 20% improvement in the UPDRS activities of daily living and motor scores in the active treatment group (29). Side effects in these investigations included nausea, somnolence, dizziness, and hallucinations (Table 4).

The Parkinson Study Group reported data comparing pramipexole to levodopa in early PD (CALM-PD) (2,29,30). In this trial, 301 subjects were randomized to pramipexole or placebo and were followed for 4 years. At the conclusion of the trial, 52% of pramipexole and 74% of levodopa subjects reached the primary endpoint of motor complications. Furthermore, dyskinesias (25% vs. 54%) and wearing off (47% vs. 67%) were present in a greater percentage of patients initiated with levodopa. However, UPDRS assessments found significantly greater improvements (approximately 4 points) in subjects receiving levodopa (30). Eighty-two subjects in the CALM-PD cohort also underwent sequential SPECT imaging with β-CIT to assess striatal uptake of this dopamine transporter molecule (2). Comparisons between the pramipexole ($n = 42$) and the levodopa ($n = 40$) groups found statistically significant differences ranging from 6.4 to 9.5% in transporter uptake at 22, 34, and 46 months, suggesting less decline in the subjects receiving the dopamine agonist (Table 4). This study differs from the PELMOPET study comparing pergolide to levodopa in that supplemental levodopa was allowed at the discretion of the investigator in either group. The dosages of pramipexole averaged 2.78 mg/day, with 48% of subjects receiving a levodopa supplement of a mean dosage of 264 mg/day, while 36% of the levodopa-treated subjects required levodopa supplementation with a mean dosage of 509 mg/day.

Two large, randomized clinical trials using pramipexole in levodopa-treated patients have demonstrated significant benefit in off time (31% and 15%), activities of daily living (22% and 27%), motor scores (25% and 35%), and levodopa dosage reduction (27%) (18,31). The mean dosage of pramipexole was 3.36 mg/day, and side effects including dyskinesias, orthostatic hypotension, dizziness, insomnia, hallucinations, nausea, confusion, and headache were seen (18,31) (Table 3).

Ropinirole

Ropinirole was approved in the United States in September 1997. This DA is a nonergot compound with affinity for the D_2 family of receptors, but not the D_1 or D_5 receptors. In addition, unlike pergolide or pramipexole, ropinirole lacks affinity for adrenergic, cholinergic, or serotonergic receptors (Table 1). This drug is also rapidly absorbed from the gut with peak plasma concentrations occurring in 1–2 hours and is 40% protein bound (1). The elimination half-life is 6 hours, and the P450 CYP1A2 hepatic enzyme pathway metabolizes the drug. Because of this, patients given ciprofloxacin may have an increase in serum ropinirole concentrations. Because of the difference in potency, when compared to pramipexole and pergolide, this agent is often underdosed. Ropinirole is available in 0.25, 0.5, 1.0, 2.0, 3.0, 4.0, and 5.0 mg tablets and is usually titrated to 12 mg/day over a 7-week period. Clinical improvement is usually not seen until patients are taking 6 mg/day (12) (Table 2). Side effects are similar to those seen with the other DA and include nausea, somnolence, hallucinations, and orthostatic hypotension (Table 3).

Ropinirole has been tested extensively in early and advanced PD populations, and its development closely mirrors that of pramipexole. Adler et al. randomized 241 untreated subjects to ropinirole ($n = 116$) or placebo ($n = 125$) arms in a 24-week trial (32). Responders were defined as subjects achieving at least a 30% improvement in UPDRS total and motor scores, the primary outcome variables. In addition, subjects were assessed for time to levodopa initiation and with a clinical global improvement scale. With an average dosage of 15.7 mg daily, 47% of ropinirole subjects were identified as responders, while only 20% of subjects responded in the placebo arm. The mean changes in UPDRS of 24% in the ropinirole group and 3% in the placebo group reached statistical significance. Time to levodopa significantly differed, with 11% of ropinirole subjects and 29% of placebo subjects requiring additional therapy. Requirement for levodopa therapy for the ropinirole subjects was 16, 27, and 40% at 1, 2, and 3 years, respectively (1).

Studies have also been completed in de novo patients randomized to ropinirole or placebo (ropinirole 056 study) and followed by PET scanning (REAL-PET) (3,33). The 5-year clinical trial randomized 268 subjects to ropinirole ($n = 179$) or placebo ($n = 89$) in a 2:1 fashion, allowing add-on levodopa at the discretion of the investigator. Eighty-five subjects in the ropinirole group (47%) and 45 subjects in the levodopa group (51%) completed the study. In the ropinirole group 29 of the 85 patients (34%) received no levodopa supplementation at 5 years. The analysis of the time to dyskinesia showed a significant difference in favor of ropinirole, and at 5 years the cumulative incidence of dyskinesias, regardless of levodopa supplementation, was 20% in the ropinirole group and 45% in the levodopa group. The mean daily dose by the end of the study was 16.5 mg of ropinirole. The average dosage for levodopa supplementation was 427 mg/ day. The subjects randomized to levodopa received an average of 753 mg/ day. Recently, the results of a PET analysis comparing ropinirole to levodopa have been reported (REAL-PET) (3). This 2-year randomized trial found a statistically significant difference in striatal uptake when comparing ropinirole 13% to levodopa 20%. Clinical evaluation of these subjects found that 14% of the ropinirole group vs. 8% of the levodopa group required levodopa, while only 3% of subjects on ropinirole and 27% on levodopa developed dyskinesias. Lang et al. (34) reviewed ropinirole data to assess whether the development of dyskinesias in subjects exposed to early DA monotherapy would have sustained benefit compared to levodopa, a gradual return to the dyskinesia of those receiving early levodopa, or a rapid return to the dyskinesias of levodopa subjects (34). In this review, no differences were seen between groups, and a parallel rate of sustained efficacy without dyskinesia was seen. A 6-month, placebo-controlled trial of 149 subjects with advanced PD randomized to ropinirole ($n = 95$) or placebo ($n = 54$) followed for levodopa dosage and off-time reduction was conducted. In this study, levodopa dosage was reduced an average of 31% in ropinirole subjects compared to 6% in placebo subjects. Off-time was reduced by 12% in the ropinirole group and 5% in the placebo group, a difference in off-time of slightly over one hour per day (36).

Other Dopamine Agonists

Cabergoline is a once-daily, ergot-derived, dopamine agonist available in the United States for the treatment of hyperprolactinemia. It has been demonstrated to be effective in PD, but is prohibitively expensive in the United States. Cabergoline has been evaluated in de novo and advanced PD populations. In a double-blind, 2:1 placebo-controlled trial of 188 subjects taking levodopa, the addition of cabergoline allowed for an 18% reduction in levodopa, with a 16% improvement in motor scores (37). Clarke and Deane have compared cabergoline to bromocriptine in a meta-analysis of five randomized, double-blind, parallel group studies in 1071 patients (35). Cabergoline produced benefits similar to bromocriptine in off-time reduction, motor impairment and disability ratings, and levodopa dose reduction over the first 3 months of therapy. Dyskinesia and confusion were increased with cabergoline, but otherwise the frequency of adverse events and withdrawals from treatment were similar with the two agonists.

Rotigotine is a novel DA that is unique in that it is delivered through a skin patch transdermal system. In one multicenter phase II b trial, 316 patients were randomized to placebo or active drug in a 1:4 ratio and followed by UPDRS for 4 weeks (38). In this dose-finding study, statistical improvement in UPDRS activity of daily living and motor scores were seen at 9, 13.5, and 18 mg/day. No changes were seen with placebo or at 4.5 mg/day. Positive responder rates (>20% UPDRS change) increased with dosage; responder rates were as follows: placebo, 29%; 4.5 mg, 38%; 9 mg, 45%; 13.5 mg, 57%; 18 mg, 53% (daily dosages) (38).

COMPARISONS BETWEEN DOPAMINE AGONISTS

At this time 15 comparative trials between DA are known: Tan and Jankovic have summarized these studies and report conversion factors of 10:1 for bromocriptine to pergolide, 1:1 for pergolide to pramipexole, 1:6 for pergolide to ropinirole, and 10:6 for bromocriptine to ropinirole (6). Hanna et al. followed 21 stable subjects on pergolide switched safely to pramipexole in a 1:1 ratio (39). Although not statistically significant, levodopa dosages were reduced by 16.5%, and 13 of the 21 (62%) subjects reported improvement with the change in regimen. Hauser et al. reported conversion of stable subjects on levodopa and pramipexole to levodopa and ropinirole in a 1:3 mg ratio. A gradual transition was somewhat better tolerated when compared to rapid change (40). However, the difficulties reported by subjects in retrospect may have been improved with a higher conversion factor for ropinirole.

Although there are obvious difficulties when making direct comparisons in studies to determine dosage equivalence, a reasonable equation of relative DA potency would suggest bromocriptine $(\times 10) =$ pergolide = pramipexole = ropinirole $(\times 6)$ on a milligram-to-milligram basis. Using the least potent and longest prescribed DA, a dosing equivalence range may provide a useful measure of the treatment dosing spectrum using these agents (Table 4). Using these assumptions, dosing ranges appear to be higher in the ergot-related compounds, suggesting a longer treatment horizon. However, at higher prescribed amounts, the dosing curves for these agents tend to become more level, and the linear improvement seen at midrange dosages may not be present at higher doses. Perhaps a better measure of treatment response is to review similar trials of DA therapy. In the early PD population, UPDRS data in similar, placebo-controlled studies using pramipexole and ropinirole found remarkably similar benefit (Table 4). Another potential comparison perspective is to evaluate trials comparing two active interventions with the DA and levodopa. In the imaging trials for pergolide, pramipexole, and ropinirole, subjects treated with the agonist demonstrated similar, but less, benefit than those with levodopa. It is unfortunate that the levodopa supplementation in the pramipexole and ropinirole trials limited long-term monotherapy assessment, so extensive direct comparisons cannot be made, but in general the three trials produced similar benefit when compared to levodopa response.

Because the data in the PELMOPET, CALM-PD, and 056/REAL-PET trials represent, perhaps, the most rigorous and careful information gathered about these compounds, it is useful to compare them as closely as possible (2–4,31,33) (Table 4). Clinically, subjects treated with pergolide at an average dosage of 3.23 mg/day demonstrated a motor scale decline of 3 points over 36 months, while subjects randomized to levodopa still demonstrated benefit of 2.5 points in the same time interval. Although the DA/levodopa trials using pramipexole and ropinirole allowed for levodopa supplementation and had different durations, it is interesting to note that, like the 5.5 point difference seen in the PELMOPET trial, the differences between pramipexole (− 3.4) and levodopa (− 7.3) at 23.5 months (difference = 3.9 points) and ropinirole (− 0.8) and levodopa (− 4.8) at 60 months (difference = 4 points) are highly similar. Furthermore, the small differences between the PELMOPET (5.5 UPDRS motor points) and the CALM-PD (3.9 points) and 056 (4.0) trials may be explained by the levodopa supplementation allowed in the latter studies. The functional imaging data from these investigations are also similar for dosages of 3.23, 2.78, and 16.5 mg/day for pergolide, pramipexole, and ropinirole, respectively (Fig. 1). F-dopa PET demonstrates ropinirole striatal decline 65.0% of levodopa at 24 months and pergolide striatal decline 54.5% of levodopa at 36 months. SPECT imaging with β-CIT demonstrates 52.6%, 55.6%, and 62.7% pramipexole to levodopa decline at 22, 34, and 46 months of treatment. The imaging impact of added levodopa in the pramipexole and ropinirole groups is unknown.

In summary, similar designs between pergolide, pramipexole, and ropinirole demonstrate similar benefits in terms of levodopa dosage reduction, levodopa percent reduction, treatment responders, and decrease in off-time in adjunctive therapy trials (Tables 3, 4). In these studies subject selection, methodological design, and data collected differed to the point that trends are less reliable than in the early patient studies, but in general similar improvements in all variables were seen.

TREATMENT WITH DOPAMINE AGONISTS

Initiation of Therapy in a New-Onset PD Patient

DA provide substantial improvement in PD symptoms while delaying the development of early morning foot dystonia, motor fluctuations, and dyskinesias (41). In addition, similar trials comparing DA (pergolide, pramipexole, ropinirole) to levodopa in a randomized fashion suggest possible long-term benefit by functional imaging measures (42). In a clinical setting of a 30-year-old patient, it is quite compelling to delay levodopa therapy in favor of DA because of the potentially long clinical horizon (43). Conversely, in an 80-year-old patient with other health concerns, treatment with levodopa may be better tolerated. The decisions regarding initial therapy in the 50 years between these two examples is dependent on the

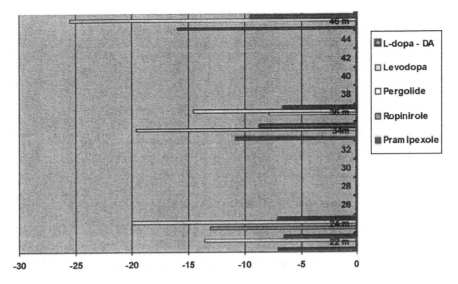

FIGURE 1   Dopamine agonist imaging data. Striatal decline by F-dopa and β-CIT in Parkinson's disease.

health of the patient, the relationship of the physician and the patient, the side effect profiles of the DA and levodopa, and, unfortunately, the cost of the drug (Table 2).

Dopaminergic medications carry similar side effect profiles, including nausea, sleepiness, confusion, orthostatic hypotension, and hallucinations (Table 3). Besides these problems, lower extremity edema, hair loss, and weight gain have also been seen with DA, and the ergoline derivatives bromocriptine, cabergoline, and pergolide also carry a slight risk of erythromelalgia (a reddish discoloration of the legs), and pulmonary and retroperitoneal fibrosis has been reported in 2–5% of subjects exposed to these agents (1). With the exception of nausea, DA are more likely than levodopa to cause these clinical difficulties, and discussion of the potential side effects at the time of prescribing will greatly aid in the tolerance of any new pharmacological agent. Because the statistical spectrum of side effects of these agents are quite similar but vary from patient to patient, it is important for any patient to understand that if he or she does not tolerate the first DA, there is no reason to expect that the other DA will not provide benefit.

Lastly, the nonergoline agonists pramipexole and ropinirole have been associated with "unexpected sleep episodes," and although this problem has been reported with pergolide and levodopa, it remains difficult to refute the observation that this symptom had not been reported prior to the use of pramipexole and ropinirole (24,25). In general, patients reporting excessive daytime sleepiness should be monitored closely with the increase of any dopaminergic therapy, especially in the first 3 months after the change.

Initiation of DA therapy is somewhat dependent on the needs and emotional state of the patient (44). Each of the DA requires a titration period of 4–8 weeks (Table 3). In the healthy patient seeking to improve quickly, initiation of a rapidly titratable agent may be preferred, while the more slowly titrated schedules may suit the needs of a patient reluctant to take any drugs. However, each patient should be reminded that the differences in titration time usually are less than 3 weeks, a brief period of time in the context of a 20-year treatment horizon (Table 2).

Initiation of Dopamine Agonists as Adjunctive Therapy

The initiation of therapy in the early patient is somewhat arbitrary with the exception of pramipexole and renal metabolism vs. the other DA and hepatic metabolism. With advancing PD, the addition of a DA should minimize the risk of aggravating further symptoms of nausea, sleepiness, orthostatic hypotension, and other problems (45) (Table 3).

CONCLUSIONS

The development of DA, particularly pergolide, pramipexole, and ropinirole, has gradually shifted treatment paradigms in PD. In the last 20 years, many parkinsonologists have moved from using DA as adjunctive therapy to levodopa to initiating antiparkinsonian therapy with one of these agents in otherwise healthy subjects (41). More recently, imaging data with SPECT and PET scanning have produced debate regarding the possible "neuroprotective" advantages of DA when compared to levodopa (2–4). In this regard some have questioned whether these agents should be initiated sooner in the disease course, perhaps before obvious disability develops. Regardless of when DA therapy is initiated, each patient benefits from the choice of several agents for treating the symptoms of PD, and it is the responsibility of the physician to provide the information regarding the reasons for using this class of drugs and for choosing one agent over another.

REFERENCES

1. Factor SA. Dopamine agonists. Med Clin North Am 1999; 83:415–443.
2. Parkinson Study Group. Dopamine transporter brain imaging to assess the effects of pramipexole vs. levodopa on Parkinson disease progression. JAMA 2002; 287:1653–1661.
3. Whone AL, Remy P, Davis MR, et al. The REAL-PET study: slower progression in early Parkinson's disease treated with ropinirole compared with l-dopa. Neurology 2002; 58(suppl 3): A82–83.
4. Oertel WH, Schwartz J, Leenders DL, et al. Results of a 3-year randomized, double-blind, PET-controlled study of pergolide vs. levodopa as monotherapy in Parkinson's disease (PELMOPET trial). J Neurol Sci 2001; 187(suppl):S444.
5. Le WD, Jankovic J. Are dopamine receptor agonists neuroprotective in Parkinson's disease? Drugs Aging 2001; 18(6):389–396.
6. Tan E-K, Jankovic J. Choosing dopamine agonists in Parkinson's disease. Clin Neuropharmacol 2001; 24:247–253.
7. Pierantozzi M, Palmieri MG, Mazzone P, Marciani MG, Rossini PM, Stefani A, Giacomini P, Peppe A, Stanzione P. Deep brain stimulation of both subthalamic nucleus and internal globus pallidus restores intracortical inhibition in Parkinson's disease paralleling apomorphine effects: a paired magnetic stimulation study. Clin Neurophysiol 2002; 113:108–113.
8. Poewe W, Wenning GK. Apomorphine: an underutilized therapy for Parkinson's disease. Mov Disord 2000; 15(5):789–794.
9. Dewey RB Jr, Hutton JT, LeWitt PA, Factor SA. A randomized, double-blind, placebo-controlled trial of subcutaneously injected apomorphine for parkinsonian off-state events. Arch Neurol 2001; 58:1385–1392.
10. Stocchi F, Vacca L, De Pandis MF, Barbato L, Valente M, Ruggieri S. Subcutaneous continuous apomorphine infusion in fluctuating patients with Parkinson's disease: long-term results. Neurol Sci 2001; 22(1):93–94.
11. Manson AJ, Hanagasi H, Turner K, Patsalos PN, Carey P, Ratnaraj N, Lees AJ. Intravenous apomorphine therapy in Parkinson's disease: clinical and pharmacokinetic observations. Brain 2001; 124(Pt 2):331–340.
12. Pahwa R, Lyons KE. Solving the puzzle of Parkinson's therapy. Pract Neurol 2002; 1:17–18,22–24.
13. Goetz CG, Tanner CM, Glantz RH, Klawans HL. Chronic agonist therapy for Parkinson's disease: a 5-year study of bromocriptine and pergolide. Neurology 1985; 85:749–751.
14. Physician's Desk Reference, 56th ed. Montvale, NJ: Medical Economics Co., 2002.
15. Factor SA, Weiner WJ. Viewpoint: Early combination therapy with bromocriptine and levodopa in Parkinson's disease. Mov Disord 1993; 8:257–262.
16. Clarke CE, Speller JM. Pergolide versus bromocriptine for levodopa-induced motor complications in Parkinson's disease. Cochrane Database Syst Rev 2000; (2):CD000236.

17. Ramaker C, van Hilten JJ. Bromocriptine versus levodopa in early Parkinson's disease. Cochrane Database Syst Rev 2000; (3):CD002258.
18. Guttman M, International Pramipexole-Bromocriptine Study Group. Double-blind comparison of pramipexole and bromocriptine treatment with placebo in advanced Parkinson's disease. Neurology 1997; 49:1060–1065.
19. Jankovic J. Long-term study or pergolide in Parkinson's disease. Neurology 1985; 35:296–299.
20. Bonuccelli U, Colzi A, Del Dotto P. Pergolide in the treatment of patients with early and advanced Parkinson's disease. Clin Neuropharmacol 2002; 25:1–10.
21. Mizuno Y, Kondo T, Narabayashi H. Pergolide in the treatment of Parkinson's disease. Neurology 1995; 45(suppl):S13–21.
22. Olanow CW, Fahn S, Muenter M, et al. A Multicenter double-blind placebo controlled trial of pergolide as adjunct to Sinemet in the treatment of Parkinson's disease. Mov Disord 1994; 9:40–47.
23. van Hilten JJ, Ramaker C, Van de Beek WJ, Finken MJ. Bromocriptine for levodopa-induced motor complications in Parkinson's disease. Cochrane Database Syst Rev 2000; (2):CD001203.
24. Frucht S, Rogers JD, Greene PE, et al. Falling asleep at the wheel; motor vehicle mishaps in persons taking pramipexole and ropinirole. Neurology 1999; 52:1908–1910.
25. Stacy MA. Sleep attacks: Is it the drug or the disease? Drugs Aging 2002; 19:733–739.
26. Samanta JES, Stacy M. Pathologic gambling in Parkinson's disease. Mov Disord 1998; 15(suppl 3):111.
27. Gschwandtner U, Astar J, Renard S, Fuhr P. Pathologic gambling in patients with Parkinson's disease. Clin Neuropharmacol 2001; 24:170–172.
28. Hubble JP, Koller WC, Cutler NR, et al. Pramipexole in patients with early Parkinson's disease. Clin Neuropharmacol 1995; 18:338–347.
29. Parkinson Study Group. Pramipexole vs. levodopa as and initial treatment for Parkinson disease. JAMA 2000; 284:1931–1938.
30. Holloway RG and the Parkinson Study Group. Pramipexole versus levodopa as initial treatment for Parkinson's disease: a four-year randomized controlled trial. Neurology 2002; 58(suppl 3):A81–82.
31. Lieberman AN, Ranhosky A, Korts D. Clinical evaluation of pramipexole in advanced Parkinson's disease: results of a randomized, placebo-controlled, parallel group study. Neurology 1997; 49:162–168.
32. Adler CH, Sethi KD, Hauser RA, et al. Ropinirole for the treatment of early Parkinson's disease. Neurology 1997; 49:393–399.
33. Rascol O, Brooks DJ, Korczyn AD, De Deyn PP, Clarke CE, Lang AE. A five-year study of the incidence of dyskinesia in patients with early Parkinson's disease who were treated with ropinirole or levodopa. 056 Study Group. N Engl J Med 2000; 342:1484–1491.

34. Lang AE, Rascol O, Brooks DJ, et al. The development of dyskinesias in Parkinson's disease patients receiving ropinirole and given supplemental l-dopa. Neurology 2002; 58(suppl 3):A82.

35. Lieberman A, Olanow CW, Sethi K, et al. A multicenter trial of ropinirole as adjunct treatment for Parkinson's disease. Neurology 1998; 51:1057–1061.

36. Hutton JT, Koller WC, Ahlskog JE, et al. Multicenter, placebo-controlled trial of cabergoline taken once daily in Parkinson's disease. Neurology 1996; 46:1062–1065.

37. Clarke CE, Deane KD. Cabergoline versus bromocriptine for levodopa-induced complications in Parkinson's disease. Cochrane Database Syst Rev 2001; (1):CD001519.

38. Bianchine J, Poole K. Efficacy and dose response of the novel transdermally applied dopamine agonist rotigotine CDS in early Parkinson's disease. Neurology 2002; 58(suppl 3):A162–163.

39. Hanna PA, Ratkos L, Ondo WG, et al. A comparison of the therapeutic efficacy of pergolide and pramipexole in Parkinson's disease. J Neural Transm 2001; 108:63–70.

40. Hauser R, Reider C, Stacy M, et al. Acute vs. gradual pramipexole to ropinirole switch. Mov Disord 1998; 15(suppl):133.

41. Olanow CW, Koller WC. An algorithm for the management of Parkinson's disease. Neurology 1998; 50(suppl):S10–14.

42. Hubble JP. Long-term studies of the dopamine agonists. Neurology 2002; 58(suppl):S42–51.

43. Poewe W. Should treatment of Parkinson's disease be started with a dopamine agonist? Neurology 1998; 51(suppl):S21–24.

44. Hauser R, Zesiewicz TA. Management of early Parkinson's disease. Med Clin North Am 1999; 393–414.

45. Olanow CW. The role of dopamine agonists in the treatment of early Parkinson's disease. Neurology 2002; 59(suppl):S33–41.

19

Monoamine Oxidase Inhibitors in Parkinson's Disease

Daryl Victor and Cheryl Waters
Columbia University, New York, New York, U.S.A

HISTORY

Monoamine oxidase (MAO) is an enzyme involved in the breakdown of catecholamines including dopamine, norepinephrine, and serotonin. MAO inhibitors were discovered in the late 1950s and were first utilized in the treatment of depression. In 1962 Bernheimer showed that MAO inhibitors could potentiate the antiparkinsonian effect of levodopa but caused severe hypertensive crisis (1). In 1968, Johnston identified two types of monoamine oxidase: A and B (2). Each has a separate affinity for various catecholamines and works in different parts of the body. MAO-B is found predominantly in the human brain (3) and platelets and has an affinity for dopamine and benzylamine. MAO-A is found predominantly in the intestinal tract and has an affinity for serotonin and norepinephrine. Both types can oxidize tyramine, though MAO-B does so only at higher concentrations.

In 1972, Knoll and Maygar described selegiline (Deprenyl®) as a selective irreversible MAO-B inhibitor (4). They also showed that at low doses selegiline did not potentiate the pressor effect of tyramine also known as the "cheese effect." That same year Squires (3) reported that 80% of

MAO activity in the brain is MAO-B. In autopsied brains, 10 mg of selegiline was found to be sufficient to selectively inhibit 90% of MAO-B in such areas as the caudate, substantia nigra, globus pallidus, and thalamus (5). Hence, it was shown that selective MAO-B inhibitors such as selegiline could inhibit the MAO that has strong affinity for the basal ganglia. This may augment the concentration of dopamine in areas in which it is deficient.

For over two decades MAO-B inhibitors have been used in Parkinson's disease (PD). They were originally developed as antidepressants but were later found to have benefit in patients with PD. Knoll's study showed that selegiline, a selective nonreversible MAO-B inhibitor, lengthened the life span of rodents by 50% (6). The neuroprotective properties of MAO inhibitors were evaluated over the next two decades. There was much interest in their ability to protect neurons against neurodegenerative processes such as PD. The bulk of the scientific interest revolves around selegiline, while more recent studies have looked at rasagiline (a selective irreversible MAO-B inhibitor) and lazabemide (a selective reversible, competitive inhibitor of MAO-B). In clinical practice, selegiline is used as monotherapy or as adjunctive therapy to levodopa.

MECHANISMS OF ACTION

In PD there is a loss of dopaminergic neurons in the substantia nigra pars compacta. The mechanisms involved in the destruction of these cells are complex. Abnormalities found in PD include abnormal iron metabolism (7), increased free radical production (8), and decreased scavenging systems such as reduced glutathione (GSH). The latter two comprise the "oxidative stress" theory. Some mechanisms appear paradoxical. For instance, Mytilineou et al. (9) demonstrated both deleterious and beneficial effects from levodopa. Levodopa can produce free radicals, but it can also increase the rate of reduced GSH synthesis and protect against toxins such as L-buthionine sulfoximine (L-BSO) an inhibitor of GSH synthesis. There are three theories to justify the use of MAO inhibitors to slow progression of PD: oxidative stress, neurotoxicity, and potential regenerative properties of MAO-B inhibitors.

Oxidative Stress Theory

This theory proposes that the parkinsonian brain is under oxidative stress (10): there is an overabundance of free radicals or oxygen species in the brain causing damage to the dopaminergic cells. This skewed proportion of reactive oxygen species may be due to an increased production or a decreased clearing of these products due to an impaired GSH system or abnormal iron cycling (7,11). One pathway in the degradation of dopamine is through MAO-B or autooxidation. This degradative process can produce free radicals such as hydrogen peroxide and hydroxyl radicals that in turn may cause cellular damage. A solution is to reduce formation of these free oxygen species by inhibiting the degradation of dopamine. Selegiline slows the rate of dopamine degradation and, hence, the rate of free radical production. Selegiline also allows for an increase in GSH that helps clear free radicals from the system (8).

MPTP and Neurotoxicity

Studies have shown that various chemicals including dopamine, levodopa, and 6-hydroxydopamine act as neurotoxins (12,13). Selegiline has been shown to protect against these neurotoxins through mechanisms other than MAO-B inhibition.

In 1982, Tetrud and Langston (14) reported that 1-methyl-4-phenyl-1,2,3,6-tetrahydropyridine (MPTP) produced a parkinsonism indistinguishable from PD in young drug addicts. This was later found to be due to its oxidative byproduct 1-methyl-4-phenylpyridinium ion (MPP$^+$). Others have demonstrated MPTP's toxic properties on dopaminergic neurons (15). MAO-B inhibitors successfully prevent the conversion of MPTP to MPP$^+$ (16) and protect dopaminergic neurons from this toxicity (15,17). MAO-B inhibitors were originally thought to prevent this conversion via MAO inhibition. Since then, MPTP has been shown to inhibit mitochondrial respiration via complex I, through free radical synthesis (18). In a study by Vizuete et al. (19), selegiline protected cells from MPP$^+$ toxicity, but not through inhibition of the conversion of MPTP to MPP$^+$. Matsubara and others (20) showed selegiline prevented mitochondrial toxicity elicited by MPTP and 2,9-Me$_2$NH$^+$, which is an N-methylated β-carbolinium cation and an analog of MPTP with protoxic activity. They hypothesized that selegiline impacts mitochondrial electron transport, resulting in membrane potential stabilization.

Tatton and Greenwood (21) exposed rats to MPTP for 72 hours. Selegiline or saline was then given. These rats were sacrificed and the substantia nigra compacta stained with tyrosine hydroxylase (TH +) immunostain to measure the amount of dopaminergic cells. Selegiline was shown to prevent 50% of the loss due to MPTP. The importance of this observation was the absence of MAO-B activity in those regions implying a different mechanism for selegiline's action.

Maygar et al. (22) showed that selegiline and other MAO-B inhibitors were effective in blocking N-(2-chloroethyl-)-N-ethyl-2-bromobenzylamine

(DSP-4) toxicity. DSP-4 is a neurotoxin that inhibits ^{3}H-noradrenaline uptake into central and peripheral noradrenergic neurons in rodents. Knoll (23) found that selegiline could protect striatal dopaminergic cells from 6-hydroxydopamine (6-OHDA) neurotoxicity. These studies suggest that MAO-B inhibitors may have other neuroprotective properties besides that of MAO inhibition.

Potential Regenerative Properties

Li et al. (24) reported that selegiline and other irreversible MAO-B inhibitors decreased the messenger RNA for glial fibrillary acidic protein (GFAP), a biological marker of cell injury, in C6 rat glomeruli cells. Increased GFAP expression contributes to tissue scarring and creates a physical barrier near damaged neurons. Presumably, MAO-B inhibitors either inhibit the physical barrier, prohibiting vital repairs to damaged neurons, or they protect neurons from damage directly, thus producing less GFAP expression. In the PC12 cell apoptosis model, Tatton et al. (25) documented increased cell survival with selegiline. In this study, selegiline induced new protein synthesis. These experiments give credence to neuronal protection. De Girolamo et al. (26) reported that selegiline not only protected N2a cells from MPTP but also reversed the toxic effects on axonal growth, suggesting that selegiline may help regenerate damaged neurons. The possible mechanisms include direct neuronal survival, regeneration, or indirect induction of cellular changes.

BIOCHEMICAL PROPERTIES

Selegiline is a selective irreversible MAO-B inhibitor. Taken orally, it is readily absorbed from the intestine and reaches plasma levels in 30–120 minutes. It has a mean half-life of 2 hours. Its major metabolites, L-methamphetamine and L-amphetamine, have half-lives of 20.5 and 17.7 hours, respectively. At doses of 5 and 10 mg it has mild antiparkinsonian effects without causing pressor effects. At higher doses such as 30 and 60 mg it has greater antidepressant effects but is associated with an increased pressor effect via tyramine, requiring patients to adhere to a low-tyramine diet. It has an extremely long half-life as confirmed with positron emission tomography (PET) imaging (27,28). Withdrawal from selegiline is not associated with an amphetamine-like withdrawal. Selegiline also significantly increases phenylethylamine (PEA) output. PEA is a strong dopamine uptake inhibitor and induces dopamine release (29). The reader is referred to Heinonen et al.'s article on the pharmacokinetics and metabolism of selegiline for further details (30).

CLINICAL APPLICATIONS

Selegiline is primarily used in patients with early PD as monotherapy or as adjunctive therapy to levodopa. It is usually used as 5 mg every morning or 5 mg twice a day, in the morning and afternoon. It is not given at night to avoid insomnia from methamphetamine metabolites. Hubble et al. (31) did not find a significant difference using 10 mg versus 5 mg daily in patients with moderately advanced PD.

The Quality Standards Subcommittee of the American Academy of Neurology (32) confirmed that selegiline has only mild symptomatic antiparkinsonian effects when used as monotherapy. Compared to placebo, selegiline improves motor scores in PD patients (33–35). Withdrawal of selegiline results in a worsening of the Unified Parkinson's Disease Rating Scale (UPDRS) tremor and bradykinesia scores (36). These scores recover with resumption of this drug.

Selegiline decreases the amount of disability in early PD. Palhagen et al. (34) noted patients on selegiline had better UPDRS scores over time and had a delay to reach disability or need for levodopa. Myllyla et al. (37) described a slowing of disability in PD patients on selegiline and a delay in the need for levodopa therapy.

DATATOP STUDY

The DATATOP study was a large prospective double-blind, four-arm study that included over 800 patients. It compared the effects of placebo, selegiline, tocopherol (vitamin E), and selegiline plus tocopherol in early PD. Endpoints were the need to start levodopa therapy and the onset of disability. Patients were evaluated by clinical exams and cerebrospinal fluid analysis (38). Selegiline delayed the onset of levodopa therapy and slowed parkinsonian disability. Patients on placebo demonstrated a 50% faster decline than those on drug. However, this phenomenon occurred largely in the first year and was not sustained (39). A 53% reduction in the development of freezing of gait (FOG) was also observed with selegiline (40). Benefit with selegiline on FOG waned after selegiline was discontinued. The mechanism behind selegiline's protection against FOG is unknown. A potential benefit in FOG would be important because there are no proven treatments to help FOG. However, the clinical significance of the reduction in FOG with selegiline is questionable.

ADJUNCTIVE THERAPY

As adjunctive therapy MAO-B inhibitors decrease motor fluctuations, improve UPDRS scores, and allow for a reduction in levodopa dosing. In the late 1970s, Lee et al. (41) and Rinne et al. (42) reported that selegiline added to levodopa therapy reduced the "on-off" episodes in PD patients. However, Golbe (43) found that selegiline added to levodopa therapy only reduced "off" time without an increase in "on" time. This benefit was lost after about one year. Lieberman (44) showed that selegiline added to levodopa improved UPDRS scores in early PD patients without motor fluctuations more than in patients with fluctuations. In various studies selegiline allows a reduction in the total dosage of levodopa. Both Myllyla et al. (45) and Larsen et al. (46) showed in double-blind trials that selegiline use in early PD delays the need for levodopa, decreases the amount of levodopa needed, and decreases the rate of escalation of levodopa compared with placebo. The Parkinson's Disease Research Group of the United Kingdom found no clinical delay in disability with adjunctive therapy (47).

ADVERSE EFFECTS

Most of the common side effects of selegiline are due to its dopaminergic properties, such as nausea, constipation, diaphoresis, hallucinations, and dyskinesias (43). Often these effects are found in patients using selegiline in conjunction with levodopa. Reducing the levodopa dosage may diminish these side effects. The average reduction in levodopa needed to alleviate side effects seen in combination therapy has been estimated at 20% (48,49). Nausea may be ameliorated in many cases by taking the medication postprandially.

Selegiline and levodopa can produce orthostatic hypotension (45,48). Churchyard et al. (33) found that 30% of patients on long-term selegiline therapy (in combination with levodopa or other antiparkinsonian agents) had postural hypotension. Other concerns with MAO-B inhibitors are drug interactions and hepatic toxicity. Golbe (43) reported that, although there was a trend for liver function tests to rise, none of the patients had levels outside the normal range.

Serotonin syndrome may develop with the combined use of selective serotonin reuptake inhibitors (SSRIs) and MAO-B inhibitors. The serotonin syndrome consists of diaphoresis, hypertension, and confusion. Richard et al. (50) reviewed over 4000 cases in which both drugs were used together, including case reports and adverse events reported to the U.S. Food and Drug Administration and the manufacturer of selegiline. Of 4000 patients, only 11 fulfilled criteria for this syndrome. They concluded that if the interaction does exist, it is extremely rare. In this report the one death was in a patient without PD (FDA report). This is consistent with a previous report by Waters (51).

MORTALITY

The Parkinson's Disease Research Group of the United Kingdom found a significantly higher rate of mortality in patients treated with selegiline and levodopa than levodopa alone. The study was criticized for technical reasons: half of the participants did not complete the study, the study was not double-blind, and patients were rerandomized into a different trial arm. Another retrospective study by Thorogood et al. (52) found an increase in mortality in patients on selegiline, especially in younger patients on selegiline alone and in elderly patients with combined therapy.

The DATATOP study was reviewed to examine mortality (53). There was a 2.1% death rate per year found in all patients for the 10 years of observation. This was unaffected by selegiline or tocopherol or both combined. The initial selegiline patients and tocopherol patients had slightly higher mortality, but the numbers were not found to be statistically significant. Statistical analysis found no differences between early and late users of selegiline. Hence, the investigators did not find a significant increase or decrease in mortality with selegiline.

A meta-analysis done by Olanow et al. in 1998 (54) concluded that there was no evidence for increased mortality with selegiline use. Recently the Quality Standards Subcommittee of the American Academy of Neurology also concluded that there was no convincing evidence for an increased mortality with selegiline (32).

LAZABEMIDE

The Parkinson Study Group investigated the clinical use of lazabemide at various strengths in a double-blind study (55). It showed that at a single oral dose of 200 mg, lazabemide inhibited MAO-B for 24 hours. However, it gave only a modest benefit in activities of daily living (ADL) scores and none in motor scores. At 400 mg it caused asymptomatic elevations of liver enzymes and creatinine. A later study in 1996 (56) showed that 43.9% of patients on placebo reached the endpoint of requiring symptomatic therapy versus 31.4% of patients on varying doses of lazabemide. UPDRS scores were not significantly different between those on lazabemide and placebo. The study was not able to distinguish a true neuroprotective property of lazabemide. Lazabemide will not be marketed because of its mild symptomatic efficacy and concerns regarding possible liver and renal toxicity.

RASAGILINE

Rasagiline is an irreversible selective MAO-B inhibitor that is five times more potent than selegiline. Its major metabolite is 1-(R)-aminoidan. Rasagiline is devoid of amphetamine properties, and thus, it does not have a pressor effect. It is currently in Phase III studies. It is said to have symptomatic dopaminergic effects. It is purported to have neuroprotective effects seen in mouse models, in which it rescues dopaminergic neurons from neurotoxins (57).

Finberg et al. (58) investigated rasagiline, an isomer of N-propargyl-1-aminoindane, in rat fetal mesencephalic cells containing 95% neurons, 20% of which were tyrosine hydroxylase positive. Rasagiline was shown in the mitochondria to have selective MAO-B inhibitory properties similar to selegiline but with greater potency in a single oral preparation. Both increased the striatal dopamine level after chronic ingestion. In another experiment selegiline and rasagiline increased the percentage of positive tyrosine hydroxylase neurons. Rasagiline increased the number of surviving cells in serum medium and the number of surviving cells in the absence of serum.

Rabey et al. (59) studied rasagiline given at various strengths (0.5, 1, and 2 mg) versus placebo as adjunctive therapy to levodopa for 12 weeks with evaluation at 12 and 18 weeks. Rasagiline had greater improvement in UPDRS scores than placebo, particularly for motor and ADL scores at all strengths and time points. However, due to a strong placebo effect, the difference was deemed insignificant.

Kieburtz et al. (57) studied 400 patients with early PD on rasagiline at either 1 or 2 mg versus placebo for 26 weeks. A subset of 55 patients received a challenge of 75 mg oral dose of tyramine. The study showed improved UPDRS scores in the rasagiline group versus controls. There was no significant increase in mean systolic blood pressure in either group. None of the patients who received the tyramine challenge had an adverse reaction. They concluded that rasagiline was safe and useful as monotherapy in early PD.

CONCLUSION

The role of MAO-B inhibitors for treatment of PD continues to be explored. It is possible that with its modest symptomatic effect, selegiline will be replaced by other MAO-B inhibitors. Rasagiline has a stronger potency and a possible role as a neuroprotective agent. Selegiline continues to be used as monotherapy and as an adjunctive agent to levodopa for motor fluctuations. When adding selegiline to levodopa, it must be remembered that the dopaminergic side effects of levodopa can be enhanced. MAO-B inhibitors will continue to be studied in the laboratory as potential neuroprotective agents.

REFERENCES

1. Bernheimer H, Birkmayer W, Hornykiewicz O. Verhalten der Monoanioxydase im Gehirn des Menschen nach Therapie mit Monoaminoxydase Hemmer. Wien Klin Wschr 1962; 74:558–559.
2. Johnston JP. Some observations upon a new inhibitor of monoamine oxidase in brain tissue. Biochem Pharmacol 1968; 17:1285–1297.
3. Squires JP. Multiple forms of monoamine oxidase in intact mitochondria as characterized by selective inhibitors and thermal stability: a comparison of eight mammalian species. Adv Biochem Psychopharmacol 1972; 5:355–370.
4. Knoll J, Maygar K. Some puzzling pharmacological effects of monoamine oxidase inhibitors. Adv Biochem Psychopharm 1972; 5:393–408.
5. Riederer P, Youdim MBH, Rausch WD, Birkmayer W, Jellinger K, Seemann D. On the mode of action of L-deprenyl in the human central nervous system. J Neural Transm 1978; 43:217–226.
6. Knoll J. The striatal dopamine dependency of life span in male rats. Longevity study with (-) deprenyl. Mech Ageing Dev 1998; 46:237–262.
7. Dexter DT, Carayon A, Javoy-Agid F, Agid Y, Wells FR, Daniel SE, Lees AJ, Jenner P, Marsden CD. Alterations in the levels of iron, ferritin and other trace metals in Parkinson's disease and other neurodegenerative diseases affecting the basal ganglia. Brain 1991; 14:1953–1975.
8. Cohen G, Spina M. Deprenyl suppresses the oxidant stress associated with increased dopamine turnover. Ann Neurol 1989; 26:689–690.
9. Mytilineou C, Han S, Cohen G. Toxic and protective effects of L-DOPA on mesencephalic cell cultures. J Neurochem 1993; 61:1470–1478.
10. Fahn S, Cohen G. The oxidant stress hypothesis in Parkinson's disease: evidence supporting it. Ann Neurol 1992; 32:804–812.
11. Riederer P, Sofie E, Rausch W, Schmidt B, Gavin PR, Jellinger K, Youdim MBH. Transition metals, ferritin, glutathione, and ascorbic acid in parkinsonian brains. J Neurochem 1989; 52:515–520.
12. Michel PP, Hefti F. Toxicity of 6-hydroxydopamine and dopamine for dopaminergic neurons in culture. J Neurosci Res 1990; 26:428–435.
13. Mylitineou C, Danias P. 6-Hydroxydopamine toxicity to dopamine neurons in culture: potentiation by the addition of superoxide dismutase and N-acetylcysteine. Biochem Pharmacol 1989; 38(11):1872–1875.
14. Tetrud JW, Langston JW. Chronic parkinsonism in humans due to a product of meperidine-analog synthesis. Science 1982; 219:979–980.

15. Heikkila RE, Manzino L, Cabbat FD, Duvoisin RC. Protection against the dopaminergic neurotoxicity of 1-methyl-4-phenyl-1,2,5,6-tetrahydropyridine by monoamine oxidase inhibitors. Nature 1984; 311:467–469.
16. Langston JW, Irwin I, Langston EB, Forno LS. 1-Methyl-4-phenylpyridinium ion (MPP+): identification of a metabolite of MPTP, a toxin selective to the substantia nigra. Neurosci Lett 1984; 48:87–92.
17. Cohen G, Pasik P, Cohen B, Leist A, Mytilineou C, Yahr M. Pargyline and deprenyl prevent the neurotoxicity of 1-methyl-4-phenyl-1,2,5,6-tetrahydro-pyridine (MPTP) in monkeys. Eur J Pharm 1985; 106:209–210.
18. Cleeter MWJ, Cooper JM, Schapira AHV. Irreversible inhibition of mitochondrial complex I by 1-methyl-4-phenylpyridinium: evidence for free radical involvement. J Neurochem 1992; 58:786–789.
19. Vizuete MI, Steffen V, Ayala A, Cano J, Machado A. Protective effect of deprenyl against 1-methyl-4-phenylpyridinium neurotoxicity in rat striatum. Neurosci Lett 1993; 152:113–116.
20. Matsubara K, Senda T, Uezono T, Awaya T, Ogawa S, Chiba K, Shimizu K, Hayase N, Kimura K. L-Deprenyl prevents the cell hypoxia induced by dopaminergic neurotoxins, MPP+ and β-carbolinium: a microdialysis study in rats. Neurosci Lett 2001; 302:65–68.
21. Tatton WG, Greenwood CE. Rescue of dying neurons: a new action for deprenyl in MPTP parkinsonism. J Neurosci Res 1991; 30:666–672.
22. Magyar K, Szende B, Lengyel J, Tekes K. The pharmacology of B-type selective monoamine oxidase inhibitors; milestones in (-) deprenyl research. J Neural Transm 1996; 48:29–41.
23. Knoll J. The pharmacology of (-) deprenyl. J Neural Transm 1986; (suppl 22):75–89.
24. Li XM, Qi J, Juorio AV, Boulton AA. Reduction in glial fibrillary acidic protein mRNA Abundance induced by (-)-deprenyl and other monoamine oxidase B inhibitors in C6 glioma cells. J Neurochem 1993; 63:1572–1576.
25. Tatton WG, Ju WYL, Holland DP, Tai C, Kwan M. (-)-Deprenyl reduces PC12 cell apoptosis by inducing new protein synthesis. J Neurochem 1994; 63:1572–1575.
26. De Girolamo LA, Hargreaves AJ, Billett EE. Protection from MPTP-induced neurotoxicity in differentiating mouse N2a neuroblastoma cells. J Neurochem 2001; 76:650–660.
27. Arnett CD, Fowler JS, MacGregor RR, Schlyer DJ, Wolf AP, Langstrom B, Halldin C. Turnover of brain monoamine oxidase measured in vivo by positron emission tomography using L-[11C] deprenyl. J Neurochem 1987; 49:522–527.
28. Fowler JS, Volkow ND, Logan J, Wang GJ, MacGregor RR, Schlyer D, Wolf AP, Pappas N, Alexoff D, Shea C, Dorflinger E, Kruchowy L, Yoo K, Fazzini E, Patlak C. Slow recovery of human brain MAO B after L-deprenyl (selegiline) withdrawal. Synapse 1994; 18:86–93.
29. Youdim MBH. Pharmacology of MAO B inhibitors: mode of action of (-) deprenyl in Parkinson's disease. J Neural Transm 1986; (suppl 22):91–105.

30. Heinonen EH, Myllyla V, Sotaniemi K, Lammintausta R, Salonen JS, Anttila M, Savijarvi M, Kotila M, Rinne UK. Pharmacokinetics and metabolism of selegiline. Acta Neuro Scand 1989; 311:467–469.

31. Hubble JP, Koller WC, Waters C. Brief report: effects of selegiline dosing on motor fluctuations in Parkinson's disease. Clin Neuropharmacol 1993; 16(1):83–87.

32. Miyasaki JM, Martin W, Suchowersky O, Weiner WJ, Lang AE. Practice parameter: initiation of treatment for Parkinson's disease: an evidence-based review (Report of the Quality Standards Subcommittee of the American Academy of Neurology). Neurology 2002; 58:11–17.

33. Churchyard A, Mathias CJ, Phil D, Lees AJ. Selegiline-induced postural hypotension in Parkinson's disease: a longitudinal study on the effects of drug withdrawal. Mov Disord 1999; 14:246–251.

34. Palhagen S, Heinonen EH, Hagglund J, Kaugesaar T, Kontants H, Maki-Ikola O, Palm R, Turunen J, and the Swedish Parkinson Study Group. Selegiline delays the onset of disability in de novo parkinsonian patients. Neurology 1998; 51:520–525.

35. Allain H, Pollack P, Neukirch HC, and members of the French Selegiline Multicenter Trial. Symptomatic effect of selegiline in de novo Parkinson's patients. Mov Disord 1993; 8(suppl 1):S36–S40.

36. Negrotti A, Bizzari G, Calzetti S. Long-term persistence of symptomatic effect of selegiline in Parkinson's disease. A two-months placebo-controlled withdrawal study. J Neural Transm 2001; 108:215–219.

37. Myllyla VV, Sotaniemi KA, Vuorinen JA, Heinonen EH. Selegiline in de novo Parkinson's patients: The Finnish Study. Mov Disord 1993; 8(suppl 1):S41–S44.

38. Parkinson Study Group. DATATOP: a multicenter controlled clinical trial in early Parkinson's disease. Arch Neurol 1989; 46:1052–1060.

39. Shoulson I. On behalf of the Parkinson Study Group. DATATOP: a decade of neuroprotective inquiry. Ann Neurol 1998; 44(suppl 1):S160–S166.

40. Giladi N, McDermott MP, Fahn S, Przedborski S, Jankovic J, Stern M, Tanner C, and the Parkinson Study Group. Freezing of gait in PD: prospective assessment in the DATATOP cohort. Neurology 2001; 56:1712–1721.

41. Lee AJ, Shaw KM, Kohout LJ. Deprenyl in Parkinson's disease. Lancet 1977; 2:791–796.

42. Rinne UK, Siirtola T, Sonninen V. L-Deprenyl treatment of on-off phenomena in Parkinson's disease. J Neural Transm 1978; 43:253–262.

43. Golbe LI. Long-term efficacy and safety of deprenyl (selegiline) in advanced Parkinson's disease. Neurology 1989; 39:1109–1111.

44. Leiberman A. Long-term experience with selegiline and levodopa in Parkinson's disease. Neurology 1992; 42(suppl 4):32–36.

45. Myllyla VV, Heinonen EH, Vuorinen JA, Kilkku OI, Sotaniemi KA. Early selegiline therapy reduces levodopa dose requirement in Parkinson's disease. Acta Neurol Scand 1995; 91:177–182.

46. Larsen JP, Boas J. and the Norwegian-Danish Study Group. The effects of early selegiline therapy on long-term levodopa treatment and parkinsonian disability: an interim analysis of a Norwegian-Danish 5-year study. Mov Disord 1997; 12:175–182.

47. Parkinson's Disease Research Group of United Kingdom. Investigation by Parkinson's Disease Research Group of the United Kingdom into excess mortality seen with combined levodopa and selegiline treatment in patient with early, mild Parkinson's disease: further results of randomized trial and confidential inquiry. BMJ 1998; 316:1191–1196.

48. Brodersen P, Philbert G, Stigard GA. The effect of L-deprenyl on on-off phenomena in Parkinson's disease. Acta Neurol Scand 1985; 71:494–497.

49. Myllyla VV, Sotaniemi KA, Hakulinen P, Maki-Ikola O, Heinonen EH. Selegiline as the primary treatment of Parkinson's disease—a long-term double blind study. Acta Neurol Scand 1997; 95:211–218.

50. Richard IH, Kurlan R, Tanner C, Factor S, Hubble J, Suchowersky O, Waters C, and the Parkinson Study Group. Serotonin syndrome and the combined use of deprenyl and an antidepressant in Parkinson's disease. Neurology 1998; 48:1070–1077.

51. Waters CH. Fluoxetine and selegiline-lack of significant interaction. Can J Neurol Sci 1994; 21:259–261.

52. Thorogood M, Armstrong B, Nichols T, Hollowell J. Mortality in people taking selegiline: observational study. BMJ 1998; 317:252–254.

53. Parkinson Study Group. Mortality in DATATOP: A Multicenter Trial in Early Parkinson's Disease. Ann Neurol 1998; 43:318–325.

54. Olanow CW, Myllyla VV, Sotaniemi KA, Larsen JP, Palhagen S, Przuntek H, Heinonen EH, Kilkku O, Lammintausta R, Maki-Ikola O, Rinne UK. Effect of selegiline on mortality in patients with Parkinson's disease: a meta analysis. Neurology 1998; 51:825–830.

55. Parkinson Study Group. A controlled trial of lazabemide (RO19-6327) in untreated Parkinson's disease. Ann Neurol 1993; 33:350–356.

56. Parkinson Study Group. Effect of lazabemide on the progression of disability in early Parkinson's disease Ann Neurol 1996; 40:99–107.

57. Kieburtz K, on behalf of the Parkinson Study Group. Efficacy and safety of rasagiline as monotherapy in early Parkinson's disease. Abstracts/Parkinsonism Rel Disord 2001; (suppl 7):S60.

58. Finberg JPM, Lamensdorf I, Commissiong JW, Youdim MBH. Pharmacology and neuroprotective properties of rasagiline. J Neural Transm 1996; 48:95–101.

59. Rabey JM, Sagi I, Huberman M, Melamed E, for the Rasagiline Study Group. Rasagiline mesylate, a new MAO-B inhibitor for the treatment of Parkinson's disease: a double-blind study as adjunctive therapy to levodopa. Clin Neuropharm 2000; 23:324–330.

20

Catechol-O-Methyltransferase in Parkinson's Disease

Ronald F. Pfeiffer
University of Tennessee Health Science Center, Memphis, Tennessee, U.S.A.

The introduction of levodopa therapy for Parkinson's disease (PD), initially by Birkmayer and colleagues in 1961 and Barbeau and colleagues in 1962, and in its ultimately successful form by Cotzias and colleagues in 1967, still represents the defining landmark in the treatment of PD (1–3). This dramatic advance was preceded by methodical basic laboratory research in the late 1950s and early 1960s, which formed a groundwork documenting the presence of striatal dopamine deficiency in PD (4–8) and paved the road for the application of this knowledge in the clinical arena.

These developments took place against a broader backdrop in which both the role of catecholamines and their metabolic pathways in body and brain were being unraveled (9). As part of this panorama, Axelrod, in 1957, first suggested that one of the metabolic pathways for catecholamines might be via O-methylation (9–11), and in the same year Shaw and colleagues proposed that catechol-O-methyltransferase (COMT) might be important in the inactivation of dihydroxyphenylalanine (DOPA) and dopamine (12). By 1964 the metabolic pathways for DOPA and dopamine had been delineated and the involved enzymes identified. Aromatic amino acid decarboxylase (AAAD) and COMT were identified as being responsible for converting

DOPA to dopamine and 3-O-methyldopa (3-OMD), respectively, while monoamine oxidase (MAO) and COMT were documented as being responsible for converting dopamine to 3,4-dihydroxyphenylacetic acid (DOPAC) and 3-methoxytyramine (3-MT), respectively. As early as 1964 it was suggested that agents inhibiting COMT might potentiate the effects of DOPA (13).

COMT is found throughout the body, with highest concentrations in the liver, kidneys, gastrointestinal tract, spleen, and lungs (14–17). It is also present in the brain, where it resides primarily in nonneuronal cells, such as glia. There is little COMT in neurons, and none has been identified in nigrostriatal dopaminergic neurons (18). It is principally a cytoplasmic enzyme, although a membrane-bound component has also been identified (11). A number of substrates are acted upon by COMT, including catecholamines such as epinephrine, norepinephrine, and dopamine and their hydroxylated metabolites, but all known substrates have a catechol configuration (11). COMT mediates the transfer of a methyl group from S-adenosylmethionine to a hydroxyl group on the catechol molecule. Its actions, especially in peripheral structures such as intestinal mucosa, seem to be primarily directed toward protecting the body by inactivating biologically active or toxic catechol compounds (11,18,19). Both levodopa and dopamine are examples of such biologically active compounds.

Recognition of the wretched bioavailability of orally administered levodopa in the treatment of PD, with perhaps only 1% of the levodopa actually reaching the brain because of extensive peripheral metabolism by both AAAD and COMT (18,20), fueled the search for drugs that might inhibit the two enzymes and improve levodopa therapeutic efficacy. This led relatively quickly to the introduction of two inhibitors of AAAD, carbidopa and benserazide, as adjunctive agents administered concomitantly with levodopa to PD patients (21,22). This approach of administering levodopa in conjunction with an AAAD inhibitor remains the standard today. However, use of these agents only expands the amount of levodopa reaching the brain to an estimated 10% of an administered dose, primarily because blocking AAAD simply shunts levodopa into the COMT metabolic pathway, with increased peripheral formation of 3-OMD (20).

FIRST-GENERATION COMT INHIBITORS

During the 1960s and 1970s a number of COMT inhibitors were identified and studied. Pyrogallol (1,2,3-trihydroxybenzene) was perhaps the first COMT inhibitor to be identified (23,24), but its short duration of action, toxicity (methemoglobinemia and renal impairment), and probable lack of COMT specificity precluded its clinical use (11). The list of additional "first-generation" COMT inhibitors that were studied and subsequently abandoned as potential therapeutic agents is long. Catechol itself, adnamine and noradnamine, various flavonoids, tropolone and its derivatives, 8-hydroxyquinolines, S-adenosylhomocysteine, sulfhydryl binding agents, pyrones and pyridones, papaveroline, methylspinazarin, 2-hydroxylated estrogens, and 3-mercaptotyramine represent only a partial listing of such compounds (11). Even the two agents that are primarily recognized as inhibitors of AAAD, carbidopa and benserazide, have some modest COMT-inhibiting properties, although not enough to be clinically relevant (11).

Several of these early COMT inhibitors did undergo pilot testing in humans. N-Butyl gallate (GPA 1714), a derivative of gallic acid, was found to be effective in alleviating signs and symptoms of PD when administered to 10 patients in a pilot study (25). The dose of levodopa was reduced by an average of 29%, and the drug was also noted to alleviate nausea and vomiting in affected patients. No significant adverse effects were noted in this initial study, but testing was eventually abandoned because of toxicity (26). Another compound, 3,4-dihydroxy-2-methylpropiophenone (U-0521), demonstrated significant COMT inhibition in animal studies in the laboratory, but when it was administered orally to a single human in progressively increasing doses it demonstrated no effect on erythrocyte COMT activity (26).

SECOND-GENERATION COMT INHIBITORS

Little literary attention was devoted to the subject of COMT inhibitors for the treatment of PD during the mid-1980s, but the dawning of the 1990s ushered in renewed interest in the potential clinical usefulness of these compounds. This attention was prompted by the development of a "second generation" of COMT inhibitors, substances that were more potent, more selective, and less toxic than their predecessors. Several nitrocatechol compounds, eventually bearing the names nitecapone, entacapone, and tolcapone, became the favored subjects of laboratory, and eventually clinical, focus.

Nitecapone

Nitecapone (OR 462) was demonstrated to be well tolerated and modestly effective when administered to mice, rats, and monkeys (27–29). Its actions were confined to the periphery since it did not cross the blood-brain barrier (30), and, in fact, its primary action appeared to be in the intestinal mucosa (31,32). In subsequent human studies it was noted to "slightly but significantly" increase the relative bioavailability of levodopa and to reduce plasma 3-OMD (33), but it eventually ceded its place in clinical PD development to entacapone (OR 611), which was judged to be the more effective compound.

Entacapone

Entacapone is readily absorbed across the intestinal mucosa and does not seem to be significantly affected by first-pass metabolism in the liver. The bioavailability of an oral dose of entacapone ranges from 30 to 46% (18,34–37). It is highly (98%) protein bound and metabolized via glucuronidation. The elimination half-life of entacapone is generally reported to be 0.4–0.7 hours (18,34–36). Entacapone does not cross the blood-brain barrier to any significant extent and is generally considered to exert its action exclusively in the periphery (38), although some inhibition of striatal COMT activity following entacapone administration in rats has been described (38,39). When administered to humans, the inhibition of COMT activity by entacapone is dose dependent. Soluble COMT is reduced by 82% with an entacapone dose of 800 mg, the maximum amount that has been administered (40). In multiple dose studies, 100 mg of entacapone given 4–6 times daily with levodopa reduced COMT activity by 25% compared to placebo, while 200 mg produced a 33% reduction and 400 mg generated a 32% diminution in COMT activity (35).

Entacapone also has a dose-related effect on both levodopa and 3-OMD pharmacokinetics. In the same group of patients noted above, the elimination half-life ($T_{1/2}$) of levodopa was prolonged by 23, 26, and 48% at entacapone doses of 100, 200, and 400 mg, respectively, while the area under the levodopa plasma curve (AUC) was increased by 17, 27, and 37% (35). Investigators in two earlier studies, however, had noted a leveling off of the levodopa AUC increase between entacapone doses of 200 and 400 mg and suggested that this might be due to interference with carbidopa absorption by entacapone at the higher dose (41,42). In other studies utilizing an entacapone dose of 200 mg, increases in the levodopa AUC ranged between 23 and 48%, and prolongation of the levodopa $T_{1/2}$ hovered around 40% (18). Despite these rather dramatic alterations, no significant increase in the time to reach the maximum plasma levodopa concentration (T_{max}) or the maximum plasma levodopa concentration itself (C_{max}) is seen following concomitant administration of levodopa and entacapone. The T_{max} remains between 30 and 60 minutes (18,31,43–46). Nutt notes that the absence of an effect on the levodopa T_{max} and C_{max} is, strictly speaking, true only for the initial dose of the day and that some modest progressive elevation of the levodopa C_{max} develops with repeated doses during the day (47). This does not carry over to the next day and progressive escalation of COMT inhibition does not occur (18,43). Concomitant with these changes in levodopa pharmacokinetics, entacapone also induces a significant reduction in the plasma AUC of 3-OMD, reflecting reduced COMT-mediated peripheral metabolism of levodopa to 3-OMD (18,35,37). It was predicted that the clinical correlate of these pharmacokinetic alterations would be extended efficacy of a levodopa dose. This is due to a combination of the prolonged $T_{1/2}$ and increased AUC of levodopa and the reduced AUC of 3-OMD, possibly without an increase in levodopa-related toxicity, in light of the absence of change in levodopa C_{max}. Subsequent full-scale clinical trials have largely validated these predictions and confirmed the safety and efficacy of entacapone.

The SEESAW study, a double-blind, placebo-controlled trial conducted by the Parkinson Study Group, evaluated the safety and efficacy of entacapone over a 6-month period in 205 PD patients on levodopa with motor fluctuations (48,49). A statistically significant 5% increase in "on" time per day (translating to approximately 1 hour) was documented in patients receiving entacapone, compared to the placebo group. Motor function, as measured by the Unified Parkinson's Disease Rating Scale (UPDRS) (50), improved slightly in the entacapone-treated group, while it deteriorated during the 6 months of the trial in the placebo group. Average daily levodopa dosage diminished by 12% (from 791 to 700 mg/day) in the entacapone-treated group but did not change in the placebo group. Adverse effects were generally mild and manageable, consisting primarily of symptoms consistent with enhanced dopaminergic activity, such as dyskinesia, nausea, and dizziness. Dyskinesia was reported as an adverse effect by 53% (55/103) of patients on entacapone, compared to 32% (33/102) of individuals on placebo. Yellow discoloration of the urine also occurred in 37% of those receiving entacapone, but diarrhea was infrequent (7%).

A second, large multicenter study, NOMECOMT, had a trial design similar to the SEESAW study with similar results (47,49,51). This trial, also 6 months in duration, included 171 PD patients on levodopa who were experiencing motor fluctuations. In the entacapone-treated group, mean "on" time increased by 1.4 hours, compared to an increase of 0.2 hours in the placebo group. This relative increase of 13% in the treatment group was statistically significant. The mean benefit from an individual levodopa dose increased by 24 minutes in the group receiving entacapone. Average daily levodopa dosage diminished by 12% in the entacapone group, compared to a 2% increase in the placebo group. Adverse effects in this study were similar to those in the SEESAW study, except that worsening of dyskinesia was reported by only 8.2% of entacapone-treated participants (vs. 1.2% of those on placebo), while diarrhea was reported by 20%.

More recent studies have augmented the findings of the SEESAW and NOMECOMT studies. Two additional large multicenter trials have investigated the safety and efficacy of entacapone in PD patients (52,53). In an open-label study of 8 weeks duration 489 patients were administered entacapone in conjunction with each dose of levodopa up to a maximum of 10 doses per day (52). Some reduction in "off" time was experienced by approximately 41% of patients and quality of life, as measured by the Parkinson's Disease Questionnaire (PDQ-39), was also improved. In a double-blind study of 301 PD patients, most of whom were experiencing motor fluctuations, significant improvement in both motor function and activities of daily living was documented in the group receiving entacapone compared to the placebo group (53). Concerns that the efficacy of entacapone might be reduced when used in conjunction with controlled-release levodopa preparations, because of a potential "mismatch" in absorption and metabolism of the two drugs, led several groups of investigators to address the issue (42,53,54). The effect of entacapone was, for the most part, found to be comparable between standard and controlled-release levodopa preparations.

Drug interactions are not a prominent problem with entacapone, although the capability of entacapone to chelate iron in the GI tract has been noted (55), and it has been suggested that a 2- to 3-hour interval be allowed between entacapone and iron ingestion (18).

Genetic polymorphism has been demonstrated with COMT. The gene on chromosome 22 is regulated by two co-dominant alleles, one of which codes for a high-activity thermostable COMT and one for a low-activity thermolabile COMT (56,57). It appears, however, that this dichotomy has little or no effect on the clinical response to entacapone (56).

Tolcapone

Tolcapone (Ro 40-7592), like entacapone, is rapidly absorbed after oral administration and reaches T_{max} in approximately 1.5–2 hours (18,58,59). The bioavailability of an oral dose is about 60% (60). Tolcapone is very highly (99.9%) protein bound (61). Metabolism of tolcapone is primarily, but not exclusively, via glucuronidation (62) since both methylation and oxidation also occur (63). The elimination $T_{1/2}$ of tolcapone is between 2 and 3 hours, which is distinctly longer than that of entacapone (58). At doses above 200 mg three times per day (TID), some accumulation of tolcapone can occur, but this appears to be of no practical significance since levels, even at doses of 800 mg TID, remain well below those associated with toxicity in animals (58).

Unlike entacapone, tolcapone is sufficiently lipophilic to cross the blood-brain barrier to some degree (64). While tolcapone-induced inhibition of COMT within the brain has clearly been demonstrated in animal experiments (63,65), it has been less convincingly demonstrated that similar central COMT inhibition takes place in humans receiving tolcapone in clinically relevant doses. Fluorodopa position emission tomography (PET) studies have provided some evidence that such central COMT inhibition does, indeed, take place with tolcapone doses of 200 mg (66). Tolcapone has also been identified in the cerebrospinal fluid (CSF) of patients with PD 1–4 hours after oral intake of 200 mg, concentrations sufficient to reduce CSF COMT activity by 75% (67). Inhibition of COMT within both peripheral and CNS structures provides some theoretical advantages over peripheral inhibition alone since, in addition to the peripheral levodopa-sparing capability, concomitant central COMT inhibition would not only reduce metabolism of levodopa to 3-OMD within the striatum, but would also block one route of metabolism of dopamine itself.

Single-dose studies demonstrated tolcapone to be a noticeably more potent COMT inhibitor than entacapone. At a dose of 200 mg, tolcapone increases the levodopa AUC by anywhere from 50 to 100%, prolongs the levodopa $T_{1/2}$ by 60–80%, and reduces the AUC of 3-OMD by 64% (18,47,68,69). No appreciable increase in C_{max} or T_{max} is seen with 200 mg of tolcapone, although some delay in the T_{max} becomes evident at higher doses (68).

A number of double-blind, placebo-controlled clinical trials have confirmed the efficacy of tolcapone in reducing motor fluctuations in individuals with PD (70–73). In each of these multicenter trials, which varied in length from 6 weeks to 6 months, significant increases in "on" time and reductions in "off" time were documented in the tolcapone-treated groups compared to the placebo groups. Reduction in both total daily levodopa dosage and number of levodopa doses taken was often evident in the tolcapone-treated groups.

In these four multicenter studies, in which 517 patients (out of 745 enrolled), received tolcapone in various doses ranging from 50 to 400 mg TID, adverse effects were generally mild and most often felt to be dopaminergic in character (70–73). In the three studies where the treatment groups consisted of placebo vs. 100 mg TID vs. 200 mg TID, dyskinesia was reported as an adverse event in 19–21%, 37–62%, and 53–66%, respectively (71–73). Diarrhea, at times unresponsive to medication and of sufficient severity to warrant drug discontinuation, was reported in a relatively small percentage of individuals receiving tolcapone, possibly in a dose-related pattern (47,72,73). The mechanism of the diarrhea is uncertain, although tolcapone has been noted to trigger intestinal fluid and electrolyte secretion, albeit not actual diarrhea, in dogs (18,74). As with entacapone, yellowish urine discoloration also occurred in some individuals.

In these initial multicenter trials, elevation of liver transaminase levels occurred in a small number of individuals, but all were clinically asymptomatic and the laboratory abnormalities sometimes returned to normal despite continued treatment. In all clinical trials of tolcapone the reported incidence of transaminase elevations greater than three times the upper limit of normal was approximately 1% at a dose of 100 mg TID and 3% at a dose of 200 mg TID (75). However, following introduction of tolcapone into routine clinical use, three cases of fulminant hepatic failure with a fatal outcome occurred, which led regulatory agencies in Europe and Canada to withdraw tolcapone from the market and the Food and Drug Administration in the United States to severely limit its use to situations in which other drugs have not provided sufficient benefit. Baseline liver function tests must be normal, and monitoring of liver function studies must be performed on a regular basis in patients receiving tolcapone. Similar hepatotoxicity has not occurred with entacapone.

CURRENT STATUS OF COMT INHIBITORS

Two COMT inhibitors are currently available for use as adjunctive therapy in PD, to be used in conjunction with levodopa and an AAAD inhibitor in patients who have developed motor fluctuations with end of dose failure. Tolcapone is the more potent of the two and, with its longer $T_{1/2}$, can be given on a TID basis. However, its potential to produce hepatic failure has severely restricted its clinical utility. Because of this, the field has largely been ceded to entacapone, which is a somewhat less potent, but a safer alternative. Because of its short $T_{1/2}$, entacapone must be administered with each dose of levodopa. The additional 1–2 hours of "on" time per day a COMT inhibitor typically affords to a fluctuating patient can be beneficial. A recent cost-effectiveness analysis of entacapone concluded that the additional drug costs when entacapone is employed are offset by reductions in other costs and improvement (6%) in "quality-adjusted life years" (76).

While it is clear that COMT inhibitors provide quantifiable improvement in function for PD patients with motor fluctuations, their potential benefit in stable PD patients who have not yet developed motor fluctuations has received much less attention. Two clinical trials have addressed this question with tolcapone (77,78). In the larger of the two trials (77), statistically significant improvement in both Part II (activities of daily living) and Part III (motor exam) of the UPDRS were documented. Improvement was most evident in more severely affected patients. Fewer patients in the tolcapone-treated group developed motor fluctuations during the duration of the trial, which extended to a maximum of 12 months for some participants (average 8.5 months). Adverse events were similar to those encountered in earlier trials described above. The second, smaller trial actually did not examine nonfluctuating PD patients, but rather evaluated individuals who had previously experienced wearing-off of levodopa efficacy, which had been successfully controlled by levodopa dosage adjustment (78). A greater reduction of levodopa dosage was achieved in the tolcapone-treated group, but this did not achieve statistical significance. A single tolcapone trial in levodopa untreated patients demonstrated no clinical benefit (79). Studies in nonfluctuating patients have not yet been reported with entacapone. Therefore, at the present time the adjunctive role for COMT inhibitors still seems most appropriate.

THE FUTURE OF COMT INHIBITORS

The pathogenesis of motor fluctuations in individuals with PD receiving levodopa has been the subject of much speculation, but little certainty, over the years. Both peripheral and central mechanisms have been hypothesized. Both may actually be active, but it appears that most often the predominant mechanisms driving the pathogenic process are within the CNS. Evidence has begun to accumulate that with PD progression the dwindling number of surviving nigrostriatal dopaminergic neurons are unable to maintain the normal synaptic atmosphere of constant dopaminergic stimulation; instead, the environment becomes one in which dopamine receptor stimulation is intermittent, characterized by pulses of dopaminergic stimulation coincident with levodopa administration. It appears that this pulsatile stimulation, in turn, incites a cascade of changes within the postsynaptic striatal spiny neurons that produces sensitization of glutamate receptors and altered motor responses (80,81).

If this is correct, providing and maintaining a synaptic environment of more constant dopaminergic stimulation from the beginning of treatment might forestall the development of the postsynaptic alterations and delay or prevent the appearance of motor fluctuations. This has led to the proposal that a COMT inhibitor, such as entacapone, be administered along with levodopa and carbidopa right from the initiation of therapy (82). To bolster this hypothesis, Jenner and colleagues recently reported that in marmosets with MPTP-induced parkinsonism, initiation of treatment with levodopa combined with entacapone resulted in less frequent and less severe dyskinesia than that which developed in animals treated with levodopa alone (83). If a reduction or delay in the development of motor fluctuations with such treatment is demonstrated, in humans the role for COMT inhibitors in the treatment of PD may expand dramatically.

REFERENCES

1. Birkmayer W, Hornykiewicz O. Der 1–3,4 Dioxyphenylalanin (=DOPA)-Effekt bei der Parkinson-Akinese. Wien J Klin Wochenschr 1961; 73:787–788.
2. Barbeau A, Sourkes TL, Murphy CF. Les catecholamines dans la maladie de Parkinson. In: Ajuriaguerra J de, ed. Monoamines et Systeme Nerveaux Central. Geneva: Gerog, 1962:247–262.
3. Cotzias GC, Van Woert MH, Schiffer LM. Aromatic amino acids and modification of parkinsonism. N Engl J Med 1967; 276:374–379.
4. Carlsson A, Lindquist M, Magnusson T. 3,4-Dihydroxyphenylalanine and 5-hydroxytryptophan as reserpine antagonists. Nature 1957; 180:200.
5. Bertler A, Rosengren E. Occurrence and distribution of catecholamines in brain. Acta Physiol Scand 1959; 47:350–361.
6. Ehringer H, Hornykiewicz O. Verteilung von Noradrenalin und Dopamin (3-Hydroxytyramin) im Gehirn des Menschen und ihr Verhalten bei Erkrankungen des extrapyramidalen Systems. Wien Klin Wochenschr 1960; 38:1236–1239.
7. Anden NE, Carlsson A, Dahlstrom A, Fuxe J/K, Hillarp N-A, Karlsson K. Demonstration and mapping of nigroneostriatal dopamine neurons. Life Sci 1964; 3:523–530.
8. Poirier LJ, Sourkes TL. Influence of the substantia nigra on the catecholamine content of the striatum. Brain 1965; 8:181–192.
9. Axelrod J. Catecholamine neurotransmitters, psychoactive drugs, and biological clocks. J Neurosurg 1981; 55:669–677.
10. Axelrod J. The O-methylation of epinephrine and other catechols in vitro and in vivo. Science 1957; 126:1657–1660.
11. Guldberg HC, Marsden CA. Catechol-O-methyl transferase: pharmacological aspects and physiological role. Pharmacol Rev 1975; 27:135–206.
12. Shaw KNF, McMillan A, Armstrong MD. The metabolism of 3,4-dihydroxyphenylalanine. J Biol Chem 1957; 226:255–266.
13. Carlsson A. Functional significance of drug-induced changes in brain monoamine levels. In: HE Himwich, WA Himwich, eds. Biogenic Amines. Amsterdam: Elsevier, 1964:9–27.
14. Nissinen E, Tuominen R, Perhoniemi V, Kaakkola S. Catechol-O-methyltransferase activity in human and rat small intestine. Life Sci 1988; 42:2609–2614.
15. Schultz E, Nissinen E. Inhibition of rat liver and duodenum soluble catechol-O-methyltransferase by a tight-binding inhibitor OR-462. Biochem Pharmacol 1989; 38:3953–3956.
16. Mannisto PT, Ulmanen I, Lundstrom K, Taskinen J, Tenhunen J, Tilgmann C, Kaakkola S. Characteristics of catechol-O-methyltransferase (COMT) and properties of selective COMT inhibitors. Prog Drug Res 1992; 39:291–350.
17. Ding YS, Gatley SJ, Fowler JS, Chen R, Volkow ND, Logan J, Shea CE, Sugano Y, Koomen J. Mapping catechol-O-methyltransferase in vivo: initial studies with [18F] Ro41-0960. Life Sci 1996; 58:195–208.

18. Teravainen H, Rinne U, Gordin A. Catechol-O-methyltransferase inhibitors in Parkinson's disease. In: Calne D, Calne S, eds. Parkinson's Disease. Philadelphia: Lippincott Williams Wilkins, 2001:311–325.
19. Huotari M, Gogos JA, Karayiorgou M, Koponen O, Forsberg M, Raasmaja A, Hyttinen J, Mannisto PT. Brain catecholamine metabolism in catechol-O-methyltransferase (COMT)-deficient mice. Eur J Neurosci 2002; 15:246–256.
20. Olanow CW, Schapira AHV, Rascol O. Continuous dopamine-receptor stimulation in early Parkinson's disease. Trends Neurosci 2000; 23(suppl):S117–S126.
21. Rinne UK, Sonninen V, Siirtola T. Treatment of parkinsonian patients with levodopa and extracerebral decarboxylase inhibitor, Ro 4-4602. In: Calne D, ed. Progress in the Treatment of Parkinsonism. New York: Raven Press, 1973:59–71.
22. Porter CC. Inhibitors of aromatic amino acid decarboxylase—their biochemistry. In: Yahr MD, ed. Treatment of Parkinsonism—The Role of Dopa Decarboxylase Inhibitors. New York: Raven Press, 1973:37–58.
23. Bacq AM, Gosselin L, Dresse A, Renson J. Inhibition of O-methyltransferase by catechol and sensitization to epinephrine. Science 1959; 130:453–454.
24. Axelrod J, LaRoche MJ. Inhibitor of O-methylation of epinephrine and norepinephrine in vitro and in vivo. Science 1959; 130:800.
25. Ericsson AD. Potentiation of the L-Dopa effect in man by the use of catechol-O-methyltransferase inhibitors. J Neurol Sci 1971; 14:193–197.
26. Reches A, Fahn S. Catechol-O-methyltransferase and Parkinson's disease. In: Hassler RG, Christ JF, eds. Parkinson-Specific Motor and Mental Disorders. New York: Raven Press, 1984:171–179.
27. Linden IB, Nissinen E, Etemadzadeh E, Kaakkola S, Mannisto P, Pohto P. Favorable effect of catechol-O-methyltransferase inhibition by OR-462 in experimental models of Parkinson's disease. J Pharmacol Exp Ther 1988; 247:289–293.
28. Tornwall M, Mannisto PT. Acute toxicity of three new selective COMT inhibitors in mice with special emphasis on interactions with drugs increasing catecholaminergic neurotransmission. Pharmacol Toxicol 1991; 69:64–70.
29. Cedarbaum JM, Leger G, Reches A, Guttman M. Effect of nitecapone (OR-462) on the pharmacokinetics of levodopa and 3-O-methyldopa formation in cynomolgus monkeys. Clin Neuropharmacol 1990; 13:544–552.
30. Marcocci L, Maguire JJ, Packer L. Nitecapone: a nitric oxide radical scavenger. Biochem Mol Biol Int 1994; 34:531–541.
31. Nissinen E, Linden IB, Schultz E, Kaakkola S, Mannisto PT, Pohto P. Inhibition of catechol-O-methyltransferase activity by two novel disubstituted catechols in the rat. Eur J Pharmacol 1988; 153:263–269.
32. Schultz E, Tarpila S, Backstrom AC, Gordin A, Nissinen E, Pohto P. Inhibition of human erythrocyte and gastroduodenal catechol-O-methyltransferase activity by nitecapone. Eur J Clin Pharmacol 1991; 40:577–580.
33. Kaakkola A, Gordin A, Jarvinen M, Wikberg T, Schultz E, Nissinen E, Pentikainen PJ, Rita H. Effect of a novel catechol-O-methyltransferase

inhibitor, nitecapone, on the metabolism of L-Dopa in healthy volunteers. Clin Neuropharmacol 1990; 13:436–447.

34. Najib J. Entacapone: a catechol-O-methyltransferase inhibitor for the adjunctive treatment of Parkinson's disease. Clin Ther 2001; 23:802–832.

35. Heikkinen H, Nutt JG, LeWitt PA, Koller WC, Gordin A. The effects of different repeated doses of entacapone on the pharmacokinetics of L-Dopa and on the clinical response to L-Dopa in Parkinson's disease. Clin Neuropharmacol 2001; 24:150–157.

36. Keranen T, Gordin A, Karlsson M, Korpela K, Pentikainen PJ, Rita H, Schultz E, Seppala L, Wikberg T. Inhibition of soluble catechol-O-methyltransferase and single-dose pharmacokinetics after oral and intravenous administration of entacapone. Eur J Clin Pharmacol 1994; 46:151–157.

37. Keranen T, Gordin A, Harjola V-P, Karlsson M, Korpela K, Pentikainen PJ, Rita H, Seppala L, Wikberg T. The effect of catechol-O-methyl transferase inhibition by entacapone on the pharmacokinetics and metabolism of levodopa in healthy volunteers. Clin Neuropharmacol 1993; 16:145–156.

38. Nissinen E, Linden I-B, Schultz E, Pohto P. Biochemical and pharmacological properties of a peripherally acting catechol-O-methyltransferase inhibitor entacapone. Naunyn Schmiedebergs Arch Pharmacol 1992; 346:262–266.

39. Brannan T, Prikhojan A, Yahr MD. Peripheral and central inhibitors of catechol-O-methyl transferase: effects on liver and brain COMT activity and L-DOPA metabolism. J Neural Transm 1997; 104:77–87.

40. Keranen T, Gordin A, Karlsson M, Korpela K, Pentikainen P, Schultz E, Seppala L, Wikberg T. Effect of the novel catechol-O-methyltransferase inhibitor OR-611 in healthy volunteers. Neurology 1991; 41(suppl):213.

41. Ruottinen HM, Rinne UK. A double-blind pharmacokinetic and clinical dose-response study of entacapone as an adjuvant to levodopa therapy in advanced Parkinson's disease. Clin Neuropharmacol 1996; 19:283–296.

42. Ahtila S, Kaakkola S, Gordin A, Korpela K, Heinavaara S, Karlsson M, Wikberg T, Tuomainen P, Mannisto PT. Effect of entacapone, a COMT inhibitor, on the pharmacokinetics and metabolism of levodopa after administration of controlled-release levodopa-carbidopa in volunteers. Clin Neuropharmacol 1995; 18:46–57.

43. Rouru J, Gordin A, Huupponen R, Huhtala S, Savontaus E, Korpela K, Reinikainen K, Scheinin M. Pharmacokinetics of oral entacapone after frequent multiple dosing and effects on levodopa disposition. Eur J Clin Pharmacol 1999; 55:461–467.

44. Heikkinen H, Saraheimo M, Antila S, Ottoila P, Pentikainen PJ. Eur J Clin Pharmacol 2001; 56:821–826.

45. Kaakkola S, Teravainen H, Ahtila S, Rita H, Gordin A. Effect of entacapone, a COMT inhibitor, on clinical disability and levodopa metabolism in parkinsonian patients. Neurology 1994; 44:77–80.

46. Schapira AHV, Obeso JA, Olanow CW. The place of COMT inhibitors in the armamentarium of drugs for the treatment of Parkinson's disease. Neurology 2000; 55(suppl 4):S65–S68.

47. Nutt JG. Effect of COMT inhibition on the pharmacokinetics and pharmacodynamics of levodopa in parkinsonian patients. Neurology 2000; 55(suppl 4):S33–S37.
48. Parkinson Study Group. Entacapone improves motor fluctuations in levodopa-treated Parkinson's disease patients. Ann Neurol 1997; 42:747–755.
49. Kieburtz K, Hubble J. Benefits of COMT inhibitors in levodopa-treated parkinsonian patients: results of clinical trials. Neurology 2000; 55(suppl 4):S42–S45.
50. Fahn S, Elton RL, Members of the UPDRS Development Committee. Unified Parkinson's disease rating scale. In: Fahn S, Marsden CD, Goldstein M, Calne DB, eds. Recent Developments in Parkinson's Disease, Vol 2. New York: Macmillan, 1987:153–163.
51. Rinne UK, Larsen JP, Siden A, Worm-Petersen J, and the Nomecomt Study Group. Entacapone enhances the response to levodopa in parkinsonian patients with motor fluctuations. Neurology 1998; 51:1309–1314.
52. Durif F, Devaux I, Pere JJ, Delumeau JC, Bourdeix I, F-01 Study Group. Efficacy and tolerability of entacapone as adjunctive therapy to levodopa in patients with Parkinson's disease and end-of-dose deterioration in daily medical practice: an open, multicenter study. Eur Neurol 2001; 5:111–118.
53. Poewe WH, Deuschl G, Gordin A, Kultalahti ER, Leinonen M, the Celomen Study Group. Efficacy and safety of entacapone in Parkinson's disease patients with suboptimal levodopa response: a 6-month randomized placebo-controlled double-blind study in Germany and Austria (Celomen Study). Acta Neurol Scand 2002; 105:245–255.
54. Piccini P, Brooks DJ, Korpela K, Pavese N, Karlsson M, Gordin A. The catechol-O-methyltransferase (COMT) inhibitor entacapone enhances the pharmacokinetic and clinical response to Sinemet CR in Parkinson's disease. J Neurol Neurosurg Psychiatry 2000; 68:589–594.
55. Orama M, Tilus P, Taskinen J, Lotta T. Iron (III)-chelating properties of the novel catechol O-methyltransferase inhibitor entacapone in aqueous solution. J Pharm Sci 1997; 86:827–831.
56. Lee MS, Kim HS, Cho EK, Lim JH, Rinne JO. COMT genotype and effectiveness of entacapone in patients with fluctuating Parkinson's disease. Neurology 2002; 58:564–567.
57. Tai CH, Wu RM. Catechol-O-methyltransferase and Parkinson's disease. Acta Med Okayama 2002; 56:1–6.
58. Jorga KM. Pharmacokinetics, pharmacodynamics, and tolerability of tolcapone: a review of early studies in volunteers. Neurology 1998; 50(suppl 5):S31–S38.
59. Dingemanse J, Jorga K, Zurcher G, Schmitt M, Sedek G, Da Prada M, Van Brummelen P. Pharmacokinetic-pharmacodynamic interaction between the COMT inhibitor tolcapone and single-dose levodopa. Br J Clin Pharmacol 1995; 40:253–262.
60. Jorga K, Fotteler B, Heizmann P, Zurcher G. Pharmacokinetics and pharmacodynamics after oral and intravenous administration of tolcapone,

a novel adjunct to Parkinson's disease therapy. Eur J Clin Pharmacol 1998; 54:443–447.

61. Dingemanse J. Issues important for rational COMT inhibition. Neurology 2000; 55(suppl 4):S24–S27.

62. Jorga K, Fotteler B, Heizmann P, Gasser R. Metabolism and excretion of tolcapone, a novel inhibitor of catechol-O-methyltransferase. Br J Clin Pharmacol 1999; 48:513–520.

63. Da Prada M, Borgulya J, Napolitano A, Zurcher G. Improved therapy of Parkinson's disease with tolcapone, a central and peripheral COMT inhibitor with an S-adenosyl-L-methionine-sparing effect. Clin Neuropharmacol 1994; 17(suppl 3):S26–S37.

64. Dingemanse J. Catechol-O-methyltransferase inhibitors: clinical potential in the treatment of Parkinson's disease. Drug Dev Res 1997; 42:1–25.

65. Zurcher G, Dingemanse J, Da Prada M. Potent COMT inhibition by Ro 40-7592 in the periphery and in the brain. Preclinical and clinical findings. In Narabayashih H, Nagatsu T, Yanagisawa N, Mizuno Y, eds. Parkinson's Disease. From Basic Research To Treatment. New York: Raven Press, 1993:641–647.

66. Ceravolo R, Piccini P, Bailey DL, Jorga KM, Bryson H, Brooks DJ. 18F-dopa PET evidence that tolcapone acts as a central COMT inhibitor in Parkinson's disease. Synapse 2002; 43:201–207.

67. Russ H, Muller T, Woitalla D, Rahbar A, Hahn J, Kuhn W. Detection of tolcapone in the cerebrospinal fluid of parkinsonian subjects. Naunyn Schmiedebergs Arch Pharmacol 1999; 360:719–720.

68. Sedek G, Jorga K, Schmitt M, Burns RS, Leese P. Effect of tolcapone on plasma levodopa concentrations after coadministration with levodopa/ carbidopa to healthy volunteers. Clin Neuropharmacol 1997; 20:531–541.

69. Kurth MC, Adler CH. COMT inhibition: a new treatment strategy for Parkinson's disease. Neurology 1998; 50(suppl 5):S3–S14.

70. Kurth MC, Adler CH, St. Hilaire M, Singer C, Waters C, LeWitt P, Chernik DA, Dorflinger EE, Yoo K, and the Tolcapone Fluctuator Study Group I. Tolcapone improves motor function and reduces levodopa requirement in patients with Parkinson's disease experiencing motor fluctuations: a multi-center, double-blind, randomized, placebo-controlled trial. Neurology 1997; 48:81–87.

71. Adler CH, Singer C, O'Brien C, Hauser RA, Lew MF, Marek KL, Dorflinger E, Pedder S, Deptula D, Yoo K, for the Tolcapone Fluctuator Study Group III. Randomized, placebo-controlled study of tolcapone in patients with fluctuating Parkinson's disease treated with levodopa-carbidopa. Arch Neurol 1998; 55:1089–1095.

72. Rajput AH, Martin W, Saint-Hilaire M-H, Dorflinger E, Pedder S. Tolcapone improves motor function in parkinsonian patients with the "wearing-off" phenomenon: a double-blind, placebo-controlled, multicenter trial. Neurology 1997; 49:1066–1071.

73. Baas H, Beiske AG, Ghika J, Jackson M, Oertel WH, Poewe W, Ransmayr G, on behalf of the study investigators. Catechol-O-methyltransferase inhibition with tolcapone reduces the "wearing-off" phenomenon and levodopa requirements in fluctuating parkinsonian patients. J Neurol Neurosurg Psychiatry 1997; 63:421–428.

74. Larsen KR, Dajani EZ, Dajani NE, Dayton MT, Moore JG. Effects of tolcapone, a catechol-O-methyltransferase inhibitor, and Sinemet on intestinal electrolyte and fluid transport in conscious dogs. Dig Dis Sci 1998; 43:1806–1813.

75. Watkins P. COMT inhibitors and liver toxicity. Neurology 2000; 55(suppl 4).S51–S52.

76. Nuijten MJ, van Iperen P, Palmer C, van Hilten BJ, Snyder E. Cost-effectiveness analysis of entacapone in Parkinson's disease: a Markov process analysis. Value Health 2001; 4:316–328.

77. Waters CH, Kurth M, Bailey P, Shulman LM, LeWitt P, Dorflinger E, Deptula D, Pedder S, and the Tolcapone Stable Study Group. Tolcapone in stable Parkinson's disease: efficacy and safety of long-term treatment. Neurology 1997; 49:665–671.

78. Dupont E, Burgunder J-M, Findley LJ, Olsson J-E, Dorflinger E, and the Tolcapone in Parkinson's Disease Study Group II (TIPS II). Tolcapone added to levodopa in stable parkinsonian patients: a double-blind placebo-controlled study. Mov Disord 1997; 12:928–934.

79. Hauser RA, Molho E, Shale H, Pedder S, Dorflinger EE, and the Tolcapone De Novo Study Group. A pilot evaluation of the tolerability, safety and efficacy of tolcapone alone and in combination with oral selegiline in untreated Parkinson's disease patients. Mov Disord 1998; 13:643–647.

80. Chase TN. Levodopa therapy: consequences of the nonphysiologic replacement of dopamine. Neurology 1998; 50(suppl 5):S17–S25.

81. Chase TN, Oh JD. Striatal dopamine- and glutamate-mediated dysregulation in experimental parkinsonism. Trends Neurosci 2000; 23(suppl):S86–S91.

82. Olanow CW, Obeso JA. Pulsatile stimulation of dopamine receptors and levodopa-induced motor complications in Parkinson's disease. Implications for the early use of COMT inhibitors. Neurology 2000; 55(suppl 4):S72–S77.

83. Jenner P, Al-Barghouthy G, Smith L, Kuoppamaki M, Jackson M, Rose S, Olanow W. Initiation of entacapone with L-dopa further improves antiparkinsonian activity and avoids dyskinesia in the MPTP primate model of Parkinson's disease. Neurology 2002; 58(suppl 3):A374–A375.

21

Investigational Pharmacological Treatments for Parkinson's Disease

William Ondo
Baylor College of Medicine, Houston, Texas, U.S.A.

Effective therapy for Parkinson's disease (PD) has existed for 40 years. Currently, levodopa, the precursor to dopamine, remains the most consistently effective medication. Most other pharmacologic treatments, such as dopamine agonists, augment and replace the endogenous dopamine loss that causes PD symptoms. Other treatments such as anticholinergic medications and amantadine often help symptoms through nondopaminergic mechanisms. Numerous other medications such as antidepressants and antipsychotics are used to treat specific symptoms in PD.

Conceptually, there are two major shortcomings to our current pharmacological armamentarium: loss of effect and lack of effect. Dopaminergic medications often initially improve symptoms, but as the disease progresses, patients develop motor fluctuations. Initially, the duration of medication action shortens. The subsequent development of dyskinesia and on/off phenomenon complicates dosing and markedly worsens quality of life. This is particularly problematic in younger patients. Certain aspects of PD never respond well to dopaminergic drugs, such as cognition, mood, balance, gait freezing, gastroenterological and urological symptoms, and bulbar symptoms. Finally, no available medication can definitely claim to offer anything other than symptomatic benefit. Therefore, despite a recent increase in available medications and the tremendous advances in surgical treatments, the overall treatment of PD remains wanting.

New medications can be broadly classified into three categories: 1) improved versions of drugs that employ similar mechanisms of action as currently available medications, 2) drugs with novel mechanisms of action, and 3) drugs designed to treat only a particular aspect of the disease (psychosis, dementia, etc.). In this chapter we will only discuss new drugs designed to treat the motor features of PD.

NEW DOPAMINERGIC AGENTS

The general goals of new dopaminergic therapies are to maximize the therapeutic effect while minimizing typical adverse events (AEs), including sedation, nausea, hallucinations, edema, and hypotension. Clinically, a rapid onset to action is also desirable. Furthermore, there is increasing evidence that continuous dopaminergic stimulation may delay the appearance of fluctuations and potentially retard neuronal degeneration. The new dopaminergics generally achieve one of these goals.

Ropinirole (Requip®) controlled-release (CR) capsules (Glaxo-SmithKline) are currently undergoing Phase II/III trials for PD. The dopamine agonist component (ropinirole) is identical to the currently available drug. The CR tablet employs a Geomatrix® technology involving altering layers of active drug and erodible hydroxypropyl methylcellulose polymers, which slow absorption of the drug. This formulation is already used in medications marketed in the United States including diltiazem hydrochloride (Dilacor XR®) and paroxetine hydrochloride (Paxil CR®). The ropinirole Geomatrix system differs slightly from previous systems in that it employs a carboxymethylcellulose sodium. Pharmacokinetic studies show that this safely slows absorption without any dose dumping. Two Phase II trials are ongoing with doses ranging from 0.75 to 3.0 mg tablets. No unexpected AEs have been reported to date.

Rotigotine CDS® (constant delivery system), (-)-5,6,7,8-tetrahydro-6-[propyl-[2-(2-thienyl-ethyl) amino]-1-naphthalenolis (Schwarz Pharma, Mannheim, Germany) is a silicone-based lipophilic D2 agonist patch designed to deliver constant drug levels over a 24-hour period (1). Detectable serum levels are achieved 2–3 hours after initial application and a serum steady state is achieved after approximately 24 hours. In the current formulation, the 9 mg (20 cm^2) patch delivered approximately 5 mg of drug over a 24-hour period. Increased dermal sizes appear to proportionally increase serum drug levels. Pharmacokinetic studies demonstrate that the drug (N-0923) has a half-life ($T_{1/2}$) of about 5 hours but maintains steady-state levels while the patch is worn. There were no measurable metabolites.

Phase I and II studies have shown efficacy and a similar adverse event profile to that of other dopamine agonists (DAs) (2,3). The most common AEs included nausea, hypotension, drowsiness, and dizziness. AEs were generally dose dependent. Many patients also reported some skin irritation after repetitive administration to the same location. Between 1.4 and 3.6% withdrew from studies due to skin irritation. Subsequent studies allowing for placement on different skin areas have reduced this problem.

Phase IIa dose finding studies showed a linear dose-response curve, as measured by the Unified Parkinson's Disease Rating Scale (UPDRS), from 4.5 to 54 mg/day. A Phase IIb study of early PD patients found significant improvement compared to placebo at doses from 9 to 40 mg (4).

Sumanirole maleate (PNU-95666E; Pharmacia) is a novel oral D2 agonist, which differs from existing dopamine agonists secondary to its low affinity for the D3 receptor. In PD, the positive motor features elicited by DAs appear to be modulated primarily by D2 receptors. The role of D3 receptors in PD is not clear, but in animal models, pure D3 agonists may actually slow movement (5). All existing DAs have strong affinity for both receptors, so it is impossible to segregate the contributions of each receptor type in human disease. Nevertheless, 6-OHDA rat models of PD treated with sumanirole improved more robustly than those treated with traditional DAs.

Sumanirole has a relatively short $T_{1/2}$, but several preparations, including an extended release and a combination extended release/immediate release, have also been tested in Phase II trials. Therefore, dosing varies from two to four times daily depending on the preparation.

Phase II trials in early and advanced PD patients have generally reported efficacy similar to that of other DAs at doses ranging from 2 to 48 mg/day. No unexpected serious AEs have been reported. Sedation and hallucinations may occur less frequently than what is historically reported in DA trials, but this awaits head-to-head confirmation. The drug is also being tested for restless legs syndrome, hyperprolactinemia, and sexual dysfunction.

Etilevodopa (TV-1203/carbidopa), TEVA Pharmaceuticals, is an ethyl ester derivative of levodopa. The prodrug is designed to be absorbed more rapidly and reliably in the gut than levodopa, primarily because it is more soluble in aqueous solutions. It is rapidly and almost completely hydrolyzed to levodopa by pancreatic enzymes in the gastric tract, and only negligible amounts of etilevodopa are detected in serum. Several animal and human pharmacokinetic studies have confirmed that peak plasma levels of levodopa are achieved more rapidly after ingestion of etilevodopa compared to equimolar amounts of levodopa. Some of these have also demonstrated slightly higher peak levels than seen with equimolar concentrations of oral levodopa, without any difference in the total levodopa absorbed.

To date, Phase I and Phase II trials of etilevodopa, in combination with a decarboxylase inhibitor have demonstrated good efficacy and AEs comparable to levodopa compounds. No meaningful unexpected AEs have been reported. Phase III trials are ongoing to test etilevodopa in patients with fluctuating PD.

MONOAMINE OXIDASE INHIBITORS

Rasagiline (N-propargyl-1R-aminoindan) mesylate (TEVA Pharmaceuticals) is a potent irreversible inhibitor of monoamine oxidase B (MAO-B). In addition to improving motor symptoms in animal models of PD, rasagiline improved cognitive impairment in animals resulting from hypoxia (6) and trauma (7) and improved cell survival in a variety of in vitro and in vivo models of cell death (7,8). Rasagiline has several potential advantages over oral selegiline, including its superior ability to inhibit MAO-B, better penetration into the central nervous system (CNS), and lack of potentially pro-oxidant and amphetamine-like metabolites.

Several Phase I and II trials have reported good efficacy and excellent tolerability in early- and late-stage PD patients (9). A 404-patient, 26-week, double-blind Phase III study showed that both 1 and 2 mg/day of rasagiline improved UPDRS scores compared to placebo in subjects with early PD (10). AEs were similar to those of placebo. Over the subsequent 6 months, all subjects received rasagiline. At the end of 12 months, subjects who were originally assigned to rasagiline maintained relatively better UPDRS scores (11). Given the potential interaction between tyramine and MAO inhibition, a subset of patients also underwent uneventful tyramine challenge tests (12). Blood pressures were generally unchanged after a 75 mg tyramine ingestion. Phase III trials in fluctuating PD are ongoing.

Zydis® selegiline (Elan Pharmaceuticals) is formulated as a sublingually absorbed preparation. The Zydis preparation is a drug-impregnated, water-soluble polymer matrix that is rapidly absorbed through oral mucosa. Oral selegiline undergoes extensive first-pass hepatic metabolism to amphetamine compounds that could potentially counteract the theoretical reduction in oxidative stress and inhibit any neuroprotective effect of the parent drug. Mucosal absorption bypasses most of the metabolism such that much smaller doses equally inhibit CNS MAO-B without compromising systemic MAO-B specificity or accumulating amphetamine metabolites.

Phase I and II trials did not show any unexpected AEs. Pooled data from two identical placebo controlled trials (1.25 mg/day for 6 weeks followed by 2.5 mg/day for 6 weeks) in fluctuating PD showed that the drug reduced the percentage of "off" time and improved UPDRS motor "off" examinations (13). It was well tolerated. Specifically, stomatitis and ulcerations were not seen more than in placebo.

AGENTS WITH NOVEL MECHANISMS OF ACTION

KW-6002 [(E)-1,3-diethyl-8-(3,4-dimethoxystryl)-7-methyl-3,7-dihydro-1H-purine-2,6-dione; Kyowa Pharmaceuticals, Princeton, NJ] is a novel adenosine 2A antagonist. Adenosine receptors are found throughout the CNS, but type 2A receptors are seen almost exclusively on gamma-aminobutyric acid (GABA), enkephalin, and cholinergic (ACh) spiny neurons in the striatum. These neurons receive inhibitory dopaminergic input from the substantia nigra and then project to inhibit pallidal neurons as part of the indirect pathway of the basal ganglia. Therefore, in PD, dopaminergic cell loss results in disinhibition of striatal spiny neurons that subsequently overly inhibit the globus pallidus externus (GPe), which in turn overly stimulate the subthalamic nucleus (STN) and globus pallidus internus (GPi).

Antagonism of the adenosine A_2 receptor appears to modulate GABA and ACh release in a manner that could counteract the deleterious effects of reduced dopaminergic stimulation. In fact, nonspecific adenosine antagonists such as caffeine have been known to counteract motor retardation caused by dopaminergic blockade (14). Specific affinity for the striatal A_2 receptors could significantly reduce the numerous other effects mediated by gross manipulation of adenosine systems.

Animal studies using KW-6002 with 6-OH-dopa rodents and 1-methyl-4-phenyl-1,2,3,6-tetrahydropyridine (MPTP) primates have consistently shown beneficial motor effects (15,16). A single dose typically improved locomotion for about 10 hours. Interestingly, motor hyperactivity (dyskinesia) did not develop with long-term administration of KW-6002. When used in combination with dopaminergic drugs in these models, KW-6002 potentiated the duration and also allowed for dose reduction and improved dyskinesia, while maintaining improved locomotion.

Several Phase I trials in humans have not identified any serious AEs. A completed Phase II trial using three doses of KW-6002 (10, 20, 40 mg) in fluctuating PD patients found that the drug group reported less "off" time without any increase in dyskinesia (17,18). AEs were minimal, and additional studies are ongoing.

CEP-1347 (Cephalon Inc.) is a 5,16-bis[(ethylthio)methyl] derivative of indolocarbazole, k252a, which is being tested for neurodegenerative disease including PD. The drug inhibits proteins in the mixed-lineage kinase family (MLK) (19–21). These proteins activate c-Jun N-terminal kinase (JNK), which is a key kinase in the stress-activated protein kinase (SAPK) pathway. Therefore, the drug is thought to inhibit programmed cell death. A variety of animal models, including MPTP primates, support this.

The terminal $T_{1/2}$ of CEP-1347 averages about 30 hours in humans. Metabolism is predominately oxidation and hydrolysis with biliary excretion. Phase I and IIa trials have not demonstrated any consistent AEs at doses ranging from 5 to 150 mg/day, although gastrointestinal irritation has been reported in some series. Two 28-day trials in PD did not show any symptomatic clinical effect or change on [^{123}I] B-CIT single photon emission computed tomography (SPECT). Longer studies designed to look at possible neuroprotective effects in PD are ongoing.

THC346 (dibenzo[b,f]oxepin-10-ylmethyl-prop-2-ynyl-amine, hydrogen maleate salt; Novartis Pharmaceuticals) is a novel compound being studied for the treatment of neurodegenerative diseases such as PD. The drug is structurally similar to selegiline but has only a negligible effect on MAO. The mechanism of action is not entirely known, but the drug appears to interact with the glycolytic enzyme glyceraldehyde 3-phosphate dehydrogenase (GAPDH), which is involved with programmed cell death. Furthermore, the drug maintains mitochondrial membrane potential, which may reduce oxidative damage.

Pharmacokinetic studies have demonstrated variable oral bioavailability and extensive first-pass metabolism that results in multiple metabolites of uncertain significance, which are predominately excreted in the urine. To date, multiple Phase I trials and a single Phase II trial in PD patients have not demonstrated any consistent meaningful AEs. Efficacy trials are ongoing.

Sarizotan (Merck KGaA, Darmstadt, Germany) is a novel compound belonging to the aminomethyl chromane chemical group, which was initially developed as an atypical antipsychotic, but is now being evaluated to treat dopaminergic-induced dyskinesia in PD. The drug has affinity for $5HT_{1A}$, D2, D3, and D4 receptors. After oral ingestion, it is rapidly absorbed and highly protein bound, but readily crosses the blood-brain barrier. The terminal serum $T_{1/2}$ is approximately 7 hours, and the drug is extensively metabolized by N-dealkylation and hydroxylation.

In animal models of PD, including MPTP primates, sarizotan improved drug-induced dyskinesia without worsening motor function (22). In a Phase IIa open-label trial of 64 dyskinetic PD subjects, the drug, at doses ranging from 2 to 10 mg BID, prolonged the amount of "on" time without dyskinesia. PD symptoms were not worsened, as assessed by "off" time or UPDRS examinations, although some patients did list "worsening of parkinsonism" as an AE. Additional AEs reported in tolerability studies included sedation and nausea. Higher doses have been associated with suppression of the cortisol response to adrenocorticotrophic hormone (ACTH) challenge, but this was not seen in PD.

Glial-derived neurotrophic factor (GDNF) (Amgen Inc., Thousand Oaks, CA) is a recombinant neuropeptide, which may promote survival of or regenerate dopaminergic neurons. When delivered directly into the CNS of animal PD models, GDNF improved pathological dopaminergic systems and clinical signs. Determining the best CNS delivery system in humans has been problematic. A single large controlled trial delivered between 25 and 4000 µg in monthly doses directly into the cerebral spinal fluid via intraventricular catheter (23). Overall, those receiving drug did not improve clinically compared to placebo. Furthermore, GDNF infusion was often complicated by nausea and headache. Some subjects also suffered from an infusion-associated chemical meningitis. Other AEs included weight loss and hyponatremia. It was postulated that the lack of symptom improvement might have resulted from failure of the drug to reach target tissues. In contrast, a recent five-subject, open-label trial that directly delivered GDNF to the putamen reported robust improvement in UPDRS scores, improved "on" time, and reduced dyskinesia (24). Alternative methods of delivery, including viral vector delivery systems, are also under development (25).

AMG-474-00 (aka GP-1046) (Amgen, Thousand Oaks, CA) is a synthetic drug that binds to intracellular neuro-immunophilin receptor proteins. Neuro-immunophilin drugs, through unknown mechanisms, possess neurotrophic properties, which may restore cell viability. Chemically, the drug is related to immunological drugs such as cyclosporine and FK-506, but lacks any immunosuppressive actions. AMG-474-00 is highly orally bioavailable and readily crosses the blood-brain barrier. When administered after MPTP lesioning in animal models of PD, oral AMG-474-00 resulted in robust reinnervation by dopaminergic terminals at doses ranging from 0.01 to 50 mg/kg/day. Clinically, motor function also improved.

CONCLUSION

The past 10 years have seen a marked acceleration in therapeutic research for PD. In addition to novel pharmacological agents, novel surgical approaches and drug-delivery systems are under development to address the unmet needs of PD management. Continued research into disease pathogenesis and continued integration of governmental, academic, and pharmaceutical industrial resources will no doubt continue to foster innovative treatment strategies and hopefully cure PD altogether.

REFERENCES

1. Konitsiotis S, Oh JD, Metman LV. Continuous transdermal dopaminergic stimulation in advanced Parkinson's disease. Adv Neurol 2001; 86:355–360.
2. Metman LV, Gillespie M, Farmer C, Bibbiani F, Konitsiotis S, Morris M, et al. Continuous transdermal dopaminergic stimulation in advanced Parkinson's disease. Clin Neuropharmacol 2001; 24:163–169.
3. Hutton JT, Metman LV, Chase TN, Juncos JL, Koller WC, Pahwa R, et al. Transdermal dopaminergic D(2) receptor agonist therapy in Parkinson's disease with N-0923 TDS: a double-blind, placebo-controlled study. Mov Disord 2001; 16:459–463.
4. Bianchine J, Poole K, Woltering F. Efficacy and dose response of the novel transdermally applied dopamine agonist rotigotine CDS in early Parkinson's disease. Neurology 2002; 58(suppl 3):A162–A163.
5. Svensonn K, Carlsson A, Huff R, Kling P, Waters N. Behavioural and neurochemical data suggests functional differences between dopamine D2 and D3 receptors. Eur J Pharmacol 1994; 263:235–243.
6. Veinberg A, Lerner D, Goldenberg W, Levy R, Youdim M, Finberg J, et al. Sparing by rasagiline (TVP-1012) of cholinergic functions and behavior in the postnatal anoxia rat. J Neural Transm Suppl 1998; 52:301–305.
7. Katzir O, Rehavi M, Zabarski T, Cohen S, Huang W. Neuroprotective effect of rasagiline, a selective monoamine oxidase-B inhibitor, against closed head injury in the mouse. Pharmacol Biochem Behav 1998; 60:387–393.
8. Kirschbaum-Slager N, Lazarovici P, Bejar C, Youdim MB, Shoham S, Maruyama W. Antiapoptotic properties of rasagiline, N-propargylamine-1(R)-aminoindan, and its optical (S)-isomer, TV1022. NY Acad Sci 2001; 939:148–161.
9. Akao Y, Youdim MB, Davis BA, Naoi M, Rabey JM. Rasagiline mesylate, a new MAO-B inhibitor for the treatment of Parkinson's disease: a double-blind study as adjunctive therapy to levodopa. J Neurochem 2001; 78:727–735.
10. Parkinson Study Group. A controlled trial of early Parkinson's disease. Ann Neurol 2000; 48(suppl):489.
11. Parkinson Study Group. Earlier treatments with rasagiline may attenuate (UPDRS) progression of PD. Mov Disord 2001; 16:981.
12. Parkinson Study Group. Tyramine challenge to assess the safety of rasagaline monotherapy in a placebo-controlled multicenter trial for early Parkinson's disease (the TEMPO study). Neurology 2001; 56(suppl 3):A345.
13. Shellenberger M, Clarke A, Donoghue S. Zydis selegiline reduces time and improves symptoms in patients with Parkinson's disease. Mov Disord 2001; 15(suppl 2):116–117.

14. Daly J, Butts-Lamb P, Padgett W. Subclass of adenosine receptors in the central nervous system: interaction with caffeine and related methylxanthines. Cell Mol Neurobiol 1983; 8:69–74.

15. Jackson MJ, Smith LA, Pearce RK, Nakamura J, Kase H, Kuwana Y, et al. Adenosine A2A receptors modify motor function in MPTP-treated common marmosets. Ann Neurol 1998; 43:507–513.

16. Sakamaki T, Kanda T, Ito Y, Sumino H, Masuda H, Ohyama Y, et al. Adenosine A2A receptors modify motor function in MPTP-treated common marmosets. Res Commun Mol Path Pharmacol 1998; 101:25–34.

17. Hubble J, Hauser R. A novel adenosine antagonist (KW-6002) as a treatment for advanced Parkinson's disease with motor complications. Neurology 2002; 58(suppl 3):A162.

18. Sherzai A, Bara-Jimenez W, Gillespie M, et al. Adenosine Aza antagonist treatment of Parkinson's disease. Neurology 2002; 58(suppl 3):A467.

19. Harris CA, Deshmukh M, Tsui-Pierchala B, Maroney AC, Johnson EM, Jr, Ylikoski J. Inhibition of the c-Jun N-terminal kinase signaling pathway by the mixed lineage kinase inhibitor CEP-1347 (KT7515) preserves metabolism and growth of trophic factor-deprived neurons. J Neurosci 2002; 22:103–113.

20. Le S, Connors TJ, Maroney AC. c-Jun N-terminal kinase specifically phosphorylates p66ShcA at serine 36 in response to ultraviolet irradiation. J Bio Chem 2001; 276:48332–48336.

21. Maroney AC, Glicksman MA, Basma AN, Walton KM, Knight E, Jr, Murphy CA, et al. Motoneuron apoptosis is blocked by CEP-1347 (KT 7515), a novel inhibitor of the JNK signaling pathway. J Neurosci 1998; 18:104–111.

22. Bibbiani F, Oh JD, Chase TN. Serotonin 5-HT1A agonist improves motor complications in rodent and primate parkinsonian models. Neurology 2001; 57:1829–1834.

23. Nutt J, Brownstein J, Carter J, Comella C. Intraventricular administration of GDNF in the treatment of Parkinson's disease. Neurology 2001; 56(suppl 3):A375.

24. Gil S, Patel N, O'Sullivan K, Brooks D. Intraparenchymal putaminal administration of glial-derived neurotrophic factor in the treatment of advanced Parkinson's disease. Neurology 2002; 58(suppl 7):A241.

25. Kordower JH, Emborg ME, Bloch J, Ma SY, Chu Y, Leventhal L, et al. Neurodegeneration prevented by lentiviral vector delivery of GDNF in primate models of Parkinson's disease. Science 2000; 290:767–773.

22

Lesion Surgeries

Michael Samuel and Anthony E. Lang
The Toronto Western Hospital, University of Toronto,
Toronto, Ontario, Canada

EARLY SURGICAL EXPERIMENTS AND SUCCESS OF SURGERY FOR MOVEMENT DISORDERS

The following description is of case VI from James Parkinson's 1817 essay on paralysis agitans (1):

> About a year since, on waking at night, he found that he had nearly lost the use of the right side, and that his face was much drawn to the left side. His medical attendant saw him the following day, when he found him languid, with a small and quick pulse and without pain in the head or disposition of sleep. Nothing more therefore was done ... and in about a fortnight the limbs had entirely recovered from their palsied state. During the time of their having remained in this state, neither the arm nor the leg of the paralytic side was in the least affected with the tremulous agitation; but as the paralyzed state was recovered, the shaking returned.

This may be the first description of a cerebral insult that alleviated an extrapyramidal sign. Interestingly, 175 years later this phenomenon is still being described (2). Early attempts to treat tremor by open resection of motor and premotor cortex resulted in the substitution of disabling extrapyramidal symptoms with disabling hemiparesis (3,4). A major advance came about with the publications of Russell Meyers in 1942 and 1951, showing that surgical resection of the head of the caudate nucleus and pallidofugal fibers (5,6) could resolve tremor and rigidity without inducing paresis. This paved the way for the next 20 years of experimental basal ganglia lesion surgery as treatment for extrapyramidal syndromes. Surgical precision was improved and comorbidity reduced with the development of the stereotaxic technique (7). Subsequently, stereotaxic chemopallidectomy using procaine oil (8), alcohol (9), and pallidal electrocoagulation (10,11) were reported to effectively improve tremor and rigidity.

It is important to note that at this time results were not reported in an objective manner and lesion locations within the pallidum were not precisely documented. The target was the anterodorsal pallidum, a target now proposed to be part of the associative circuits involved in motor control (12). The benefit of a more ventral lesion had already been documented with lesions, which included the ansa lenticularis (13). This group also reported the benefit from more posterior lesions by showing that five patients, who had gained only temporary relief from tremor from anterodorsal pallidotomy, gained sustained antitremor benefits when their lesions were extended by 4–6 mm posteriorly (14).

In an attempt to study and improve outcomes, Svennilson et al. varied the position of their lesions in the first 32 cases from their cohort of 81 patients between 1953 and 1957 and showed sustained improvements in rigidity and tremor by 79 and 82%, respectively, when the lesion was in the posteromedial aspect of the pallidum (15). They also reported additional benefit to general motor function, as assessed by their patients' ability to return to work (25%) or become independent in activities of daily living (37%).

During this era, other surgical groups were varying lesion locations not just within the pallidum but within the basal ganglia. Some early evidence suggested the superiority of thalamotomy in resolving tremor and rigidity (9,16). These reports were later extended to specify ventrolateral and ventral intermediate thalamotomy (17,18). In 1967, the introduction of levodopa as effective antiakinetic and antitremor therapy for parkinsonism (19) led to a major worldwide reduction in the use of pallidotomy and thalamotomy to treat parkinsonism. In today's practice, lesion surgery has reemerged with a new role as a result of identification of new indications and new targets within the basal ganglia (20–22). We shall review some general principles that apply to all patients considered for lesion surgery of the pallidum, thalamus, and subthalamus before discussing the merits of lesions at each target site. This chapter will not consider gamma-knife lesions.

PATIENT SELECTION

Modern Indications for Surgery for Parkinson's Disease

The modern incentive to reevaluate surgical therapy for Parkinson's disease (PD) has been driven by the realization of the inadequacy of chronic dopaminergic replacement as a main strategy of treatment, namely that:

1. Levodopa treatment is associated with the development of motor fluctuations and dyskinesia (23,24) in about 50% of patients after 5 years of treatment (25). In early PD, these side effects are generally associated with peak plasma levels of drugs and so can usually be controlled by adjusting dose size and frequency. With disease progression, the "therapeutic window" narrows and dyskinesia may develop during any period of benefit or biphasically and cannot be controlled by dosing changes. At this stage, neither parkinsonism (akinesia and tremor) nor drug-related side effects (dyskinesia and fluctuations) can be managed optimally and surgery is warranted. In this scenario, the primary objective of surgery is to alleviate dyskinesia and fluctuations. The post-operative dose of dopaminergic medication will be determined by the patient's clinical needs. This may be less than that required before surgery. However, in some patients (depending on the procedure) it may be unchanged or even higher.

2. Some patients show effective initial response to dopaminergic medication, which becomes less effective with disease progression, such that in time the dose of levodopa or dopamine agonists required to provide symptomatic relief from akinesia or tremor is associated with the development of unacceptable peak dose effects, such as postural hypotension or behavioral disturbances and psychosis. Other unresponsive symptoms can include painful cramps and dystonia. In this scenario, the objective of surgery is to act as an adjunct to antiparkinsonian medication to allow the patients to obtain effective antiparkinsonian relief from the combination of surgery and lower doses of dopaminergic drugs that do not induce undesirable side effects.

Often patients present with a mixture of these two indications.

Entering a Patient for a Surgical Procedure

Prior to enrolling a patient into a surgical program, it is generally recommended that patients be assessed by a neurologist with experience in movement disorders since it is essential to document that the patient does indeed have **PD** and not a parkinson-plus syndrome, such as multiple system atrophy, progressive supranuclear palsy, or vascular parkinsonism. There have been a few case reports of the use of lesion surgery in the management of these parkinson-plus syndromes, and their success rates are generally disappointing (26,27). Additionally, it is necessary to show that a patient has a good response to dopaminergic drugs (see Fig. 1), since the antiparkinsonian benefit from levodopa correlates with the antiparkinsonian response to surgery (with the exception of tremor). A standard levodopa challenge test, as described in the Core Assessment Program for Intracerebral Transplantations (CAPIT) (28) or Core Assessment Program for Surgical Interventional Therapies in Parkinson's Disease (CAPSIT-PD) (29), is one prognostic indicator of a patient's short-term response to a successful surgical procedure (30). A history of unresponsiveness to levodopa may also be an indicator that the patient is suffering from a parkinson-plus syndrome.

Some patients or physicians seek referral for surgery before adequate trials of available medication have been carried out. At times this is due to inadequate experience in the management of PD, and at other times it is due to a misguided desire to avoid complications of dopaminergic medication. Patients should receive appropriate trials of available medication before considering invasive and potentially complicated surgery.

Many patients in late-stage disease may have cognitive or active psychiatric symptoms. These patients should be excluded from surgery. There are no absolute contraindications to lesion surgery over and above those of general surgery as determined by the patient's general medical state. However, patients with a significant dementia or cortical atrophy may have less benefit from surgery and may cognitively decompensate postoperatively (27,31). Centers should obtain formal neuropsychometric testing prior to surgery and utilize these results in considering surgical candidacy.

Speech, swallowing, and gait disturbances are common in advanced PD. Although these symptoms are less likely to improve following surgery and indeed may deteriorate postoperatively, especially following bilateral procedures (32–35), they should be recognized as relative, and not absolute, contraindications. For example, a patient who already has a percutaneous feeding gastrostomy, should not be denied a surgical therapy solely on the basis of the severity of the dysphagia, which may deteriorate postoperatively, since it is likely that the feeding tube will still remain in situ postoperatively.

Considering Lesion Surgery over Deep Brain Stimulation

Several open trials have demonstrated the efficacy of deep brain stimulation (DBS) of the basal ganglia nuclei in the treatment of parkinsonism and the

1) Does the patient have idiopathic Parkinson's disease?
2) What is the best antiparkinsonian response to levodopa?
3) Has the patient failed on established optimal medical therapy?
4) Does the patient's general medical condition permit neurosurgery?
5) What is the degree of dementia?
6) Are there any relative contraindications?

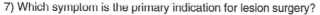

7) Which symptom is the primary indication for lesion surgery?
- Parkinsonism, responding to medical therapy but accompanied by side effects
- Parkinsonism, previously responding to medical therapy, but now inadequately so
- Dyskinesia that invariably accompanies the antiparkinsonian effect
- Tremor, unresponsive to medical therapy

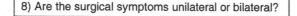

8) Are the surgical symptoms unilateral or bilateral?

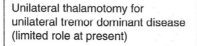

Unilateral thalamotomy for
unilateral tremor dominant disease
(limited role at present)

Unilateral pallidotomy for unilateral
dyskinetic dominant disease

Unilateral subthalamotomy
- role uncertain

Bilateral – consider deep brain
stimulation

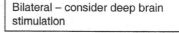

Bilateral thalamotomy – high risk of
dysarthria/cognitive deficits

Bilateral pallidotomy – uncertain,
possibly risk of dysarthria/abulia

Bilateral subthalamotomy – role
uncertain

FIGURE 1 Factors in deciding on lesion surgery for a patient with Parkinson's disease.

resolution of levodopa-induced dyskinesia (36–38). Only one included a double-blind evaluation of symptoms (39). Although there are no direct comparative trials of the safety of DBS and lesion surgery, it is generally accepted that DBS is effective, allows patients to lower the overall drug requirement, and may involve less permanent risk since the target is not electrocoagulated. This makes the consequences of a misplaced target reversible with DBS, but irreversible with lesion surgery. This is most important when considering bilateral procedures, since the risks of dysphasia, dysarthria, dysphagia, and cognitive deficits are increased in bilateral procedures (32–35). Although there are no blinded, evidence-based trial data to indicate which type of surgery to offer, the following guidelines can be considered:

1. If a patient requires a bilateral procedure from the outset, then bilateral DBS is usually preferred over bilateral lesion surgery. This is the case for most patients with advanced PD.
2. If a patient has already had a unilateral procedure (whether a lesion or DBS) and requires a second procedure in the other hemisphere, then DBS should be considered in preference to a lesion since any new side effects from the second procedure are more likely to be reversible.
3. If a patient is considered for a unilateral procedure from the outset, then lesion surgery and DBS should be considered according to the preference of the patient and the surgical center.

The longest reported results are 10 years for pallidotomy (40) and 13 years for thalamotomy (18). Despite the untested longer-term safety of either lesion surgery or DBS, there are some general advantages of lesions compared with DBS. First, when health resources of either an individual or a health care provider are limited, it is usual to adopt the more economical option. Lesion surgery avoids the cost of the hardware, the potential cost of repeatedly replacing the implantable pulse generators due to battery failure, and the manpower expenses for programming the stimulators. Second, for patients who live in areas that have no local expertise in maintenance of deep brain stimulators, the placement of a lesion may avoid frequent journeys to a neurosurgical center for stimulator programming. Programming is required periodically throughout the time the stimulators are in place. Third, it is possible that with time we shall discover more unique but disastrous complications of stimulators interacting with other electrical systems, such as diathermy for dental treatment (41). Finally, DBS electrodes can fracture, become infected, cause skin erosion, or the battery lifetime may become impractically short. In these instances, a lesion may be the only alternative for patients for whom DBS is no longer suitable for technical reasons. Oh et al. described two patients in whom therapy was changed from DBS to a lesion because one patient needed four battery replacements in 5 years while the other developed skin erosions over the electrode leads (42).

PRACTICAL ISSUES IN THE CHOICE OF A TARGET

The three main basal ganglia targets are the pallidum, thalamus, and subthalamic nucleus, and each has been lesioned unilaterally and bilaterally. In considering the results from different reports, it should be emphasized that the methods of clinical assessment, site of target, method of target localization, and method of target confirmation have varied widely among centers. These factors probably account for the differences in clinical outcome across centers. The most comprehensive assessment would have to include:

1. Pre- and postoperative blinded evaluation of objective rating scales, such as the Unified Parkinson's Disease Rating Scale (UPDRS) Hoehn and Yahr, timed motor tests (28,29), dyskinesia rating scales (43), and cognitive rating scales.
2. Identification of the anatomical target by computed tomography (CT), magnetic resonance imaging (MRI), or CT-MRI fusion.
3. Identification of the physiological target by microrecordings and macrostimulation.
4. Verification of lesion size and location postoperatively by volumetric MRI.
5. Long-term follow-up.

It is no wonder, therefore, that reports originating from different centers are rarely directly comparable. The method of target localization can be primarily based on anatomical landmarks, such as stereotaxic CT or MRI coordinates or combined CT-MRI fusion. Most groups will also use macrostimulation at the target site prior to lesioning to check for adverse effects, which most commonly manifest as contraction of the face, arm, or foot, sensory changes, ocular deviations, phosphenes, or speech arrest.

Some centers also rely on intraoperative microelectrode recordings from the target site. For thalamotomy, this is used to demonstrate oscillations synchronous with tremor ("tremor cells"), which aid the surgeon in finding the correct target and avoiding the ventral caudal (VC, sensory) nucleus. For pallidotomy and "subthalamotomy," tremor may not be the primary indication for surgery and these oscillations may not be detectable. In these instances, there are other advantages of using intraoperative microelectrode recordings. First, the identification of cells that change their firing rates in response to active or passive movements will confirm that the tip of the electrode is at the sensorimotor region of the target zone. This method of electrophysiological mapping increases the probability that the lesion is placed in the sensorimotor region of the pallidum or subthalamus and decreases the probability that the lesion is placed in the nonmotor region of the target, where there may be less clinical benefit and potentially greater adverse effects. Second, identification of the boundaries of the pallidum and subthalamus allows the lesion to be placed away from the optic tract and internal capsule, reducing the likelihood of undesirable effects. This is especially important for placement of very ventral pallidal lesions where CT alone, MRI alone, or CT-MRI fusion may not be sufficiently accurate to avoid the optic tract (44). Third, recording the response rates of neurons in these nuclei has aided our understanding of PD (45–47) by providing direct human evidence that the overactivity of internal pallidal and subthalamic neurons contributes to the pathophysiology of parkinsonism.

UNILATERAL PALLIDOTOMY

Posteroventrolateral, Posteroventromedial, or Pallidoansotomy?

The era of modern pallidotomy started when Laitinen reexplored Leksell's pallidotomy for patients who were refractory to medical therapy (48). In this first study of 38 patients, he confirmed that the optimal target should be in the posteroventral, rather than anterodorsal, pallidum. He showed that there was complete or almost complete relief of rigidity and hypokinesia (92% of patients), tremor (81% of patients), and an improvement in levodopa-induced dyskinesia. These lesions were placed 16–24 mm lateral to the midline but were associated with a 14% risk of damage to the optic tract, which could be located as far as 21 mm lateral to the midline. In his subsequent series, the laterality was increased to 24–27 mm from the midline in the posteroventrolateral pallidum, with particular attention paid to "minimizing damage to the medial pallidum" (27). It is hypothesized that the beneficial effect is the result of interruption of the direct striatopallidal and indirect pallidosubthalamic afferents to the internal pallidum. In this manner it is argued that pallidotomy "releases the medial pallidum" from abnormal regulation by the external pallidum and subthalamus. These series should be considered distinct from other contemporary series, in which the objective of pallidotomy is to ablate and reduce the overactivity of the medial pallidum.

Many groups have generally reproduced the clinical findings in open studies in which the anatomical target was located within the posteroventral pallidum by anatomical guidance (49–52). Other groups have extended the understanding of the pathophysiology of parkinsonism by using microelectrode recordings to map the sensorimotor region of the internal pallidum during functional neurosurgery and have argued that optimal clinical response is best achieved by placing the lesion at the neurophysiological target (45,46,53–57). The caudal internal pallidum has been shown to contain cells that directly respond to active and passive manipulation of limb movements (45,58) and is thought to represent the sensorimotor region of the internal pallidum. The location of the human sensorimotor region of the internal pallidum is in general agreement with that from the parkinsonian primate (59). It is somatotopically arranged (60), although the boundaries between one area and the next are less distinct than in the cortex. However, there is some controversy whether clear somatotopy can be demonstrated in parkinsonian humans at the time of pallidal microrecording. Successful lesions should theoretically encompass the sensorimotor region of the internal pallidum. Bakay et al. reported that they have increased the mediolateral extent of their pallidotomy to maximize benefit (61). As mentioned below, some authors have argued that the ideal lesion should be made in the extreme ventral pallidum attempting to include the ansa lenticularis (62) (i.e., pallidoansotomy). However, in the nonhuman primate it has been shown that most of the sensorimotor output of the internal pallidum to the thalamus comes directly across the internal capsule via the lenticular fasciculus (63), and so purposefully lesioning the ansa may be both ineffective and unnecessarily risky since it is very close to the optic tract.

Trial Results

The results of only one randomized, single-blind trial of pallidotomy have been published (64). In this study, 37 patients, who were matched for age and severity of PD, were randomized to receive either unilateral pallidotomy within one month ($n = 19$) or maximal medical therapy for 6 months ($n = 18$). While the nonoperated group showed an 8% deterioration of median UPDRS motor scores and no change in dyskinesias, the operated group showed 31% and 50% improvements in parkinsonism and dyskinesia scores, respectively.

There have been two nonblinded studies of patients treated by pallidotomy compared with a medically treated group (53,65), with each study demonstrating the benefits of pallidotomy. The numerous other open-label nonrandomized trials (30,46,48,49,51,52,66–77) have generally drawn the same conclusion (Table 1, Fig. 2), indicating that the most dramatic response is the reduction in contralateral dyskinesia by 80–95%, which is sustained for up to 5.5 years (77). The off UPDRS score improves by 24–

TABLE 1 Summary of Large Pallidotomy Series in Order of Study Size[a]

Author	n	Surgical method	Main clinical assessment	Follow-up interval	Akinesia (Δ%)	Tremor (Δ%)	Gait (Δ%)	Dyskinesias (Δ%)	Overall mortality (%)	Overall morbidity (%)
Laitinen, 1995 (73)	259[b]	CT/MRI + MES	"Fair, good, poor"	<48 hours	82% "good"		Not given	Not given	0	7
Kondziolka et al., 1999 (51)	58	MRI + MES	UPDRS	6–24 months	24	50	0	40	0	7
Iacono et al., 1994 (49)	55	MRI + ventriculography + MES	"Minor, good or excellent"	1–24 months	"Excellent"	"Good"	"Excellent"	"Excellent"	0	7
Jankovic et al., 1999 (71)	41	MRI + μER + MES	MT	3 months	24	Not given	Not given	Not given	Not given	Not given
Lang et al., 1999 (74)	40	MRI + μER + MES	UPDRS + Goetz	3–24 months	43	54	42 transient	83	0	38
Alterman and Kelly, 1998 (66)	34	MRI + μER + MES	UPDRS + timed motor tests	6 months	50%	Not given	Not given	"Effectively relieved"	0	10
Masterman et al., 1998 (75)	32	MRI + μER + MES	UPDRS	3–6 months	23 B	43 B	30	61 B	0	16
Hirai et al., 1999 (70)	28	MRI + μER + MES	"Fair, good or excellent"	6 months		Improved B	Dramatic in 8	Improved B	0	0
de Bie et al., 1999 (68)	26	Ventriculography	UPDRS + Goetz	5 months	33	83	38	50	0	50
Shannon et al., 1998 (76)	26	MRI + μER + MES	UPDRS	6 months	26 A + T + R		0	73	4	30
Samuel et al., 1998 (30)	26	CT + μER + MES	UPDRS	3 months	24[c]	33[c]	7	67	8	58
Johansson et al., 1997 (72)	22	CT/MRI + MES	UPDRS v/VAS PLM	12 months	0	0	0	33	0	19[d]
Samii et al., 1999 (52)	20	CT + MES	UPDRS + GOETZ + PPT	24 months	0	90	0	83	5[e]	5[f]
Dalvi et al., 1999 (67)	20	CT-MRI fusion + μER + MES	UPDRS	3–12 months	22 + R	62	0	71	0	45
Fine et al., 2000 (77)	20	MRI + μER + MES	UPDRS + Goetz	66 months	18%	65%	43%	71%	Not given	Not given
Baron et al., 1996 (46)	15	CT/MRI + μER + MES	UPDRS	12 months	≥50[g]	100 in 7/8 cases	Not given	100 in 9/10 cases	0	20
Fazzini et al., 1997 (69)	11	CT/MRI + μER + MES	UPDRS	12–48 months	43	Not given	Not given	"Did not return"	Not given	Not given
Laitinen et al., 1992 (48)	38	CT + MES	Writing, drawing, walking in a circle	2–71 months	≥40[g] in 35/36	Excellent in 26/32	≥23[*]	"Greatly improved"	0	22

[a] For comparison, the original series of Laitinen is the final entry. n = number of patients; MES = macroelectrode stimulation at target site; μER = microelectrode recording at target site; MT = finger movement time between two adjacent targets; Goetz = the Goetz dyskinesia rating scale; Δ% = % change; A + T + R = combined score for akinesia, tremor and rigidity; + R = combined score with rigidity reported; PPT = Purdue Pegboard test; v/VAS = video and visual assessment scale; PLM = electronic recording of posturolocomotion manual test; B = assumed bilateral as no distinction made between contralateral and ipsilateral assessment.

[b] Some patients had Parkinson-plus syndromes and others had combined pallidotomy and thalamotomy.

[*] Marginally significant result.

[c] 1 patient developed anarthria and 2 patients require reoperation as they had no benefit from the first pallidotomy.

[d] 1 death two weeks post-operatively secondary to ipsilateral intracerebral haemorrhage.

[e] 1 patient required re-operation as had no benefit from the first.

[f] Figure calculated from a graph in manuscript.

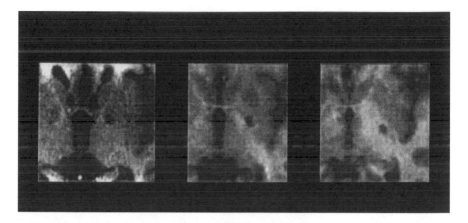

FIGURE 2 MRI scan of unilateral posteroventromedial pallidotomy. (Courtesy of Dr. A. M. Lozano, Toronto Western Hospital, Ontario, Canada.)

37% and declines thereafter to about 18%, although this continues to remain significantly improved at 5.5 years from baseline (57,77). Individual items of contralateral tremor, rigidity, and akinesia generally mirror this response, although the magnitude of the antitremor effect (up to 65%) appears greater and more sustained than that of rigidity (43%) or akinesia (46% at 6 months to 17% at 5.5 years). Despite these sustained differences in UPDRS subset scores, an initial improvement in activity of daily living of 37% is not sustained (77), but results from patient self-assessments imply that patients continue to benefit generally (57). In contrast to contralateral off scores, ipsilateral off scores and both contralateral and ipsilateral on scores are not significantly sustained, although an initial improvement of up to 27% may occur. Ipsilateral on dyskinesia scores appear to be improved initially by 30%. This effect is also decreased with time and is not significant 12 months postsurgery (57).

Despite the reported differences in lesion location, the 10-year effects of Leksell's original series of posteroventrolateral pallidotomy (using anatomical targeting methods and intending to lesion lateral pallidum while causing minimal damage to internal pallidum) are remarkably similar to the long-term responses of posteroventromedial pallidotomy (using anatomical and electrophysiological targeting methods and intending to avoid lateral pallidum while causing maximum damage to the sensorimotor region of internal pallidum).

The responses of axial symptoms and gait are variable. Complex analysis of posturography has shown that an improvement in gait and posture may be maintained for up to 12 months (78). Three-dimensional motion capture analysis of walking suggests that the effect is mainly due to an improvement in speed of walking (79). More traditional UPDRS gait/ postural instability subset scores, however, show only an initial modest improvement (26–37%), which is lost within subsequent years (57,77). It is possible that the effect of pallidotomy on gait may be mediated in part via descending influences on the brainstem, as well as ascending influences on thalamo-cortical circuits (78). Longer follow-up of complex gait analyses is required before reliable conclusions can be drawn.

Complication rates are generally quoted as approximately 5% with transient facial and limb paresis the most common. Hemianopsia or quadrantanopsia are potential complications of lesioning the nearby optic tract. There is a well-documented consistent feature of a mild but asymptomatic decrease in verbal fluency (34), mostly following left-sided unilateral pallidotomy (80). Postoperative weight gain has been described (81). This "side effect" was found in 23% of patients in one study (82). It was highly correlated with the improvement in off motor UPDRS scores but not with changes in energy intake or dyskinesia scores. This suggests that the effect is not purely related to less dyskinesia postoperatively. Some series have reported a higher overall incidence of major complications. In the controlled trial of de Bie et al. (64), 9 of the 19 (47%) operated patients had surgical morbidity (2 major, 4 minor persistent, and 3 minor transient). Lesion locations were not presented, but this level of high morbidity has also been documented by other independent groups (30,76). It is likely that the variability of lesion locations and surgical techniques account for these differences, and this remains one area in need of refinement and agreement across international centers.

Variability of Trial Results

A systematic attempt to correlate outcome with lesion location has been made. Gross et al. studied the variability in lesion location within the ventral pallidum in 33 patients with PD (83,84). Lesions were not distributed randomly within internal pallidum but were distributed along a line running anteromedially-posterolaterally, parallel to the lateral border of the posterior limb of the internal capsule. In this cohort, anteromedial lesions were associated with a greater improvement in dyskinesias while central lesions led to a greater improvement in akinesia scores and gait disturbance (84). This result may partly explain the variable results in resolution of dyskinesia/akinesia among different neurosurgical centers and clearly demonstrates the precision required to perform pallidotomy. This notion is also supported by studies of internal pallidal DBS. Since the clinical effects of electrode activation are similar to pallidotomy, it is commonly believed that DBS acts by locally inhibiting target nuclei. Studies (85,86) have shown that ventral stimulation leads to resolution of dyskinesias and rigidity with concurrent worsening of akinesia, while stimulation of the most dorsal contacts leads to opposite clinical effects.

Furthermore, both human and primate studies have shown that the discharge rate of the parkinsonian internal pallidal neurons is sustained at a high rate (80 Hz) (45,87). The internal pallidal output via the ansa lenticularis and lenticular fasciculus terminates in the ventral anterior and lateral thalamic nuclei (88) and uses the inhibitory neurotransmitter γ-aminobutyric acid. On the basis of these observations, it is hypothesized that medial pallidotomy would be most effective if the lesion were large enough to include the sensorimotor arm and leg areas and include the neurons that give rise to the ansa lenticularis and lenticular fasciculus (Fig. 3). Such a lesion would interrupt the overactive inhibitory "noisy" outflow of clinically relevant sensorimotor regions of the internal pallidum, thereby disinhibiting the motor thalamus (12). Direct evidence for this is still lacking, but in a retrospective analysis it was documented that lesions were more effective when located within the internal pallidum, and the efficacy was reduced when the lesion encroached on the external pallidum (61). Although now it is generally accepted that the lesion should be in the posterior and ventral pallidum, whether lateral pallidum should be included in the lesion is still controversial. This is likely to remain so until a large data set of clinicopathological cases is gathered worldwide.

There has been recent quantitative evidence supporting the rationale for use of microelectrode recording in guiding lesion placement in pallidotomy. Guridi et al. compared the theoretical target location (obtained from MRI alone) with actual target location (obtained from microelectrode mapping of GPi) in 50 patients who underwent microelectrode-guided internal pallidotomy (56). They showed a maximum discrepancy of 2.3 ± 1.6 mm mediolaterally and 3.0 ± 1.9 mm anteroposteriorly between the anatomical and electrophysiological targets. In only 45% of the patients did the electrophysiological and anatomical targets overlap. Similar posterior and lateral misregistration of the actual target from the electrophysiological target has been described by Tsao et al. (89). These findings imply that surgery based solely on anatomical landmarks may miss the physiological target, even when the lesion is in the correct nucleus.

There remain concerns that the increased number of needle tracts necessary for intraoperative microelectrode recordings increase the overall length of the procedure without clear added benefit and also may increase the overall risk of surgical morbidity from hemorrhage or by increasing the overall lesion volume (the summation of multiple microlesions). To date

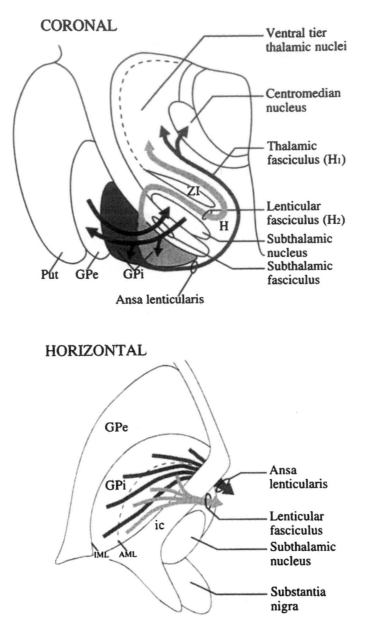

FIGURE 3 Drawing of the coronal and horizontal sections through the human basal ganglia showing the output pathways from the pallidum. Put = putamen, GPe = external pallidum, GPi = internal pallidum, H, H1, H2 = fields of Forel, IC = internal capsule, ZI = zona incerta. (From Ref. 125.)

there are no clinical trials demonstrating an additional benefit from the use of intraoperative microelectrode recordings, although there are reports of patients who have undergone a second procedure with intraoperative microelectrode recordings and achieved a better result than from the first procedure, in which a lesion was placed outside the sensorimotor region of the internal pallidum (90). Conversely, there are no studies demonstrating additional morbidity from intraoperative recordings, and so the choice of method of target identification is still largely determined by individual preferences, available equipment, and local expertise.

Another group has specifically targeted only the most ventral region of the posterior pallidum and attempted to produce pallidotomy and ansotomy (62). They have performed 31 pallidotomy/ansotomy operations just 0.5 mm above the optic tract with the entire lesion being situated below the commissural plane. In this series, they described a 63% reduction in "off" parkinsonism and the cessation of contralateral dyskinesia in 21 of 23 patients who had disabling dyskinesias preoperatively. These reports, however, require further validation before general acceptance. It is clear from these variable lesion locations that the optimal target for unilateral pallidotomy remains a matter of controversy and that neither the ventroposterolateral pallidotomy of Laitinen (73), nor pallidoansotomy of Iacono (62), nor the more extensive internal pallidotomy (46,69,74) can fully explain the clinical findings of alleviation in parkinsonism and levodopa-induced dyskinesia concurrently.

BILATERAL PALLIDOTOMY

Laitinen (73) and Iacono et al. (62) reported early good outcomes in 12 and 10 bilaterally operated patients, respectively. There are, however, concerns regarding permanent cognitive and bulbar side effects of bilateral pallidotomy, which have been confirmed in a study of 4 patients in whom contemparous bilateral pallidotomy was performed (91). Despite a 40% improvement in motor UPDRS scores and resolution of dyskinesias, one patient developed dysarthria, dysphagia, and eyelid opening apraxia, another developed abulia, and a third developed mental automatisms. Scott et al. described hypophonia, increased salivation, and reduced verbal fluency following bilateral simultaneous pallidotomy (34). An open-label trial of bilateral simultaneous pallidotomy compared with unilateral pallidotomy plus DBS had to be halted early as all three patients with bilateral lesions developed deterioration in speech, swallowing, salivation, depression, apathy, freezing, and falling (92). In another recent series, staged bilateral pallidotomy was associated with a deficit in speech in four patients, one patient had a decline in memory, and there were three cases of infarction

(93). Further, a reduced response to levodopa has been documented in a small number of patients undergoing bilateral staged pallidotomy (93).

These results are in contrast to the milder side effects reported in one series of 14 patients who underwent staged bilateral pallidotomy, in whom no overall effect on speech and cognitive function was detected 6 months postoperatively, but in whom five had mild hypophonia, two had transient confusion, two had deterioration of gait, and one had deterioration of a preexisting dysarthria postoperatively (94). A series of 53 bilaterally operated patients was presented with a follow-up of 17 patients for 12 months (95). Major deterioration in speech (defined as a 2 point decline on the UPDRS subset score) occurred in 8% of bilaterally operated patients compared with 4% of unilaterally operated patients, although the study was not specifically designed to compare the two procedures. Similarly, postoperative major deterioration in salivation occurred in 13% and 10% of bilaterally and unilaterally operated patients, respectively. Gait freezing while on and handwriting each deteriorated with a frequency of 11% in the bilaterally operated group, and medically unresponsive eyelid opening apraxia occurred in 6%. Dysphagia was not reported. The authors suggest that these relatively low rates of complications may be attributable to the placement of a smaller lesion ($100\,mm^3$) in the medial pallidum contributing to the lesser affected hemibody, compared with the medial pallidum contributing to the worse affected hemibody ($150\,mm^3$). Complications were only defined according to their occurrence on the UPDRS rather than by using specific questions designed to assess their presence and severity. Additionally, precise lesion locations and cognitive results were omitted. The question of safety and timing of bilateral pallidotomy remains controversial, and this procedure has not been undertaken by many groups. It is likely to continue to fall out of favor, especially where bilateral DBS is available as an alternative.

UNILATERAL THALAMOTOMY

Vim Thalamotomy

Thalamotomy has been performed since the 1950s, when some surgeons noted the excellent relief of tremor compared to anterodorsal pallidotomy. Hassler et al. reported the successful treatment of a patient by making a lesion in the ventrolateral (VL) region of the thalamus (96), and Cooper too advocated that this was the optimal target (16). The ventrolateral region of the thalamus contains at least three important nuclei; from anterior to posterior, these are the Voa (ventral oralis anterior), Vop (ventral oralis posterior), and Vim (ventral intermediate). Hassler subsequently refined the target to the Vop (by his nomenclature) for tremor and Voa for rigidity (97). It is now generally agreed that the optimal target for tremor control is the Vim nucleus, which receives its input primarily from the cerebellum. Although most surgeons now target Vim, in the past subthalamic sites were also targeted including the zona incerta and fields of Forel. These "subthalamotomies" were distinct from the subthalamic nucleus lesions (subthalamic nucleotomy) discussed in the next section.

The method of target selection is similar in principle to that of pallidotomy, namely that anatomical coordinates are derived from CT or MRI, and electrophysiological recording or stimulation can be used to further identify "tremor cells" and avoid the sensory nucleus (VC) and internal capsule. Lesion sizes tend to be smaller (about $60\,mm^3$) (98) compared with pallidotomy (about $220\,mm^3$) (27).

There have been four long-term open-label reports of thalamotomy in PD. Kelly and Gillingham reported the 10-year follow-up of 60 parkinsonian patients who had thalamotomy between 1965 and 1967 and showed sustained improvement in tremor and rigidity, but continued progression of bradykinesia (99). Later, 12 patients were reported who also had a marked improvement or cessation in contralateral tremor without complications (17). A larger series of 103 operated patients between 1964 and 1969, also followed-up for 10 years, showed that, overall, 87 patients had "good" effect, and in only 7 patients were tremor or rigidity not alleviated completely (33). Only a proportion of these patients had CT confirmation of lesion location. In a more recent series from 1984 to 1989, all 36 patients underwent CT and microelectrode-guided VL thalamotomy and 86% showed complete cessation of tremor, with the remainder showing a significant improvement up to 68 months (100). The antitremor effect was shown to be maintained in one blinded retrospective study following thalamotomy alone, subthalamotomy alone, or combined thalamotomy and subthalamotomy (101). These studies used the terminology "ventrolateral" thalamotomy.

More recently, the records of 42 patients with PD who underwent thalamotomy were reviewed, and 86% had cessation of or moderate-to-marked improvement in their contralateral tremor, with a concomitant improvement in function which persisted for as long as 13 years. The mean daily dose of levodopa was reduced by 156 mg and lesion location was in the Vim (102). Postoperatively, rigidity improved by 30%, ipsilateral tremor worsened, and there was no significant change in other features of parkinsonism.

The complication rates of unilateral thalamotomy range from 10% transient confusion and 8% facial weakness or numbness (33), to 58% transient and 23% persistent complications of contralateral weakness, dysarthria, and blepharospasm (18). Twenty-two of the 36 (61%) in the series of Fox et al. experienced complications. Half of these cleared by 7 days and only 6% were permanent or bothersome, including dysarthria, dyspraxia, or cognitive dysfunction (100). Deficits of verbal memory are more common after left thalamotomy compared with right thalamotomy (103).

One study compared the short-term safety and efficacy of Vim thalamotomy with Vim stimulation (104). Cessation or improved tremor resolution was detected in 79% of the lesioned group compared with 90% in the stimulated group. These results were not statistically different, but only 18% of the lesioned group had an improved functional status compared with 55% of the stimulated group. Additionally, the complication rate for the stimulated group was 16% compared with 47% in the lesioned group, but there was one death in the stimulated group. These positive and negative effects of thalamotomy and thalamic DBS are very similar to a retrospective report comparing the two treatments (105), in which it was additionally shown that tremor recurrence occurred in 15% of patients with thalamotomy, but only in 5% of patients with DBS. Consequently, 15% of patients with thalamotomy required reoperation. These studies show the expected improved morbidity of DBS compared with irreversible lesioning. However, long-term follow-up (up to 40 months) has highlighted the potential hardware complications of DBS, which include lead fracture, erosion or migration, infection, cerebral spinal fluid (CSF) leak, short or open circuits, or other system malfunctions (106). In one study the mean time to the first complication was 10 months (107). From these studies it is estimated that 25–40% of patients with deep brain stimulators may require further surgery to maintain good clinical outcome (106–108). Further long-term comparative studies are necessary to define whether the potential short-term reduction of side effects of DBS outweighs the higher long-term need for re-operation as a result of hardware failure.

The Vim nucleus is proposed to be the cerebellar recipient nucleus of the thalamus, and so the effect on tremor may have a different physiological basis from the improvement of bradykinesia and dyskinesia that accompany internal pallidotomy. It is proposed that internal pallidotomy affects the thalamic nuclei that receive inputs from the basal ganglia (Voa and Vop). One factor that therefore continues to confound our understanding of thalamotomy is the variability of lesion locations across series. This is more problematic than with pallidotomy since the boundaries of the thalamic nuclei are not as well demarcated anatomically as in the pallidal complex and the nomenclature of the thalamic nuclei varies across series and also from human to primate (Figs. 4, 5).

The above studies support a role for Vim thalamotomy in patients whose predominant symptom is medically intractable asymmetrical tremor

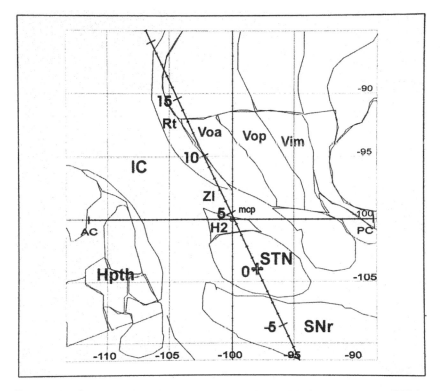

FIGURE 4 Stereotactic trajectory targeting the subthalamic nucleus (STN) and showing the relative positions of the thalamic nuclei Voa, Vop and Vim, the Zona incerta (ZI), the substantia nigra (SNr) and the commissural plane. AC = anterior commissure, PC = posterior commissure, mcp = mid commissural point, Hpth = hypothalamus, IC = internal capsule. (From Ref. 125.)

and who are not suitable for DBS. The majority of patients with PD are, however, likely to have progressive bradykinesia, even if this is not present at the time of presentation for surgery. This symptom is not modified by Vim thalamotomy, and so thalamotomy (and Vim DBS) in the treatment of PD has largely been replaced by alternative therapies.

Thalamic Targets Other Than Vim

It would not be predicted from the known anatomical circuits that Vim thalamotomy would improve dyskinesia, and yet there are reports of this. Five patients in the series of Jankovic et al. had considerable improvement in levodopa-induced dyskinesia following Vim thalamotomy (18). The location of these antidyskinetic lesions may not have been confined to Vim

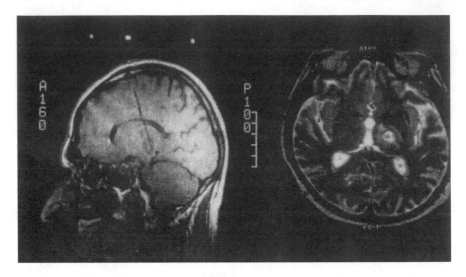

FIGURE 5 MRI scan of unilateral Vim thalamotomy. (Courtesy of Dr. A. M. Lozano, Toronto Western Hospital, Ontario, Canada.)

and may have included more anterior regions in ventrolateral thalamus. One patient in the series of Fox et al. had improved levodopa-induced dyskinesia following ventrolateral thalamotomy (100). The antidyskinetic findings have also been replicated in experimental monkeys in which thalamotomy was stereotaxically tailored to the thalamic nuclei that receive afferents from the internal pallidum (109) and shown to abolish contralateral chorea but not dystonia. Interestingly, Vim thalamotomy did not affect these dyskinesias and thalamotomy encroaching on the centromedian nuclei reduced, but did not abolish, chorea.

These findings have been reproduced in humans (110). In an older series, Vim thalamotomy was performed via one needle tract, and another lesion was deliberately placed more anteriorly via another needle tract in the Voa/Vop complex specifically to relieve rigidity. Patients in whom the Voa/Vop region was also targeted had almost complete resolution of contralateral dyskinesia as well as tremor, and those whose lesions were restricted to Vim did not experience a reduction in dyskinesia (111). Recently there has been a retrospective correlation of the location of the tip of thalamic deep brain stimulators (stereotaxically aimed at the Vim) with clinical outcome. It was shown that electrode tips placed more medially and ventrally were more likely to be associated with the resolution of levodopa-induced dyskinesia (112). It was concluded that these electrode tips lay within the centromedian (CM) and parafascicular (PF) thalamic nucleus and not in the Vim. Interestingly, however, they were equally effective in the resolution of tremor. It has been suggested that CM/PF thalamic stimulation may lead to reduction of dyskinesia by reducing internal pallidal input to these nuclei, in contrast to Vim stimulation, which interrupts the cerebellar-thalamic circuits. These findings are, however, at odds with a single case report of a CM/PF thalamotomy, which was inadvertently placed during an attempt to treat a tremulous patient with PD with DBS of the Vim (113). Postoperatively, this patient had suboptimal contralateral tremor control and a progressive worsening of contralateral parkinsonism. The patient died from an unrelated illness 12 years later, with exhausting dyskinesia present. Postmortem examination showed that one of the electrode tracts was associated with a cavity within the CM/PF nucleus, which was marginally larger than the volume of the electrode tip, but the entire surrounding CM/PF nucleus showed marked astrocytosis and neuronal loss. There has not been a direct comparison of the positive and negative effects of lesions of different thalamic nuclei, nor of ventrolateral thalamotomy with internal pallidotomy. Further clinical trials with precise imaging of Vim, Voa, Vop, VL, CM, and PF thalamotomy would, therefore, be required before clinical-pathological correlations can be made reliably.

BILATERAL THALAMOTOMY

The clinical efficacy of bilateral thalamotomy in terms of resolution of bilateral tremor is as effective as unilateral thalamotomy for unilateral tremor (102). However, a high incidence of speech disturbance has been noted in several series: 18% (33), 44%, (32), and 60% (114). The high rate of speech and cognitive deficits following bilateral thalamic lesions has persuaded most surgeons to offer patients an alternative to bilateral thalamotomy if bilateral surgical treatment is required.

UNILATERAL SUBTHALAMIC NUCLEOTOMY

The realization that the neurons of the subthalamic nucleus (STN) in parkinsonian monkeys are overactive led to interest in this nucleus as a possible target for therapy for PD (115). It is postulated that overactivity of the STN leads to excessive excitatory drive to the medial pallidum. The occurrence of cognitive deficits reported with thalamotomy and pallidotomy has driven the interest in trying to find alternative targets to lesion, especially for patients who require bilateral procedures and who are not suitable for DBS. The most recent development in lesion surgery is the reevaluation of "subthalamotomy." Surgeons previously avoided the STN given the longstanding awareness that lesions of the normal STN in normal primates can have a deleterious effect by causing hemiballism (116), and this is a well-known consequence of infarcts and hemorrhages in this region in humans. In contrast, it has been shown that excitotoxic (117) or thermocoagulation (118) lesions of the pathological STN in MPTP-treated primates can alleviate parkinsonism. It should be realized that these thermocoagulation lesions involved the internal capsule, ansa lenticularis, and globus pallidus (118,119), and so the clinical benefit in these cases may not have been solely due to deactivation of the STN.

Early studies of deactivation of the subthalamic area by lesioning cannot be used to provide good quality evidence by today's standards because the lesions in this eloquent region of the brain were not anatomically well defined (120). Indeed, as mentioned above, "subthalamic" lesions usually purposefully avoided the STN proper in an attempt to prevent hemiballism. When the STN became a logical target in the surgical treatment of PD, concern over the possibility of introducing chorea led neurosurgeons to apply DBS rather than electrocoagulation to this site, since the former can be successful and yet is more reversible (39,121). However, the relatively high technological demands and costs of DBS have recently encouraged some groups to attempt subthalamic nucleotomy in patients with PD. Data on the safety and efficacy of this approach are very limited.

There have been only three open-label, nonrandomized reports of the use of unilateral subthalamic nucleotomy in PD. The target in one study was the sensorimotor region of the dorsal STN, defined by semimicrorecordings and stimulation (20). These authors showed a sustained reduction in off motor UPDRS by 50% in 10 of 11 patients, and this effect was maintained in 4 of 11 patients for 2 years. UPDRS on scores and ADL scores also improved "drastically." Ipsilateral bradykinesia improved by 20%, but this effect was not sustained at 12 months. Axial scores for gait and postural instability showed marked and sustained improvements. Dyskinesias were seen in the contralateral limbs of 5 patients during lesioning and lasted up to 12 hours before abating spontaneously. One patient developed transient delayed chorea. Another patient developed a post-operative infarction affecting the area of the lesioned STN, zona incerta, and ventral thalamus. This resulted in severe contralateral dyskinesia that persisted despite cessation of all levodopa and eventually required treatment with a pallidotomy on the same side as the "subthalamotomy." It is interesting to note that, apart from this patient, the dose of medication was maintained for 12 months, unlike cases of bilateral subthalamic DBS in which medication doses can be reduced significantly.

In the second series, the target was the central area of the subthalamus in nine patients and lesioning was guided by macrostimulation (21). Efficacy results were not reported, but only one patient developed chorea post-operatively, which initially required medical treatment but then subsided spontaneously to only mild movements. Four subjects had their medication doses reduced. In the series of Gill and Heywood, five patients had unilateral and five had bilateral small subthalamotomies with improved parkinsonism, and only one case had mild dyskinesia (122). These early studies showed that the risk of significant chorea after unilateral "subthalamotomy" is about 10% and that medication doses may not be significantly reduced, possibly because the ipsilateral side is minimally affected by the lesion.

The precise location of lesions in the subthalamic area needs further confirmation of exactly where the optimal target should be placed. It could be hypothesized, for example, that discrete small lesions confined to the nucleus (i.e., subthalamic nucleotomy) may be more likely to lead to chorea, whereas lesions that include the subthalamic nucleus but also extend dorsally (i.e., subthalamic nucleotomy with additional interruption of the ansa lenticularis, zona incerta, lenticular fasciculus) may be less likely to induce chorea since any potential to induce chorea may be counteracted by the concurrent interruption of these efferent fibers from the internal pallidum. However, the experience of Alvarez et al. (20), in which the one patient with the large infarct involving the more extensive area had the most severe persistent hemiballism, suggests that this prediction may not be correct. Therefore, the exact location and role of unilateral lesions of the subthalamic region remains unclear in clinical practice.

BILATERAL "SUBTHALAMOTOMY"

The effects of bilateral subthalamic nucleotomy were reported earlier than unilateral "subthalamotomy." There has only been one report of two patients dedicated to this subject, showing that small lesions in the dorsolateral STN could reduce the off motor UPDRS scores by over 68% without inducing dyskinesia (123). Both patients were reported to have no complications and to have medication withdrawn. This group later reported in abstract that bilateral "subthalamotomy" had been accomplished safely in five subjects (122). There is one other report of a stereotaxic "subthalamotomy" performed for dystonia, which was associated with bilateral apraxia of eyelid opening (124). It is premature to comment on the place of such surgery in clinical practice.

CONCLUSION

The single most consistent result of unilateral pallidotomy is the resolution of contralateral dyskinesia, and this therapy is best reserved for those few patients who exhibit asymmetrical disabling dyskinesia when on medication and whose level of parkinsonism is unacceptable when the medication is reduced. In general, the thalamic target has been largely abandoned in the surgical management of PD. Unilateral thalamotomy could be considered for those few patients who exhibit asymmetrical longstanding tremor that is unresponsive to maximum tolerated doses of medication and who have few or nonprogressive signs of parkinsonism, or for patients who have required multiple battery changes following unilateral stimulation of the ventralintermediate nucleus. These groups comprise only a small minority of patients with advanced PD in whom the signs are typically bilateral and progressive. In this situation, the optimal therapy at the moment is bilateral DBS of the STN or internal pallidum, although the STN is generally favored. Bilateral pallidotomy and thalamotomy are rarely performed due to concerns about postoperative speech and cognitive decline. The role of unilateral and bilateral lesions of the subthalamic region remains to be established. Few data are available on long-term follow-up. Lesion site, size, the inclusion of external pallidum, ansa lenticularis, Voa/Vop, STN, peri-STN structures, the need for microelectrode recordings, and the safety and efficacy of bilateral lesions all remain important and controversial issues in lesion surgeries.

ACKNOWLEDGMENT

Michael Samuel is supported by the Peel Medical Research Trust, London, England.

REFERENCES

1. Parkinson J. An Essay on the Shaking Palsy. London: Whittingham and Roland, 1817.
2. Sellal F, Hirsch E, Lisovoski F, Mutschler V, Collard M, Marescaux C. Contralateral disappearance of parkinsonian signs after subthalamic hematoma. Neurology 42:255–256, 1992.
3. Bucy JC, Case TJ. Tremor: physiological mechanisms and abolition by surgical means. Arch Neurol Psychiatry 41:721, 1939.
4. Bucy JC, Case TJ. Cortical extirpation in the treatment of involuntary movements. Arch Neurol Psychiatry 21:551, 1942.
5. Meyers R. The modification of alternating tremors, rigidity and festination by surgery of the basal ganglia. Res Publ Nerv Ment Dis Proc 20:602–665, 1942.

6. Meyers R. Surgical experiments in the therapy of certain "extrapyramidal" disease: A current evaluation. Acta Psychiat Neurol Suppl 67:3–42, 1951.
7. Spiegel EA, Wycis HT, Marks M, Lee AST. Stereotaxic apparatus for operations on the human brain. Science 106:349–350, 1947.
8. Narabayashi H, Okuma T. Procaine-oil blocking of the globus pallidus for the treatment of rigidity and tremor of parkinsonism. Proc Jpn Acad 29:134–137, 1953.
9. Cooper IS, Bravo G. Chemopallidectomy and chemothalamectomy. J Neurosurg 15:244–250, 1958.
10. Guiot G, Brion S. Traitement des mouvements anormaux par la coagulation pallidale. Technique et résultats. Rev Neurol 89:578–580, 1953.
11. Guiot G. Le traitement des syndromes parkinsoniens par la destruction du pallidum interne. Neurochirurgia 1:94–98, 1958.
12. Alexander GE, Crutcher MD, DeLong MR. Basal ganglia-thalamocortical circuits: parallel substrates for motor, oculomotor, "prefrontal" and "limbic" functions. Prog Brain Res 85:119–146, 1990.
13. Spiegel EA, Wycis HT. Ansotomy in paralysis agitans. Arch Neurol 71:598–614, 1954.
14. Spiegel E, Wycis H, Baird H. Long-range effects of electropallidoansotomy in extrapyramidal and convulsive disorders. Neurology:734–740, 1958.
15. Svennilson E, Torvik A, Lowe R, Leksell L. Treatment of parkinsonism by stereotactic thermolesions in the pallidal region. Acta Psychiatr Neurol Scand 35:358–377, 1960.
16. Cooper IS, Bravo G. Implications of a 5-year study of 700 basal ganglia operations. Neurology 8:701–707, 1958.
17. Kelly PJ, Ahlskog JE, Goerss SJ, Daube JR, Duffy JR, Kall BA. Computer-assisted stereotactic ventralis lateralis thalamotomy with microelectrode recording control in patients with Parkinson's disease. Mayo Clin Proc 62:655–664, 1987.
18. Jankovic J, Cardoso F, Grossman RG, Hamilton WJ. Outcome after stereotactic thalamotomy for parkinsonian, essential, and other types of tremor. Neurosurgery 37:680–686, 1995.
19. Cotzias GC, Van Woert MH, Schiffer LM. Aromatic amino acids and modification of parkinsonism. N Engl J Med 276:374–379, 1967.
20. Alvarez L, Macias R, Guridi J, Lopez G, Alvarez E, Maragoto C, Teijeiro J, Torres A, Pavon N, Rodriguez-Oroz MC, Ochoa L, Hetherington H, Juncos J, DeLong MR, Obeso JA. Dorsal subthalamotomy for Parkinson's disease. Mov Disord 16:72–78, 2001.
21. Barlas O, Hanagasi HA, Imer M, Sahin HA, Sencer S, Emre M. Do unilateral ablative lesions of the subthalamic nucleus in parkinsonian patients lead to hemiballism? Mov Disord 16:306–310, 2001.
22. Su PC, Ma Y, Fukuda M, Mentis MJ, Tseng HM, Yen RF, Liu HM, Moeller JR, Eidelberg D. Metabolic changes following subthalamotomy for advanced Parkinson's disease. Ann Neurol 50:514–520, 2001.

23. Fahn S. "On-off" phenomenon with levodopa therapy in Parkinsonism. Clinical and pharmacologic correlations and the effect of intramuscular pyridoxine. Neurology 24:431–441, 1974.

24. Marsden CD, Parkes JD. "On-off" effects in patients with Parkinson's disease on chronic levodopa therapy. Lancet 1:292–296, 1976.

25. Stocchi F, Nordera G, Marsden CD. Strategies for treating patients with advanced Parkinson's disease with disastrous fluctuations and dyskinesias. Clin Neuropharmacol 20:95–115, 1997.

26. Fazzini E, Dogali M, Aea Breic. The effects of unilateral ventral posterior medial pallidotomy in patients with Parkinson's disease and Parkinson's plus syndromes. In: Koller WC, Paulson G, eds. Therapy of Parkinson's Disease. New York: Marcel-Dekker, 1994, pp 353–379.

27. Laitinen L. Optimal target of pallidotomy; A controversy. In: Krauss J, Grossmann R, Jankovic J, eds. Pallidal Surgery for the Treatment of Parkinson's Disease and Movement Disorders. Philadelphia: Lippincott-Raven, 1998, pp 285–289.

28. Langston JW, Widner H, Goetz CG, Brooks D, Fahn S, Freeman T, Watts R. Core assessment program for intracerebral transplantations (CAPIT). Mov Disord 7:2–13, 1992.

29. Defer GL, Widner H, Marie RM, Remy P, Levivier M. Core assessment program for surgical interventional therapies in Parkinson's disease (CAPSIT-PD). Mov Disord 14:572–584, 1999.

30. Samuel M, Caputo E, Brooks DJ, Schrag A, Scaravilli T, Branston NM, Rothwell JC, Marsden CD, Thomas DG, Lees AJ, Quinn NP. A study of medial pallidotomy for Parkinson's disease: clinical outcome, MRI location and complications. Brain 121:59–75, 1998.

31. Trepanier LL, Kumar R, Lozano AM, Lang AE, Saint-Cyr JA. Neuropsychological outcome of GPi pallidotomy and GPi or STN deep brain stimulation in Parkinson's disease. Brain Cogn 42:324–347, 2000.

32. Matsumoto K, Asano T, Baba T, Miyamoto T, Ohmoto T. Long-term follow-up results of bilateral thalamotomy for parkinsonism. Appl Neurophysiol 39:257–260, 1976.

33. Matsumoto K, Shichijo F, Fukami T. Long-term follow-up review of cases of Parkinson's disease after unilateral or bilateral thalamotomy. J Neurosurg 60:1033–1044, 1984.

34. Scott R, Gregory R, Hines N, Carroll C, Hyman N, Papanasstasiou V, Leather C, Rowe J, Silburn P, Aziz T. Neuropsychological, neurological and functional outcome following pallidotomy for Parkinson's disease. A consecutive series of eight simultaneous bilateral and twelve unilateral procedures. Brain 121:659–675, 1998.

35. Ghika J, Ghika Schmid F, Fankhauser H, Assal G, Vingerhoets F, Albanese A, Bogousslavsky J, Favre J. Bilateral contemporaneous posteroventral pallidotomy for the treatment of Parkinson's disease: neuropsychological and neurological side effects. Report of four cases and review of the literature. J Neurosurg 91:313–321, 1999.

36. Limousin P, Pollak P, Benazzouz A, Hoffmann D, Le Bas JF, Broussolle F, Perret JE, Benabid AL. Effect of parkinsonian signs and symptoms of bilateral subthalamic nucleus stimulation. Lancet 345:91–95, 1995.

37. Moro E, Scerrati M, Romito LM, Roselli R, Tonali P, Albanese A. Chronic subthalamic nucleus stimulation reduces medication requirements in Parkinson's disease. Neurology 53:85–90, 1999.

38. Bejjani BP, Gervais D, Arnulf I, Papadopoulos S, Demeret S, Bonnet AM, Cornu P, Damier P, Agid Y. Axial parkinsonian symptoms can be improved: the role of levodopa and bilateral subthalamic stimulation. J Neurol Neurosurg Psychiatry 68:595–600, 2000.

39. Kumar R, Lozano AM, Kim YJ, Hutchison WD, Sime E, Halket E, Lang AE. Double-blind evaluation of subthalamic nucleus deep brain stimulation in advanced Parkinson's disease. Neurology 51:850–855, 1998.

40. Hariz MI, Bergenheim AT. A 10-year follow-up review of patients who underwent Leksell's posteroventral pallidotomy for Parkinson disease. J Neurosurg 94:552–558, 2001.

41. Nutt JG, Anderson VC, Peacock JH, Hammerstad JP, Burchiel KJ. DBS and diathermy interaction induces severe CNS damage. Neurology 56:1384–1386, 2001.

42. Oh MY, Hodaie M, Kim SH, Alkhani A, Lang AE, Lozano AM. Deep brain stimulator electrodes used for lesioning: proof of principle. Neurosurgery 49:363–367, 2001.

43. Goetz CG, Stebbins GT, Shale HM, Lang AE, Chernik DA, Chmura TA, Ahlskog JE, Dorflinger EE. Utility of an objective dyskinesia rating scale for Parkinson's disease: inter- and intrarater reliability assessment. Mov Disord 9:390–394, 1994.

44. Carlson JD, Iacono RP. Electrophysiological versus image-based targeting in the posteroventral pallidotomy. Comput Aided Surg 4:93–100, 1999.

45. Hutchison WD, Lozano AM, Davis KD, Saint-Cyr JA, Lang AE, Dostrovsky JO. Differential neuronal activity in segments of globus pallidus in Parkinson's disease patients. Neuroreport 5:1533–1537, 1994.

46. Baron MS, Vitek JL, Bakay RAE, Green J, Kaneoke Y, Hashimoto T, Turner RS, Woodard JL, Cole SA, McDonald WM, DeLong MR. Treatment of advanced Parkinson's disease by posterior GPi pallidotomy: 1-year results of a pilot study. Ann Neurol 40:355–366, 1996.

47. Hutchison WD, Allan RJ, Opitz H, Levy R, Dostrovsky JO, Lang AE, Lozano AM. Neurophysiological identification of the subthalamic nucleus in surgery for Parkinson's disease. Ann Neurol 44:622–628, 1998.

48. Laitinen LV, Bergenheim AT, Hariz MI. Leksell's posteroventral pallidotomy in the treatment of Parkinson's disease [see comments]. J Neurosurg 76:53–61, 1992.

49. Iacono RP, Lonser RR, Mandybur G, Morenski JD, Yamada S, Shima F. Stereotactic pallidotomy results for Parkinson's exceed those of fetal graft. Am Surg 60:777–782, 1994.

50. Sutton JP, Couldwell W, Lew MF, Mallory L, Grafton S, DeGiorgio C, Welsh M, Apuzzo MLJ, Ahmadi J, Waters CH. Ventroposterior medial pallidotomy in patients with advanced Parkinson's disease. Neurosurgery 36:1112–1117, 1995.

51. Kondziolka D, Bonaroti E, Baser S, Brandt F, Kim YS, Lunsford LD. Outcomes after stereotactically guided pallidotomy for advanced Parkinson's disease. J Neurosurg 90:197–202, 1999.

52. Samii A, Turnbull IM, Kishore A, Schulzer M, Mak E, Yardley S, Calne DB. Reassessment of unilateral pallidotomy in Parkinson's disease. A 2-year follow-up study [see comments]. Brain 122:417–425, 1999.

53. Dogali M, Fazzini E, Kolodny E, Eidelberg D, Sterio D, Devinsky O, Beric A. Stereotactic ventral pallidotomy for Parkinson's disease. Neurology 45:753–761, 1995.

54. Tsao K, Wilkinson S, Overman J, Koller WC, Batnitzky S, Gordon MA. Pallidotomy lesion locations: significance of microelectrode refinement. Neurosurgery 43:506–512, 1998.

55. Alterman RL, Sterio D, Beric A, Kelly PJ. Microelectrode recording during posteroventral pallidotomy: impact on target selection and complications. Neurosurgery 44:315–321, 1999.

56. Guridi J, Gorospe A, Ramos E, Linazasoro G, Rodriguez MC, Obeso JA. Stereotactic targeting of the globus pallidus internus in Parkinson's disease: imaging versus electrophysiological mapping. Neurosurgery 45:278–287, 1999.

57. Baron MS, Vitek JL, Bakay RA, Green J, McDonald WM, Cole SA, DeLong MR. Treatment of advanced Parkinson's disease by unilateral posterior GPi pallidotomy: 4-year results of a pilot study. Mov Disord 15:230–237, 2000.

58. Beric A, Sterio D, Dogali M, Fazzini E, Eidelberg D, Kolodny E. Characteristics of pallidal neuronal discharges in Parkinson's disease patients. Adv Neurol 69:123–128, 1996.

59. DeLong MR, Crutcher MD, Georgopoulos AP. Primate globus pallidus and subthalamic nucleus: functional organization. J Neurophysiol 53:530–543, 1985.

60. Sterio D, Beric A, Dogali M, Fazzini E, Alfaro G, Devinsky O. Neurophysiological properties of pallidal neurons in Parkinson's disease. Ann Neurol 35:586–591, 1994.

61. Bakay A, Starr P. Optimal target of pallidotomy; a controversy. In: Krauss J, Grossmann R, Jankovic J, eds. Pallidal Surgery for the Treatment of Parkinson's Disease and Movement Disorders. Philadelphia: Lippincott-Raven, 1998, pp 275–283.

62. Iacono RP, Carlson JD, Mohamed AS, Kuniyoshi SM. Reversal of levodopa failure syndrome by posteroventral-ansa pallidotomy. Adv Neurol 80:619–622, 1999.

63. Baron MS, Sidibe M, DeLong MR, Smith Y. Course of motor and associative pallidothalamic projections in monkeys. J Comp Neurol 429:490–501, 2001.

64. de Bie RM, de Haan RJ, Nihssen PC, Rutgers AW, Beute GN, Bosch DA, Haaxma R, Schmand B, Schuurman PR, Staal MJ, Speelman JD. Unilateral

pallidotomy in Parkinson's disease: a randomised, single-blind, multicentre trial. Lancet 354:1665–1669, 1999.

65. Merello M, Nouzeilles MI, Cammarota A, Betti O, Leiguarda R. Comparison of 1-year follow-up evaluations of patients with indication for pallidotomy who did not undergo surgery versus patients with Parkinson's disease who did undergo pallidotomy: a case control study. Neurosurgery 44:461–467, 1999.

66. Alterman RL, Kelly P, Sterio D, Fazzini E, Eidelberg D, Perrine K, Beric A. Selection criteria for unilateral posteroventral pallidotomy. Acta Neurochir Suppl Wien 68:18–23, 1997.

67. Dalvi A, Winfield L, Yu Q, Cote L, Goodman RR, Pullman SL. Stereotactic posteroventral pallidotomy: clinical methods and results at 1-year follow up. Mov Disord 14:256–261, 1999.

68. de Bie R, Schuurman PR, Haan PS, Bosch A, Speelman JD. Unilateral pallidotomy in advanced Parkinson's disease: A retrospective study of 26 patients. Mov Disord 14:951–957, 1999.

69. Fazzini E, Dogali M, Sterio D, Eidelberg D, Beric A. Sterotactic pallidotomy for Parkinson's disease: a long-term follow-up of unilateral pallidotomy. Neurology 48:1273–1277, 1997.

70. Hirai T, Ryu H, Nagaseki Y, Gaur MS, Fujii M, Takizawa T. Image-guided electrophysiologically controlled posteroventral pallidotomy for the treatment of Parkinson's disease: a 28-case analysis. Adv Neurol 80:585–591, 1999.

71. Jankovic J, Ben Arie L, Schwartz K, Chen K, Khan M, Lai FC, Krauss JK, Grossman R. Movement and reaction times and fine coordination tasks following pallidotomy. Mov Disord 14:57–62, 1999.

72. Johansson F, Malm J, Nordh E, Hariz M. Usefulness of pallidotomy in advanced Parkinson's disease. J Neurol Neurosurg Psychiatry 62:125–132, 1997.

73. Laitinen LV. Pallidotomy for Parkinson's disease. Neurosurg Clin N America 6:105–112, 1995.

74. Lang AE, Lozano AM, Montgomery EB, Tasker RR, Hutchison WD. Posteroventral medial pallidotomy in advanced Parkinson's disease. Adv Neurol 80:575–583, 1999.

75. Masterman D, DeSalles A, Baloh RW, Frysinger R, Foti D, Behnke E, Cabatan Awang C, Hoetzel A, Intemann PM, Fairbanks L, Bronstein JM. Motor, cognitive, and behavioral performance following unilateral ventro-posterior pallidotomy for Parkinson disease. Arch Neurol 55:1201–1208, 1998.

76. Shannon KM, Penn RD, Kroin JS, Adler CH, Janko KA, York M, Cox SJ. Stereotactic pallidotomy for the treatment of Parkinson's disease. Efficacy and adverse effects at 6 months in 26 patients. Neurology 50:434–438, 1998.

77. Fine J, Duff J, Chen R, Chir B, Hutchison W, Lozano AM, Lang AE. Long-term follow-up of unilateral pallidotomy in advanced Parkinson's disease. N Engl J Med 342:1708–1714, 2000.

78. Roberts-Warrior D, Overby A, Jankovic J, Olson S, Lai EC, Krauss JK, Grossman R. Postural control in Parkinson's disease after unilateral posteroventral pallidotomy. Brain 123 (Pt 10):2141–2149, 2000.

79. Siegel KL, Metman LV. Effects of bilateral posteroventral pallidotomy on gait of subjects with Parkinson disease. Arch Neurol 57:198–204, 2000.

80. Trepanier LL, Saint Cyr JA, Lozano AM, Lang AE. Neuropsychological consequences of posteroventral pallidotomy for the treatment of Parkinson's disease. Neurology 51:207–215, 1998.

81. Lang AE, Lozano A, Tasker R, Duff J, Saint-Cyr J, Trepanier L. Neuropsychological and behavioral changes and weight gain after medial pallidotomy. Ann Neurol 41:834–836, 1997.

82. Ondo WG, Ben Aire L, Jankovic J, Lai E, Contant C, Grossman R. Weight gain following unilateral pallidotomy in Parkinson's disease. Acta Neurol Scand 101:79–84, 2000.

83. Gross RE, Lombardi WJ, Hutchison WD, Narula S, Saint Cyr JA, Dostrovsky JO, Tasker RR, Lang AE, Lozano AM. Variability in lesion location after microelectrode-guided pallidotomy for Parkinson's disease: anatomical, physiological, and technical factors that determine lesion distribution. J Neurosurg 90:468–477, 1999.

84. Gross RE, Lombardi WJ, Lang AE, Duff J, Hutchison WD, Saint Cyr JA, Tasker RR, Lozano AM. Relationship of lesion location to clinical outcome following microelectrode-guided pallidotomy for Parkinson's disease [see comments]. Brain 122:405–416, 1999.

85. Bejjani B, Damier P, Arnulf I, Bonnet AM, Vidailhet M, Dormont D, Pidoux B, Cornu P, Marsault C, Agid Y. Pallidal stimulation for Parkinson's disease. Two targets? Neurology 49:1564–1569, 1997.

86. Krack P, Pollak P, Limousin P, Hoffmann D, Benazzouz A, Le Bas JF, Koudsie A, Benabid AL. Opposite motor effects of pallidal stimulation in Parkinson's disease. Ann Neurol 43:180–192, 1998.

87. Bergman H, Wichmann T, Karmon B, DeLong MR. The primate subthalamic nucleus. II. Neuronal activity in the MPTP model of parkinsonism. J Neurophysiol 72:507–520, 1994.

88. Carpenter MB. Anatomical organization of the corpus striatum and related nuclei. In: Yahr MD, ed. The Basal Ganglia. New York: Raven Press, 1976, pp 1–36.

89. Tsao K, Wilkinson S, Overman J, Kieltyka J, Tollefson T, Koller WC, Pahwa R, Troster AI, Lyons KE, Batznitzky S, Wetzel L, Gordon MA. Comparison of actual pallidotomy lesion location with expected stereotactic location. Stereotact Funct Neurosurg 71:1–19, 1998.

90. Vitek JL, Bakay RA, Hashimoto T, Kaneoke Y, Mewes K, Zhang JY, Rye D, Starr P, Baron M, Turner R, DeLong MR. Microelectrode-guided pallidotomy: technical approach and its application in medically intractable Parkinson's disease. J Neurosurg 88:1027–1043, 1998.

91. Ghika J, Villemure JG, Fankhauser H, Favre J, Assal G, Ghika Schmid F. Efficiency and safety of bilateral contemporaneous pallidal stimulation (deep

brain stimulation) in levodopa-responsive patients with Parkinson's disease with severe motor fluctuations: a 2-year follow-up review. J Neurosurg 89:713–718, 1998.

92. Merello M, Starkstein S, Nouzeilles MI, Kuzis G, Leiguarda R. Bilateral pallidotomy for treatment of Parkinson's disease induced corticobulbar syndrome and psychic akinesia avoidable by globus pallidus lesion combined with contralateral stimulation. J Neurol Neurosurg Psychiatry 71:611–614, 2001.

93. Intemann PM, Masterman D, Subramanian I, DeSalles A, Behnke F, Frysinger R, Bronstein JM. Staged bilateral pallidotomy for treatment of Parkinson disease. J Neurosurg 94:437–444, 2001.

94. Counihan TJ, Shinobu LA, Eskandar EN, Cosgrove GR, Penney JB, Jr. Outcomes following staged bilateral pallidotomy in advanced Parkinson's disease. Neurology 56:799–802, 2001.

95. Oh MY, Abosch A, Kim SH, Lang AE, Lozano AM. Long-term hardware-related complications of deep brain stimulation. Neurosurgery 2002; 50:1268–1274.

96. Hassler R, Mundinger F, Riechert T. Correlations between clinical and autopic findings in steroeotaxic operations of parkinsonism. Confin Neurol 26:282–290, 1965.

97. Hassler R, Mundinger F, Riechert T. Pathophysiology of tremor at rest derived from the correlation of anatomical and clinical data. Confin Neurol 32:79–87, 1970.

98. Perry VL, Lenz FA. Ablative therapy for movement disorders. Thalamotomy for Parkinson's disease. Neurosurg Clin North Am 9:317–324, 1998.

99. Kelly PJ, Gillingham FJ. The long-term results of stereotaxic surgery and L-dopa therapy in patients with Parkinson's disease. A 10-year follow-up study. J Neurosurg 53:332–337, 1980.

100. Fox MW, Ahlskog JE, Kelly PJ. Stereotactic ventrolateralis thalamotomy for medically refractory tremor in post-levodopa era Parkinson's disease patients. J Neurosurg 75:723–730, 1991.

101. Diederich N, Goetz CG, Stebbins GT, Klawans HL, Nittner K, Koulosakis A, Sanker P, Sturm V. Blinded evaluation confirms long-term asymmetric effect of unilateral thalamotomy or subthalamotomy on tremor in Parkinson's disease. Neurology 42:1311–1314, 1992.

102. Jankovic J, Hamilton WJ, Grossman RG. Thalamic surgery for movement disorders. Adv Neurol 74:221–233, 1997.

103. Ojemann GA, Hoyenga KB, Ward AA, Jr. Prediction of short-term verbal memory disturbance after ventrolateral thalamotomy. J Neurosurg 35:203–210, 1971.

104. Schuurman PR, Bosch DA, Bossuyt PM, Bonsel GJ, van Someren EJ, de Bie RM, Merkus MP, Speelman JD. A comparison of continuous thalamic stimulation and thalamotomy for suppression of severe tremor. N Engl J Med 342:461–468, 2000.

105. Tasker RR. Deep brain stimulation is preferable to thalamotomy for tremor suppression. Surg Neurol 49:145–153, 1998.
106. Lyons KE, Koller WC, Wilkinson SB, Pahwa R. Long term safety and efficacy of unilateral deep brain stimulation of the thalamus for parkinsonian tremor. J Neurol Neurosurg Psychiatry 71:682–684, 2001.
107. Parkin SG, Gregory RP, Scott R, Bain P, Silburn P, Hall B, Boyle R, Joint C, Aziz TZ. Unilateral and bilateral palidotomy for idiopathic Parkinson's disease: a case series of 115 patients. Mov Disord 2002; 17:682–692.
108. Pahwa R, Lyons KE, Wilkinson SB, Troster AI, Overman J, Kieltyka J, Koller WC. Comparison of thalamotomy to deep brain stimulation of the thalamus in essential tremor. Mov Disord 16:140–143, 2001.
109. Page RD, Sambrook MA, Crossman AR. Thalamotomy for the alleviation of levodopa induced dyskinesia—experimental study in the 1-methyl-4-phenyl-1,2,3,6-tetrahydropyridine treated parkinsonian monkey. Neuroscience 55:147–165, 1993.
110. Miyamoto T, Bekku H, Moriyama E, Tsuchida S. Present role of stereotactic thalamotomy for parkinsonism. Retrospective analysis of operative results and thalamic lesions in computed tomograms. Appl Neurophysiol 48:294–304, 1985.
111. Narabayashi H, Yokochi F, Nakajima Y. Levodopa-induced dyskinesia and thalamotomy. J Neurol Neurosurg Psychiatry 47:831–839, 1984.
112. Caparros-Lefebvre D, Blond S, Feltin MP, Pollak P, Benabid AL. Improvement of levodopa induced dyskinesias by thalamic deep brain stimulation is related to slight variation in electrode placement: possible involvement of the centre median and parafascicularis complex. J Neurol Neurosurg Psychiatry 67:308–314, 1999.
113. Henderson JM, O'Sullivan DJ, Pell M, Fung VS, Hely MA, Morris JG, Halliday GM. Lesion of thalamic centromedian—parafascicular complex after chronic deep brain stimulation. Neurology 56:1576–1579, 2001.
114. Rossitch E, Jr, Zeidman SM, Nashold BS, Jr, Horner J, Walker J, Osborne D, Bullard DE. Evaluation of memory and language function pre- and postthalamotomy with an attempt to define those patients at risk for postoperative dysfunction. Surg Neurol 29:11–16, 1988.
115. Wichmann T, Bergman H, DeLong MR. The primate subthalamic nucleus. I. Functional properties in intact animals. J Neurophysiol 72:494–506, 1994.
116. Carpenter M, Whittier J, Mettler F. Analysis of choreic hyperkinesia in the rhesus monkey. Surgical and pharmacological analysis of hyperkinesia resulting form lesions in the subthalamic nucleus of Luys. J Comp Neurol 92:293–331, 1950.
117. Bergman H, Wichmann T, DeLong MR. Reversal of experimental parkinsonism by lesions of the subthalamic nucleus. Science 249:1436–1438, 1990.
118. Aziz TZ, Peggs D, Sambrook MA, Crossman AR. Lesion of the subthalamic nucleus for the alleviation of 1-methyl-4-phenyl-1,2,3,6-tetrahydropyridine (MPTP)-induced parkinsonism in the primate. Mov Disord 6:288–292, 1991.

119. Aziz IZ, Peggs D, Agarwal E, Sambrook MA, Crossman AR. Subthalamic nucleotomy alleviates parkinsonism in the 1-methyl-4-phenyl-1,2,3,6-tetrahydropyridine (MPTP)-exposed primate. Br J Neurosurg 6:575–582, 1992.
120. Fager CA. Evaluation of thalamic and subthalamic surgical lesions in the alleviation of Parkinson's disease. J Neurosurg 28:145–149, 1968.
121. Limousin P, Pollak P, Benazzouz A, Hoffmann D, Broussolle E, Perret JE, Benabid AL. Bilateral subthalamic nucleus stimulation for severe Parkinson's disease. Mov Disord 10:672–674, 1995.
122. Gill S, Heywood P. Bilateral subthalamic nucleotomy can be accomplished safely. Mov Disord 13 (suppl 2):201, 1998.
123. Gill SS, Heywood P. Bilateral dorsolateral subthalamotomy for advanced Parkinson's disease. Lancet 350:1224, 1997.
124. Klostermann W, Vieregge P, Kompf D. Apraxia of eyelid opening after bilateral stereotaxic subthalamotomy. J Neuroophthalmol 17:122–123, 1997.
125. Lozano AM, ed. Movement Disorder Surgery. Basel: Karger, 2000.

23

Deep Brain Stimulation in Parkinson's Disease

Rajesh Pahwa and Kelly E. Lyons
University of Kansas Medical Center, Kansas City, Kansas, U.S.A.

Stereotactic surgeries for movement disorders were introduced in the 1950s (1,2) but were not widely accepted due to significant morbidity, mortality, and limited knowledge in target selection for symptomatic benefit. In the late 1950s and early 1960s there was an increase in the number of stereotactic surgeries performed. With advances in pharmacological therapy, particularly the availability of levodopa, these surgeries were rarely performed until the late 1980s. Currently, based on the recognition of the limitations of drug treatments for Parkinson's disease (PD) and a better understanding of the physiology and circuitry of the basal ganglia, there has been a marked increase in surgical therapies for PD. In addition, advances in surgical techniques, neuroimaging, and improved electrophysiological recordings allow stereotactic procedures to be done more accurately, leading to reduced morbidity. Over the last decade, deep brain stimulation (DBS) is increasingly replacing lesion surgery as the preferred procedure. DBS in PD is associated with three targets: the ventral intermediate nucleus (VIM) of the thalamus, the globus pallidus interna (GPi), and the subthalamic nucleus (STN).

HISTORY

Benabid and coworkers were the pioneers of DBS surgery. In the late 1980s, Benabid and colleagues (3), during thalamic lesioning, observed that stimulation at the site of the lesion could induce either an increase or a reduction in tremor amplitude. They noted that low-frequency stimulation increased tremor and frequencies above 100 Hz were able to alleviate tremor. They extended these observations by implanting an electrode in the contralateral motor thalamus of a patient who had undergone thalamotomy and needed surgery on the second side. This was done due to the higher rate of complications known to occur with bilateral lesion surgeries. These results were satisfactory, and soon thalamic stimulation was increasingly used instead of thalamotomy even in patients undergoing unilateral procedures. These methods have been now used in the GPi and STN to deliver high-frequency stimulation instead of creating lesions in those nuclei.

DEEP BRAIN STIMULATION HARDWARE

The Activa® Tremor Control therapy and the Activa® Parkinson Control therapy are approved therapies in the United States and Europe. These devices and other hardware have undergone multiple changes since they were first introduced. Presently the implanted hardware is manufactured by Medtronic, Inc. (Minneapolis, MN). The Activa Tremor Control and Parkinson Control therapies consist of a DBS lead, an extension wire that connects the DBS lead to an implantable pulse generator (IPG), and the neurostimulator. There are two DBS leads available. The intracranial end of both leads has four platinum-iridium contacts. One lead has contacts that are separated by 1.5 mm (Model 3387 DBS lead) and the second lead has contacts that are separated by 0.5 mm (Model 3389 DBS lead). The DBS leads are connected to the neurostimulator by the extension wire that is tunneled under the skin. There have been multiple models of stimulators that have been used for Activa therapy. The Itrel II® Neurostimulator, Model 7424 was initially used. The Soletra® Model 7426 and Kinetra® are the two neurostimulators presently available. The Kinetra has the advantage of using one stimulator to control both sides, instead of two separate Soletra neurostimulators, one for each side. The neurostimulators are typically implanted subcutaneously in the infraclavicular area. The neurostimulators can be programmed for monopolar stimulation or bipolar stimulation. Adjustable parameters include pulse width, amplitude, stimulation frequency, and the choice of active contacts. The patient can turn the stimulator on or off using a hand-held magnet or using Access Review®, which also has a feature to tell the patient if the neurostimulator is on or off. The typical stimulation parameters are stimulation frequency of 135–185 Hz, pulse width of 60–120 µs, and amplitude of 1–3 v.

ADVANTAGES AND DISADVANTAGES OF DBS

The advantages of the DBS system include no destructive lesion in the brain, adjustment of stimulation parameters to increase efficacy or reduce adverse effects, bilateral operations with relative safety and reduced adverse effects, and the potential use of future neuroprotective therapies when available. The disadvantages include cost of the system, time and effort involved in programming the system, repeat surgeries related to device problems, use of general anesthesia to implant the stimulator, and battery replacement every 3–7 years.

DEEP BRAIN STIMULATION OF THE THALAMUS

Efficacy Studies

DBS of the thalamus is increasingly replacing thalamotomy as the preferred surgery for the treatment of medication resistant PD tremor. There are multiple reports regarding the efficacy of these procedures for parkinsonian tremor (Table 1) (4–17). The majority of the studies have reported that even though tremor is markedly improved, this often does not result in improvement in activities of daily living. As DBS of the thalamus does not improve bradykinesia, rigidity, or drug-induced dyskinesias, this procedure should be restricted to PD patients whose major disability is tremor.

TABLE 1 Selected Studies of Deep Brain Stimulation of the Thalamus

Author	Number of implants	Tremor improvement (%)	Follow-up (months)
Benabid et al. (7)	111	63	6
Blond et al. (5)	10	70	17
Albanese et al. (14)	31	68	8
Koller et al. (10)	24	91	12
Ondo et al. (11)	9	95	3
Limousin et al. (9)	74	85	12
Albanese et al. (14)	27	92	9
Lyons et al. (17)	9	87	40

There are very few randomized, controlled trials of thalamic DBS in PD. Open-label evaluations have indicated that 65–95% of patients have improvement in tremor (5,6,8,9). Studies with randomized, blinded evaluations have confirmed the results of unblinded studies. (10,11). The majority of the studies evaluated the efficacy of unilateral thalamic stimulation. The usual outcome variable was the clinical tremor rating scale with severity ratings of 0–4, where 0 is no tremor and 4 is severe tremor.

Benabid and colleagues have had the most experience with DBS of the thalamus. In 1997, they reported 80 PD patients who had DBS of the thalamus for drug-resistant tremor (12). The tremor was predominant at rest but persisted during posture holding and action. Bradykinesia and rigidity were mild in the majority of the patients. At the last follow-up (up to 7 years, mean 3 years) global evaluations showed the best control for parkinsonian rest tremor and the least satisfactory control for action tremor. There was no dramatic effect on other symptoms like bradykinesia, rigidity, or dyskinesias.

Koller et al. (10) reported the results of a double-blind multicenter study in 24 PD patients who had undergone unilateral thalamic stimulation. At 1 year there was a significant tremor improvement, although activities of daily living as measured by the Unified Parkinson's Disease Rating Scale (UPDRS) were not significantly changed. Results of blinded evaluations performed at 3 months were similar to the open-label evaluations.

In another multicenter trial, Limousin et al. (9) reported 57 PD patients who had undergone unilateral implant and 16 PD patients who had undergone bilateral implants. At 12 months, tremor and bradykinesia were significantly reduced by stimulation as compared to baseline. There was a 74% reduction in tremor, 16% reduction in rigidity, and 34% reduction in bradykinesia on the treated side. These improvements in rigidity and bradykinesia are not consistently reported in other studies. They did not observe any improvements in axial symptoms. Speech, postural instability, and gait were not affected by unilateral or bilateral surgery. Levodopa-induced dyskinesias were slightly but not significantly reduced. Adverse effects were reported for the entire cohort of patients, including essential tremor (ET) patients. Three patients had subdural hematomas, one of whom also had a thalamic hematoma. Two patients had infection of the system, and in five patients the electrode was replaced because of unsatisfactory results. Stimulation-related adverse effects were mild.

Ondo et al. (11) reported 19 PD patients with severe tremor, PD patients reported an 82% reduction in contralateral tremor and significant improvement in disability and global impressions. They did not find any meaningful improvement in other motor aspects of the disease, and the activities of daily living did not change. They also performed blinded PD assessments, which resembled the unblinded outcomes. There were no significant surgical complications, and two patients had breakage of the extension wire.

Bilateral Studies

There is a lack of adequate data regarding bilateral thalamic stimulation in PD. Ondo et al. (13) reported eight patients who underwent bilateral thalamic stimulation for PD. The main cause of disability in the patients was tremor with relatively little bradykinesia and rigidity. After the second implantation, three patients reported marked improvement, two reported moderate improvement, one reported mild improvement, one patient had no change, and one patient was mildly worse. Although there was a significant improvement in tremor after the second procedure, bradykinesia, gait, and balance scores were worse. Similarly, activities of daily living scores and adverse effects were worse after the second procedure.

Long-Term Studies

Long-term results of DBS of the thalamus are not widely reported. Albanese et al. (14) reported 27 PD patients (6 with bilateral implants) with DBS of the thalamus. The longest follow-up was 2 years with a mean follow-up of 0.9 years. Tremor was completely or almost completely suppressed in 78%, unchanged in 15%, and slightly reduced in 7% of the patients. Moderate relief of bradykinesia was reported in three patients, and antiparkinsonian medications were reduced in 26% of the patients. There was one intracranial hemorrhage, one skin erosion, one electrode breakage, two infections, and two lead replacements. Kumar et al. (15) described seven PD patients with a mean follow-up of 16.2 months, and Hariz et al. (16) reported 22 PD patients with a mean follow-up of 21 months. Both studies reported long-term improvement in tremor scores. Lyons et al. (17) reported the results of 12 PD patients with a mean follow-up of 40 months and a maximum follow-up period of 66 months. Although tremor scores continued to be improved by 87%, there was a worsening of the motor UPDRS scores, suggesting the worsening of other parkinsonian symptoms. Lead repositioning occurred in two patients, and neurostimulator and extension wire replacement in one patient due to shocking sensation.

Tremor Rebound

Some authors have reported frequent tremor rebound upon turning the stimulation off (7,16,18), while others denied occurrence of such rebound

(19). Albanese et al. (14) reported a paradoxical increase of tremor in 22% of the patients when the stimulation was turned off. Similarly, Hariz et al. (16) reported that persistent tremor rebound occurred in 32% of the PD patients. Kumar et al. (15) reported tremor rebound in 57% when turning the devices off, and these patients had to continuously use stimulation. Although the cause of rebound is not known, it could be related to disease progression or tolerance to stimulation. Kumar et al. (15) speculated that rebound could be due to the removal of the inhibitory effect on the VIM nucleus provided by stimulation and likely represents habituation.

Tolerance to Chronic Stimulation

A gradual loss of tremor benefit over time when the stimulation parameters are kept constant suggests tolerance to chronic stimulation (15). Although increases in parameters can initially result in benefit, in patients with a true tolerance phenomenon the increased stimulation parameters lead to adverse effects without further benefit. Occasionally, a stimulation holiday may improve the tolerance phenomenon, but in the majority of patients this is a temporary improvement. Although the exact mechanism of tolerance is not known, Kumar et al. (15) postulated that tolerance could be secondary to progression of the underlying disease, loss of a microthalamotomy effect over time, habituation of the neuronal network, and an increase in impedance at the stimulating tip.

Patient Selection

With the advent of other target sites for PD, the role of thalamic stimulation in PD has been reduced significantly. Presently, thalamic stimulation should be restricted in PD patients with a combination of PD and essential tremor, elderly patients (greater than 80 years of age) in whom the major disability is tremor, and patients with medication-resistant tremor in whom a definitive diagnosis of PD cannot be established. In general, patients should not have any significant cognitive impairment, significant comorbidities, or a cardiac pacemaker.

DEEP BRAIN STIMULATION OF THE GLOBUS PALLIDUS

Efficacy Studies

Surgery targeting the internal segment of the GPi improves the cardinal features of PD. Lesion surgery and DBS of the GPi appear to improve tremor, bradykinesia, rigidity, and dyskinesias. Due to concerns about severe complications related to bilateral lesions, DBS of the GPi is preferred to pallidotomy.

Siegfried and Lippitz were among the first to report the use of DBS for continuously stimulating the ventroposterolateral pallidum. They implanted bilateral GPi electrodes in three PD patients. Follow-up in these three patients ranged from 3 months to 1 year. They reported improvement in Webster Rating Scale scores and on-off motor fluctuations.

Since then, multiple studies have reported the efficacy of GPi stimulation for PD (see Table 2). All studies reported a small number of patients, and follow-up has ranged from days to a maximum of 30 months. The patients have been implanted unilaterally and bilaterally. The improvement in the off medication state in activities of daily living ranged from 19 to 68%, and the UPDRS Motor score improvement ranged from 24 to 50%. The improvement in activities of daily living in the on medication state ranged from 22 to 60%, and UPDRS Motor scores ranged from 1 to 60%. All studies reported significant reductions in dyskinesias, resulting in improvement in on time during the day.

Pahwa et al. (22) reported five PD patients who underwent pallidal stimulation. Three patients had bilateral implants, and two had unilateral implants. Four patients were markedly improved, and one was moderately improved after surgery. The activities of daily living subscores of the UPDRS improved by 19% in the off-medication state and by 42% in the on-

TABLE 2   Selected Studies of Deep Brain Stimulation of the Globus Pallidus

Author	Number of patients	Follow-up	UPDRS improvement
Pahwa et al. (22)	3 unilateral 2 bilateral	3 months	off scores: ADL 19%, Motor 24% on scores: ADL 41%, Motor 60%
Gross et al. (54)	7 unilateral	1–3 years	off scores: Motor 30% on scores: Motor 43%
Krack et al. (55)	5 bilateral	3–6 months	motor 39%
Kumar et al. (56)	4 unilateral/4 bilateral	3–6 months	off scores: ADL 26%, Motor 27%
Ghika et al. (26)	6 bilateral	24 months	off scores: ADL 68%, Motor 50% on scores: ADL 60%, Motor 26%
Volkmann et al. (57)	9 bilateral	12 months	off scores: Motor 44%
Merello et al. (58)	6 unilateral	3 months	off scores: ADL 58%, Motor 29% on scores: ADL 22%, Motor 8%
DBS for PDSG (37)	38 bilateral	6 months	off scores: ADL 36%, Motor 33% on scores: ADL 31%, Motor 32%
Kumar et al. (24)	17 bilateral 5 unilateral	6 months	off scores: ADL 40%, Motor 32% on scores: ADL 30%, Motor 1%

UPDRS = Unified Parkinson's Disease Rating Scale; ADL = activities of daily living;
DBS = deep brain stimulation; PDSG = Parkinson's Disease Study Group.

medication state. Patient diaries demonstrated an increase in on-time with a decrease in both off-time and on-time with dyskinesias.

A review by the American Academy of Neurology identified reports on 64 patients who had undergone DBS of the globus pallidus (23). An approximately equal number of patients underwent unilateral and bilateral implantations. Benefit was reported in all aspects of PD with a marked attenuation of motor fluctuations and dyskinesias. In unilateral implants, the benefits were most pronounced on the contralateral side.

Kumar et al. (24) reported 22 PD patients who were treated with either unilateral ($n = 5$) or bilateral ($n = 17$) GPi stimulation. Evaluations performed in the off-medication state at 6 months reported a 32% improvement in UPDRS motor scores, 40% improvement in UPDRS activities of daily living scores, and 23% improvement in dyskinesias. When the evaluations were repeated in the medication "on state," UPDRS motor scores improved by 1%, UPDRS activities of daily living scores improved by 30%, and dyskinesias improved by 68%.

The Deep Brain Stimulation for Parkinson's Disease Study Group reported a multinational, prospective study of bilateral GPi stimulation in PD (25). Forty-one patients were enrolled; electrodes were implanted in 38 patients (two patients had cerebral hemorrhage and one patient had intraoperative confusion). In comparison to baseline, there was a significant improvement in the UPDRS motor scores in the off-medication state and a smaller improvement in the on-medication state. In the off-medication state, all the subscales of the UPDRS also improved. Tremor scores improved by 59%, rigidity improved by 31%, bradykinesia improved by 26%, gait by 35%, and postural instability by 36%. In the on-medication state, tremor scores improved by 85%, rigidity and bradykinesia by 22%, gait by 33%, and postural instability by 50%. Patient diaries revealed that the percentage of on time without dyskinesias during the awake time increased from 28 to 64%, and the off time reduced from 37 to 24%. The mean daily dose in levodopa equivalents was unchanged between baseline and 6 months.

Long-term results of DBS of the globus pallidus have been lacking. Ghika et al. (26) reported six PD patients with a mean age of 55 years and disease duration of 16 years with a minimum follow-up of 24 months. The mean improvement in the UPDRS motor "off" scores and the ADL scores was more than 50%. The mean "off" time decreased from 40 to 10%, and the dyskinesia scores were reduced by 30%. Although the improvements persisted beyond 2 years after surgery, signs of decreased efficacy were seen after 12 months.

In summary, DBS of the globus pallidus results in improvement of the cardinal features of PD including tremor, bradykinesia, rigidity, and gait and a marked reduction of levodopa-induced dyskinesias. There is an improvement in daily motor fluctuations. The daily levodopa dosage or antiparkinsonian medication dosage is not reduced.

Optimal Pallidal Electrode Location

Studies of GPi stimulation have reported variable and sometimes opposite effects by using different electrode contacts (27–29). Bejjani et al. (27) investigated the effect of stimulation on different sites of the globus pallidus (GP) in five PD patients. Stimulation in the dorsal GP (upper contact) significantly improved gait, akinesia, and rigidity and could induce dyskinesia when the patients were in the off-state. In contrast, stimulation of the posteroventral GP (lower contact) significantly worsened gait and akinesia. Krack et al. (28) reported similar results and suggested using an intermediate contact between the dorsal and the posteroventral contacts as a good compromise between these opposite effects.

DEEP BRAIN STIMULATION OF THE SUBTHALAMIC NUCLEUS

The STN has gained importance in PD. Although it is believed that subthalamic lesions induce ballism, patients who undergo subthalamotomy or subthalamic stimulation usually do not have these involuntary movements. In a study by Carpenter et al. (30) it was shown that in animals ballism was induced on the contralateral side if more than a minimal percentile volume of the nucleus, greater than 20%, was destroyed or the lesion was not too large or if it did not involve the adjacent structures. Hence if the lesions extend beyond the STN, and in particular if they involve the internal segment of the globus pallidus or the pallidal fugal pathways, then no involuntary movements are seen (31).

There are multiple reports of the antiparkinsonian effects of STN DBS (Table 3) (32–38). Limousin et al. (39) reported results of bilateral STN and found improvements of 58–88% in the activities of daily living subscores and 42–84% in the motor subscores of the UPDRS. Kumar et al. (40) conducted evaluations in a double-blind fashion and reported improvements of 30% in the activities of daily living and a 58% improvement in motor scores of the UPDRS. They also reported a mean reduction of 40% of antiparkinsonian medications and 83% improvement in dyskinesias.

Other studies have duplicated these results with STN stimulation. All studies have consistently reported improvement in the UPDRS scores in the off-medication state. The improvement in the ADL scores ranged from 30 to 72%, and the UPDRS Motor score improvements ranged from 42 to 74% in the off-medication state (Table 3). Irrespective of the percentage of

TABLE 3   Selected Studies of Deep Brain Stimulation of the Subthalamic
Nucleus

Author	Number of patients	Follow-up	Improvement
Krack et al. (55)	8	3–6 months	UPDRS off scores: Motor 71% Medication reduction 56%
Limousin et al. (39)	24	12 months	UPDRS off scores: ADL 58%, Motor 60%, Dyskinesias 63%, Meds reduced 50%
Kumar et al. (40)	7	6–12 months	UPDRS off scores: ADL 30%, Motor 58% Dyskinesias 83%, Meds reduced 40%
Maro et al. (36)	7	16 months	UPDRS off scores: ADL 52%, Motor 42% Medication reduction 65%, UPDRS on scores: ADL 7%, Motor 5%
Molinuevo et al. (59)	15	6 months	UPDRS off scores: ADL 72%, Motor 66% Dyskinesia reduction 81%, Medication reduction 80%
Houeto et al. (60)	23	6 months	UPDRS off scores: ADL 66%, Motor 67% Dyskinesia reduction 77%, Meds reduced 61%
Rodriguez et al. (38)	15	12–36 months	UPDRS off scores: ADL 70%, Motor 74% Meds reduced 55%
Romito et al. (42)	22	1–3 years	UPDRS off scores: ADL 68%, Motor 50% Meds reduction 69%
Thobois et al. (61)	18	6–12 months	UPDRS off scores: ADL 53%, Motor 55% Dyskinesias reduction 66%, Med reduced 76%
DBS for PDSG (37)	96	6 months	UPDRS off scores: ADL 44%, Motor 51% Dyskinesia reduction 70%, Meds reduced 37%

improvement in the motor scores, these improvements are similar to those
observed with the levodopa challenge. In other words, if the patient is
evaluated 12 hours after not taking antiparkinsonian medications (off-
medication state) and the evaluations are repeated after the patient has
taken antiparkinsonian medications and the medications have started
working (on-medication state), the percentage improvement would be
similar to that seen after surgery with stimulation alone. This levodopa
challenge predicts the response to surgery if the electrodes are in the correct
position and programming of the stimulators is optimized.

The other consistent finding with STN stimulation is the reduction in
antiparkinsonian medications after surgery, which results in a marked
reduction in dyskinesias. Antiparkinsonian medications are usually reduced
by 37–80% after surgery, resulting in a 63–81% reduction in dyskinesias
(Table 3). The improvement in the off-medication UPDRS Motor scores
also results in a reduction in off-time during the day.

One of the largest studies of STN stimulation is a prospective study that was performed in 18 countries (37). One hundred and two patients were enrolled, 96 of whom had electrodes implanted in both subthalamic nuclei. Bilateral procedures were not performed in 6 patients due to complications with the first procedure (intracranial hemorrhage in two, hemiparesis in one, confusion in one, lack of response in one, and improper lead placement in one). In the off-medication state there was a mean improvement of 44% in the activities of daily living and a mean improvement of 51% in the UPDRS Motor scores. All subscores of the UPDRS (off medication state) also improved—tremor scores by 79%, rigidity by 58%, bradykinesia by 42%, gait by 56%, and postural instability by 50%. Patient home diaries revealed that the off-state during the day decreased by 61%, on-state increased by 64%, and on-state with dyskinesias decreased by 70%. Although there was some improvement in the on-state UPDRS scores, it was not as robust.

Long-term follow-up results for STN DBS are limited. Benabid et al. (41) followed more than 50 patients for one year who maintained the benefit. Thirty patients were assessed at 2 years, 16 patients at 3 years, 9 patients at 4 years, and 4 patients at 5 years. They observed adequate control of the cardinal features of PD and the reduced levodopa requirement persisted. They observed a tendency towards increased hypophonia and axial motor features. Rodriquez et al. (38) reported initial results in 15 patients after 12 months and in 9 patients between 30 and 36 months after surgery. They reported a 74% improvement in the UPDRS motor scores in the off state with a 55% reduction in the levodopa daily dose. Nine patients with long-term follow-up continued to have a 61% improvement in UPDRS motor scores and a 38% reduction in levodopa dosage. Romito et al. (42) reported on 22 patients, 7 of whom were followed up at 36 months. In the off-medication state, the UPDRS activities of daily living scores were improved by 59%, UPDRS Motor scores by 49%, and the antiparkinsonian medications were reduced by 70%.

In summary, studies of STN stimulation indicate that stimulation induces a 40–75% improvement in UPDRS motor scores in the off medication condition and all cardinal features of PD improve. UPDRS on medication motor scores are not significantly improved, but there is a 40–80% reduction in antiparkinsonian medication. Off periods and dyskinesias are also significantly improved. Activities of daily living and patient quality of life scales have also shown significant improvements in multiple studies.

PATIENT SELECTION FOR GPi AND STN SURGERY

The criteria for patient selection for these targets in PD are similar. The ideal candidate for DBS of the GPi and STN is a patient with idiopathic levodopa-responsive PD. We recommend that patients undergo a levodopa challenge 12 hours after not taking any antiparkinsonian medications. The patients should have improvement of at least 30% in the UPDRS Motor scores after the levodopa challenge to be candidates for surgery. Patients should be under 75 years as older patients may have difficulty tolerating the procedure. Patients should have been tried on combinations of different antiparkinsonian medications, including all those currently available. Patients with disabling medication-resistant tremor or an inability to tolerate antiparkinsonian medications should be excluded. Patients should exhibit no evidence of dementia or significant cognitive abnormalities. Patients should undergo detailed neuropsychological testing. Patients should have no behavioral problems and a realistic expectation of surgery. Unfortunately, there are no tests available that would predict what kind of behavior problems would interfere with the outcome of surgery, but close evaluation by the neurologist and neuropsychologist can help exclude unsuitable patients.

WHICH LOCATION—DEEP BRAIN STIMULATION OF THE GPi OR STN?

The criteria for patient selection for GPi and STN targets are similar. A few studies have compared patients who have undergone surgeries at these targets, but most of these are not randomized studies and the number of patients in these studies is small. Krack et al. (34) retrospectively compared eight patients who were operated on the STN and five patients who were operated on the GPi. In the off-state, the UPDRS Motor score improved by 71% with STN stimulation and by 39% with GPi stimulation. Rigidity and tremor showed good improvement in both groups, but bradykinesia was more improved in the STN group. There was a reduction in levodopa dosage only in the STN group. Burchiel et al. (35) performed a randomized blinded prospective study in 10 PD patients with 5 patients randomized to GPi and 5 to STN stimulation. At 12 months in the off-state both groups demonstrated a 40% improvement in the UPDRS Motor scores. Dyskinesias were reduced in both groups, although the antiparkinsonian medications were only reduced in the STN group. In another study, Scotto di Luzio and colleagues (43) compared nine patients who had undergone bilateral STN stimulation to five who had undergone GPi stimulation. STN stimulation was superior to GPi stimulation in the reduction of the clinical features and the decrease in medication off-state. There was a reduction in levodopa dose only in the STN group. Volkmann et al. (44) retrospectively compared 16 patients who had undergone STN stimulation with 11 patients who had undergone GPi stimulation. There was a 54% improvement in the UPDRS Motor scores with GPi stimulation as compared to 67%

improvement with STN. Medication was reduced only in the STN group, and they required less electrical power compared to the GPi group. Finally Krause et al. (45) prospectively compared 6 GPi patients with 12 STN patients. Although STN stimulation improved Schwab and England scores, GPi stimulation did not improve these scores. GPi stimulation directly reduced the dyskinesias, whereas STN stimulation reduced the dyskinesias due to reduction in antiparkinsonian medications. STN stimulation improved the UPDRS Motor scores; GPi stimulation did not have a similar effect. These and other noncomparative studies show a greater improvement in patients who have undergone STN stimulation as compared to GPi stimulation, hence the majority of the surgery centers favor STN stimulation over GPi stimulation.

ADVERSE EFFECTS OF DBS

Complications of DBS are relatively similar in the three groups (VIM, GPi, and STN) and can be divided into those related to the surgical procedure, those associated with the device, and those associated with stimulation. These complications are also related to the expertise of the personnel, the proper patient selection, and the mechanical failure of the equipment.

Surgical

Surgical complications are those that occur within 30 days of surgery. These complications are typical of those seen with other intracranial stereotactic procedures and occur in less than 5% of the patients. These complications include hemorrhage, ischemic lesions, seizures, and infections. Pollack et al. (46) assessed 212 patients who had undergone STN, GPi, or VIM DBS. Two patient deaths could be indirectly related to surgery. One occurred 2 weeks after surgery and was due to pulmonary embolism, and another occurred 3 years after surgery in a patient who developed a frontal hematoma during surgery. In this series, permanent severe morbidity occurred in seven patients (2.3%): three patients who had intracerebral hematoma during surgery, three patients who had worsening of cognitive status leading to dementia, and one patient due to an unrelated traumatic hematoma. Intracranial hematoma is one of the most severe complications of stereotactic surgery. In the series by Pollack et al. (46) there was a 4.2% risk of intracranial hemorrhage. In another large series there was a 4.8% risk of intracranial hemorrhage (37). The risk of infection is usually less than 5%. Other transient events include seizures, confusion, subcutaneous bleeding, dysarthria, nonhemorrhagic hemiparesis, and brachial plexus injury. The majority of these events are transient and resolve within 30 days.

Hardware-Related

Device-related events include misplacement or displacement of the electrode, skin erosion, fracture of electrode or its components, and mechanical problems with the electrical system. These device-related events can occur in up to 25% of the patients (47). Oh et al. (47) reported 79 patients who had received 124 electrode implants. Overall, 20 patients (25.3%) had hardware complications. These included four lead fractures, four lead migrations, three short or open circuits, 12 erosions or infections, and two foreign body reactions. The most frequent complication was related to electrode connectors. Pollack et al. (46) in their series of 300 patients reported that infection or cutaneous erosion occurred in 10 patients, breakage of lead connection in 7 patients, and stimulator repositioning in 5 patients. In another series (37), out of a total of 143 patients, lead migration occurred in 5 patients, infection in 4 patients, lead breakage in 2 patients, lead erosion in one patient, and intermittent function in one patient.

Stimulation-Related

Stimulation-related adverse effects depend on the exact location of the active electrode contact and the intensity of stimulation. The majority of these adverse effects can be reduced by either using another electrode contact or reducing the stimulation intensity. These adverse effects include eye lid closure, double vision, dystonic posturing, dysarthria, dyskinesias, paresthesia, limb and facial muscle spasms, depression, mood changes, visual disturbances, and pain. Occasionally nonspecific sensations like anxiety, panic, palpitations, nausea, and strange sensations can also occur. If these adverse effects persist, this usually indicates that the electrode is not in the ideal position.

MECHANISM OF ACTION

The exact mechanism of action of DBS is unknown. As the effects observed after stimulation are similar to those observed after ablation in the thalamus, GPi, and STN it was believed that DBS acts by suppressing neuronal activity and decreasing the output from the stimulated site. In addition, DBS of the GPi or pallidotomy produce similar changes in the cortical metabolic activity as measured by positron emission tomography (48,49). Electrophysiological studies such as those of Benazzouz et al. (50) reported that after 5 seconds of stimulation of the STN nucleus in rats at the usual parameters used in humans, the STN neurons were inhibited for several hundred seconds and the entopeduncular nucleus (corresponds to

GPi in humans) is strongly depressed and the GP (corresponds to GPe in humans) is excited. They believed that inhibition of the STN occurs due to local inhibitory effect of the high-frequency stimulation.

Although the above data might suggest that electrical stimulation inhibits neuronal activity and decreases neuronal output from the stimulated structure, other data support the hypothesis that electrical stimulation leads to increased output from the stimulated structure, suggesting that activation plays a role. Windels et al. (51) studied the effects of STN stimulation in rats and found that there were increased levels of glutamate suggesting activation of glutamatergic output from the STN. Hashimoto et al. (52) also demonstrated increased discharge rates of neurons in the GPi during chronic STN stimulation with resultant improvement in motor signs. In addition, it has been shown that there is an irregular pattern of neuronal activity present before stimulation, which changes to a tonic activation pattern of the GPi during STN stimulation. Also, Montgomery and Baker (53) used computer simulations that modeled the effect of different frequencies and regularity of neuronal activity. The simulations suggested that irregular activity in the neurons converging with other neurons could result in a loss of information transfer. They suggested that the therapeutic effect of DBS could be due to driving neurons at higher and perhaps more importantly at regular frequencies that result in improvement of the symptoms due to regularity of the neurons.

CONCLUSION

DBS of the thalamus is indicated for PD patients with medication-resistant tremor with minimal bradykinesia or rigidity. DBS of the GPi or STN is indicated for patients with motor fluctuations and dyskinesias. All cardinal signs and symptoms of PD improve with DBS of the GPi and STN. The PD medications can be reduced with DBS of the STN but not with DBS of the GPi. All these procedures have very low risk of morbidity, although device-related events could lead to repeat surgery in some patients.

REFERENCES

1. Fenelon F, Thiebant F. Resultats du traitement neurochirurgical d'une rigidte parkinsonienne par intervention striopallidale unilaterale. Rev Neurol 1950; 83:280.
2. Guiot BS. Traitment des mouvements anormaux par la coagulation pallidale. Rev Neurol 1953; 89:578.

3. Benabid AL, Pollak P, Louveau A, et al. Combined (thalamotomy and stimulation) stereotactic surgery of the VIM thalamic nucleus for bilateral Parkinson disease. Appl Neurophysiol 1987; 50:344–346.

4. Blond S, Siegfried J. Thalamic stimulation for the treatment of tremor and other movement disorders. Acta Neurochir Suppl 1991; 52:109–111.

5. Blond S, Caparros-Lefebvre D, Parker F, et al. Control of tremor and involuntary movement disorders by chronic stereotactic stimulation of the ventral intermediate thalamic nucleus. J Neurosurg 1992; 77:62–68.

6. Alesch F, Pinter MM, Helscher RJ, et al. Stimulation of the ventral intermediate thalamic nucleus in tremor dominated Parkinson's disease and essential tremor. Acta Neurochir 1995; 136:75–81.

7. Benabid AL, Pollak P, Goa D, et al. Chronic electrical stimulation of the ventralis intermedius nucleus of the thalamus as a treatment of movement disorders [see comments]. J Neurosurg 1996; 84:203–214.

8. Benabid AL, Pollak P, Hoffmann D, et al. Chronic high-frequency thalamic stimulation in Parkinson's disease. In: Koller WC, Paulson G, eds. Therapy of Parkinson's Disease. New York: Marcel Dekker, 1995:381–401.

9. Limousin P, Speelman JD, Gielen F, Janssens M. Multicentre European study of thalamic stimulation in parkinsonian and essential tremor. J Neurol Neurosurg Psychiatry 1999; 66:289–296.

10. Koller W, Pahwa R, Busenbark K, et al. High-frequency unilateral thalamic stimulation in the treatment of essential and parkinsonian tremor. Ann Neurol 1997; 42:292–299.

11. Ondo W, Jankovic J, Schwartz K, et al. Unilateral thalamic deep brain stimulation for refractory essential tremor and Parkinson's disease tremor. Neurology 1998; 51:1063–1069.

12. Pollak P, Benabid AL, Limousin P, Benazzouz A. Chronic intracerebral stimulation in Parkinson's disease. Adv Neurol 1997; 74:213–220.

13. Ondo W, Almaguer M, Jankovic J, Simpson RK. Thalamic deep brain stimulation: comparison between unilateral and bilateral placement. Arch Neurol 2001; 58:218–222.

14. Albanese A, Nordera GP, Caraceni T, Moro E. Long-term ventralis intermedius thalamic stimulation for parkinsonian tremor. Italian Registry for Neuromodulation in Movement Disorders. Adv Neurol. 1999; 80:631–634.

15. Kumar K, Kelly M, Toth C. Deep brain stimulation of the ventral intermediate nucleus of the thalamus for control of tremors in Parkinson's disease and essential tremor. Stereotact Funct Neurosurg 1999; 72:47–61.

16. Hariz MI, Shamsgovara P, Johansson F, et al. Tolerance and tremor rebound following long-term chronic thalamic stimulation for Parkinsonian and essential tremor. Stereotact Funct Neurosurg 1999; 72:208–218.

17. Lyons KE, Koller WC, Wilkinson SB, Pahwa R. Long term safety and efficacy of unilateral deep brain stimulation of the thalamus for parkinsonian tremor. J Neurol Neurosurg Psychiatry. 2001; 71:682–684.

18. Fogel W, Kronenbuerger M, Tronnier V, et al. Tremor rebound as a side-effect of thalamic stimulation for suppression of tremor (abstr). Mov Disord 1997; 13:139–140.
19. Villagra F, Lyons K, Koller W, et al. Lack of rebound effect on tremor in Parkinson's disease and essential tremor patients that have undergone VIM thalamic stimulation (abstr). Neurology 1996; 6:A372–A373.
20. Siegfried J, Lippitz B. Bilateral chronic electrostimulation of ventroposterolateral pallidum: a new therapeutic approach for alleviating all parkinsonian symptoms. Neurosurgery 1994; 85:1126–1129; discussion 1129–1130.
21. Siegfried J, Lippitz B. Chronic electrical stimulation of the VL-VPL complex and of the pallidum in the treatment of movement disorders: personal experience since 1982. Stereotact Funct Neurosurg 1994; 62:71–75.
22. Pahwa R, Wilkinson S, Smith D, et al. High-frequency stimulation of the globus pallidus for the treatment of Parkinson's disease. Neurology 1997; 49:249–253.
23. Hallett M, Litvan I. Evaluation of surgery for Parkinson's disease: a report of the Therapeutics and Technology Assessment Subcommittee of the American Academy of Neurology. The Task Force on Surgery for Parkinson's Disease. Neurology 1999; 53:1910–1921.
24. Kumar R, Lang AE, Rodriguez-Oroz MC, et al. Deep brain stimulation of the globus pallidus pars interna in advanced Parkinson's disease. Neurology, 2000; 55:S34–39.
25. The Deep Brain Stimulation for Parkinson's Disease Study Group. Deep-brain stimulation of the subthalamic nucleus or the pars interna of the globus pallidus in Parkinson's disease. N Engl J Med 2001; 345:956–963.
26. Ghika J, Villemure JG, Fankhauser H, et al. Efficiency and safety of bilateral contemporaneous pallidal stimulation (deep brain stimulation) in levodopa-responsive patients with Parkinson's disease with severe motor fluctuations: a 2-year follow-up review. J Neurosurg 1998; 89:713–718.
27. Bejjani B, Damier P, Arnulf I, et al. Pallidal stimulation for Parkinson's disease. Two targets? Neurology 1997; 49:1564–1569.
28. Krack P, Pollak P, Limousin P, et al. Opposite motor effects of pallidal stimulation in Parkinson's disease. Ann Neurol 1998; 43:180–192.
29. Krack P, Pollak P, Limousin P, et al. Inhibition of levodopa effects by internal pallidal stimulation. Mov Disord 1998; 13:648–652.
30. Carpenter M, Whittier J, Mettler F. Analysis of choreoid hyperkinesia in the rhesus monkey. J Comp Neurol 1950; 92:293–322.
31. Lozano AM. The subthalamic nucleus: myth and opportunities. Mov Disord 2001; 16:183–184.
32. Kumar R, Lozano AM, Sime E, et al. Comparative effects of unilateral and bilateral subthalamic nucleus deep brain stimulation. Neurology 1999; 53:561–566.
33. Kumar R, Lozano AM, Kim YJ, et al. Double-blind evaluation of subthalamic nucleus deep brain stimulation in advanced Parkinson's disease. Neurology 1998; 51:850–855.

34. Krack P, Pollak P, Limousin P, et al. Subthalamic nucleus or internal pallidal stimulation in young onset Parkinson's disease. Brain 1998; 121:451–457.

35. Burchiel KJ, Anderson VC, Favre J, Hammerstad JP. Comparison of pallidal and subthalamic nucleus deep brain stimulation for advanced Parkinson's disease: results of a randomized, blinded pilot study. Neurosurgery 1999; 45:1375–1382; discussion 1382–1384.

36. Moro E, Scerrati M, Romito LM, et al. Chronic subthalamic nucleus stimulation reduces medication requirements in Parkinson's disease. Neurology 1999; 53:85–90.

37. Bilateral deep brain stimulation (DBS) of the subthalamic nucleus (STN) or the globus pallidus interna (GPi) for treatment of advanced Parkinson's disease. Technologica MAP Suppl 2001; 1–8.

38. Rodriguez-Oroz MC, Gorospe A, Guridi J, et al. Bilateral deep brain stimulation of the subthalamic nucleus in Parkinson's disease. Neurology 2000; 55:S45–51.

39. Limousin P, Krack P, Pollak P, et al. Electrical stimulation of the subthalamic nucleus in advanced Parkinson's disease. N Engl J Med 1998; 339:1105–1111.

40. Kumar R, Lozano AM, Kim YJ, et al. Double-blind evaluation of subthalamic nucleus deep brain stimulation in advanced Parkinson's disease. Neurology 1998; 51:850–855.

41. Benabid AL, Krack PP, Benazzouz A, et al. Deep brain stimulation of the subthalamic nucleus for Parkinson's disease: methodologic aspects and clinical criteria. Neurology 2000; 55:S40–44.

42. Romito LM, Scerrati M, Contarino MF, et al. Long-term follow up of subthalamic nucleus stimulation in Parkinson's disease. Neurology 2002; 58:1546–1550.

43. Scotto di Luzio AE, Ammannati F, Marini P, et al. Which target for DBS in Parkinson's disease? Subthalamic nucleus versus globus pallidus internus. Neurol Sci 2001; 22:87–88.

44. Volkmann J, Allert N, Voges J, et al. Safety and efficacy of pallidal or subthalamic nucleus stimulation in advanced PD. Neurology 2001; 56:548–551.

45. Krause M, Fogel W, Heck A, et al. Deep brain stimulation for the treatment of Parkinson's disease: subthalamic nucleus versus globus pallidus internus. J Neurol Neurosurg Psychiatry 2001; 70:464–470.

46. Pollak P, Fraix V, Krack P, et al. Treatment results: Parkinson's disease. Mov Disord 2002; 17:S75–83.

47. Oh MY, Abosch A, Kim SH, et al. Long-term hardware-related complications of deep brain stimulation. Neurosurgery 2002; 50:1268–1274; discussion 1274–1276.

48. Limousin P, Greene J, Pollak P, et al. Changes in cerebral activity pattern due to subthalamic nucleus or internal pallidum stimulation in Parkinson's disease. Ann Neurol 1997; 42:283–291.

49. Davis KD, Taub E, Houle S, et al. Globus pallidus stimulation activates the cortical motor system during alleviation of parkinsonian symptoms. Nat Med 1997; 3:671–674.

50. Benazzouz A, Piallat B, Pollak P, Benabid AL. Responses of substantia nigra pars reticulata and globus pallidus complex to high frequency stimulation of the subthalamic nucleus in rats: electrophysiological data. Neurosci Lett 1995; 189:77–80.

51. Windels F, Bruet N, Poupard A, et al. Effects of high frequency stimulation of subthalamic nucleus on extracellular glutamate and GABA in substantia nigra and globus pallidus in the normal rat. Eur J Neurosci 2000; 12:4141 4146.

52. Hashimoto T, Elder C, DeLong M, Vitek J. Responses of pallidal neurons to electrical stimulation of the subthalamic nucleus is experimental primates. Mov Disord 2000; 15:31.

53. Montgomery EB, Jr, Baker KB. Mechanisms of deep brain stimulation and future technical developments. Neurol Res 2000; 22:259–266.

54. Gross C, Rougier A, Guehl D, et al. High-frequency stimulation of the globus pallidus internalis in Parkinson's disease: a study of seven cases. J Neurosurg 1997; 87:491–498.

55. Krack P, Pollak P, Limousin P, et al. Subthalamic nucleus or internal pallidal stimulation in young onset Parkinson's disease. Brain 1998; 121:451–457.

56. Kumar R, Lozano AM, Montgomery E, Lang AE. Pallidotomy and deep brain stimulation of the pallidum and subthalamic nucleus in advanced Parkinson's disease. Mov Disord 1998; 13:73–82.

57. Volkmann J, Sturm V, Weiss P, et al. Bilateral high-frequency stimulation of the internal globus pallidus in advanced Parkinson's disease. Ann Neurol 1998; 44:953–961.

58. Merello M, Nouzeilles MI, Kuzis G, et al. Unilateral radiofrequency lesion versus electrostimulation of posteroventral pallidum: a prospective randomized comparison. Mov Disord 1999; 14:50–56.

59. Molinuevo JL, Valldeoriola F, Tolosa E, et al. Levodopa withdrawal after bilateral subthalamic nucleus stimulation in advanced Parkinson disease. Arch Neurol 2000; 57:983–988.

60. Houeto JL, Damier P, Bejjani PB, et al. Subthalamic stimulation in Parkinson disease: a multidisciplinary approach. Arch Neurol. 2000; 57:461–465.

61. Thobois S, Mertens P, Guenot M, et al. Subthalamic nucleus stimulation in Parkinson's disease: clinical evaluation of 18 patients. J Neurol 2002; 249:529–534.

24

Neural Transplantation in Parkinson's Disease

Elmyra V. Encarnacion and Robert A. Hauser
University of South Florida and Tampa General Healthcare,
Tampa, Florida, U.S.A.

INTRODUCTION

Parkinson's disease (PD) is a chronic, degenerative disease characterized by a progressive loss of mesencephalic dopaminergic cells in the substantia nigra pars compacta (SNc) resulting in a loss of dopaminergic innervation to the striatum (caudate and putamen). Parkinsonian signs appear after approximately 50% of nigral cells are lost and striatal dopamine levels are reduced 80% (1). The administration of the dopamine precursor levodopa remains the cornerstone of long-term symptomatic medical management. Patients initially experience satisfactory improvement but as the disease progresses, the clinical response is frequently complicated by motor fluctuations and dyskinesias. Increased disability over time also arises in part due to nondopaminergic-responsive symptoms, including balance and cognitive dysfunction. Better treatments are needed to improve the long-term outcome of patients with PD. One approach is the transplantation of cells that might replace those that have been lost due to the disease process.

In the 1970s, Bjorklund et al. demonstrated that transplanted fetal catecholaminergic and cholinergic neurons can survive, extend processes, establish synaptic connections, and enhance the release of neurotransmitters

(2–5). Since that time, more than 300 PD patients have undergone cell transplantation under various clinical protocols. To date, insufficient clinical benefit has been demonstrated for this procedure for it to be made available as a therapeutic modality (6). New research is focusing on ways to improve the methodology of transplantation to provide meaningful clinical benefit for PD patients.

This chapter discusses the rationale for transplantation, results in animal models, results in human clinical trials, methodological issues, and prospects for the future.

RATIONALE

The basic principle underlying neural transplantation is tantalizingly simple. Functional restoration in the human brain should be achievable if lost or diseased neurons can be replaced by healthy ones (7). To be effective, transplanted cells must survive the procedure, establish lost connections, and function normally.

PD is a rational candidate for cell transplantation for several reasons:

1. PD is predominantly associated with a relatively well-defined and specific neuronal degeneration, specifically mesencephalic dopaminergic neurons.
2. The main anatomical target of degenerating neurons, the striatum, is well-defined and accessible to surgery (8).
3. Dopamine-replacement medications provide dramatic clinical benefits (9), thereby demonstrating the potential capacity of downstream response.
4. Animal models are available to test the safety, efficacy, and side effects of the procedure (10).

Commonly used animal models use 6-hydroxydopamine (6-OHDA) or 1-methyl-4-phenyl-1,2,3,6-tetrahydropyridine (MPTP) to create lesions in the dopaminergic pathways. These models have been proven to have good predictive value regarding the efficacy of potential new therapies (see Chapter 12).

6-OHDA is a specific neurotoxin for catecholaminergic neurons. In 1970, Ungerstedt and Arbuthnott showed that the dopamine agonist apomorphine induces contralateral turning and amphetamine induces ipsilateral turning in the unilateral 6-OHDA rat model (11). Denervation by 6-OHDA renders the lesioned side "supersensitive" to dopamine agonists, and the number of turns in a given time provides a quantitative assessment of the severity of the denervation. The ability of grafts transplanted into the lesioned side to reduce rotations in response to apomorphine or amphetamine reflects normalization of dopamine innervation.

MPTP was discovered when several drug abusers accidentally injected themselves with it and subsequently developed parkinsonian symptoms (12). MPTP administration has been shown to be toxic to dopamine neurons and produce parkinsonian signs in rodents and primates. Monkeys given MPTP unilaterally in the carotid artery or after systemic treatment show signs analagous to PD, including limb and head tremor, delayed initiation of movements, difficulty eating, and freezing (13,14). Improvement in parkinsonian signs can be used to evaluate the efficacy of transplantation in this model.

The discovery of animal models that mimic the cardinal features of PD allowed more rigorous preclinical evaluation of neural transplantation. However, these are static models that do not mirror the progression of PD or its pathogenic mechanisms. It is hoped that newer transgene models of PD will more accurately reflect both the pathogenic mechanisms and progressive nature of the human disease.

RESULTS IN ANIMAL MODELS

Fetal Mesencephalic Cells

Using 6-OHDA–lesioned rats, Perlow et al. (15) demonstrated in 1979 that rat fetal mesencephalic substantia nigra (SN) dopaminergic grafts implanted into the lateral ventricle adjacent to the caudate could establish appropriate functional input to the denervated adult caudate. The reduction in turning was significantly greater for rats transplanted with SN grafts compared to those transplanted with sciatic nerve grafts (controls). Histochemical studies revealed survival, growth, and proliferation of the fetal SN grafts, while control grafts degenerated. All but one SN graft survived without rejection for at least 2 months.

A few months later, Bjorklund and Stenevi (16) used the same model to demonstrate that transplantation of rat fetal SN into the dorsal surface of denervated striatum in adult rats resulted in a reduction of amphetamine-induced turning. Long-term cell survival (up to 7 months) was good, and there was growth of dopamine fibers into the striatum from the transplant. The number of fibers formed was proportional to the number of surviving transplanted neurons. In the case with the largest number of surviving transplanted neurons and the most extensive ingrowth of fibers to the striatum, there was gradual reversal and then complete elimination of amphetamine-induced turning.

Additional studies confirmed that rat embryonic SN implanted into denervated rat striatum can result in a substantial or complete recovery of ampetamine- and apomorphine-induced turning (17–20), and biochemical and histochemical studies demonstrated that the degree of recovery was proportional to the extent of dopamine restoration and nigrostriatal reinnervation (18–20). Similar results were obtained transplanting embryonic monkey SN grafts into MPTP-lesioned monkeys, as parkinsonian signs were ameliorated and graft survival, fiber outgrowth and graft-derived dopamine production were demonstrated (21–24).

Adrenal Medulla

The chromaffin cells of the adrenal medulla normally produce epinephrine and norepinephrine, and a small amount of dopamine. However, when separated from the overlying adrenal cortex and placed under the influence of corticosteroids, their metabolism is altered so that they produce increased amounts of dopamine (9).

When grafted to the lateral ventricle or into the striatum of 6-OHDA–lesioned rats, adrenal chromaffin cells attenuated apomorphine-induced turning but not contralateral sensorimotor inattention (25–27). The behavioral effects were limited and not as great in magnitude or duration as those observed with fetal SN grafts (28).

RESULTS IN HUMAN TRIALS

Adrenal Medulla

Ethical and immunological issues regarding the use of human fetal allografts resulted in a quest for alternative cells. Although the behavioral benefits of adrenal medullary tissue transplantation in animals were modest, early human investigations focused on transplantation of adrenal medulla cells.

Direct stereotactic implantation of autologous adrenal medullary tissue into the caudate (29) and putamen (30) failed to show long-term changes. Revising the surgical procedure by placing the adrenal grafts into the intraventricular surface of the right caudate, Madrazo et al. (31) in 1987 observed impressive, sustained improvements in two patients. Preoperatively, Patient 1 was wheelchair-bound and had bilateral rigidity, bradykinesia, resting tremor, and speech impairment. At 5 months postsurgery, he was reported to be speaking more clearly, ambulating and performing routine activities independently, and had less tremor and virtually no rigidity or akinesia on either side. Improvement persisted, and at 10 months, the patient visited the clinic independently, was playing soccer with his son, and was considering returning to work. Likewise, Patient 2, who was severely disabled prior to transplantation, exhibited impressive improvement at 3 months postsurgery, as he had no tremor, was ambulating independently, and was speaking clearly with almost normal facial expression (31). Both patients were able to discontinue antiparkinsonian medications postoperatively. Unfortunately, these results were not replicated by subsequent studies using the same techniques (32–34).

Goetz et al. (35) performed a multicenter trial utilizing the same procedure wherein 18 patients received unilateral adrenal medullary grafts into the right caudate. Evaluation at 6 months postsurgery revealed that the mean duration of on time increased from 48 to 75%, on time without dyskinesias increased from 27 to 59%, and off time decreased from 53 to 25%. Off Unified Parkinson's Disease Rating Scale (UPDRS) Activities of Daily Living (ADL) and Schwab and England scores showed significant improvement during off time. Off UPDRS motor subscale scores showed a trend toward improvement, while off Hoehn and Yahr scores did not change. Overall, the benefits observed in this study were quite modest compared to those of Madrazo et al. (31). Long-term evaluations found that benefits were maximal at 6 months and progressively and gradually declined thereafter with deterioration in most parameters by 18 months. Nonetheless, off UPDRS motor and ADL and Hoehn-Yahr scores were still statistically improved compared with baseline (36). Another study noted no benefits that could be ascribed to bilateral adrenal medulla graft placement (37).

Autopsy results from one patient whose performance level improved at 4 months postsurgery revealed necrotic adrenal tissue and no definite viable cells (38). Autopsy of another patient (who experienced marked and persistent benefit for 18 months) at 30 months postsurgery revealed that within the graft site there was a paucity of tyrosine hydroxylase (TH) immunoreactive (IR) cells, which lacked neurite extension into the host striatum (39). However, located lateral and ventral to the few surviving grafts was an enhanced fiber network of TH-IR terminals and processes, thought to represent sprouting by residual host dopaminergic neurons mediated by the host striatal response to injury (39). Similar observations have been noted in both rat (40) and monkey models (41–45). The poor survival of adrenal medullary grafts following transplantation suggests other factors are responsible for the clinical benefits observed. It has been hypothesized that the secretion of trophic factors from the graft or reactive host cells may be responsible for transplant-related functional improvement (39). However, these were uncontrolled studies, and some or all of the observed benefits could have been due to placebo effects or examiner or patient bias.

The use of adrenal autografts has been abandoned as only modest improvement was observed. Significant morbidity was associated with the surgery, including procedure-related deaths and medical and neuropsychiatric complications. The failure of adrenal cells to produce significant benefit caused investigators to turn again to fetal mesencephalic cells, as these had produced greater benefit in animal models.

Human Fetal Mesencephalic Cells

Lindvall et al. published a series of reports describing results in PD patients who received fetal mesencephalic cell transplants (46). The first report described two patients who received fetal grafts aged 7–9 weeks postconception (PC) unilaterally in the caudate and putamen. Patients received immunosuppression with cyclosporine, azothioprine, and steroids. Evaluation 6 months after surgery revealed no major therapeutic benefit in most outcome measures, but a small yet significant improvement in motor performance during off time, specifically in movement speed for pronation-supination, fist clenching, and foot lifting. There was no increase in the duration of levodopa benefit, and there was also no significant increase in fluorodopa (FD) uptake by positron emission tomography (PET) at the graft site (46).

Due to minimal benefit from the initial procedures, the same team performed subsequent transplantation studies under a modified protocol (implantation cannula was thinner, storage medium was a balanced PH-stable solution and not saline, time of storage was shorter, transplantation was solely in the putamen). In subsequently transplanted patients, there was a significant reduction in rigidity and bradykinesia, a significant decrease in off time and a reduction in the number of daily off periods (47–49). These benefits were maximal at 3–5 months (47,48) and were maintained through the first (48) and third year (49) postsurgery. Other investigations of unilateral intrastriatal fetal implantation with (50–52) or without (50,53,54) immunosuppression demonstrated similar effects on reducing disability in PD (50–55), with evidence of sustained clinical improvement as long as 46 months postsurgery (51). FD-PET assessments showed that grafts restored dopamine synthesis and storage in the grafted area (47,49–53,55), with evidence of survival even after 3 years (49). Unilateral transplantation provided benefit that was more pronounced on the side contralateral to transplantation, and thus investigations of bilateral transplantation were undertaken in an effort to increase clinical benefit.

Freeman et al. (56) noted significant improvement at 6 months postsurgery in patients who received bilateral grafts of tissue from embryos aged 6.5–9 weeks PC implanted into the posterior postcommisural putamen.

Improvements were seen in total UPDRS score during off time, in the Schwab and England disability score during off time, and in the percentage of on time with and without dyskinesias. FD-PET uptake increased bilaterally, with some patients attaining normal striatal FD uptake (56,57). Hauser et al. (58) reported results in six patients [including the four reported by Freeman et al. (56)], noting long-term benefits at clinical evaluations 12–24 months following surgery, including a significant reduction in off time, improved function in the off state, and increased on time without dyskinesias. All patients received immunosuppression, and FD uptake was significantly increased at 6 (48%) and 12 months (61%) (58). In other studies, bilateral implantation without immunosuppression also provided clinical benefit (51). In addition, sequential bilateral grafting demonstrated moderate to marked improvement after the second procedure and did not compromise the survival and function of either the first or second graft as assessed by FD-PET (59).

A retrospective review by Hagell et al. regarding bilateral putamenal transplantation studies (58–63) reported that FD-PET uptake increased from 55 to 107% at 10–23 months postsurgery for patients receiving tissue from three to five donors per putamen. These patients experienced a 30–40% overall improvement in off UPDRS motor scores and a 43–59% decrease in off time. A majority of patients also had a reduced need for antiparkinsonian medication (64). Patients with MPTP-induced parkinsonism also demonstrated substantial and sustained clinical improvement after bilateral graft implantation (65).

Freed et al. (66) performed the first double-blind, placebo-controlled trial using embryonic grafts aged 7–8 weeks PC, transplanted bilaterally into the putamen without immunosuppression. Evaluation at one year revealed significant improvement in off UPDRS motor and Schwab and England scores in subjects 60 years and younger, while the older group did not show any significant improvement as compared to the sham-surgery (control) group. At 5.5 years postsurgery, patients who demonstrated a good response to levodopa preoperatively also experienced significant improvement during off time postoperatively, regardless of age. The maximum postoperative benefit correlated with the preoperative "best on" levodopa response (66). Increased FD-PET uptake was detected after one year with no laterality (63) and was sustained for as long as 4 years after transplantation (67). Dystonia and dyskinesias occurred in 5 out of 33 patients who ultimately received transplants, even after levodopa was decreased or eliminated (63). Three of these five patients received deep brain stimulation of the globus pallidus interna (GPi) combined with medical treatment with a TH inhibitor and carbidopa/levodopa, while the other two received medication alone (66). Autopsy results from a patient who died 3 years after transplantation revealed surviving dopamine neurons in all transplant sites that contained neuromelanin granules that became more dense by 8 years after transplant (66). Each transplant site had dopamine-neuron outgrowth throughout the putamen (63). Another double-blind, controlled study is underway (68). Although some ethicists still challenge the idea of sham surgery (69,70), it seems clear that to expose a small number of patients to sham surgery in order to accurately assess safety and efficacy is preferable to exposing a large number of patients to a surgical treatment in which the safety and efficacy are largely unknown.

In summary, human clinical trials have shown that implanted embryonic dopaminergic neurons can exhibit short- and long-term survival as evidenced by increased FD-PET uptake. In most cases, symptomatic improvement has been observed during off periods, and the percentage of off time during the day decreased. Improved health-related quality of life and ability to resume full-time work has also been observed (71). Nonetheless, in spite of the significant symptomatic benefit that has been observed, the improvement is incomplete, both in the degree and pattern of functional recovery (6). Some patients have developed severe dyskinesias postoperatively.

ISSUES

Experience with fetal cell transplantation has suggested that many factors can affect the functional benefit derived from transplantation.

Maximizing Survival and Reinnervation

The Donor

Age. TH-IR neurons first appear in the subventricular layer at 5.5–6.5 weeks PC, while neuritic processes are first identified at 8 weeks PC and reach the striatum at 9 weeks (8,9). The optimal time for grafting is between the time when dopamine-containing cells first appear and prior to their extension of neuritic process. This time is between 5.5 and 8 weeks postconception for suspension grafts, and 6.5–9 weeks postconception for solid grafts (8,9).

Spontaneous vs. Elective Abortion. Fetal nigral tissue from elective abortions is preferable to tissue from spontaneous abortions because tissue from spontaneous abortions may contain genetic or central nervous system (CNS) defects, infections, nonviable cells, and disrupted structure, thereby providing low-quality tissue and making staging and dissection difficult (8). Relatively few spontaneous abortions occur during the optimal time for tissue transplantation.

Volumetric Issues

The amount of transplanted tissue has been variable at each center, and outcomes from clinical trials and autopsy studies have shown that to produce a clinical effect, a minimum number of neurons is needed to survive grafting. Approximately 100,000 surviving grafted dopamine neurons per putamen may be sufficient to produce clinical benefit (64). The survival of embryonic neurons after grafting is only 5–20% in both animal experiments and clinical trials (5). This makes it difficult to achieve a large number of surviving transplanted neurons and is a limiting factor in neural transplantation.

It has been estimated that mesencephalic tissue from at least three to four human embryos per side are needed to induce a therapeutically significant improvement (5). Nguyen et al. (62) noted a difference in clinical outcome after 2 years comparing patients receiving bilateral implants from 2–3 embryos (1–1.5 per putamen) to those patients receiving 6 embryos (3 per putamen). Those who received 2–3 donors showed only mild benefit, with a 6% improvement in off UPDRS motor scores and a 15% increase in off time. Those who received 6 embryos exhibited a 33% improvement in off UPDRS motor scores and a 66% decrease in off time (62). Overall results suggest that enhanced functional recovery can be better achieved by a larger number of transplanted cells.

Transplantation Technique

The choice of medium for tissue dissection and separation is potentially important, and special media have now been proposed for storage instead of the glucose-saline solution used in the past (71).

In human trials, both solid (50,51,53,56,58) and suspension (46–49) grafts have been used with apparent functional benefit. Clarkson and Freed (72) conducted a retrospective analysis of 35 patients and characterized the clinical benefits as none, mild, or moderate. They concluded that recipients of solid grafts experienced greater improvement in motor function and were able to reduce their levodopa dose more than the cell suspension groups (38% vs. 8%) (72), suggesting that solid grafts produce better outcome than suspension grafts. Forceful titrations through a pipette tip until a single cell suspension is obtained may cause mechanical injury that can result in irreversible damage to embryonic cells (73).

A delay between cannula insertion and the injection of cells into the striatum may maximize the number of surviving neurons; a 1- or 3-hour delay resulted in two to three times the number of surviving cells, while a 20-minute delay had no effect (74).

Autopsy results have shown that the territory of reinnervation surrounding graft deposits is between 2.5 and 7 mm (75,76). This suggests it is necessary to transplant cells at a 5 mm interval in three-dimensional space.

Cytoprotection

Animal studies have demonstrated that a majority of grafted neurons die within the first week (77–80) after transplantation, and neuronal death occurs as early as within 24 hours (81) to as late as the second week after transplantation (82). Apoptosis or programmed cell death (PCD) is a process wherein a cell dies through activation of genetically determined processes. Apoptosis appears to be the predominant mechanism of cell death in transplanted neurons. Activation of caspases initiates a cascade of events that lead to apoptosis. Conversely, growth factors have a protective effect on neurons (83). Pretreatment of neural grafts with caspase inhibitors and growth factors may reduce apoptosis and enhance survival; the combination may also act synergistically against PCD (83).

Oxidative stress and free radical formation also contribute to PCD. Graft treatment with antioxidants (84) and with lazaroids, compounds that inhibit the radical-mediated process of lipid peroxidation, have also been noted to improve survival (85). Neuronal injury is commonly associated with sustained elevation of intracellular calcium, and the addition of flunarizine, a calcium channel antagonist, has been shown to be protective against oxidative stress and lipid peroxidation in vitro (86).

Immunosuppression

The brain has been considered an immunologically privileged site due to the presence of the blood-brain barrier and poorly developed lymphatic system (87,88). However, some investigators have noted that the CNS is relatively immunologically responsive, and this may significantly threaten intracerebral graft survival (89–93). The presence of immune markers for microglia, macrophages, and B and T cells within the grafted region 18 months postsurgery has been reported, but the significance of this immunological response is unknown (58). In human trials, both immunosuppressed and nonimmunosuppressed patients have shown clinical benefit after transplantation. Continued benefit and increased FD uptake on PET have been observed from 6 to 12 months after withdrawal of immunosuppressive drugs (58) and up to 4 years without immunosuppression (67). The use of encapsulated cells for transplantation can provide an immunoprotective barrier (94) but allow nutrients to pass. Microcarrier beads cotransplanted with cells may provide protection by establishing a matrix for the cells to attach to and grow in a cell culture (95).

Location of Graft

Caudate vs. Putamen. Rat studies have demonstrated that dopamine in the striatal complex and nucleus accumbens subserves various types of behavior, and nigral transplants placed in various parts of the forebrain have a strong regional specificity of function (96,97). In humans, the putamen is most important for motor function (98,99) and is associated with the most extensive dopamine depletion in PD (100). The posterior or postcommissural putamen is the most crucial striatal region for nigral grafting (101). There is no clear FD-PET evidence for survival of dopaminergic grafts in the caudate, as the conditions for survival may be more favorable in the putamen (6).

Unilateral vs. Bilateral. Most studies have noted more clinical benefit with bilateral grafts, correlating with increased FD-PET uptake on both sides.

Alternative Target Areas. Grafting solely in the striatum, whether unilateral or bilateral, does not reinnervate the other structures such as the substantia nigra or subthlamic nucleus (STN). Therefore, intrastriatal transplantation fails to reconstruct the basal ganglia circuitry. One study of intrastriatal and intranigral graft implantation (double grafts) resulted in numerous TH-IR axons from the SN grafts, which reinnervated the ipsilateral striatum. This resulted in not only a greater striatal innervation, but also a faster and more complete rotational recovery to an amphetamine challenge compared to standard intrastriatal grafts (102). Similarly, one study demonstrated that intrastriatal, intranigral, and intrasubthalamic nucleus dopaminergic transplants resulted in improvement of complex sensorimotor behavior in hemiparkinsonian rats with evidence of dense TH-IR cells and neuritic outgrowth from all three grafted regions (103).

Age of Recipient

In aged rats, implanted grafts have been noted to be smaller and less effective, and neuronal survival significantly diminished (104,105) as compared to transplantation in younger rats. Symptomatic benefit was more delayed following surgery and no significant improvement in off UPDRS motor and Schwab and England scores was seen in older subjects compared to younger subjects in the double-blind controlled study after one year postsurgery (63). In contrast, some investigators found that clinical benefit did not correlate with age (72).

Alternative Cells

Human fetal neurons have been used to test "proof of principle" that neural transplantation is feasible and can provide clinical benefit. New cells are being considered for possible testing and others are in development. Greater clinical benefit is the primary goal.

Carotid Cell Bodies

Carotid body cells are derived from the neural crest and have the highest dopamine content in the body. Intrastriatal grafting of these cells in 6-OHDA lesioned rats resulted in complete disappearance of motor asymmetries and deficits in sensorimotor orientation (106). This functional recovery started within a few days postsurgery and progressively increased during the 3-month study. The behavioral effects were correlated with long-term survival of the glomus cells in the host tissue, where they retained their ability to secrete dopamine and were organized in clusters containing fibers extending outside the graft (106). There are no trials to date of carotid cell bodies transplantation in humans.

Sertoli Cells and Teratocarcinoma

Sertoli cells secrete a wide variety of nutritive, trophic, regulatory, and immunosuppressive factors. Transplantation of rat and porcine Sertoli cells survived in a normal rat brain without immunosuppression (107). Cotransplantation of these cells with dopamine fetal neural cells in parkinsonian rats improved parkinsonian features significantly and enhanced the survival and fiber outgrowth of the transplanted neurons (108).

Teratocarcinoma is a malignant tumor that contains a variety of parenchymal cell types that arise from totipotential cells and are principally found in the gonads. Neurons from human teratocarcinoma (hNT) were implanted alone or in combination with rat Sertoli cells; hNT cells cotransplanted with Sertoli cells showed increased graft survival and were associated with an increase in graft size and fewer microglia, suggesting persistent immunosuppressive effects of Sertoli cells (109). Neural transplantation of hNT into ischemic rats has been shown to produce amelioration of behavioral symptoms (110), but intrastriatal and intranigral transplantation of hNT neurons in 6-OHDA rats showed a low number of TH-IR neurons, which was not sufficient to produce significant functional recovery (111).

Porcine Cells

Intrastriatal implantation of embryonic porcine mesencephalic grafts in immunosuppressed 6-OHDA–lesioned rats resulted in a significant, sustained reversal of amphetamine-induced turning (113). Histological analyses showed graft survival and fiber outgrowth with immunosuppression (113,114).

An initial open-label study of 10 patients who received unilateral intrastriatal transplantation demonstrated no major complications. Off UPDRS scores at 12 months improved 19% and in several patients improved more than 30% (115). A double-blind, randomized, controlled study of bilateral transplantation into the caudate and putamen (with immunosuppression) demonstrated a 25% and a 22% mean improvement of off total UPDRS score in the transplant and control groups, respectively, at 18 months postsurgery ($p = 0.599$). There were no differences seen in change in off time. FD-PET showed no changes 12 months postsurgery. Based on this study, there is no evidence that porcine cell transplantation has clinical efficacy in PD patients (116). Autopsy results of one patient from the initial open-label study at 7 months demonstrated survival of 642 surviving porcine TH neurons, with extensive growth of porcine axons within the grafts and a large number of porcine axons extending from the graft sites into the host striatum (117). Immunological concerns and risk of viral transfer still needs to clarified.

Retinal Cells

Human retinal pigment cells (hRPE) are derived from the inner layer of the neural retina located between the photoreceptors and choriocapillaries (118). They also synthesize and secrete dopamine (119) and secrete several trophic factors (120). Animal studies have shown that intrastriatal implantation of these cells on microcarriers into 6-OHDA rats reduced apomorphine-induced turning (119,121) and behavioral deficits were reversed in MPTP-lesioned monkeys (122,123) with minimal host immune response (124). An open-label study of the unilateral intrastriatal transplantation of hRPE on microcarriers (Spheramine) in 6 patients without immunosuppression showed that off UPDRS motor scores improved 33% at 6 months, 42% at 9 months, and 44% at 12 months postsurgery. Follow-up at 15 months showed continued clinical efficacy with a 44% improvement in off UPDRS motor scores. Bilateral improvement was seen, with greater effect on the contralateral side. There was a 37–53% reduction in off time, and half of the patients had lower Dyskinesia Rating Scale scores than at baseline (124). Double-blind studies are underway.

Stem Cells

Stem cells (SCs) are multipotential precursor cells that have the capability to self-replicate under environmental stimulation. Various stem cell types have been isolated from mice, including adult and fetal neural SCs, lineage-restricted precursor cells, neural crest SCs, embryonic cells, embryonic carcinoma cells, and immortalized multipotent cell lines (126). Human fetal and adult neural SCs, lineage-restricted precursor cells, and embryonic cells have also been isolated (126). In vitro methods have recently been developed that allow neuronal growth and differentiation from SCs. Transplantation of these cells in rats has demonstrated that they can migrate and integrate into the neural networks and reconstitute the three neural lineages, namely neurons, astrocytes, and oligodendrocytes.

Proposed therapeutic strategies for cell replacement in PD include the use of embryonic mesencephalic progenitors (127,128), neural SCs (129–131), and engineered neural SCs ready to differentiate into dopaminergic neurons (132) and embryonic SCs (133,134) that can produce growth factors (135). Implementation and testing of these proposed strategies is limited by the poor survival of dopaminergic neurons (136). The oncogenic potential or "tumorigenesis" of SCs needs to be addressed further.

THE FUTURE

PD is a chronic, degenerative disease characterized mainly by dopamine depletion in the nigrostriatal system. Cell transplantation has the potential of restoring function in PD patients by replacing lost neurons. After two decades of research, there is much hope, but no transplantation strategy has yet been proven to provide PD patients consistent and meaningful benefit. However, the obstacles to achieving this goal have become more clearly defined. New cells are being developed and tested in animal models. Some of these are genetically modified to increase their own survival or to help protect host neurons. There is great hope that stem cells may be able to migrate to areas of injury or degeneration, transform into multiple lost cell types, and restore normal neuronal function. Transgene animal models may be helpful to predict long-term outcome following transplantation. Double-blind clinical trials have now become accepted as a means of clearly defining the safety and efficacy of transplantation.

REFERENCES

1. Riederer P, Wuketich S. Time course of nigrostriatal degeneration in Parkinson's disease. J Neural Transm Park Dis Dement Sect 38:277–301, 1976.

2. Bjorklund A, Kromer LF, Stenevi U. Cholinergic reinnervation of the rat hippocampus by septal implants is stimulated by perforant path lesion. Brain Res 173:57–64, 1979.

3. Bjorklund A, Stenevi U. Reformation of the severed septohippocampal cholinergic pathway in the adult rat by transplanted septal neurons. Cell Tissue Res 85:289, 1977.

4. Bjorklund A, Stenevi U. Reconstruction of the nigrostriatal dopamine pathway by intracerebral nigral transplants. Brain Res 177:555–560, 1979.

5. Bjorklund A, Stenevi U, Svendgaard NA. Growth of transplanted monoaminergic neurons into the adult hippocampus along the perforant path. Nature 262:787, 1976.

6. Lindvall O. Neural transplantation: can we improve the symptomatic relief? Parkinson's Dis Advances Neurol (80).635–649, 1999.

7. Lindvall O. Neural transplantation in Parkinson's Disease. In: Novartis Foundation Symposium. Neural Transplantation in Neurodegenerative Disease: Current Status and New Directions. Chichester, NY: John Wiley & Sons, Ltd, 2000, pp 110–128.

8. Bjorklund A. Cell replacement strategies for neurodegenerative disorders. In: Novartis Foundation Symposium. Neural Transplantation in Neurodegenerative Disease: Current Status and New Directions. Chichester, NY: John Wiley & Sons, Ltd, 2000, pp 7–20.

9. Olanow CW, Kordower JH, Freeman TB. Fetal nigral transplantation as a therapy for Parkinson's disease. Trends Neurosci 19:102–109, 1996.

10. Hauser RA, Olanow CW. Neural transplantation. In: Jankovic T, Tolosa E, eds. Parkinson's Disease and Movement Disorders. Baltimore: Williams & Wilkins, 1992, pp 549–568.

11. Ungerstedt U, Arbuthnott GW. Quantitative recording of rotational behavior in rats after 6-hydroxy-dopamine lesions of the nigrostriatal dopamine system. Brain Res 24(3):485–493, 1970.

12. Langston JW, Ballard P, Tetrud JW, Irwin I. Chronic Parkinsonism in humans due to a product of meperidine-analog synthesis. Science 219(4587):979–980, 1983.

13. Bakay RAE, Barrow DL, Fiandaca MS, et al. Biochemical and behavioral correction of MPTP Parkinsonian-like syndrome by fetal cell transplantation. Ann NY Acad Sci 495:623–640, 1987.

14. Bankiewicz KS, Plunkett RJ, Jacobowitz DM, et al. The effect of fetal mesencephalon implants on primate MPTP-induced parkinsonism. J Neurosurg 72:231–244, 1990.

15. Perlow MJ, Freed WJ, Hoffer BJ, Wyatt RJ. Brain grafts reduce motor abnormalities produced by destruction of nigrostriatal dopamine system. Science 204:643–647, 1979.

16. Bjorklund A, Stenevi U. Reconstruction of the nigrostriatal dopamine pathway by intracerebral transplants. Brain Res 177:555–560, 1979.

17. Dunnett SB, Bjorklund A, Stenevi U, Iversen SD. Behavioral recovery following transplantation of substantia nigra in rats subjected to 6-OHDA

lesions of the nigrostriatal pathway. I. Unilateral lesions. Brain Res 215:147–161, 1981.

18. Bjorklund A, Dunnett SB, Stenevi U, Lewis ME, Iversen SD. Reinnervation of the denervated striatum by substantia nigra transplants: functional consequences as revealed by pharmacological and sensorimotor testing. Brain Res 199:307–333, 1980.

19. Freed WJ, Perlow MJ, Karoum F, et al. Restoration of dopaminergic function by grafting of fetal rat substantia nigra to the caudate nucleus: long-term behavioral, biochemical and histochemical studies. Ann Neurol 8:510–519, 1980.

20. Dunnett SB, Hernandez TD, Summerfield A, Jones JH, Arbuthott G. Graft-derived recovery from 6-OHDA lesions: specificity of ventral mesencephalic graft tissue. Exp. Brain Res 71:411–424, 1988.

21. Bakay RAE, Barrow DL, Fiandaca MS, et al. Biochemical and behavioral correction of MPTP-Parkinson-like syndrome by fetal cell transplantation. Ann NY Acad Sci 495:623–640, 1987.

22. Redmond DE, Sladek JR, Roth RH. Fetal neuronal grafts in monkeys given MPTP. Lancet 1:1125–1127, 1986.

23. Sladek JR Jr, Collier TC, Haber SN, et al. Survival and growth of fetal catecholamine neurons transplanted into the primate brain. Brain Res Bull 17:809–817, 1986.

24. Fine A, Hunt SB, Oertel WH, et al. Transplantation of embryonic dopaminergic neurons to the corpus striatum of marmosets rendered parkinsonian by 1-methyl-4-phenyl-1,2,3,6-tetrahydropyridine. In: Gash DM, Sladek JR, eds. Transplantation into the Mammalian CNS. Prog Brain Res 78:479–490, 1988.

25. Freed WJ, Morihisa JM, Spoor E, et al. Transplanted adrenal chromaffin cells in rat brain reduce lesion-induced rotational behavior. Nature 292:351–352, 1981.

26. Freed WJ, Cannon-Spoor HE, Krauthmer E. Intrastriatal adrenal medulla grafts in rats: long-term survival and behavioral effects. J Neurosurg 65:664–670, 1986.

27. Stromberg I, Herrera-Marschitz M, Ungerstedt U, et al. Chronic implants of chromaffin tissue into the dopamine-denervated striatum. Effects of NGF on graft survival, fiber growth and rotational behavior. Exp Brain Res 60:335–349, 1985.

28. Herrera-Marschitz M, Stromberg I, Olsson D, et al. Adrenal medullary implants in the dopamine-denervated rat striatum. II, Acute behavior as a function of graft amount and location and its modulation by neuroleptics. Brain Res 297:53–61, 1984.

29. Backlund EO, Granberg PO, Hamberger B, et al. Transplantation of adrenal medullary tissue to striatum in parkinsonism. J Neurosurg 62:169–173, 1985.

30. Lindvall O, Backlund E, Farde L, et al. Transplantation in Parkinson's disease: two case of adrenal medullary grafts to the putamen. Ann Neurol 22:457–468, 1987.

31. Madrazo I, Drucker-Colin R, Diaz V, et al. Open microsurgical autografts of adrenal medulla to right caudate nucleus in 2 patients with intractable Parkinson's disease. N Engl J Med 316:831–834, 1987.

32. Penn RD, Christopher CG, Tanner CM, et al. The adrenal medullary transplant operation for Parkinson's disease: Clinical observations in five patients. Neurosurgery 22(6):999–1004, 1988.

33. Kelly PJ, Ahlskog JE, Van Herdeen JA, et al. Adrenal medullary autograft transplantation into the striatum of patient's with Parkinson's disease. Mayo Clin Proc 64:282–290, 1989.

34. Ahlskog JE, Kelly PJ, Van Herdeen JA, et al. Adrenal medullary transplantation into the brain for treatment of Parkinson's disease: clinical outcome and neurochemical studies. Mayo Clin Proc 65:305–328, 1990.

35. Goetz CG, Olanow CW, Koller WC, et al. Multicenter study of autologous adrenal medullary transplantation to the corpus striatum in patients with advanced Parkinson's disease. N Eng J Med 320:337–341, 1989.

36. Olanow CW, Koller W, Goetz CG, et al. Autologous transplantation of adrenal medulla in Parkinson's disease. Arch Neurol 47:1286–1289, 1990.

37. Apuzzo MLJ, Neal JH, Waters CH, et al. Utilization of unilateral and bilateral stereotactically placed adrenomedullary-striatal autografts in parkinsonian humans: rationale, techniques, and observations. Neurosurgery 26(5):746–757, 1990.

38. Peterson DI, Price ML, Small CS. Autopsy findings in a patient who had an adrenal-to-brain transplant for Parkinson's disease. Neurology 39:235–238, 1989.

39. Kordower JH, Cochran E, Penn RD, Goetz CG. Putative chromaffin cell survival and enhanced host-derived TH-fiber innervation following a functional adrenal medulla autograft for Parkinson's disease. Ann Neurol 29:405–412, 1991.

40. Bohn C, Cupit L, Marciano F, et al. Adrenal medulla grafts enhance recovery of striatal dopaminergic fibers. Science 237:913–916, 1987.

41. Bankiewicz KS, Plunket RJ, Kopin IJ, et al. Transient behavioral recovery in hemiparkinsonian primates after adrenal medullary allografts. Prog Brain Res 78:543–550, 1988.

42. Fiandaca MS, Kordower JH, Jiao S-S, et al. Adrenal medullary autografts into the basal ganglia of Cebus monkeys: injury-induced regeneration. Exp Neurol 102:427–442, 1988.

43. Kordower JH, Fiandaca MS, Niotter MFD, et al. Peripheral nerve provides NGF-like trophic support for grafted Rhesus adrenal chromaffin cells. J Neurosurg 73:418–428, 1990.

44. Bankiewicz KS, Plunkett RJ, Jacobowitz DM, et al. Fetal nondopaminergic neural implants in parkinsonian primates: histochemical and behavioral studies. J Neurosurg 72:231–244, 1990.

45. Plunkett RJ, Bankiewicz KS, Cummings AC, et al. Evaluation of hemiparkinsonism monkeys after adrenal medullary autografting or cavitation alone. J Neurosurg 73:918 926, 1990.

46. Lindvall O, Rehncrona S, Brundin P, et al. Human fetal dopamine neurons grafted into the striatum in two patients with severe Parkinson's disease. A detailed account of methodology and a 6-month follow-up. Arch Neuro 46:615–631, 1989.
47. Lindvall O, Brundin P, Widner H, et al. Grafts of fetal dopamine neurons and improve motor function in Parkinson's disease. Science 247:574–577, 1990.
48. Lindvall O, Widner H, Rehncrona S, et al. Transplantation of fetal dopamine neurons in Parkinson's disease: one-year clinical and neurophysiological observations in two patients with putaminal implants. Ann Neurol 35:172–180, 1992.
49. Lindvall O, Sawle G, Widner H, et al. Evidence for long-term survival and function of dopaminergic grafts in progressive Parkinson's disease. Ann Neurol 35:172–180, 1994.
50. Freed CR, Breeze RE, Rosenberg NL, et al. Survival of implanted fetal dopamine cells and neurologic improvement 12 to 46 months after transplantation for Parkinson's disease. N Engl J Med 327:1549–1555, 1992.
51. Spencer DD, Robbins RJ, Naftolin F, et al. Unilateral transplantation of human fetal mesencephalic tissue into the caudate nucleus of patients with Parkinson's disease. N Engl J Med 327 (22):1521–1548, 1992.
52. Peschanski M, Defer G, Nguyen JP, et al. Bilateral motor improvement and alteration of L-dopa effect in two patients with Parkinson's disease following intrastriatal trrasnplantation of foetal ventral mesencephalon. Brain 117:487–499, 1994.
53. Freed CR, Breeze RE, Rosenberg NL, et al. Transplantation of human fetal dopamine cells for Parkinson's disease: Results at 1 year. Arch Neurol 47:505–512, 1990.
54. Henderson BTH, Clough CG, Hughes TC, et al. Implantation of human fetal ventral mesencephalon to right caudate nucleus in advanced Parkinson's disease. Arch Neurol 48:822–827, 1991.
55. Wenning GK, Odin P, Morrish P, et al. Short- and long-term survival and function of unilateral intrastriatal dopaminergic grafts in Parkinson's disease. Ann Neurol 42:95–107, 1997.
56. Freeman TB, Olanow CW, Hauser RA, et al. Bilateral fetal nigral transplantation into the postcommisural putamen as a treatment for Parkinson's disease. Ann Neurol 38:379–388, 1995.
57. Olanow CW, Kordower JH, Freeman TB. Fetal nigral transplantation as a therapy for Parkinson's disease. Trends Neurosci 19:102–109, 1996.
58. Hauser RA, Freeman TB, Snow BJ, et al. Long-term evaluation of bilateral fetal nigral transplantation in Parkinson's Disease. Arch Neurol 56:179–197, 1999.
59. Haggell P, Schrag A, Piccini P, et al. Sequential bilateral transplantation in Parkinson's disease: effects of second graft. Brain 122:1121–1132, 1999.
60. Brundin P, Pogarell O, Hagell P, et al. Bilateral caudate and putamen grafts of embryonic mesencephalic tissue treated with lazaroids in Parkinson's disease. Brain 123:1380–1390, 2000.

61. Mendez I, Dagher A, Hong M, et al. Enhancement of survival of stored dopaminergic cells and promotion of graft survival by exposure of human fetal nigral tissue to glial cell line-derived neurotrophic factor in patients with Parkinson's disease. Report of two cases and technical considerations. J Neurosurg 92:863–869, 2000.

62. Nguyen JP, Remy P, Palfi S, et al. Bilateral intrastriatal grafts of fetal mesencephalic neurons in Parkinson's disease: long-term results in 9 patients. Mov Disord 15:53–54, 2000.

63. Freed CR, Greene PE, Breeze RE, et al. Transplantation of embryonic dopamine neurons for severe Parkinson's disease. N Engl J Med 344:710–719, 2001.

64. Hagell P, Brundin P. Cell survival and clinical outcomes following intrastriatal transplantation in Parkinson's disease. J Neuropath Exp Neurol 60(8), 2001.

65. Widner H, Tetrud J, Rehncrona S, et al. Bilateral fetal mesencephalic grafting in two patients with parkinsonism induced by 1-methyl-4-phenyl-1, 2,3,6-tetrahydropyridine (MPTP). N Engl J Med 327:1556–1563, 1992.

66. Freed CR, Breeze RE, DeMasters BK, et al. Transplants of embryonic dopamine cells show progressive histologic maturation for at least 8 years and improve signs of Parkinson up to the maximum benefit of 1-dopa preoperatively. Abstract American Academy of Neurology, Annual Conference, S31.006, 2002.

67. Pillai V, Ma Y, Dhawan V, et al. Pet imaging in Parkinson's disease four years following embryonic dopamine cell transplantation. Abstract American Academy of Neurology, Annual Conference, S31.005, 2002.

68. Freeman TB, Vawter DE, Leaverton PE, et al. Use of placebo surgery in controlled trails of a cellular-based therapy for Parkinson's disease. N Engl J Med 341:988–991, 1999.

69. Macklin R. The ethical problems with sham surgery in clinical research. N Engl J Med 341:992–996, 1999.

70. Dekkers W, Boer G. Sham neurosurgery in patients with Parkinson's disease: Is it morally acceptable?. J Med Ethics 271:151–156, 2001.

71. Brundin P, Karlsson J, Emgard M, et al. Improving the survival of grafted dopaminergic neurons: a review over current approaches. Cell Transplant 9:179–195, 2000.

72. Clarkson ED, Freed CR. Development of fetal neural transplantation as a treatment for Parkinson's disease. Life Sci 65(23):2427–2437, 1999.

73. Barker RA, Fricker RA, Abrous DN, et al. A comparative study of preparation techniques for improving the viability of nigral grafts using vital stains, in vitro cultures, and in vivo grafts. Cell Transplant 4:173–200, 1995.

74. Sinclair SR, Fawcett JW, Dunnett SB. Delayed implantation of nigral grafts improves survival of dopamine neurons and rate of functional recovery. Neuroreport 10:1263–1267, 1999.

75. Kordower JH, Freeman TB, Snow BJ, et al. Neuropathological evidence of graft survival and striatal reinnervation after transplantation of fetal

mesencephalic tissue in a patient with Parkinson's disease. N Engl J Med 332:1118–1124, 1995.

76. Kordower JH, Rosenstein JM, Collier T, et al. Functional fetal nigral grafts in a patient with Parkinson's disease. Comp Neurol 379:203–230, 1996.

77. Barker RA, Dunnett SB, Faissner A, et al. The time course of loss of dopaminergic neurons and the gliotic reaction surrounding grafts of embryonic mesencephalon to the striatum. Exp Neurol 141:79–93, 1996.

78. Duan WM, Widner H, Brundin P. Temporal pattern of host responses against intrastriatal grafts of syngeneic, allogeniec or xenogeneic embryonic neuronal tissue in rats. Exp Brain Res 104:227–242, 1995.

79. Emgard M, Karlsson J, Hansson O, et al. Patterns of cell death and dopaminergic neuron survival in intrstriatal nigral grafts. Exp Neurol 160:279–288, 1999.

80. Nikkah G, Olsson M, Eberhard J, et al. A microtransplantation approach for cell suspension grafting in the rat Parkinson model: a detailed account of the methodology. Neuroscience 63:57–72, 1994.

81. Zawada WM, Zastrow DJ, Clarkson ED, et al. Growth factors improve immediate survival of embryonic dopamine neurons after transplantation into rats. Brain Res 786:96–103, 1998.

82. Mahalik TJ, Hahn WE, Clayton GH, Owens GP. Programmed cell death in developing grafts of fetal substantia nigra. Exp Neurol 129:27–36, 1994.

83. Boonman Z, Isacson O. Apoptosis in neuronal development and transplantation: role of caspases and trophic factors. Exp Neurol 156:1–15, 1999.

84. Nakao N, Frodl Em, Widner H, et al. Overexpressing CU/Zn superoxide dismutase enhances survival of transplanted neurons in rat model of Parkinson's disease. Nat Med 1:226–231, 1995.

85. Nakao N, Frodl M, Duan WM, et al. Lazaroids improve the survival of grafted rat embryonic dopamine neurons. Proc Natl Acad Sci USA 91:12408–12412, 1994.

86. Takei M, Hiramatsu M, Mori A. Inhibitory effects of calcium antagonists on mitochondrial swelling induced by lipid peroxidation or arachidonic acid in the rat brain in vitro. Neurochem Res 19:1199–1206, 1994.

87. Braker CF, Billingaham RE. Immunologically privileged sites. Adv Immunol 25:1–54, 1977.

88. Scheinberg LC, Edelman FL, Levy AW. Is the brain an immunologically privileged site? Arch Neurol 11:248–264, 1964.

89. Finsen BR, Sorensen T, Gonzales B, et al. Immunological reactions to neural grafts in the central nervous system. Restor Neurol Neurosci 2:271–282, 1991.

90. Hudson JL, Hoffman A, Sromberg I, et al. Allogeneic grafts of fetal dopamine neurons: behavioral indices of immunological interactions. Neurosci Lett 171:32–36, 1994.

91. Sloan DJ, Wood MJ, Charlton HM. The immune response to intracerebral grafts. Trends Neurosci 14:341–346, 1991.

92. Widner H, Brundin P. Immunological aspects of grafting in the mammalian central nervous system: a review and speculative synthesis. Brain Res Rev 13:287–324, 1988.

93. Widner H, Brundin P, Bjorklund A, Moller E. Survival and immunogenicity of dissociated allogeneic fetal neural dopamine-rich grafts when implanted into the brains of adult mice. Exp Brain Res 76:187–197, 1989.

94. Emerich DF, Winn SR, Christenson L, et al. A novel approach to neural transplantation in Parkinson's disease: use of a polymer-encapsulated cell therapy. Neurosci Biobehav Rev 16:437–447, 1992.

95. Cherkey BD. Microcarrier pre-adhesion enhances long term survival of adult cells implanted into the mammalian brain. Exp Neurol 129:20, 1994.

96. Brundin P, Duan WM, Sauer H. Functional effects of mesencephalic dopamine neurons and adrenal chromaffin cells grafted to the rodent striatum. In: Dunnett SB, Bjorklund A, eds. Functional Neural Transplantation. New York: Raven Press, 1994, pp 9–46.

97. Reading RJ. Neural transplantation in the ventral striatum. In: Dunnett SB, Bjorklund A, eds. Functional Neural Transplantation. New York: Raven Press, 1994, pp 197–216.

98. Morrish P, Sawle GV, Brooks DJ. An (18F) dopa-PET and clinical study of rate of progression in Parkinson's disease. Brain 119:585–591, 1996.

99. Holthoff-Detto VA, Kessler J, Herholz K, et al. Functional effects of striatal dysfunction in Parkinson's disease. Arch Neurol 54:145–150, 1997.

100. Kish SJ, Shannak K, Hornykiewicz O. Uneven pattern of dopamine loss in the striatum of patients with idiopathic Parkinson's disease. Pathophysiology and clinical implication. N Engl J Med 318:876–880, 1988.

101. Olanow CW, Kordower JH, Freeman TB. Fetal nigral transplantation as a therapy for Parkinson's disease. Trends Neurosci 19:102–109, 1996.

102. Mendez I, Sadi D, Hong M. Reconstruction of the nigrostriatal pathway by simultaneous intrastriatal and intranigral dopaminergic transplants. J Neurosci 16(22):7216–7227, 1996.

103. Mukhida K, Baker KA, Mendez I. Enhancement of sensorimotor behavioral recovery in hemiparkinsonian rats with intrastriatal, intranigral and intra-subthalamic nucleus dopaminergic transplants. J Neurosci 21(10):3521–3530, 2001.

104. Collier TJ, Sortwell CE, Daley BF. Diminished viability, growth and behavioral efficacy of fetal dopamine neuron grafts in aging rats with long-term dopamine depletion: an argument for neurotrophic supplementation. J Neurosci 19:5563–5573, 1999.

105. Carvey PM, Ptak LR, Sierens DK, et al. Striatal-derived growth promoting activity is decreased in the aged rat: implications in Parkinson's disease. Soc Neurosci Abstr 18:934, 1992.

106. Espejo EF, Montoro RJ, Armengol JA, Lopez-Barneo J. Cellular and functional recovery of parkinsonian rats after intrastriatal transplantation of carotid body cell aggregates. Neuron 20:197–206, 1998.

107. Saporta S, Cameron DF, Borlongan CV, Sanberg PR. Survival of rat and porcine Sertoli cell transplants in the rat striatum without cyclosporine-A immunosuppression. Exp Neurol 146(2):299–304, 1997.
108. Willing AE, Othberg AI, Saporta S, et al. Sertoli cells enhance the survival of co-transplanted dopamine neurons. Brain Res 822(1–2):246–250, 1999.
109. Willing AE, Sudberry JJ, Othberg AI, et al. Sertoli cells decrease microglial response and increase engraftment of human hNT neurons in the hemi-parkinsonian rat striatum. Brain Res Bull 48(4):441–444, 1999.
110. Saporta S, Borlongan CV, Sndberg PR. Neural transplantation of human neuroteratocarcinoma (hNT) neurons into ischemic rats. A quantitative dose-response analysis of cell survival and behavioral recovery. Neuroscience 9(2):519–525, 1999.
111. Baker KA, Hong M, Sadi D, Mendez I. Intrastriatal and intranigral grafting of hNT neurons in the 6-OHDA rat model of Parkinson's disease. Exp Neurol 162(2):350–360, 2000.
112. Sinden JD, Stroemer P, Grigoryan G, et al. Functional repair with neural stem cells. In: Novartis Foundation Symposium. Neural Transplantation in Neurodegenerative Disease. Chichester: Wiley, 2000, pp. 270–288.
113. Galpern WR, Burns LH, Deacon TW, et al. Xenotransplantation of porcine fetal ventral mesencephalon in a rat model of Parkinson's disease: functional recovery and graft morphology. Exp Neurol 140:1–13, 1996.
114. Freeman TB, Wojak JC, Brandeis L, et al. Cross-species intracerebral grafting of embryonic swine dopaminergic neurons. Prog Brain Res 78:473–477, 1988.
115. Fink JS, Schumacher JM, Ellias JL, et al. Porcine xenografts in Parkinson's disease and Huntington's disease patients: preliminary results. Cell Transplant (2):273–278, 2000.
116. Hauser RA, Watts R, Freeman TB, et al. A double-blind, randomized, controlled, multicenter clinical trial of the safety and efficacy of transplanted fetal porcine ventral mesencephalic cells versus imitation surgery in patients with Parkinson's disease. Movement Disorders 16:983–984, 2001.
117. Deacon T, Schumacher J, Dinssmore J, et al. Histological evidence of fetal pig neural cell survival and transplantation into a patient with Parkinson's disease. Nature Med 3(3):350–353, 1997.
118. Marmor MF, Wolfensberger TJ. The Retinal Pigment Epithelium: Function and Disease. New York: Oxford University Press, 1998.
119. Chersky BD. Microcarrier preadhesion enhances long term survival of adult cells implanted into the mammalian brain. Exp Neurol 129:S18, 1994.
120. Campochiaro PA. Growth factors in the retinal pigment epithelium and retina. In: Marmor MF, Wolfensberger TJ, eds. The Retinal Pigment Epithelium: Function and Disease. New York: Oxford University Press, 1998.
121. Potter BM, Kidwell W, Cornfeldt M. Functional effects of intrastriatal HRPE grafts in hemiparkinsonian rats is enhanced by adhering to microcarriers. Abstract Soc for Neurosci, 27th annual meeting, 778.10, 1997.
122. Subramanian T, Bakay RAE, Burnette B, et al. Effects of stereotactic intrastriatal transplantation for human retinal pigment epithelial (hRPE) cells

attached to gelatin microcarriers on parkinsonian motor symptoms in hemiparkinsonian monkeys. Abstract Amer Soc for Neural Trans, 5th Annual Conference, 2–5, 1998.

123. Submaranian T, Burnette B, Bakay RAE, et al. Intrastriatal transplantation of human retinal pigment epithelial cells attached to gelatin carriers (hRPE-GM) improves parkinsonian motor signs in hemiparkinsonian (HP) monkeys. Abstract 5th Int Cong Parkinson's Disease and Movement Disorders, New York, October 10–14, 1998.

124. Watts RL, Raiser CD, Stover NP, et al. Stereotaxic intrastriatal implantation of retinal pigment epithelial cells attached to microcarriers in advanced Parkinson's disease (PD) patients: long term follow-up (abstr). American Academy of Neurology, 54th Annual Conference, 2002.

125. Mansergh RF, Wride MA, Rancourt DE, et al. Neurons from stem cells: implications for understanding nervous system development and repair. Biocem Cell Ciol 78:613–628, 2000.

126. Ling ZD, Potter ED, Lipton JW, Carvey PM. Differentiation of mesencephalic progenitor cells into dopaminergic neurons by cytokines. Exp Neurol 149:411–423, 1998.

127. Studer L, Csete M, Lee SH, et al. Enhanced proliferation, survival and dopaminergic differentiation and CNS precursors in lowered oxygen. J Neurosci 20(19):7377–7383, 2000.

128. Carpenter MK, Cui X, Hu Z, et al. In vitro expansion of a mutlipotent population of human neural progenitor cells. Exp Neurol 158:265–278, 1999.

129. Daadi MM, Weiss S. Generation of tyrosine hydroxylase-producing neurons from precursors of the embryonic and adult forebrain. J Neurosci 19(11):4484–4497, 1999.

130. Ostenfeld T, Caldwell MA, Prowse KR, et al. Human neural precursor cells express low level of telomerase in vitro and show diminishing cell proliferation with extensive axonal outgrowth following transplantation. Exp Neurol 164:215–226, 2000.

131. Wagner J, Akerud P, Castro DS, et al. Induction of a midbrain dopaminergic phenotype in nurrl1-overexpressing neural stem cells by type 1 astrocytes. Nat Biotech 17:653–659, 1999.

132. Kawasaki H, Mizuseki K, Nishikawa S, et al. Induction of midbrain dopaminergic neurotechnique neurons from ES cells by stromal cell-derived inducing activity. Neuron 28:31–40, 2000.

133. Lee SH, Lumelsky N, Studer L, et al. Efficient generation of midbrain and hindbrain neurons from mouse embryonic stem cells. Nat Biotech 18:675–679, 2000.

134. Akerud P, Canals JM, Snyder EY, Arenas E. Neuroprotection through delivery of glial cell line-derived neurotrophic factor by neural stem cells in a mouse model of Parkinson's disease. J Neurosci 21(20):8108–8118, 2001.

135. Bjorklund A, Lindvall O. Cell replacement therapies for central nervous system disorders. Nat Neurosci 6:537–544, 2000.

25

Parkinson's Disease Symptom Management: An Interdisciplinary Approach

Ruth Hagestuen
The National Parkinson Foundation, Miami, Florida, U.S.A.

Rosemary L. Wichmann and Marjorie L. Johnson
Struthers Parkinson's Center, Minneapolis, Minnesota, U.S.A.

INTRODUCTION

The complexity of Parkinson's disease (PD) symptoms and their physical, emotional, social, and financial impact presents a significant treatment challenge, even for the most expert and sensitive practitioner. An integrated, interdisciplinary team approach offers the skills and support necessary to ensure the highest quality of care for patients and their caregivers (Table 1). Patients derive maximum benefit from access to a full complement of professional services, including rehabilitation therapies, emotional and psychological support. This includes the provision of appropriate information and education at each stage of the disease process. Caregivers also need timely and appropriate information, support, and resources.

TABLE 1 Sample Configuration: Interdisciplinary Teams

	Physician	Physical therapy	Speech pathology	Occupational therapy	Nurse	Social worker	Music therapy	Tai chi/ yoga	Massage	Neuro- psychology	Rehab psychology	Patient	Caregiver	Dietician
Balance loss and falls	X	X	X	X	X						X	X	X	
Gait training	X	X		X		X					X	X		
Daily self-care	X	X	X	X	X						X	X	X	X
Controlling pain	X	X	X	X							X	X		
Exercise and activity	X	X	X	X	X						X	X	X	
Carepartner education	X	X	X	X	X					X	X	X	X	
Stress management	X	X	X	X	X	X	X	X	X	X	X	X	X	
Anxiety and depression	X	X	X	X	X	X	X	X	X	X	X	X	X	X
Cognition	X	X	X	X	X				X	X	X	X	X	
Speech and voice	X		X								X	X		
Swallowing and eating	X		X	X							X	X	X	X
Saliva control	X		X	X							X	X	X	X

THE INTERDISCIPLINARY TEAM

Although patients can benefit from the services of multiple disciplines, patients and even providers sometimes lack sufficient information regarding the availability and particular expertise of each of the rehabilitation and complementary therapies. This can be addressed through the referral process and an education program for patients that not only provides the right information about the disease at the right time, but informs them of multidisciplinary treatment options. This information, combined with prompt team recognition of changing patient and family needs through periodic reassessment, allows "best practice" management throughout the continuum of care.

Coordination of care through regular communication is essential among team members to ensure a comprehensive plan that addresses all areas of concern. It is essential for all team members to have a basic understanding of PD, specialized skills in treating patients with PD, and access to ongoing staff education to foster the expertise needed to manage these complicated patients effectively.

Together with the neurologist and primary care physician, nurses and social workers are at the hub of the referral process, providing and coordinating patient care and support along the disease continuum, from the time of diagnosis through the challenges of managing the complexities of advanced disease.

One of the most difficult situations faced by practitioners in the current healthcare system is the limited amount of time available for evaluation and treatment. There is often not enough time to adequately and completely discuss the disease process, goals of treatment, medications, to say nothing of the broader psychosocial and spiritual issues.

The availability of professionals who are well informed and prepared to listen and offer support and referral is important at the time of diagnosis and throughout the disease process. The emotional impact of dealing with the diagnosis combined with the need for early-stage information, developing a plan of self-care, and making appropriate connections for support are all areas that can best be addressed by the nurse and the social worker.

Registered nurses with a strong background in the treatment of PD play a key role in managing clinical aspects of patient care, providing education regarding self-care strategies and medication management. Nurses serve as a primary resource and contact for patients and caregivers throughout the continuum of care, initiating or assisting with referrals to appropriate therapies.

Dealing with the diagnosis, addressing issues of ambiguous loss, maintaining a balance in family relationships, communication, work concerns, and early-stage feelings of isolation are just some of the concerns that can be addressed early through one-on-one counseling, peer counseling, support groups, referrals to community resources, and community service agencies. Licensed social workers play a key role in helping patients and caregivers deal with social and emotional issues and may make referrals as needed for more specialized services. Psychologists who have an understanding of the dynamics of chronic illness and family relationships, and ideally an understanding of PD, are helpful in addressing some of the complicated dynamics that develop over time.

Nurses and social workers partner effectively as case managers, coordinating the services of allied professionals such as physical and occupational therapists, speech language pathologists, dietitians, psychologists, and other specialized service providers.

Patient and family-centered care is the goal and ideal, with both patients and caregivers as key participants in the entire process of developing and executing their plan of care and support. However, providing the right information at the right time, remaining accessible, and providing appropriate interventions that promote and maintain maximum quality of life are often challenges in our current healthcare system.

While the progression of symptoms results in the gradual onset of disability over time, independence can be prolonged for many years with a combination of quality medical care, compensatory adjustments of lifestyle, rehabilitation, education, and supportive services.

Most patients are likely to benefit from the expertise of rehabilitation therapists at various times throughout their disease progression as needs change or new problems are identified, though the type and amount of treatment interventions can vary widely with each individual. All skilled rehabilitation therapy interventions should remain focused on identified patient problems relating to functional impairment.

The following are many of the physical and psychological manifestations and challenges of PD progression, accompanied by descriptions of the therapies and professionals employed to care for patients throughout the disease process.

MANAGING DAILY SELF-CARE

Many PD patients report significant frustration and difficulty in performing the simple tasks of daily living. Symptoms, including bradykinesia, muscle rigidity, and declining balance skills, affect a patient's abilities to complete daily tasks such as eating, dressing, bathing, and homemaking in a safe and time-effective manner. Patients should be advised to consider scheduling their daily tasks in relation to when their medications are most effective. Medication adjustment is important in maximizing patient mobility but may not be completely effective in eradicating the difficulties experienced in performing activities of daily living.

Regular exercise can enhance the muscle strength and flexibility needed to perform daily tasks safely. Rehabilitation therapies and adaptive equipment can also aid patients and caregivers in the performance of these important daily activities.

Evaluation and treatment by members of a multidisciplinary rehabilitation team can offer effective compensatory strategies, e.g., improving bed mobility and facilitating transfers to a chair, tub, or car. Appropriate adaptive equipment may also enhance the patient's ability to eat, dress, and complete hygiene tasks. Individual patient needs and concerns will vary, as should the instruction in compensatory strategies for homemaking, cooking, laundry, yard work, and other functions particular to each patient.

Care partner instruction may also enhance safety and assistance with a patient's performance of regular activities. If a patient is unable to safely perform necessary daily tasks independently or with care partner help, referrals to social services are indicated to aid in accessing community resources or other assistance as needed.

ACTIVITY AND EXERCISE

Regular physical activity is an important element in the comprehensive management of PD. Physical therapy consultation is appropriate early in a patient's course of treatment to evaluate and teach appropriate home exercise programs. The rehabilitation team should be consulted periodically to reassess functional status and modify the plan of care as needed.

Objective, validated testing is recommended to assess baseline status and functional improvements resulting from participation in an exercise program or other treatment. Instructions in ongoing home exercise programs and referrals to community exercise resources are excellent ways to maintain ongoing activity after discharge from skilled therapies and should be included as part of a comprehensive care plan. Group exercise classes and adult day programs may help to foster patient motivation and follow-through.

Regular exercise can help reduce changes in motor disability, muscle strength, ambulation and quality of life (1–3). A variety of exercise methods, including water exercise, have been successfully utilized by PD patients.

Exercise programs should be based on individual ability and interest levels and must accommodate other health concerns. The program should include elements of stretching, strengthening, and conditioning activities, and caregivers may require instruction to assist as needed. Safety considerations should also be taken into account when designing the exercise program.

Approximately 30% of PD patients remain active in the workforce (4). Comprehensive assessment of daily tasks should also include assessment of work duties, and workplace evaluation may be indicated. Worksite modifications can be extremely helpful for those citing difficulty with work-related tasks.

A well-planned activity program should balance both movement and relaxation in the daily routine. Many patients seek a holistic approach to managing their PD symptoms and may wish to include complementary therapies such as tai chi, yoga, or other forms of movement. These activities can strengthen the mind-body connection, enhance wellness and relaxation, and even reduce stress, all important elements in a comprehensive program.

Other relaxation activities may include deep breathing, guided imagery, massage therapy, music, or involvement in forms of creative expression. Balancing activity and relaxation in daily life enhances quality of life and aids in helping those with PD take an active role in coping with their disease.

GAIT TRAINING

Common gait changes in PD include a narrowed base of support, en bloc turns, festination, freezing, and decreases in step size, heel strike, and arm swing. Gait may also be compromised by other disease symptoms and medication side effects, e.g., dyskinesia and dystonia. Secondary medical conditions, injuries related to falling, foot dysfunction, and vision changes all have the potential to compromise a patient's ability to walk safely or for extended distances.

Many "helpful hints" have been written for patients to use in improving their gait pattern, but these multiple cues may be impractical to maintain on a conscious level while performing functional tasks. Physical therapists skilled in gait evaluation and training ensure comprehensive evaluation and appropriate, graduated training in compensation strategies, and/or the use of assistive devices to meet the patient's particular needs.

Many patients with PD benefit from the use of gait-assistive devices, which can help improve balance, reduce joint stress, and enhance feelings of security when moving about. A narrowed base of support, reduced heel strike, and difficulty turning corners prohibit safe use of four-post walkers and quad canes for the majority of PD patients. Single-end canes, walking sticks, or wheeled walkers (with swivel casters, hand brakes, and bench seat) are usually more appropriate options, but their use should be assessed by a knowledgeable physical therapist prior to patient purchase. Inappropriate or poorly fitting devices will not maximize patient safety, and may contribute to balance problems.

Basic safety strategies, including instruction in appropriate footwear and the removal of home environmental barriers, should not be overlooked during gait instruction. Gait training should include practice on a variety of floor surfaces and with daily tasks such as reaching, turning, and carrying objects. Balance declines as the patient tries to focus on several tasks simultaneously; therefore, multitasking capabilities should also be assessed within the gait training session (5). Music therapy techniques, including rhythmic auditory stimulation, may also be effective in facilitating and optimizing ambulation (6).

PREVENTING FALLS

Balance changes are frequently seen in the moderate stages of PD. Injury related to balance loss and falling is directly related to increased mortality rates, rising health care costs, and reduced quality of life (7–9). Repeated falls can also contribute to chronic pain, heightened anxiety, and/or decreased activity levels. Unfortunately, medications currently used in PD symptom control prove less efficacious in controlling symptoms of postural instability than other primary symptoms.

A multidisciplinary approach is the most effective for assessing the many reasons falls may occur and to provide appropriate interventions that can improve patient safety. Loss of flexibility, postural changes, reduced muscle strength, joint pain, postural hypotension, dizziness, changes in vision, and other medical conditions may all contribute to loss of balance and falls. Exercise programs, medications, rehabilitation therapies, complementary therapies such as tai chi, and other treatments should all be considered within a comprehensive fall-prevention program.

Compensation strategies may be helpful for patients experiencing retropulsion or freezing. "Counterbalancing strategies" when reaching overhead, opening doorways, or turning corners can reduce the likelihood of posterior balance loss, while a variety of "tricks" (including visualization, music, projected light or laser beams and inverted walking sticks) have been documented to aid some patients affected by freezing episodes (10–12).

Thorough assessments of the home environment and the patient's performance of daily living activities are also important in the fall-prevention plan. Home modifications and use of appropriate adaptive equipment can be best identified after evaluation and treatment by an occupational therapist. Occupational therapy sessions may include practicing safety strategies in the kitchen, bathroom, and other areas in the home environment where falls are most likely to occur.

Reduced cognitive skills may also impact patient safety and contribute to falls. Cognitive screening and assessment is recommended in order to tailor patient instruction and safety strategies to an appropriate level. Family or other caregivers may need to be involved in the education process to ensure that the recommendations are understood and utilized.

An emergency plan should be devised for all patients who experience frequent falling. An emergency response system (i.e., cell phones, Lifeline, family/neighbor "check-in," or other appropriate alert systems) should be established. Caregivers should also be instructed in safe methods for helping patients get up from the ground after a fall, as they frequently provide primary assistance in these situations.

CONTROLLING PAIN

Complaints of pain are not uncommon in patients with PD and may be related to excessive rigidity, postural changes, inability to perform independent position change, dystonia, injuries sustained from falling, or other medical conditions. A complete assessment is needed to determine the source, frequency and intensity of pain. Instruction in recognizing pain behaviors (symptoms) may be required for caregivers as patients experiencing significant cognitive changes may exhibit agitation, wandering, anxiety, or increased confusion as pain-related behaviors.

While some patients require the use of prescribed medications or over-the-counter analgesics for pain control, there are a variety of other nonpharmacological interventions that may offer relief or reduce discomfort. Many patients have reported improvements as a result of complementary therapies, such as massage and acupuncture, though further research is required to assess the benefits of these treatments (13,14). Use of superficial heat, cold, or physical therapy modalities may also be effective in pain management. Instruction in proper positioning, seating systems, and posture principles is recommended to decrease discomfort resulting from improper postural alignment. Relaxation strategies and other forms of complementary medicine may also prove beneficial as part of a holistic approach to pain management.

SPEECH/VOICE/COMMUNICATION

An estimated 70–100% of people with PD experience changes in their ability to communicate effectively. Rarely, these changes are a first or very early manifestation of PD (15). The primary changes in speech and voice include soft or fading voice volume, monotone pitch, imprecise or slurred articulation of speech sounds, rapid and irregular rate of speech, "stutter-like" speech, and hoarse voice quality.

The changes in speech and voice are caused by the physiological changes that occur with PD. Muscle rigidity, tremor, freezing, slowness, and diminished coordination of movements can all have an impact on the complicated coordinations of movement needed for clear, loud speech and voice. The emotional, social, and economic impact of this decreased vocal ability can be significant—reduced self-confidence, social isolation, frustration related to communication breakdowns, and reduced ability to continue working.

Medication management of PD, while extremely important and helpful in managing symptoms, does not typically improve speech and voice skills. Intervention by a speech language pathologist, initiated early in the disease process, offers the best possible outcomes of speech therapy. Traditional speech therapy techniques, such as practice on oral motor exercises, specific speech sound drills, and techniques to control speech rate and better coordinate breathing with voice, have been shown to be helpful.

The most effective treatment, however, that has documented positive and long-lasting results is the Lee Silverman Intensive Voice Treatment (LSVT) (16,17). This treatment protocol was first published in 1989. The treatment concepts are quite simple: "Think Loud/Think Shout." The focus is on improving action of the vocal folds, using high effort to overcome muscle rigidity, and on intensity of practice and effort.

As PD progresses, it is sometimes necessary to "augment" speech and voice skills with devices such as personal amplifiers, word or picture boards, or computerized communication systems. Speech pathology intervention to maximize communication abilities may be needed at many different times during the course of PD as individual abilities change.

HEARING

While hearing loss is not caused by PD, it should be considered in any progressive neurological disease that occurs in an elderly population. Identifying hearing loss and providing amplification in the form of hearing aids can be very important in improving communication. Other adaptations that can improve communication with hearing loss are making sure the speaker is always visible to the listener, preferably face to face, and reducing background or competing noise.

EATING AND SWALLOWING

PD often has an impact on an individual's ability to eat and drink safely, requiring intervention by a number of professionals on the rehabilitation team. The speech pathologist focuses on the safety of the swallowing action, identifying underlying problems, making any necessary compensation for reduced ability and modifying the diet as needed for safety. The occupational therapist focuses on meal-preparation skills and strategies for getting the food from the plate to the mouth. The social worker's focus is on financial resources for purchasing food and assistance in getting the food to the home. The nurse and dietitian address general nutrition, constipation, hydration, and maximizing medication absorption with diet.

Warning signs of an eating- or swallowing-related problem include coughing or choking during eating, difficulty swallowing pills, weight loss, frequent respiratory infections, slowed rate of eating, and decreased pleasure in eating.

The speech pathologist's evaluation of swallowing safety typically includes a videofluoroscopic swallow evaluation. The patient is observed, using moving x-ray, eating and drinking substances with a variety of consistencies (thin and thick liquid, puree and solids) and trying a variety of safety techniques (e.g., chin tuck). This evaluation identifies the presence, absence, or risk of aspiration. Avoiding aspiration of contents into the lungs during eating and drinking is a primary goal of the intervention, since it often leads to pneumonia.

A diet modification that may reduce the risk of aspiration is thickening a patient's liquids to a nectar- or honey-like consistency. Techniques such as a chin tuck or double swallow may further reduce risk. Often a diet that consists of more "slippery" foods and avoids foods that are dry or crumbling can help with swallowing. Pills can be taken in applesauce.

Excessive saliva is often a concern related to reduced swallowing abilities. Learning cues to swallow more often, taking frequent sips of water or sucking on ice chips, keeping lips closed when not eating or talking, reducing sugar in the diet, and practicing lip-strengthening exercises may be helpful.

COGNITION

Decrease in cognitive skills occurs frequently in individuals with PD, particularly as the disease progresses. About 15% have diagnosed dementia, but many more are disabled by cognitive problems (18). These changes in cognitive abilities can affect an individual's safety, independence, and quality of life.

The primary cognitive changes include decline in memory, problem-solving abilities, visual-spatial skills, and changes in personality and language (19). The rehabilitation team, along with professionals in psychology and neuropsychology, can provide helpful insights into cognitive problems. Patients and caregivers can be taught how to cope with these changes and compensate whenever possible.

Memory changes have the greatest impact on short-term memory, particularly the ability to remember and follow through on an activity after being distracted. PD patients may have difficulty organizing and storing new information, may get distracted while trying to learn new information or skills, and may require prompts or memory aids. Learning to use a new walking device, a television remote control, or remembering medication schedules may become difficult. Simplifying tasks and providing memory aids, such as pill timers, calendars, and memo boards, may be very helpful and can also bolster a patient's confidence and self-sufficiency.

A decrease in executive function may create problems with activities such as driving, managing finances, and meal planning and preparation. Bradyphrenia further reduces problem-solving ability. Important tasks or decisions may need to be shifted to a family member, a formal driving evaluation may be needed, and other routine tasks may need to be simplified.

The visual-perceptual changes in PD, such as reduced contrast sensitivity and visual inattention, may make using walking devices, going up and down stairs, and walking outside with changes in terrain difficult and unsafe. Brightly colored tape to mark walker handholds and the edges of steps, in addition to decluttering the household, may be helpful.

PD patients often experience feelings of depression and anxiety, both of which can decrease quality of life. Mood changes are often managed with medications. Ancillary therapies, including social services, music therapy, pastoral care, and creative expression, can help restore a sense of well-being and a positive outlook. Referral to a clinical psychologist for individual and/or family counseling may be indicated.

Language deficits such as those seen after a stroke or head injury are not usually seen in PD (20). However, many individuals report difficulty in thinking of words, searching for words to express an idea, and losing their "train of thought" while talking. The speech pathologist can work with patients to recapture some expressive language skills and also help the family with successful communication. Simplifying and shortening verbal directions, reducing extraneous background noise, asking "choice" rather than open-ended questions, and giving the patient extra time to process information and to respond are all helpful with language and information processing.

The rehabilitation social worker is also a key professional in helping families cope with cognitive decline. Accessing external resources, such as Social Security Disability, grocery delivery services, handicap transportation agencies, and resources for financial assistance, may be helpful.

CAREGIVER INSTRUCTION AND SUPPORT

The National Family Caregivers Association estimates that in the past year 54 million Americans were involved in caregiving, spending an average of 73 hours a week or 10.5 hours a day providing care for a family member (21). All too often, the needs of these caregivers are not addressed until "burnout" or illness/injury occur.

Regarding PD, caregivers often lack adequate information or education and feel overwhelmed at the thought of trying to navigate the healthcare maze. Education regarding access to appropriate financial, supportive, and community resources is essential for caregivers, as is information about respite care options and self-care strategies.

Instruction in proper body mechanics for the physical aspects of caregiving can reduce the risk of injury to both the patient and the caregiver. Rehabilitation referrals regarding home modification, adaptive equipment, and assistance with daily activities can also be helpful to family caregivers.

The emotional aspects of caregiving can be extremely taxing, as families struggle with problems relating to role reversal, changing family dynamics, financial planning, and the physical changes experienced by their family member with PD. Social services and counseling can help caregivers adapt to these changes. Caregivers may also need specific recommendations, support, and resources to cope with the cognitive changes that PD patients experience.

Support groups may help caregivers to maintain balance and support through sharing common experiences with other group members. It is imperative that caregivers have the education, information, and support necessary to provide assistance for the PD patient, as well as to take appropriate care of themselves along the way.

Healthcare professionals must also recognize the value of caregivers as members of the interdisciplinary team. As the primary source of support for most people with PD, caregivers' observations and information should be considered when developing the care plan, or when a patient requires hospitalization or transition to higher levels of care. Both patient and caregiver input is essential to care plan development and should be reassessed periodically to ensure agreement and cooperation with the ongoing plan.

Information for patients, families, and healthcare professionals can be obtained from the following organizations:

National Parkinson Foundation
1501 NW 9th Avenue
Miami, FL 33136
800-327-4545
www.parkinson.org

Parkinson's Disease Foundation
William Black Medical Building
Columbia-Presbyterian Medical Center
710 W 168th St,
New York, NY 10032-9982
800-457-6676
www.pdf.org

American Parkinson Disease Association
1250 Hylan Boulevard, Suite 4B
Staten Island, NY 10305-1946
800-223-2732
www.apdaparkinson.org

The Michael J. Fox Foundation for Parkinson's Disease Research
Grand Central Station
P.O. Box 4777
New York, NY 10143

REFERENCES

1. Reuter I, Engelhardt M, Stecker K, Baas H. Therapeutic value of exercise training in Parkinson's disease. MedSci Sports Exerc 31(11):1544–1549, 1999.
2. Scandalis TA, Bosak A, Berliner JC, Helman LL, Wells MR. Resistance training and gait function in patients with Parkinson's disease. Am J Phys Med Rehabil 80(1):38–43, 2001.
3. Baatile J, Langbein WE, Weaver F, Maloney C, Jost MB. Effect of exercise on perceived quality of life of individuals with Parkinson's disease. J Rehab Res Dev 37(5):529–534, 2000.
4. Facts About Parkinson's Disease. National Parkinson Foundation Website, 2002.
5. Morris M. Movement disorders in people with Parkinson's disease: a model for physical therapy. Phys Ther J 80(6):578–597, 2000.
6. McIntosh GC, Rice RR, Thaut MH. Rhythmic-auditory facilitation of gait patterns in Patients with Parkinson's disease. J Neurol Neurosurg Psych 62:22–26, 1997.

7. Nevitt MC, Cummings SR, Hudes ES. Risk factors for injurious falls: a prospective study. J Gerontol 46(5):M1164–1170, 1991.
8. Cumming RG, Salkeld G, Thomas M, Szonyi G. Prospective study of the impact of fear of falling on activities of daily living, SF-36 scores and nursing home admission. J Gerontol A Biol Sci Med Sci 55(5):M299–305, 2000.
9. Tinetti ME, Williams CS. Falls, injuries due to falls, and the risk of admission to a nursing home. N Engl J Med 337(18):1279–1284, 1997.
10. Enzensberger W, Oberlander U, Stecker K. Metronome therapy in patients with Parkinson's disease. Nervenarzt 68(12):972–977, 1997.
11. Komplotti K, Goetz CG, Leurgans S, Morrissey M, Siegel IM. On freezing in Parkinson's disease: resistance to visual cue walking devices. Mov Disord 15(2):309–312, 2000.
12. Kenoun G, Defebvre L. Gait Disorders in Parkinson Disease: Gait freezing and falls: therapeutic management. Presse Med 30(9):460–468, Mar 2001.
13. Lyons K, Greene M, Pahwa R. Use of acupuncture in Parkinson's disease: a pilot study (abstr). Neurology 58:A466, 2002.
14. Manyam BV, Sanchez-Ramos JR. Traditional and complementary therapies in Parkinson's disease. Adv Neurol 80:565–574, 1999.
15. Ramig L, Gould W. Speech characteristics in Parkinson's disease. Neur Cons 4:1–6, 1986.
16. Ramig L, Countryman S, Pawlas A. The Lee Silverman Voice Treatment (LSVT). Wilbur James Gould Research Center, 1995.
17. Ramig L, Countryman S, O'Brien C, Hoehn M, Thompson L. Intensive speech treatment for patients with Parkinson's disease: short and long term comparison of two techniques. Neurology 47:1496–1504, 1996.
18. Levin B, Tomer R, Rey G. Cognitive impairments in Parkinson's disease. Neurol Clin 10(2):471–481, 1992.
19. Levin B, Tomer R, Rey G. Cognitive impairments in Parkinson's disease. Neurol Clin 10(2):471–481, 1992.
20. Levin B, Katzen H. Early cognitive changes and nondementing behavioral abnormalities in Parkinson's disease. In: Behavioral Neurology of Movement Disorders. New York: Raven Press, Ltd, 1995, pp 85–95.
21. Kensington MD. October Caregiver Survey—2000. National Family Caregivers Association (NFCA), 2000.

Index

About the Editors

RAJESH PAHWA is Associate Professor of Neurology and Director of the Parkinson's Disease and Movement Disorder Center, University of Kansas Medical Center, Kansas City. The author or coauthor of numerous journal articles and professional publications, he received the M.B.B.S. (M.D.) degree (1983) from the University of Bombay, India.

KELLY E. LYONS is Research Assistant Professor and Director of Research at the Parkinson's Disease and Movement Disorder Center, University of Kansas Medical Center, Kansas City. The author or coauthor of numerous journal articles and professional publications, she received the M.A. (1991) and Ph.D. (1993) degrees in cognitive and experimental psychology from the University of Kansas, Lawrence.

WILLIAM C. KOLLER is Professor of Neurology, Mount Sinai School of Medicine, New York, New York. Serving on the editorial board for the Neurological Disease and Therapy series (Marcel Dekker, Inc.), he is the author, coauthor, editor, or coeditor of numerous journal articles and several books including *Parkinsonian Syndromes*: *Therapy of Parkinson's Disease, Second Edition*; and the *Etiology of Parkinson's Disease*. Dr. Koller received the M.S. (1971) and Ph.D. (1974) degrees in pharmacology and the M.D. degree (1976) from Northwestern University Medical School, Chicago, Illinois.

ISBN 0-8247-4242-7